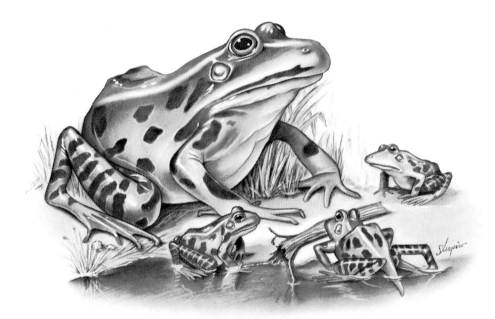

Precocious metamorphosis of the frog tadpole (*Rana pipiens*) by adding thyroid hormone (thyroxine) to the aquarium water. The mother (large frog) was caused to ovulate in September, some seven months before the normal breeding period, by subcutaneously implanting six pituitary glands from adult female donors. The eggs were artificially inseminated. When the tadpoles had developed hindlimb buds, minute amounts of thyroxine were added to the water. In about three weeks, the treated tadpoles resorbed their swimming tails, grew hindlimbs and then forelimbs, lost their horny teeth (used for plant feeding), shortened their intestinal tracts in preparation for carnivorous feeding, modified their respiratory and integumentary systems for terrestrial environments, and emerged as normal, but miniature, air-breathing adults. This experiment was first performed by Gudernatsch (1912), who fed bits of horse thyroid to young tadpoles.

Since thyroxine initiates the metamorphic changes long before they would normally occur, the resulting froglets are about one-third the size of those metamorphosing in nature. Thyroidectomized tadpoles never metamorphose, but grow to "giant" size. Drawn to scale from photographs of the living specimens.

General Endocrinology

C. DONNELL TURNER, Ph.D.
Professor of Biological Sciences
Duquesne University, Pittsburgh

JOSEPH T. BAGNARA, Ph.D.
Professor of Biological Sciences
University of Arizona, Tucson

Sixth Edition

illustrated

1976   W. B. SAUNDERS COMPANY • Philadelphia • London • Toronto

W. B. Saunders Company   West Washington Square
                          Philadelphia, Pa.   19105

                          1 St. Anne's Road
                          Eastbourne, East Sussex BN21 3UN, England

                          833 Oxford Street
                          Toronto, Ontario M8Z 5T9, Canada

Library of Congress Cataloging in Publication Data

Turner, Clarence Donnell,

General endocrinology.

First published in 1941 under title: An introduction to general endocrinology.

Includes index.

1. Endocrinology.   I. Bagnara, Joseph Thomas, joint author.   II. Title. [DNLM: 1. Endocrine glands. 2. Hormones. WK102 T945g]

QP187.T8 1976   596'.01'42   75–38156

ISBN 0–7216–8933–7

Listed here is the latest translated edition of this book together with the language of the translation and the publisher.

French (4th Edition) — Masson & Cie
                       Paris, France

Polish (3rd Edition) — Rolnicze i Lesne
                       Warsaw, Poland

Spanish (1st Edition) — Neuva Editorial Interamericana, S.A., de C.V.,
                        Mexico

Cover illustration: Micrograph from the neural lobe of a normal kangaroo rat
                     (From Scott, D. E.: Neuroendocrinology 4:347, 1969.)

General Endocrinology   ISBN 0-7216-8933-7

Last digit is the print number: 9   8   7   6   5   4   3   2   1

Preface

During the five years since the fifth edition appeared, a wealth of new information about endocrinology has emerged. In this sixth edition we have attempted to distill from this body of new knowledge those elements that are essential to the student of modern endocrinology. Consistent with the aims of the first edition, which appeared in 1948, and in keeping with the goals of all the subsequent revisions, the current version is general in its coverage of the field. We have tried to emphasize basic principles and have illustrated them with examples taken both from clinical endocrinology and from the rapidly growing field of comparative endocrinology. Attention has been devoted to invertebrate endocrine systems, not only for their own sake, but because they demonstrate analogies important to the general endocrinologist. In covering comparative aspects our attention has not been focused solely on lower vertebrates; rather, information about mammals, including man, has been integrated into the discussion through the unifying theme of evolution.

Intensive research on the mechanisms of hormone action has provided many new data. Accordingly, we have given this area strong attention not only in those chapters dealing with specific hormones, but in Chapter 2, which deals with general aspects of the science of endocrinology. To enhance this discussion we have prepared a new illustration which describes a model that includes both hormone receptor mechanisms and sites of hormone action, either at the cell membrane or at the level of the nucleus. Appropriate attention has been given to the ultrastructure of endocrine glands, mechanisms of hormone secretion and transport, and hormone assay. New biochemical information about hormones has emerged and we have presented current chemical structures of pituitary hormones, releasing hormones, and gastrointestinal hormones. This new knowledge about chemical structures has provided a cogent vehicle for the discussion of hormone evolution. Important advances have led to the recognition of new hormones such as cholecalciferol. These and many other hormone-like substances are discussed in modern context.

All of the chapters have been brought up to date and some of the changes have been extensive. In previous editions information about neuroendocrine mechanisms has been scattered among several chapters. In this revision, Professor Turner has combined this material into a new Chapter 3, Neuroendocrinology. Consequently, the last chapter, Endocrine Mechanisms in the Invertebrates, has been completely reworked since it formerly contained much information about neurosecretion and neuroendocrine mechanisms. For similar reasons, the first two introductory chapters have been modified considerably. Chapter 16 has been greatly renovated, although it still retains its role of containing miscellaneous hormone groups. Much new information about gastrointestinal hormones is presented and the endocrine role of the pineal gland is discussed. It seems likely that in subsequent editions the material covered in this chapter will form the basis for new chapters.

Just as with previous editions, an extensive bibliography is found at the end of each of the chapters. We have not documented every fact; however, the citations have been carefully chosen to assist the interested students who may wish to explore specific areas in more detail.

We are grateful to many people who have contributed to this revision. Many colleagues have generously supplied figures, and these are acknowledged in the legends. Others have offered helpful suggestions. In particular, in this regard, we acknowledge the help of Professor Hideshi Kobayashi, Dr. Mac E. Hadley, and Mr. Steve Vigna. We are also grateful to the many users of this textbook who offered suggestions that were forwarded to us by the W. B. Saunders Company. It was in response to some of these that we decided to utilize many new drawings. These were skillfully prepared by Mr. Robert Hale of the University of Arizona. Important technical support in completing various parts of the revision was kindly supplied by my wife, Mary Louise, and by my student Sally Frost. Without their help this sixth edition would have been slow in coming.

JOSEPH T. BAGNARA

Greer, Arizona
July 4, 1976

Contents

vii

Contents

CHAPTER 1

Introduction

It is not likely that endocrinology could be defined in a manner entirely acceptable to all biologists since there are many points of view and many gaps in our information. There are some who regard it as the aspect of biology dealing broadly with the chemical integration of the individual. Others, following the classic definition of Bayliss and Starling, prefer to confine its scope to the ductless glands and the adjustments that their special products facilitate. It is probable that the first position is too flexible and the second too rigid. As the field is more critically explored and more becomes known about reactions at the cellular level, it is likely that certain unifying principles will emerge. Although broad definitions are desirable and essential, they must undergo change as new information is brought to light. Endocrinology stands to be enriched by the recognition of a wide spectrum of intermediate or transitional types of chemical integrations that do not fit current definitions.[52] As comparative studies are extended, many more deviations from the conventional functional patterns will undoubtedly be revealed and these must be given ample consideration.

The term *hormone* has probably been applied too loosely to a great variety of unrelated substances. Agents emanating from injured tissues have been called "wound hormones" and growth substances in plants "phytohormones"; agents released from nerve terminals have been classified as "neurohormones"; and even carbon dioxide has been referred to as a "hormone of respiration." Some have used the term "social hormone" to describe chemical agents that are released into the external environment and serve to influence the behavior of other individuals of the same species.[66] In termites, for example, the reproductive and soldier castes prevent other individuals from becoming members of their own castes by secreting materials that are ingested and act through the corpus allatum, an endocrine gland influencing differentiation.

Some of these agents, although they perform integrative functions, probably do not fall within the scope of endocrinology. However, it must be recognized that ductless glands are present in certain invertebrates and in all vertebrates. Moreover, one would be hard pressed to give a precise definition of an endocrine gland because all cells possess some secretory capacity and contribute to the internal environment of the organism.

As research broadens and deepens our knowledge of coordinatory systems, it becomes increasingly apparent that products of these systems participate in every bodily function, and even have profound influences upon the mental states and behavioral patterns of individuals. Studies on the invertebrates and lower vertebrates suggest that chemical integration by hormones and similar agents is an overall phenomenon prevailing throughout the animal kingdom, and that important actions may be exerted during developmental stages as well as in mature organisms. Further information is urgently needed on the evolutionary history of endocrine mechanisms. Comparative endocrinologists will probably discover more clues that will be of value in helping to interpret adjustments that must be operating at the human level. Information on regulatory mechanisms is accumulating rapidly and, as in all sciences, the established data must be reevaluated as current research yields new insights; this frequently necessitates modifications in interpretation and changes in terminology. It is imperative to remember that present theories are tentative.

Biologists are beginning to realize that the nervous and endocrine systems, both functioning to integrate the organism, are not so divergent and sharply delimited as was formerly supposed. A common physiologic attribute of these two systems is their ability to synthesize and release special chemical agents that are capable of spreading for varying distances. Nerve cells produce agents that act as chemical messengers either locally (*e.g.,* acetylcholine) or at a distance (*e.g.,* oxytocin). Many endocrine glands, through their hormones, affect the nervous sytem; on the other hand, endocrine organs are frequently stimulated or inhibited by products of the nervous system. Seldom does one encounter biologic phenomena that are controlled exclusively by either the nervous sytem or the endocrine system; most are under the overlapping authority of both systems. Furthermore, studies on neurosecretion leave no doubt that the nervous system has its own endocrine specializations for the release of hormones. The functional interlocking is so remarkable that nervous and endocrine elements are now regarded as constituting a *neuroendocrine system.*

Hormones act upon *target tissues* and *organs* by regulating the rates of specific biochemical reactions in the constituent cells. These biochemical adjustments are accomplished at the cellular level by virtue of their power to augment or restrain special enzyme systems. Hormones are released at the right time and in proper amounts in the normal organism, and maladjustments of severe consequence may be precipitated if the timing is wrong or if they are deficient or present in superabundance. Obviously, hormones are without effect unless the target cells and tissues are capable of responding to them. The competence of a particular hormone within the living body may be altered by a multitude of autopharmacologic substances that are always present with it in the body fluids.

The rapid coordinations of the body are controlled by the nervous system. Since hormones are generally conveyed by the circulation and must be transmitted through intercellular tissue fluids in order to reach their target organs, we find that they regulate processes such as growth, regeneration, reproduction, blood chemistry, molting, metabolic rate, pigmentation, etc. These are adjustments that require duration rather than speed.

TYPES OF CHEMICAL MESSENGERS

Admittedly, there are many transitional situations that do not fit into the framework of formal definitions, but some agreement on terminology is essential. The suggestion of Parkes and Bruce that the term *chemical messengers* be used broadly to include both internal secretions involved in integration of the individual and external secretions concerned with the integration of populations has some merit.[48] The categorization of such chemical messengers presents certain problems, largely because demarcations between groups are not always sharp; moreover, by their nature some categories can be readily defined while others are more vague. In any event, it must be remembered that the following categories of chemical messengers were established arbitrarily with the aim of providing the most convenient means for discussion and understanding. They are: (1) hormones, (2) neurohormones and neurohumors (neurotransmitters), (3) assorted chemical messengers, (4) phytohormones, and (5) pheromones.

Hormones

According to the original use of the word, hormones are chemical agents which are synthesized by circumscribed parts of the body—generally specialized ductless glands—and are carried by the circulating blood to another part of the body where they evoke systemic adjustments by acting on specific tissues and organs. In the course of time, there has been a tendency to restrict the term *hormone* to the regulatory products of endocrine glands, and to resist the trends to broaden its meaning to include such metabolites as carbon dioxide and the large category of substances (*e.g.,* embryonic evocators) that exert localized actions. In any case, hormones facilitate integrative adjustments within the individual and must be distinguished from a growing list of exocrine gland products (pheromones) that play important roles in integrating groups of individuals.

Though often it is difficult or impossible to separate the neural and hormonal components of regulatory processes, the complex of endocrine glands in the vertebrates is quite clear-cut. This system includes the pituitary, thyroids, parathyroids, adrenals, gonads, pancreatic islets, and the hormone-producing part of the gastrointestinal tract. In certain mammals, the placenta would have to be regarded as an endocrine gland since it is the source of various steroidal and protein hormones. During the course of vertebrate evolution, there has not been much change in the position of the endocrine structures within the body. Each of these endocrine organs will be considered according to structure, synthesis of hormones, regulation of function, action of hormones, and interrelationships with other components of the regulatory system. All these glands are comparatively small, are devoid of ducts, and have access to a rich vascular supply.

The most thoroughly studied endocrine glands are multicellular, but it is quite probable that unicellular types, sometimes capable of migrating through tissues, will be recognized. Instead of releasing their products upon a free surface, as exocrine glands do, these would discharge regulatory chemicals into the body fluids.

Regarding embryonic origin, the endocrine glands differentiate from all the germ layers. Those derived from mesoderm (adrenal cortex, gonads) produce steroidal hormones; those developing from ectoderm or endoderm secrete hormones that are either modified amino acids, peptides, or proteins.

Most internal regulating agents among the invertebrates are *neuroendocrine* in nature, but circumscribed ductless glands do exist. In the latter category may be mentioned the androgenic glands of crustaceans and insects,[17] the corpora allata and prothoracic (ecdysial) glands of insects, and the Y organs of crustaceans.

Neurohormones and Neurohumors

Within the nervous systems of all animals from coelenterates and flatworms to human beings, there are nerve cells that show cytologic indications of being capable of functioning as glands.[8, 41] These cells are neurosecretory in nature and release chemical messengers called *neurohormones.* Although the neurosecretory cells are capable of conducting impulses, their principal function is the synthesis and release of neurohormones. Actually, they combine the attributes of nerve cell and gland cell, since they receive information from neural centers via ordinary afferent neurons and respond through the release of chemical messengers. The neurohormones of the vertebrate neurohypophysis (oxytocin and vasopressin) are simple peptides, and their actions have been extensively studied. The various hypophysiotrophic factors of the vertebrate median eminence are thought to be neurohormonal peptides that are delivered via a portal blood flow to the adenohypophysis, where they regulate the output of hormones. Most of the neurohormones among invertebrates are also peptides and are involved in such processes as color change (crustaceans), molting and metamorphosis (insects), the initiation of regeneration (annelids), gametogenesis, and metabolism (certain annelids and arthropods).

The ingenious experiments of Loewi in 1921 helped explain why sympathetic and parasympathetic nerves usually have opposite effects upon the effector organs they supply. He used isolated frog hearts, with nerves intact, and arranged them so that Ringer's solution perfused through one heart could be introduced into another, completely separated heart. Stimulation of the vagus nerve (parasympathetic) to the first heart caused the contraction rates of both hearts to decrease; stimulation of the sympathetic nerves caused the rates of both hearts to increase. The two kinds of nerves apparently were releasing different agents into the perfusate as it irrigated the first heart. Further studies have shown that the parasympathetic terminals release acetylcholine, whereas most of the postganglionic terminals of the sympathetic nerves release norepinephrine with perhaps traces of related compounds. The adrenergic transmitter was formerly called "sympathin," but it is now known to be norepinephrine. Depending upon the kind of neurohumor released, it is customary to classify the fibers of the autonomic system as "cholinergic" or "adrenergic." Transmission in the central nervous system probably involves a whole family of chemical agents, including acetylcholine, norepinephrine, dopamine, and serotonin.

These agents released at axonal terminals are the products of conventional nerve cells and are called *neurohumors;* they have often been thought of as "local hormones" or "diffusion hormones." Although the capacity to produce neurohumors may be regarded as providing support for the concept that secretion is a fundamental property of all nerve cells, these ordinary neurons lack the glandlike specializations of the neurosecretory cells that are the source of neurohormones. The neurohumors function at nerve terminals in minute quantities, over very short periods of time. They may be promptly inactivated by means of enzymes or, particularly in the case of adrenergic terminals, the substance seems to be rendered ineffective by being returned quickly to the presynaptic neuron that produced it, where it is temporarily stored and discharged again as the need arises.[53] The neurohumors clearly are chemical messengers of great importance, but they differ from ordinary hormones in not being transported by the circulation. They differ from neurohormones with respect to their source, coming from conventional nerve cells in general instead of from neurosecretory cells. So many intergradations are encountered that it is impossible to distinguish clearly between neurohormones and neurohumors in all instances. It is instructive to recognize such intermediate situations for they serve to emphasize the great degree of flexibility and variation that exists among the mechanisms of neurochemical communication.[53]

Assorted Chemical Messengers

This is a convenient category in which to place the large variety of chemical messengers which fail in one or more ways to satisfy the requirements generally implied by the term "hormone." The cells of all organisms, whether unicellular or multicellular, produce and release substances of some kind which change the chemistry of internal and external environments. In this sense, no cell has completely lost its glandular properties even though it has differentiated highly in another direction. Many compounds, such as carbon dioxide and urea, have general origins within the body, in contrast to the more or less specific sources of endocrine gland secretions, and perform integrative roles of great importance.

Products of dead or injured tissues, such as histamine and leukocyte attractants, are known to participate in inflammatory processes. Erythropoietin is an integrative substance released by the kidneys and perhaps other organs in response to anoxia; its action is to promote proliferation of red blood cells by the bone marrow. *Thymosin,* a hormone-like factor from the thymus, is essential for the initiation of immune reactions in response to certain particulate antigens and to skin homografts. Extracts of a variety of tissues contain substances that inhibit cell division. These have been referred to as *chalones*.[17] *Nerve growth factor (NGF),* present in a variety of tissues, notably the submaxillary glands, stimulates profound growth and development of the nervous system, especially of sensory and sympathetic cells. A similar factor, *epidermal growth factor (EGF),* is often extracted with NGF; its principal effects are epidermal growth and keratinization.[21] *Secretagogues* are extrinsic factors present in food which, after absorption into the blood, act to stimulate the glands of the gastrointestinal tract. Inductive substances are of great importance during embryonic life; they are restricted in their origin and are not effective at great distances from their source. The *prostaglandins* were originally identified in human seminal fluid, but are now known to be present in most, if not all, mammalian tissues. They have a wide range of biologic actions, but are not hormones in the strict sense. It is important to recognize all of these deviant regulatory agents without subtracting from the classic connotations generally conveyed by the term *hormone.*

The extracellular synthesis of chemical messengers may occur within body fluids, when the necessary enzymes, substrates, and energy sources are available, and this may be more widespread than is currently appreciated.[7] A clear example is the synthesis of angiotensin II, an octapeptide having powerful vasopressor effects and, at least in certain species, the capacity of eliciting the secretion of aldosterone from the adrenal cortices. Renin is a proteolytic enzyme of the mammalian kidney, probably deriving from the juxtaglomerular apparatus; it is freed into the blood. It acts upon a blood protein (substrate) to produce angiotensin I, which is then enzymatically converted to the biologically effective angiotensin II.

It is known that whole human blood contains enzymes that are capable of bringing about a variety of transformations and interconversions of steroid hormones, and of particular significance is the conversion of the less to the more biologically active compounds.[10] One study showed that 60 per cent of the plasma testosterone (potent androgen) in the human female arose from the peripheral conversion of androstenedione (weak androgen).[34] The source of the plasma enzymes is unknown.

The concept of "cooperative steroidogenesis," whereby multiple organs participate in the step-by-step synthesis of steroidal hormones, deserves consideration, especially by comparative endocrinologists.[47] The endocrine status of the corpuscles of Stannius, derived from the kidney tubules or ducts in fishes, has been debated for years; it seems now that they can effect very limited steroid transformations. Their steroidogenic ability is very meager compared with such glands as the mammalian adrenal cortex, but they may have utility in the organism if they bring about only one key transformation. The steroidal hormones (ecdysones) of insects and crustaceans are commonly regarded as being synthesized by prothoracic glands and Y organs, respectively, but this can be questioned on the grounds that these structures lack the kind of ultrastructure characteristic of steroidogenic glands of vertebrates. There is no doubt that these organs condition the synthesis of hormonal steroids from cholesterol, but they may not possess the biochemical equipment required for all of the transformations. Although it has not been demonstrated, such organs could conceivably release essential enzymes or substrates, the actual synthesis of the finished hormone occurring in the body fluids.

Phytohormones

Since plants are devoid of nervous systems, it is clear that their biologic adjustments are accomplished largely through the synthesis and dispersal of chemical messengers.[58] Great advances have been made by plant physiologists and biochemists in elucidating such regulatory substances as auxins, gibberellins, the so-called "wound hormone" (traumatic acid), leaf-growth substances, root-growth regulators, kinins, and florigens. These plant agents are principally growth regulators, and many practical applications of economic importance have been found for them. The hormones of plants and animals are similar in many ways, but there are profound differences with respect to source and method of transmission.[42] The plant cells that synthesize and release phytohormones are not sufficiently differentiated to be considered circumscribed glands of internal secretion. Moreover, the plant hormones are moved mainly from cell to cell instead of being dependent upon vascular channels for transport to distant targets. It may be discovered, however, that certain animal hormones are disseminated to a greater extent by cell-to-cell transmission than is presently appreciated.

Raper showed that the development of sex organs in the fungus *Achlya* consists of a series of steps, each being governed by particular *ectohormones* (pheromones) released by other individuals and passed through the aqueous environment.[49]

Pheromones

While acoustical and visual modes of communication are the obvious primary mechanisms of transmitting information between individuals, the use of chemical signals is also very important. Chemical signals are of two classes; those that communicate between individuals of the same species (intraspecific) are called *pheromones,* while those operating between different species (interspecific) are termed *allomones* or *kairomones.* The former refers to chemicals which favor the producer of the substance, and the latter to those that favor the recipient.[40]

The term pheromone was originally applied to the sex attractants of insects but, with the accumulation of information, the term has been broadened to include various kinds of agents released into the environment and functioning in all major groups to integrate members of the population. The pheromones are not hormones since they are generally the products of exocrine glands; however, the capacity of the exocrine glands to produce pheromones is often dependent on hormonal stimulation.[5, 45, 50] In some species, specialized receptors have evolved. The chemical structures of an array of pheromones have been established, and while no broad generalizations are yet possible, it should be noted that most of these compounds are simple ones having low molecular weights. Many are derivatives of fatty acids or terpenes. These environmental agents may be ingested, absorbed through body surfaces, or perceived by olfaction. They evoke specific behavioral, developmental, or reproductive responses and these are of great significance from the standpoint of ecology and survival of the species. The pheromones differ from hormones in several respects: (1) they are transmitted via the external environment, (2) they are typically more species-specific than are hormones and (3) they elicit adjustments in the bodies of other individuals, whereas hormones typically confine their activities to the organism that produced them. The distinctions are not always clear-cut; there are instances in which the same endocrine gland product may be active within an individual (hormone) and between individuals of a colony (pheromone). Certain hormones from the corpora allata of termites probably function in this dual manner. There are instances of host hormones influencing reproductive processes in parasites inhabiting their tissues and organs. In such situations, one and the same substance serves as a hormone for the host and as a pheromone for the parasite. Pheromones perform important roles in many symbiotic and parasitic relationships involving animals of different species.[25] It seems appropriate for endocrinologists to consider pheromones for three reasons: (1) the exocrine glands that produce pheromones are often hormone-dependent, (2) hormone metabolites being eliminated from the system may function as pheromones in some species, and (3) the "primer" pheromones initiate prolonged physiologic adjustments involving the central nervous system and multiple endocrine glands, such as the pituitary and gonads. Their actions demonstrate graphically how environmental changes impinge upon the nervous and endocrine systems to evoke functional and behavioral changes.

Pheromones are grouped broadly into two categories: (1) signaling or releaser pheromones, which produce rapid and reversible responses through the central nervous system or along quick-acting neuroendocrine channels, and (2) primer pheromones, which activate a longer series of neuroendocrine events that develop slowly and require prolonged stimulation. Sex attractants and trail and alarm substances of insects are examples of pheromones having signaling effects. Among mammals, the aggressive behavior of unfamiliar male mice may be mentioned; this is related to a pheromone of urinary origin and to another arising from the foot pads. Removal of the olfactory bulbs or destruction of the nasal epithelium removes the aggressive behavior, but these procedures do not protect the animal from attacks by intact males. Secretions from the androgen-dependent chin gland of the Australian rabbit provide repelling or inhibiting signals for other males. Subordinate males have smaller chin glands than the dominant buck, and spend less time chinning objects within their territories, including does and young animals.[13]

Reproductive life of the honey-bee colony is regulated by a pheromone from the queen's mandibular glands, and this has been chemically identified as 9-ketodecanoic acid and synthesized. The secretion has a primer effect since it is ingested by the workers and acts to inhibit the development of the ovaries, and also prevents them from constructing royal cells for the rearing of new queens. The queen substance can also produce signaling effects since it serves as a sex attractant during the nuptial flight. The females of some lycosid spiders and cockroaches secrete pheromones having aphrodisiac properties, and these are passed to the males through contact chemoreception.[16]

The primer pheromones of mice have been most carefully studied. The caging together of female mice leads to mutual disturbances of the estrous cycle: The regular periods of estrus (sexual receptivity) are interrupted by pseudopregnancies or by extended periods of diestrus (Lee-Boot effect). Since this effect on the cycles is alleviated by olfactory lobectomy, and is not dependent on audition, vision, or physical contact, it appears to result

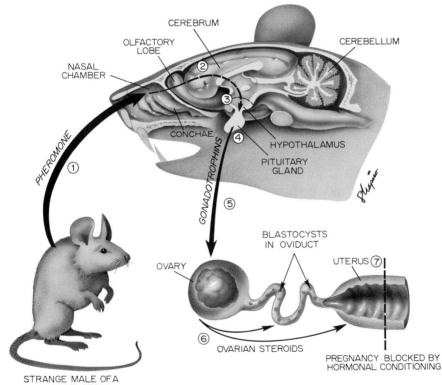

Figure 1–1. A chain of neuroendocrine reactions triggered by pheromones. Pregnancy may be blocked in a newly impregnated mouse by exposure to a strange male of a different strain (Bruce effect). 1, The volatile pheromone is perceived by the olfactory epithelium; 2, impulses are relayed through the olfactory lobes and cerebrum to the hypothalamus; 3, gonadotrophin-releasing factors in the median eminence are conveyed over the hypophysial portal veins to the anterior lobe of the pituitary; 4, the release factors regulate the output of pituitary gonadotrophins; 5, gonadotrophins condition the production of steroid hormones by the ovaries; 6, the ovarian hormones are deficient or of the wrong kind and a pregnancy-type uterus cannot be developed and maintained; 7, young embryos fail to implant, thus terminating pregnancy. (The size and shape of the pituitary gland are exaggerated in this figure for the sake of clarity.)

from an odor passed from one female to another. It is also known that the introduction of a male mouse into a group of female mice accelerates the attainment of estrus and shortens the cycle (Whitten effect). The pheromone responsible for this effect is present in male urine; castration removes the pheromone from the urine, whereas testosterone therapy in castrates of either sex causes it to appear.[15] For these reasons, the urinary factor is thought to be an androgen metabolite or the product of an androgen-dependent tissue. The odor of a strange male mouse brings about a series of neuroendocrine disturbances (Fig. 1–1) that terminates pregnancy in a newly impregnated mouse (Bruce effect). Protection against this pregnancy termination is afforded by injecting prolactin or progesterone during the period of exposure to the strange male. Endogenous prolactin supplied by ectopic pituitary grafts or induced by a suckling litter is similarly effective.[14] The administration of reserpine to the female depresses hypothalamic activity and prevents the pregnancy block. This pheromone is present in bladder urine, free from accessory gland secretions, but its source and identity remain unknown. Castration of the adult abolishes the pheromone, and it never appears if castration is accomplished before puberty. Ovariectomized females acquire the pregnancy-blocking capacity if they are given a series of androgen injections.

Mice remain vulnerable to the pregnancy-blocking pheromone for about four days after coitus, while the zygotes are developing in the oviducts. The blastocysts are moved into the uteri, but implantation is impossible because the ovaries do not produce the hormones required to build up the kind of an endometrium required for nidation. With pregnancy at an end, the female promptly returns to estrus, ovulates, and again becomes sexually receptive. Adjustments of great complexity involving both nervous and endocrine systems intervene between the olfactory stimulation and the endometrial failure (Fig. 1–1). Hypothalamic stimulation leads to a diminished release of prolactin by the anterior pituitary and a consequent failure of the ovarian corpora to secrete progesterone; the return to estrus would involve the production of two other pituitary hormones, follicle-stimulating hormone and luteinizing hormone. The sequence of events appears to be: Stimulated olfactory epithelium → ordinary neurons of CNS (neurohumors) → neurosecretory cells of the hypothalamus (3 neurohormones as releasing factors) → 3 anterior pituitary gonadotrophins → ovaries (progestogens and estrogens) → responses of accessory sex organs and behavioral changes.[16]

HISTORICAL BACKGROUND

Five points may be noted in the historical development of endocrinology: (1) It advanced as a medical specialty and the basic aspects have not yet received adequate attention. (2) In nearly all instances, a substantial amount of physiologic experimentation preceded the chemical identification of a hormone. (3) The announcement of a new hormone has usually been followed by exaggeration and oversimplification of its role in the organism. (4) The functional interrelationships of the nervous and endocrine systems are just beginning to receive proper emphasis. (5) Through the use of modern techniques, substantial progress has been made in understanding intracellular mechanisms, and this has led to a reorientation of thinking in endocrinology, especially toward a new emphasis on how hormones act at the level of target cells. The indications are that specific hormones may exert multiple actions within a particular cell, and their mechanisms of action may be different in different target tissues.

We cannot say exactly when or how the concept of internal secretion began. Perhaps the rudiments of the subject are as old as the history of man, but it is certain that the most brilliant achievements have occurred since the beginning of the present century. Scientific fields, at every stage of development, are restless with new discoveries and with changing concepts. As in a long-distance relay race, each investigator takes up the problem where someone else left off. Many of the theories advanced by nineteenth century biologists had to be rejected or modulated, but these earlier workers did succeed in laying a foundation upon which endocrinology could be built.

Early History

From ancient times there has been the general belief that organs such as the heart, gonads, or brain taken from animals or slain enemies might be eaten in order to improve one's health. This old belief appears to have been carried over to early medical practice and ultimately led to the treatment of diseased organs by administering an extract of a similar but healthy organ. In a sense, it was a crude concept of *substitution therapy.*

Hippocrates (460–357 B.C.), a Greek physician, denied that disease could be caused by the intervention of deities and demons. In his concept of the "four humors" (blood, black bile, yellow bile, and phlegm), he apparently entertained the notion that health was conditioned by the correct balance of materials in the body.

Castration of man and domesticated animals has been practiced from very early times. Aristotle (384–322 B.C.) described with remarkable accuracy the effects of castration in the bird and compared the involutionary changes with those that occur in castrated men. Although there was no understanding of the mechanism involved, experience had clearly shown that the testes are related to the sexual characteristics and reproductive capacity of the male.

John Hunter (1728–1793), a British surgeon, performed a fascinating series of experiments on the transplantation of dog and human teeth into roosters' combs. He also reported success in exchanging spurs between hens and roosters. The evidence indicates that Hunter had successfully transplanted avian testes in 1771 or earlier. He published a paper on spontaneous sex reversal in the pheasant and tried to transplant testes into female hosts but was unable to find any significant effects. There is no proof that Hunter was aware that the testes release secretions into the blood for maintenance of male sex characters.

The first clear-cut and successful experiment bearing on an endocrine gland was reported in 1849 by A. A. Berthold, a physician and professor in Göttingen.[9] He caponized cockerels and, in some of the birds, returned a single testis to the body cavity. The animals carrying testicular grafts exhibited normal sexual behavior, and the sex accessories were comparable to those of normal males. The comb became atrophic after caponization, but a testicular graft, devoid of original nervous connections, caused the comb to grow to normal proportions. He concluded that the testes release something into the blood that maintains male behavior and the secondary sex characters.

Berthold's interpretation of his results was influenced by his concept of inheritance—a variation of the theory of pangenesis. This theory held that all components of the body threw off particles that circulated freely throughout the system and finally collected in the reproductive organs, where they formed an aggregate capable of giving rise to miniature offspring resembling the parent or parents. Whatever may have been Berthold's motives for performing his experiment, he had two useful concepts at his disposal: parts of the body release specific materials into the blood, and the latter conveys them to particular sites were they are utilized for special purposes. Berthold lived for 12 years after publishing his results, and we have no idea why he apparently went no further. Forbes suggests, "Perhaps he lost interest, or perhaps his experiments were ridiculed, or perhaps he did not appreciate that he had clearly marked a path into a new field of science."[27]

Claude Bernard (1855) showed by chemical methods that the liver could release sugar directly into the blood, and referred to this function as "internal secretion." In the same year, Thomas Addison called attention to a human syndrome (now called Addison's disease) associated with deterioration of the adrenal cortex. He described the outstanding symptoms as impaired appetite, low blood pressure, extreme muscular weakness, gastrointestinal upsets, discoloration of the skin and eventual death. Although some information had accumulated by this time concerning thyroid deficiencies and excesses, Addison's disease appears to be the first clinical defect of an endocrine gland to be accurately described.

In 1889, Brown-Séquard, a French physician, aroused the scientific world by attempting self-rejuvenation, at the age of 72, by taking subcutaneous injections of aqueous extracts of dog testes. He described in intimate detail the astonishing improvement that he experienced after his treatment. Although his attempts at endocrine substitution therapy stimulated much interest, it is now known that his claimed rejuvenation was due to autosuggestion rather than to any male hormone present in the aqueous extracts. Furthermore, the year 1889 stands out in endocrinology because it saw the report by von Mering and Minkowski on the production of diabetes mellitus in the dog through surgical removal of the pancreas.

Murray (1891), an English physician, prepared a glycerin emulsion of sheep's thyroids and demonstrated that the parenteral administration of it provided a helpful replacement therapy in human subjects suffering from hypothyroidism. The parathyroid glands were regarded as small masses of accessory thyroid tissue until Gley, in the same year, demonstrated that the two tissues have separate functions.

Baumann (1895) observed an extraordinarily high concentration of iodine in the thyroid gland, the amount being hundreds of times higher than that of other tissues. He reported that thyroid glands from persons inhabiting seacoast areas contained more iodine than those from persons living further inland. Magnus-Levy (1896) discovered that thyroid deficiency leads to a marked fall in the basal metabolic rate.

The experiments of Oliver and Schäfer (1895), demonstrating the vasopressor effects of adrenal extracts, led to the isolation, purification, identification, and final synthesis of epinephrine. They also prepared extracts of the pituitary gland and found that these, upon intravenous injection, produced a rapid rise of blood pressure. A few years later, it was shown by others that this vasopressor effect could be obtained only from the "posterior lobe" of the pituitary, and that such extracts also produced powerful contractions of the uterus.

At this point the concept of internal secretion was not well established, and there was much discussion concerning the significance of iodine storage by the thyroid. Many workers alleged that the extraction of iodine from the blood by the thyroid could be interpreted as a detoxicating function. The view that iodine is an essential atom of a molecule synthesized by the thyroid began to take shape before 1900; a period of intensive interest in thyroid biochemistry was initiated and this has continued to the present time.

The Twentieth Century

By the beginning of the twentieth century the impacts of Darwin's theory of evolution and of Mendel's theory of inheritance began to be felt in all compartments of human life and thought. The rapid strides made by the biologic sciences since that time are due in large measure to the adoption of a mechanistic point of view. Investigators began to proceed on the assumption that the phenomena of living organisms — inheritance, growth, reproduction, and the like — follow the terms of natural laws that can be discovered and explained. Organic evolution, implying a genetic kinship among all organisms, suggested that the biology of the human body is best viewed in the light of its animal ancestry. It is not surprising to find that enzymatic systems appear to be similar throughout the whole biologic kingdom. The chemistry of energy exchange in bacteria and in yeast cells is not so different from that in mammalian muscles, which suggests that all living organisms are constructed according to a fundamental pattern that varies only a little from species to species. Since 1900, comparative endocrinology has slowly taken shape, and the results have already indicated that it is a fruitful avenue of approach to human problems.

The Birth of Endocrinology. The real science of endocrinology was probably born through the experiments of Bayliss and Starling (1902 to 1905).[6] Their work showed the existence and manner of action, at the level of the whole organism, of the hormone *secretin*. This secretion is released from cells of the duodenal mucosa when acidified food enters from the stomach; it is conveyed by the circulation to the pancreas, where it stimulates the rapid discharge of pancreatic juice through the pancreatic duct. Although it had been recognized before this time that a variety of endocrine glands exert influences on the body, this discovery was epoch-making because it proved unequivocally for the first time that chemical integration could occur without assistance from the nervous system. It clearly confirmed the idea that special glands elaborate chemical agents, which are freed into the blood and exert regulatory effects upon distant target organs and tissues.

Starling first used the word "hormone" (Greek *hormon,* exciting, setting in motion) in 1905 with reference to secretin. Although, if its meaning is taken literally, the term is not entirely satisfactory, it is still in common use. It is now well known that hormones may inhibit as well as excite, and they do not initiate metabolic transformations but merely alter the rate at which these changes occur. Pende introduced the term "endocrinology" (Greek *endon,* within; *krinein,* to separate) a few years later.

The twentieth century has seen the isolation and structural identification of a large number of hormones from vertebrates, and a few from invertebrates. The biochemical epoch in endocrinology began with Takamine and Aldrich (1901), who, working independently, succeeded in crystallizing epinephrine, one of the hormones from the adrenal medulla.

The Slow Growth of the Infant Science. Gudernatsch in 1912 found thyroid tissue to be an extremely potent substance in accelerating the metamorphosis of frogs and salamanders.[28] This response of the tadpole provided a sensitive test for assaying the potency of thyroid preparations. Kendall (1919) obtained pure thyroxine from the thyroid glands of swine; Harrington showed it to be an amino acid related to tyrosine and established its chemical constitution in 1926.

The isolation of insulin was a difficult undertaking because the proteolytic enzymes of the acinar portion of the pancreas destroyed its activity in the process of extraction. Banting and Best (1921, 1922), using pancreatic tissue from dogs whose acinar tissue had been caused to degenerate by ligation of the pancreatic duct, succeeded in preparing highly potent extracts.[3] The potency of the extracts was assayed on the basis of their capacity to reduce the blood sugar of experimental animals. Abel (1926) prepared insulin in crystalline form and demonstrated the protein nature of the purified hormone.

That the ovaries play a more subtle role in reproduction than the mere production of eggs had been obvious for many years. No real progress was made until it became possible to relate the cyclic changes in the ovary with those that occur in the accessory sex organs. Of paramount importance in reproductive physiology were the studies of Stockard and Papanicolaou (1917) on the estrous cycle of the guinea pig, and similar studies on the mouse by E. Allen (1922) and on the rat by Long and Evans (1922).[1, 59] Allen and Doisy, in their classic studies during the 1920's, reported that the liquor folliculi from the large follicles of swine ovaries or lipid-soluble extracts of this fluid contained an agent that induced estrous changes in the vaginae of castrated mice. All attempts at this stage to crystallize the *estrogen* (a generic term for estrus-producing compounds) met with failure.

In 1927, Aschheim and Zondek made an astonishing discovery that changed the whole face of research in this field: They reported that the urine from many pregnant animals contained two hitherto unsuspected hormones.[2] One of these was similar to the estrus-producing agent in the fluid of the graafian follicle, whereas the other caused marked growth of ovarian follicles. The latter substance is now known to be chorionic gonadotrophin (of placental origin), which forms the basis of the well-known Aschheim-Zondek test for pregnancy. Doisy and Butenandt, in 1929, independently succeeded in crystallizing the estrogenic substance from human pregnancy urine; it is now known as *estrone*. Thus, estrogens were the first steroid hormones to be isolated. The actual isolation of estrogens directly from ovarian tissue was accomplished by Doisy (1935) and MacCorquodale (1936). From 4 tons of sows' ovaries, MacCorquodale obtained some 12 mg of estradiol-17β, and this accounted for about 50 per cent of the estrogenic activity present.

Corner and W. M. Allen (1929) prepared extracts of corpora lutea that effectively maintained pregnancy in ovariectomized rabbits and worked together with estrogen to produce a proliferated uterus suitable for implantation of the blastocysts.[23] They found that the proliferative effect on the rabbit's uterus could be used as a bioassay for the hormone. Pregnanediol, a urinary metabolite of the corpus luteum hormone (progesterone), was chemically determined by Butenandt in 1932. Since pregnanediol was quite inactive biologically, no indication of the identity of progesterone was forthcoming until it was actually isolated from ovarian tissue. Four groups of workers in 1934 obtained progesterone almost simultaneously by extraction of sows' ovaries, and its structure was determined in the same year.

Hisaw (1926) presented evidence for a hormone of pregnancy which, among other effects, causes relaxation of the pelvic ligaments of guinea pigs, thus facilitating parturition.[33] This substance, called *relaxin,* is a nonsteroid and appears to be polypeptide in nature; its exact role in reproduction has not yet been revealed completely.

The first effective extracts of testicular tissue were probably prepared by Pézard in 1911. His extracts caused renewed growth of the capon's comb, and he pointed out that this effect provided a suitable bioassay for testicular secretion. Knowing that the hormone of the ovarian follicle is fat-soluble, and assuming that the male hormone was likewise fat-soluble, McGee (1927) extracted bull testes and obtained a material that was relatively potent in stimulating growth of the capon's comb.

It was discovered that, like the estrogens, androgens (substances producing masculinizing effects) are present in the urine. Butenandt (1931) extracted crystals of male sex hormone from urine and called the compound "androsterone." David and his colleagues (1935) isolated pure crystalline hormone from testicular material and named it testosterone." It was correctly assumed that androsterone is a degradation product of testosterone, and it is interesting to note that two groups of workers (Butenandt and Ruzicka) had practically synthesized testosterone before it had been obtained from testicular tissue. It was feasible to prepare testosterone synthetically from cholesterol, and large amounts promptly became available for experimental and clinical use.

Practically no progress was made in elucidating the hormones of the adrenal cortex until a satisfactory method of adrenalectomy had been perfected, and until the fat-soluble nature of these substances had become apparent, during the early 1930's. Moreover, satisfactory end-points for bioassay had to be established. The first potent extracts were made by Swingle and Pfiffner in 1930. Between the years 1936 and 1942, four groups of workers in the United States and Europe succeeded in isolating approximately 30 different steroids from the adrenal cortices of slaughterhouse animals, including six compounds that were biologically potent. The magnitude of the task is indicated by calculations from Reichstein's laboratory: It took about 20,000 cattle to give 100 kg of adrenal glands, from which 26 gm of highly fractionated material (containing all biologic activity) could be obtained; this gave a yield of approximately 300 mg each of the 29 steroid compounds obtained.

Endocrine studies on the pituitary gland were hampered for many years because of the surgical difficulties attendant upon removing the organ without injury to the brain. A landmark of great significance was the successful removal of the adenohypophysial placode of young frog tadpoles by P. E. Smith and B. M. Allen, working independently in 1916. Aschner (1910) worked out a technique for performing hypophysectomies in dogs, and Smith (1926) developed a similar method for ablating the gland in rats and other laboratory rodents.[56] A notable achievement with reference to the neural lobe was made by Kamm and his colleagues in 1928.[36] They separated the the oxytocic and vasopressor principles in sufficiently pure states for therapeutic purposes.

Since all of the pituitary hormones are polypeptides or proteins, their chemical elucidation has been understandably slow. The excellent studies of Stricker and Grueter (1928) indicated clearly that the anterior pituitary is essential for the initiation and maintenance of milk secretion. Riddle (1933) noted that the pituitary principle that induced lactation in mammals was the same as that which caused growth of the pigeon's crop gland. This discovery provided a very sensitive and useful bioassay method for this particular hormone and did much to hasten its chemical isolation. Prolactin (lactogenic hormone) was obtained in crystalline form by White and his colleagues (1937); it was the first pituitary hormone to be isolated as a pure or nearly pure protein.[63]

Many of the invertebrates lend themselves particularly well as subjects for the investigation of neuroendocrine controls. Kopeč (1917) showed that a neurohormone from the brain controlled pupation in certain insects, thereby demonstrating for the first time that central nervous structures could perform endocrine roles. Since then, various species of insects and crustaceans have been investigated intensively, and it is certain that many of the growth and differentiation, reproductive, and metabolic processes, as well as color adaptations, are under neuroendocrine control. The functional significance of neurosecretory centers became apparent in the invertebrates before it was recognized that secretion by nerve cells might be an important phenomenon in vertebrates. Clues derived from the invertebrates and lower vertebrates have appreciably influenced our interpretation of the manner in which the hypothalamic portion of the brain regulates the secretions of the mammalian pituitary gland.

The field of plant hormones began to take shape after the experiments of Boysen-Jensen (1910) on the responses of the oat coleoptile (leaf sheath) to light. The term "auxin" is applied to organic compounds that, in low concentration, cause the longitudinal growth of shoots by cell elongation, rather than by cell division. A variety of hormone-like substances have been found to influence growth, cell division, and flower formation. Indole-3-acetic acid is the best known auxin. The interesting observation has been made that a particular auxin may stimulate growth of the shoot by cell elongation, induce cell division at the site of a wound, and inhibit the growth of roots and lateral buds.

An Era of Spectacular Growth. The 1940's ushered in a period of biochemical expansion and inquiry that was unprecedented in the history of endocrinology. In 1949, Hench and his colleagues cautiously announced that a hormone of the adrenal cortex, cortisone or compound E, improved some of the clinical and biochemical symptoms of rheumatoid arthritis.[31] This study was possible because cortisone had been partially synthesized and was available in sufficient quantities for testing, whereas the other adrenal steroids could be produced only in milligram amounts. Even though this clinical announcement was followed by what now seems to have been an unwarranted outburst of enthusiasm, it immediately precipitated a period of feverish research in the field of steroid biochemistry. In attempts to manufacture large amounts of cortisone as cheaply as possible, it was found that certain microorganisms (molds such as *Rhizopus* and *Aspergillus*) could effect enzymatic changes in the steroid molecule. Some species of yam provided an organic compound from which progesterone (corpus luteum hormone) could be prepared; the latter provides a satisfactory substrate for the production of cortisone by microbial oxygenation. The manufacture of cortisone is one of the most complicated and difficult procedures ever attempted by the pharmaceutical industry.[18]

Scientific progress depends materially upon the introduction of new tools and methods. The phase and fluorescent microscopes enable us to visualize many structures in the cell that cannot be seen with the ordinary microscope; the electron microscope gives us high resolution and has contributed much to our analysis of protoplasmic structures, large chemical molecules, and viruses. Tissue culture techniques have undergone refinement, and methods are available for the perfusion of whole organs. Of great importance in endocrinology has been the widespread use of radioactive isotopes in investigations of intermediary metabolism, and in the assay of hormones by competitive protein-binding methods. Coupled with this has been the development of excellent microanalytic methods, such as paper and partition chromatography, infrared spectrophotometry, and microwave analysis.

Hechter and his co-workers studied steroid biosynthesis by means of isolated perfused adrenals of cows, pigs, dogs, and human beings.[30] After adding appropriate steroid precursors to the perfusion medium, they could study the transformation products that the adrenal tissues released into the perfusate. By perfusing C^{14}-labeled cholesterol or radioacetate, they obtained radioactive cortical steroids in the perfusate, indicating that these two substrates could act as parent compounds. Many workers contributed to this field, and the biosynthetic sequences in the adrenal proposed by Hechter and his colleagues have been confirmed as the preferred, though not obligatory, pathway. Characterization of the enzyme systems that operate in these adrenal steroid transformations has been well developed.

Very sensitive methods are now available for the quantitative determination of steroid hormones in the blood and urine. The testes and ovaries, as well as the adrenal cortices, secrete steroids into the circulation; these are metabolized along certain pathways and are excreted as urinary metabolites or degradation products. In some cases, steroid metabolites are discharged into the bile and leave the body through the feces. These patterns of steroid degradation are so constant that it is possible to determine the type of steroid that the gland is actually secreting by analysis of the metabolites found in the urine. From studies on the types of urinary metabolites released by patients suffering from certain adrenal defects, Bongiovanni and others have shown that enzymatic defects at points along the biosynthetic pathway in the adrenal are the underlying causes of the diseases of these patients.[11] The clinical consequences result from a deficiency of the usual (finished) hormones, and from an excessive accumulation of intermediate (unfinished) steroids. More than 40 steroids have been isolated from adrenocortical tissue; approximately eight of these are potent in maintaining the life of adrenalectomized animals.

Prior to 1953, it was known that the amorphous fraction of adrenocortical extracts remaining after the then known steroids had been removed was particularly potent in maintaining the lives of adrenalectomized subjects. It was suspected that the amorphous fraction contained a hormone that was highly active in regulation of water and electrolyte metabolism. The isolation and crystallization of a new adrenal steroid, called "aldosterone," by Simpson and Tait and their co-workers in 1953 was a brilliant chapter in steroid research.[55]

During the 1930's, when so many of the natural steroid hormones were being characterized, some investigators regarded them as compounds of the highest order of physiologic effectiveness, upon which man could make no further improvements. Nevertheless, we have entered an era of striking success in synthesizing compounds that not only are more potent than the natural hormones but which are also skillfully altered in molecular structure to produce desired effects.

By applying the techniques of chromatography and radioautography of compounds labeled with I^{131} (the radioactive isotope of iodine), substantial progress has been made in understanding thyroid metabolism. Using radioiodide, Pitt-Rivers, Roche, Gross, Leblond, and others (1948 to 1953) demonstrated the presence of hitherto unknown compounds in thyroid tissue, blood serum, and other tissues. Much information has accumulated on the biochemical sequences by which thyroid compounds are formed, their transportation in the blood, and their degradation and elimination from the system. Moreover, much has been learned of the mechanisms whereby the various antithyroid drugs interfere with thyroid functions.

Principally through the work of von Euler, it has been shown that the neurotransmitter released by sympathetic nerve terminals, and long referred to as "sympathin," is norepinephrine.[62] Tuller (1949) isolated crystalline L-norepinephrine from adrenal medullary tissue and provided evidence that it is normally secreted by this part of the adrenal, along with epinephrine. The predominant role of epinephrine as an emergency substance, as postulated by Cannon and Rosenblueth (1937), has been sustained.

Spectacular progress has been made since 1950 in elucidating the structure of polypeptide and protein hormones; in some instances, the natural hormone has been synthesized and analogues prepared. All of the known hormones of the pituitary gland, pancreatic islets, and parathyroids are proteins or polypeptides. Du Vigneaud and his co-workers (1953) first determined the structure of oxytocin and vasopressin, polypeptide neurohormones of the neurohypophysis. Though these principles are small molecules, their organic synthesis by du Vigneaud was a monumental achievement in this phase of chemistry. Sanger and his colleagues (1954), using the method of partition chromatography, elucidated the full chemical structure of insulin; this was the first protein for which a complete amino acid sequence was established.[61] Insulin is also the first protein to be chemically synthesized, an accomplishment of Katsoyannis and Tometsko and several other groups of workers during the 1960's.[38] Certain analogues of insulin have been prepared, and the point has been reached at which it is possible to study the relationship between molecular structure and biologic activity. There is also the possibility that compounds may be synthesized which exert highly desirable effects.

Steiner and co-workers (1967) provided evidence that the pancreatic B-cells synthesize insulin from a single-chain protein, called "proinsulin," rather than by the simultaneous synthesis of A and B chains, followed by their union into the finished molecule. After the disulfide bonds are established between the ends of the proinsulin molecule, a connecting peptide having little if any intrinsic activity is deleted.[57]

Since insulin is destroyed by the proteolytic enzymes of the intestinal tract, it is inactive when administered by mouth. Clinicians have been looking for many years for insulin substitutes that would not produce undesirable side effects.[44] Since 1954, a number of antidiabetic compounds have been tested, and some containing sulfonylurea or biguanide radicals are quite useful in lowering the blood sugar. Sulfonylureas such as tolbutamide and chlorpropamide seem to act by increasing the effectiveness of endogenous insulin. Clinicians generally agree that such compounds are valuable adjuncts to insulin in treating *selected* types of diabetic patients.

During the 1920's it became apparent that most insulin extracts contained a contaminant that antagonized the action of insulin, raising the blood sugar instead of lowering it, as insulin does. This hyperglycemic factor is called *glucagon;* it is a hormone that is elaborated by the A-cells of the islet tissue. Glucagon was obtained in crystalline form by Staub (1955), and the amino acid sequence in the polypeptide molecule was determined by Bromer and his colleagues (1957).[12]

During the 1960's it was established that the parathyroid hormone is a single polypeptide chain consisting of about 85 amino acid residues. Different laboratories have reported minor variations in the amino acid sequence. Studies on fragmentation of the molecule indicate that not all of the amino acid residues are essential for biologic potency. There are slight species differences in chemistry of the polypeptide.

Copp and Cameron (1961) presented evidence suggesting that the parathyroids are the source of a hormone (called "calcitonin"), which lowers the level of plasma calcium, an effect opposite to that of the parathyroid hormone.[22] Two years later, Hirsch and his colleagues showed that the thyroid is the source of a principle having the same action and called it "thyrocalcitonin."[32] There is strong circumstantial evidence that this hormone is secreted by a line of cells (C-cells, parafollicular cells) derived from the neural crests. The C-cells of fishes, amphibians, reptiles, and birds migrate into the ultimobranchial bodies and, in mammals, the C-cells are apparently incorporated into the thyroid and possibly into some of the parathyroids, where they constitute distinct populations.[60] It is not surprising that the ultimobranchial tissue of birds and other submammalian vertebrates possesses calcitonin-like activity (see p. 246). Thyrocalcitonin is a straight-chain polypeptide consisting of 32 amino acid residues; the molecule recently was synthesized *in vitro.*

The separate observations of Richter and Ranson during the 1930's demonstrated that experimental diabetes insipidus involved both neural and endocrine mechanisms. Ranson and his colleagues (Fisher *et al.,* 1938) produced diabetes insipidus in the cat by using a stereotaxic device to initiate electrolytic lesions at desired points in the hypothalamus.[26] Though Ranson's group believed incorrectly that the antidiuretic principle (vasopressin) originated from pituicytes within the pars nervosa, their studies stand as a landmark in neuroendocrinology. At about the same time, Harris (1937) reported that ovulation in the rabbit could be induced by electrical stimulation of the hypothalamic region.[29] Others were encouraged by these early studies to devise methods for exploring the functions of the hypothalamus and related brain areas. Techniques were found for destroying or stimulating circumscribed brain centers, for the accurate installation of hormone pellets and other agents, for the chemical testing of brain tissue, and for the use of autoradiography for detecting the affinity of neurons for particular hormones.[43] It was largely through the pioneering efforts of the Scharrers (1940) that the concept of secretion by glandlike neurons came to be appreciated.[54] Hanström, Wigglesworth, Williams, Fukuda, and others made neuroendocrine studies on a variety of arthropods during the 1940's, and their results had considerable impact upon the thinking of those who worked with higher vertebrates. The investigations and interpretations of Palay, Bargmann, and Harris were of great importance in clarifying the manner in which hypothalamic centers exert neurohormonal control of pituitary functions.

One of the most tantalizing problems in endocrinology has been that of the site of origin of the posterior pituitary principles, and the consensus has shifted several times since 1900. As an outgrowth of studies on neurosecretion, evidence has accumulated that these octapeptides are synthesized by modified neurons in certain brain nuclei. After moving along the axons of such cells the neurohormonal substances are freed into the posterior pituitary (pars nervosa) where they are stored, possibly altered, and released into the blood as needed. This concept is now well documented and is generally accepted.[4]

Another problem receiving much attention is the mechanism of release of the adenohypophysial hormones. It is generally agreed that the cells of the anterior pituitary receive very few secretory nerve fibers. Thus, it has become apparent that the gland must be regulated largely by agents that reach it through the circulation. The indications are that neurosecretory cells within the hypothalamus, in response to exteroceptive factors or to the level of hormones in the circulation, produce special *release factors,* which are delivered to the adenohypophysis via the portal vessels that course along the pituitary stalk.[51] The physiology and chemistry of these regulatory neurohormones are being pursued with great vigor. They are polypeptides of low molecular weights, and appear to be distinct from those of the neurohypophysis. While the three lobes of the pituitary gland differ markedly in their anatomic relationships with the brain, it appears that the functions of the whole gland are under direct or indirect neural control.

During the 1960's, spectacular progress was made in isolating, characterizing, and synthesizing some of the arthropod hormones. A proper balance of hormones within the insect is essential for growth, molting, metamorphosis, and reproduction, and it has become apparent that these agents may be employed as insecticides; they are effective in low concentrations, generally are specific for particular insects, probably are harmless to other animals, and there is no likelihood that an insect could survive if it built up resistance to its own hormones. Karlson and his co-workers isolated and synthesized the first invertebrate hormone, and called it "ecdysone." The natural hormone (α-ecdysone) is steroidal in nature and its production in the insect is dependent upon the prothoracic glands. It is probable that a whole family of ecdysones, slightly different in chemical structure, is present in the insect body. Beta-ecdysone (crustecdysone, ecdysterone) is the molting hormone of crustaceans, and it has also been synthesized. Fifteen or more ecdysone-like compounds (phytoecdysones) have been isolated from various weeds, ferns, and evergreen trees.[65] It is possible to modify the molecule in various ways to produce analogues for testing. Clever and Karlson (1960) proposed that insect ecdysone produces its effects by acting directly upon gene loci to stimulate the synthesis of messenger ribonucleic acid.[20, 37] This concept aroused tremendous interest, and research continues in many laboratories to determine to what extent other hormones affect gene activity.

Röller and his colleagues succeeded in 1967 in isolating and synthesizing the juvenile hormone of the silk moth *Hyalophora cecropia.*[24] This hormone is chemically related to the terpenoids and is not steroidal. Compounds similar to juvenile hormone are present in certain plants, and several analogues have been synthesized. Entomologists recognize the great potentialities of this particular hormone as a pesticide. The brain hormone (prothoracotrophin) of the silkworm *Bombyx mori* is protein-like, but its structure has not been determined.[35]

The X organ-sinus gland complex of the crustacean eyestalk contains a variety of neurohormones derived from the neurosecretory system. It is generally agreed that the chromatophorotrophins are small peptides, and some progress is being made in separating and purifying them.[39]

THE SCOPE AND POSITION OF ENDOCRINOLOGY

From the foregoing account it is clear that endocrinology, to a greater extent than most biologic studies, grew directly out of the observations and experiments of practicing physicians. In retrospect, it seems unfortunate that the hormones were studied for such a long time only from the standpoint of disease and the cure of disease. It appears that in the 1920's many investigators felt that hormones were fully understood when one became able to catalogue the signs and symptoms of their excess or deficiency. This purely clinical approach to the hormones made the subject particularly susceptible to quackery and led to considerable confusion. Not being fully aware that endocrinology is concerned with the multitude of chemical interactions occurring in health as well as with the maladjustments characterizing disease, most persons believed that endocrinologists restricted their interests to midgets, giants, bearded women, hermaphrodites, and other side-show freaks. Few if any at this period could envisage the day when endocrinologists would devote themselves to the elucidation of intracellular mechanisms in order to discover how hormones produce their organismal effects.

Happily, the tremendous impact of biochemistry, particularly with reference to intracellular controls and gene activity, felt with increasing strength during the past few decades, has led to a reorientation of thinking. With the perfusion of pure-science techniques and concepts into all phases of the subject, endocrinology has become a respected science and a dignified field of research specialization.

The Comparative Approach

There are certain parallelisms between endocrinology and anatomy. Both began at the mammalian level and progressed down the evolutionary tree. As comparative anatomy developed, largely to support or refute the theory of organic evolution, many aspects of human anatomy came to be interpreted in a new light. Advances in comparative endocrinology have necessitated the revision or deletion of numerous traditional concepts which took form when knowledge of coordinatory mechanisms was largely restricted to the higher vertebrates.

Endocrine studies have been extended to all vertebrate groups, and while they do not permit any final conclusions relative to the evolution of coordinatory systems, they do reveal a variety of unique specializations. Evaluation of the information available on the lower vertebrates (poikilotherms) makes it clear that the endocrine phenomena prevailing among mammals are far from being typical of the whole vertebrate subphylum. Even among mammals there are extreme species differences; for example, the endocrine control mechanisms responsible for the formation, functional maintenance, and loss of the ovarian corpora lutea are quite variable.[46] Invertebrate endocrinology has developed rapidly since Wigglesworth (1940), studying growth and metamorphosis in *Rhodnius* (Hemiptera), first assigned a functional role to specific groups of neurosecretory cells in the brain.[64] There is no longer any doubt that many bodily processes in insects and crustaceans are regulated through the release of neurohormones; they control many aspects of reproduction, diapause, growth, embryonic and postembryonic development, metabolism, and behavior. The concept of neurosecretion is known to find applications in many different phyla, ranging in complexity from worms to human beings. Invertebrate studies of this type had a tremendous impact on views regarding pituitary functions in vertebrates. This organ is no longer regarded as a "master gland," enjoying a high degree of autonomy, but as a structure whose output of hormones is controlled by the products of neural elements present within the central nervous system.

Endocrinology Among the Sciences

Endocrinology has many facets and, in this respect, it does not differ from most other branches of science. Its "roots" extend into various disciplines, but these roots are not one-way streets; they give as well as take. Endocrinology contributes to and draws from a large number of special fields, such as chemistry, genetics, ecology, neurology, embryology, psychology, and clinical medicine—to mention only a few. Endocrinology has both pure and applied aspects; hence, in addition to being a medical specialty, it may be properly pursued in the basic science departments as an aspect of regulatory biology.

Crystalline hormone in a test tube might hold a certain fascination for the pure chemist, but it takes on fullest meaning when studied as it operates inside a cell or organism. Although there is a large measure of overlap, biochemists and physiologists make their attacks on living protoplasm at different levels. The biochemist studies biologic systems principally at the molecular and atomic levels, whereas the physiologist is generally more concerned with the whole organism. However different these methods of attack may seem to be, application of the results to the organism itself brings unity. Investigations at all levels of biologic organization are necessary in endocrinology.

All scientists recognize that human knowledge is an entity and that sharp lines of demarcation cannot be drawn between the various disciplines. We have departments of biology, chemistry, physics, etc., simply for the practical reason that the whole is too voluminous to treat effectively. While some degree of specialization is necessary and desirable, modern science students should make every attempt to cross these departmental barriers.

The sciences have developed so rapidly that it is impossible for one person to become expert in all of the complicated techniques involved in a modern research project. It may require years to learn special surgical methods, tissue culture techniques, microchemical procedures, or the operation of complicated laboratory machines. Rapid progress, with a minimal waste of time and money, is often made when specialists from diverse areas are willing to pool their efforts and approach a research project from different angles.

REFERENCES

1. Allen, E.: The oestrous cycle of the mouse. Amer. J. Anat. *30*:297, 1922.
2. Aschheim, S., and Zondek, B.: Hypophysenvorderlappenhormon und Ovarialhormon in Harm von Schwangeren. Klin. Wschr. *6*:1322, 1927.
3. Banting, F., and Best, C. H.: The internal secretion of the pancreas. J. Lab. Clin. Med. 7: 251, 1922.
4. Bargmann, W., and Scharrer, E.: The site of origin of the hormones of the posterior pituitary. Amer. Sci. *39*:255, 1951.
5. Barth, R. H., Jr.: The endocrine control of mating behavior in the cockroach *Byrsotria fumigata* (Guérin). Gen. Comp. Endocr. *2*:53, 1962.
6. Bayliss, W.M., and Starling, E. H.: The mechanism of pancreatic secretion. J. Physiol. *28*: 325, 1902.
7. Bern, H. A.: On eyes that may not see and glands that may not secrete. Amer. Zool. 7:815, 1967.
8. Bern, H. A., and Knowles, F. G. W.: Neurosecretion. *In* L. Martini and W. F. Ganong (eds.): Neuroendocrinology, Vol. 1. New York, Academic Press, 1966, p. 139.
9. Berthold, A. A.: Trasnplantation der Hoden. Arch. Anat. Physiol. Wiss. Med. *16*:42, 1849.
10. Blaquier, J., Forchielli, E., and Dorfman, R. I.: In vitro metabolism of androgens in whole human blood. Acta Endocrinol. *55*:697, 1967.
11. Bongiovanni, A. M., Eberlein, W. R., Goldman, A. S., and New, M.: Disorders of adrenal steroid biogenesis. Rec. Progr. Horm. Res. *23*:375, 1967.
12. Bromer, W. W., Sinn, L. G., and Behrens, O. K.: The amino acid sequence of glucagon. J. Amer. Chem. Soc. *79*:2801, 1957.
13. Bronson, F. H.: Pheromonal influences on mammalian reproduction. *In* M. Diamond (ed.): Perspectives in Reproduction and Sexual Behavior. Bloomington, Indiana University Press, 1968, p. 341.
14. Bronson, F. H., Eleftheriou, B. E., and Dezell, H. E.: Strange male pregnancy block in deermice: Prolactin and adrenocortical hormones. Biol. Reprod. *1*:302, 1969.
15. Bronson, F. H., and Whitten, W. K.: Oestrus-accelerating pheromone in mice: Assay, androgen-dependency and presence in bladder urine, J. Reprod. Fert. *15*:131, 1968.
16. Bruce, H. M.: Pheromones. Brit. Med. Bull. *26*:10, 1970.
17. Bullough, W. S.: Chalone control mechanisms. Life Sciences *16*:323, 1975.
18. Callow, R. K.: The source of cortisone. Med. World *84*:477, 1956.
19. Charniaux-Cotton, H.: Androgenic gland of crustaceans. Gen. Comp. Endocr. (Suppl.) *1*: 241, 1962.
20. Clever, U., and Karlson, P.: Induktion von Puff-Veränderungen in den Speicheldrüsenchromosomen von *Chironomus tentans* durch Ecdyson. Exp. Cell Res. *20*:623, 1960.
21. Cohen, S., and Taylor, J. M.: Epidermal growth factor: Chemical and biological characterization. *In* E. J. Hay, T. J. King, and J. Papaconstantinou (eds.): Macromolecules Regulating Growth and Development. New York, Academic Press, 1974, p. 25.
22. Copp, D. H., and Cameron, E. C.: Demonstration of a hypocalcemic factor (calcitonin) in commercial parathyroid extract. Science *134*:2038, 1961.

23. Corner, G. W., and Allen, W. M.: Physiology of the corpus luteum: Production of a special uterine reaction (progestational proliferation) by extracts of the corpus luteum. Amer. J. Physiol. *88*:326, 1929.
24. Dahm, K. H., Frost, B. M., and Röller, H.: Synthesis of the racemic juvenile hormone. J. Amer. Chem. Soc. *89*:5292, 1967.
25. Davenport, D.: Specificity and behavior in symbiosis. Quart. Rev. Biol. *30*:29, 1955.
26. Fisher, C., Ingram, W. R., and Ranson, S. W.: Diabetes insipidus and the neurohormonal control of water balance: A contribution to the structure and function of the hypothalamico-hypophyseal system. Ann. Arbor, Mich., Edwards Brothers, 1938.
27. Forbes, T. R.: A. A. Berthold and the first endocrine experiment: Some speculation as to its origin. Bull. Hist. Med. *23*:263, 1949.
28. Gudernatsch, J. F.: Feeding experiments on tadpoles. Arch. Entwicklungsmech. Organ. *35*: 457, 1912.
29. Harris, G. W.: Induction of ovulation in the rabbit by electrical stimulation of the hypothalamo-hypophysial mechanism. Proc. Roy. Soc. Lond. (Suppl. B) *122*:374, 1937.
30. Hechter, O., and others: Chemical transformation of steroids by adrenal perfusion: Perfusion methods. Endocrinology *52*:679, 1953.
31. Hench, P. S., Kendall, E. C., Slocumb, C. H., and Polley, H. F.: The effect of a hormone of the adrenal cortex (17-hydroxy-11-dehydrocorticosterone: compound E) and of pituitary adrenocorticotrophic hormone on rheumatoid arthritis: Preliminary report. Proc. Staff Meet. Mayo Clin. *24*:181, 1949.
32. Hirsch, P. F., Gauthier, G. F., and Munson, P. L.: Thyroid hypocalcemic principle and recurrent laryngeal nerve injury as factors affecting the response to parathyroidectomy in rats. Endocrinology *73*:244, 1963.
33. Hisaw, F. L.: Experimental relaxation of the pubic ligament of the guinea pig. Proc. Soc. Exp. Biol. Med. *23*:661, 1926.
34. Horton, R., and Tait, J. F.: Androstenedione production and interconversion rates measured in peripheral blood and studies on the possible site of its conversion to testosterone. J. Clin. Invest. *45*:301, 1966.
35. Ishizaki, H., and Ichikawa, M.: Purification of the brain horome of the silkworm *Bombyx mori*. Biol. Bull. *133*:355, 1967.
36. Kamm, O., Aldrich, T. B., Grote, I. W., Rowe, L. W., and Bugabee, E. P.: The active principles of the posterior lobe of the pituitary gland. The separation of two principles and their concentration in the form of potent solid preparations. J. Amer. Chem. Soc. *50*:573, 1928.
37. Karlson, P., and Sekeris, C. E.: Ecdysone, an insect steriod hormone, and its mode of action. Rec. Progr. Horm. Res. *22*:473, 1966.
38. Katsoyannis, P. G., and Tometsko, A.: Insulin synthesis by recombination of A and B chains. A highly efficient method. Proc. Nat. Acad. Sci. *55*:1554, 1966.
39. Kleinholz, L. H.: Separation and purification of crustacean eyestalk hormones. Amer. Zool. *6*:161, 1966.
40. Law, J. H., and Regnier, F. E.: Pheromones. Ann. Rev. Biochem. *40*:533, 1971.
41. Lentz, T. L.: Hydra: induction of supernumerary heads by isolated neurosecretory granules. Science *150*:633, 1965.
42. Leopold, A. C., and de la Fuente, R. K.: The polarity of auxin transport. Ann. N. Y. Acad. Sci. *144*:94, 1967.
43. Lisk, R. D.: Brain investigation techniques in the study of reproduction and sex behavior. *In* M. Diamond (ed.): Perspectives in Reproduction and Sexual Behavior. Bloomington, Indiana University Press, 1968, p. 287.
44. Loubatières, A.: The hypoglycemic sulfonamides: History and development of the problem from 1942 to 1955. Ann. N. Y. Acad. Sci. *71*:4, 1957.
45. Martan, J.: Effect of castration and androgen replacement on the supracaudal gland of the male guinea pig. J. Morph. *110*:285, 1962.
46. Nalbandov, A. V.: Comparative aspects of corpus luteum functions, Biol. Repro. *2*:7, 1970.
47. Nandi, J.: Comparative endocrinology of steroid hormones in vertebrates. Amer. Zool. *7*: 115, 1967.
48. Parkes, A. S., and Bruce, H. M.: Olfactory stimuli in mammalian reproduction. Science *134*: 1049, 1961.
49. Raper, J. R.: Sexual hormones in *Achyla*. Amer. Sci. *39*:110, 1951.
50. Roth, L. M., and Barth, R. H., Jr.: The sense organs employed by cockroaches in mating behavior. Behavior *28*:58, 1967.
51. Schally, A. V., Arimura, A., Bowers, C. Y. Kastin, A. J., Sawano, S., and Redding, T. W.: Hypothalamic neurohomones regulating anterior pituitary function. Rec. Progr. Horm. Res. *24*:497, 1968.

52. Scharrer, B.: Neurohumors and neurohormones: Definitions and terminology. J. Neurovisceral Relations (Suppl.) 9:1, 1969.
53. Scharrer, B.: The spectrum of neuroendocrine communication. In S. Karger (ed.): Recent Studies of Hypothalamic Function. Int. Symp. Calgary, 1973, p. 8.
54. Scharrer, E., and Scharrer, B.: Secretory cells within the hypothalamus. Res. Pub. Ass. Res. Nerv. Ment. Dis. 20:170, 1940.
55. Simpson, S. A., Tait, J. F., Wettstein, A., Neher, R., v.Euw, J., and Reichstein, R.: Isolierung eines neuen Kristallisierten Hormons aus Nebennieren mit besonders hoher Wirksamkeit auf den Mineralstoffwechsel. Experientia 9:333, 1953.
56. Smith, P. E.: Ablation and transplantation of the hypophysis in the rat. Anat. Rec. 32:221, 1926.
57. Steiner, D. F., Cunningham, D., Spigelman, L., and Aten, B.: Insulin biosynthesis: evidence for a precursor. Science 157:697, 1967.
58. Steward, F. C.: Growth and Organization in Plants. Reading, Mass., Addison-Wesley Co., 1968, p. 132.
59. Stockard, C. R., and Papanicolaou, G. N.: The existence of a typical oestrous cycle in the guinea-pig with a study of its histological and physiological changes. Amer. J. Anat. 22: 225, 1917.
60. Taylor, S. (ed.): Calcitonin: Symposium on Thyrocalcitonin and the C Cells. London, Heineman, 1968.
61. Thompson, E. O. P.: The insulin molecule. Sci. Amer. 192(5): 36, 1955.
62. von Euler, U. S.: Adrenergic neurohormones. In U. S. vonEuler and H. Heller (eds.): Comparative Endocrinology, Vol. 2. New York, Academic Press, 1963, p. 209.
63. White, A., Catchpole, H. B., and Long, C. N. H.: A crystalline protein with high lactogenic activity. Science 86:82, 1937.
64. Wigglesworth, V. B.: The determination of characters at metamorphosis in Rhodnius prolixus (Hemiptera). J. Exp. Biol. 17:201, 1940.
65. Williams, C. M., and Robbins, W. E.: Conference on insect-plant interactions. BioScience 18:791, 1968.
66. Wilson, E. O., and Bossert, W. H.: Chemical communication among animals. Rec. Progr. Horm. Res. 19:673, 1963.

SOME BOOKS OF IMPORTANCE IN COMPARATIVE ENDOCRINOLOGY

Altschule, M. D. (ed.): Frontiers of Pineal Physiology. Cambridge, Mass., The MIT Press, 1975.
Bagnara, J. T., and Hadley, M. E.: Comparative Physiology of Animal Pigmentation. Englewood Cliffs, N. J., Prentice-Hall, 1973.
Bargmann, W., and Scharrer, B., (eds.): Aspects of Neuroendocrinology. New York, Springer-Verlag, 1970.
Barrington, E. J. W. (ed.): Trends in Comparative Endocrinology. American Zoologist Supplement. Utica, N. Y., T. J. Griffiths Sons, Inc., 1975.
Barrington, E. J. W.: An Introduction to General and Comparative Endocrinology. Oxford, Clarendon Press, 1975.
Eakin, R. M.: The Third Eye. Berkeley, University of California Press, 1973.
Etkin, W., and Gilbert, L. I. (eds.): Metamorphosis: A Problem in Developmental Biology. New York, Appleton-Century-Crofts, 1968.
Frieden, E., and Lipner, H.: Biochemical Endocrinology of the Vertebrates. Englewood Cliffs, N. J., Prentice-Hall, Inc., 1971.
Ganong, W. F., and Martini, L. (eds.): Frontiers in Neuroendocrinology. New York, Oxford University Press, Inc., 1969.
Gorbman, A., and Bern, H. A.: A Textbook of Comparative Endocrinology. New York, John Wiley & Sons, 1962.
Greep, R. O. (vol. ed.): Reproductive Physiology, Vol. 8. Baltimore, University Park Press, 1974.
Greep, R. O. and Astwood, E. B. (sect. eds.): Handbook of Physiology, Section 7: Endocrinology. Vols. I–IV. Washington, D. C., American Physiological Society, 1974.
Hamburgh, M., and Barrington, E. J. W. (eds.): Hormones in Development. New York, Appleton-Century-Crofts, 1971.
Harris, G. W., and Donovan, B. T. (eds.): The Pituitary Gland (3 vols.). Berkeley, University of California Press, 1966.
Highnam, K. C., and Hill, L.: The Comparative Endocrinology of the Invertebrates. London, Edward Arnold Ltd., 1969.

Hoar, W. S., and Bern, H. A. (eds.): Progress in Comparative Endocrinology. General and Comparative Endocrinology *Supplement 3*. New York, Academic Press, 1972.

Hoar, W. S., and Randall, D. J. (eds.): Fish Physiology (3 vols.). New York, Academic Press, 1969.

Holmes, R. L., and Ball, J. N.: The Pituitary Gland. A Comparative Account. New York, Cambridge University Press, 1974.

King, R. J. B., and Mainwaring, W. I. P.: Steroid-Cell Interactions. Baltimore, University Park Press, 1974.

Knowles, F., and Vollrath, L. (eds.): Neurosecretion—The Final Neuroendocrine Pathway. New York, Springer Verlag, 1974.

Li, C. H. (ed.): Hormonal Proteins and Peptides, Vols. 1 & 2. New York, Academic Press, 1973.

Litwack, G. (ed.): Biochemical Actions of Hormones (3 vols.). New York, Academic Press, 1975.

Long, J. A., and Evans, H. M.: The Oestrus Cycle in the Rat and Its Associated Phenomena. Men. Univ. Calif. *6*: 1–148, 1922.

Martini, L., and Ganong, W. F. (eds.): Neuroendocrinology (2 vols.). New York, Academic Press, 1966–1967.

McCann, S. M. (ed.): Endocrine Physiology, Vol. 5. Baltimore, University Park Press, 1974.

Rickenberg, H. V. (ed.): Biochemistry of Hormones, Vol. 8. Baltimore, University Park Press, 1974.

Robison, G. A., Butcher, R. W., and Sutherland, E. W.: Cyclic AMP. New York, Academic Press, 1971.

Scharrer, E., and Scharrer, B.: Neuroendocrinology. New York, Columbia University Press, 1963.

Stumpf, W. E., and Grant, L. D. (eds.): Anatomical Neuroendocrinology. Basel, Karger, 1975.

Tepperman, J.: Metabolic and Endocrine Physiology: An Introductory Text, 2nd ed. Chicago, Year Book Medical Publishers, Inc., 1968.

Thomas, J. A., and Sengel, R. L. (eds.): Molecular Mechanisms of Gonadal Hormone Action. Advances in Sex Hormone Research, vol. 1. Baltimore, University Park Press, 1975.

Williams, R. H. (ed): Textbook of Endocrinology, 5th Ed. Philadelphia, W. B. Saunders Co., 1974.

Young, W. C. (ed.): Sex and Internal Secretions, 3rd ed. (2 vols.). Baltimore, The Williams & Wilkins Co., 1961.

CHAPTER 2

The Science of Endocrinology

Just as with so many disciplines in the life sciences, our knowledge of all aspects of endocrinology, both vertebrate and invertebrate, increases every day. It is fortunate that nature has provided such consistent and well-organized endocrine systems that allow us to assimilate readily this wealth of new material. Among vertebrates, endocrine homologies are obvious, and studies of invertebrates have revealed the existence of numerous analogies with the vertebrate endocrine system. Thus, as we consider various problems and concepts in endocrinology, such as methods of study, synthesis and release of hormones, hormone transport, receptor mechanisms, mechanisms of hormone action, and hormonal interrelations, it is a happy circumstance that discoveries made on one organism may have ready application to our knowledge of others. Because our understanding of the vertebrate endocrine system is more profound than it is for that of invertebrates, and because it seems that a greater consistency exists with the former, it seems appropriate to initiate our discussion of the science of endocrinology with the vertebrate endocrine system.

GENERAL ORGANIZATION OF THE VERTEBRATE ENDOCRINE SYSTEM

The approximate positions of the best known endocrine glands of the human body are indicated in Figure 2–1. Since little positional change has occurred in these structures during evolution, this diagram would serve for almost any vertebrate.

At the center of the endocrine system is the hypophysis, or pituitary gland, a relatively small, unpaired organ attached by a slender stalk to the floor of the brain. The pituitary consists of an *adenohypophysis* and a *neurohypophysis,* and these two subdivisions are distinctly different in embryonic origin and in histologic composition. The adenohypophysis includes the anterior lobe (pars distalis) with its pars tuberalis, and the intermediate lobe (pars intermedia). The so-called "posterior lobe" is only a part of a unit that should be termed the neurohypophysis. The latter consists of the median eminence of the tuber cinereum; certain nuclei in the hypothalamus; their axons, which descend along the stalk; and the neural lobe (pars nervosa) in which many of the axons terminate. The hypophysial portal venules are of great functional importance since they convey blood from the primary capil-

28

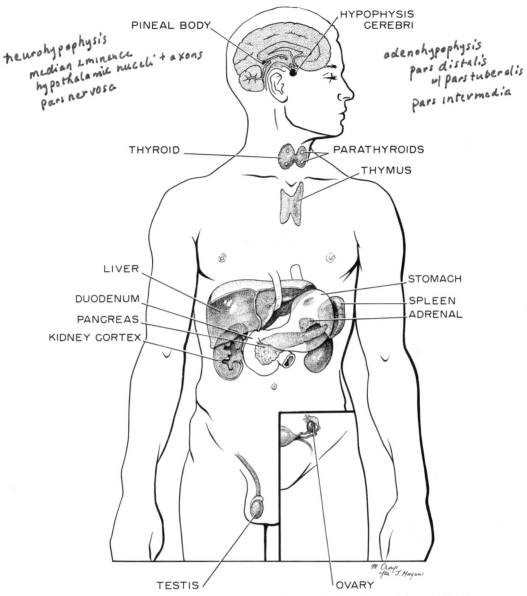

PINEAL BODY

HYPOPHYSIS
CEREBRI

neurohypophysis
median eminence
hypothalamic nuclei + axons
pars nervosa

adenohypophysis
pars distalis
w/ pars tuberalis
pars intermedia

THYROID

PARATHYROIDS

THYMUS

LIVER
DUODENUM
PANCREAS
KIDNEY CORTEX

STOMACH
SPLEEN
ADRENAL

TESTIS

OVARY

M. Craig
after J. Magan

Figure 2–1. Approximate locations of the endocrine glands of man. Though the liver, kidneys, and spleen add important materials to the blood they are not definitely known to be organs of internal secretion.

lary plexus of the median eminence to the sinusoidal spaces (secondary plexus) of the anterior lobe. An awareness of these vascular and neural connections is essential to an understanding of current concepts regarding the manner in which the hypothalamus controls the release of pituitary hormones (Fig. 2–2). There is substantial evidence that neurosecretory products (release factors) are discharged around the capillary loops of the median

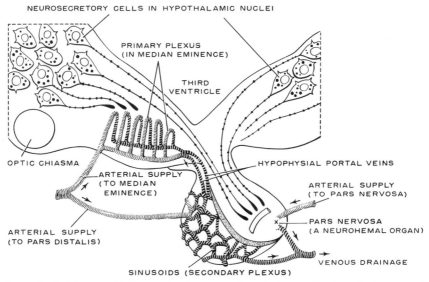

Figure 2-2. Diagram of the anatomic connections between the hypothalamus and the pituitary gland. Neurosecretory cells are present in certain hypothalamic nuclei: Some of the secretory axons pass down the infundibular stalk and terminate near blood vessels in the pars nervosa; others terminate in close proximity to the capillary loops of the median eminence. The hormones of the neurohypophysis (vasopressin and oxytocin) are the products of hypothalamic neurosecretory cells and are stored and released from the pars nervosa (a neurohemal organ). The hypophysial portal venules start as the primary plexus of the median eminence and convey blood downward to the sinusoids of the anterior lobe. There are strong indications that the hypothalamic axons of the median eminence liberate multiple releasing factors (probably peptide in nature) into the portal vessels and that these neural factors are concerned with the regulation of anterior pituitary functions. It is apparent that the whole pituitary gland is predominantly subservient to and has partly evolved from the hypothalamic portion of the brain.

eminence and that these factors condition the release of anterior pituitary hormones by virtue of the final common path of the hypophysial portal venules. Ectopic pituitary grafts, persisting without direct hypothalamic connections, function very abnormally.

Using the electron microscope and fluorescence techniques, a high content of catecholamine, thought to be mainly dopamine, has been demonstrated in the median eminence.[11] Adrenergic fibers may impinge on the capillary plexus of the median eminence, or form synaptic contacts with the perikarya and axons of neurosecretory cells. There is very little information on the precise cells that secrete the releasing factors or on how such cells are regulated. At the moment, there is uncertainty regarding the types of vesicles seen with the electron microscope in the axonal endings, and final conclusions must await further research.

The pituitary is the source of at least nine hormones, all being protein or polypeptide in nature. Six hormones arise from the pars distalis, at least one from the intermediate lobe, and two from the neurohypophysis (Table 2-1). Some of the anterior lobe hormones exert their effects indirectly by

Table 2–1 HORMONES OF THE PITUITARY GLAND

HORMONES	CELLULAR SOURCE	PRINCIPAL ACTIONS
1. Pars distalis Somatotrophin (STH, growth hormone)	Somatotrophs	Growth of bone and muscle; promotes protein synthesis; affects lipid and carbohydrate metabolism
Adrenocorticotrophin (ACTH)	Corticotrophs	Stimulates secretion of adrenal cortical steroids; certain extra-adrenal actions
Thyrotrophin (TSH)	Thyrotrophs	Stimulates thyroid gland to form and release thyroid hormones
Gonadotrophins (a) Luteinizing or interstitial cell-stimulating hormone (LH or ICSH)	Gonadotrophs (luteotrophs or interstitiotrophs)	Ovary: formation of corpora lutea; secretion of progesterone; probably acts in conjunction with FSH Testis: stimulates the interstitial cells of Leydig, thus promoting the secretion of androgen
(b) Follicle-stimulating hormone (FSH)	Gonadotrophs (folliculotrophs)	Ovary: growth of follicles; functions with LH to cause estrogen secretion and ovulation Testis: possible action on seminiferous tubules to promote spermatogenesis
(c) Prolactin (lactogenic hormone, luteotrophin)	Lactotrophs (mammotrophs)	Initiation of milk secretion; acts on crop sacs of some birds; maternal behavior in birds; resembles STH in affecting many tissues
2. Pars intermedia Melanophore-stimulating hormone (intermedin, MSH)	Melanotrophs	Expansion of amphibian melanophores; contraction of iridophores and xanthophores; melanin synthesis; darkening of skin
3. Neurohypophysis Vasopressin (ADH, antidiuretic hormone)	Hypothalamic neurons	Elevates blood pressure through action on arterioles; promotes reabsorption of water by kidney tubules
Oxytocin	Hypothalamic neurons	Affects postpartum mammary gland, causing ejection of milk; promotes contraction of uterus; possible action in parturition and in sperm transport in female tract

[margin note: adenoh.]
[margin note: adenoh.]

stimulating the functional activities of other endocrine glands; these are called *trophic* hormones. The main target organs affected by the trophic hormones are the thyroid, adrenal cortex, testis, and ovary. Secretion of both trophic hormones and hormones released by the target glands are regulated by mutual feedback mechanisms. Thus, when blood titers of target gland hormones are elevated, trophic hormone secretion is inhibited and *vice versa*. Somatotrophin (growth hormone) is a general metabolic hormone and has a variety of actions, no single endocrine organ serving as its target.[31] The MSH peptides (intermedin) of the pars intermedia have pigment cells as their main targets. Apparently, feedback mechanisms do not operate in the control of release of somatotrophin and MSH. The neuro-

Table 2–2 HORMONES OTHER THAN THOSE OF THE PITUITARY

HORMONES	CELLULAR SOURCE	PRINCIPAL ACTIONS
Thyroxine; triiodothyronine	Thyroid	Growth; amphibian metamorphosis; molting; metabolic rate in birds and mammals
Thyrocalcitonin (calcitonin)	Thyroid; ultimo-branchial bodies; parathyroids(?)	Lowers blood calcium and phosphate
Parathyroid hormone (PTH)	Parathyroids	Elevates blood calcium; lowers blood phosphate
Epinephrine	Adrenal medulla; other chromaffn cells	Mobilization of glycogen; increased blood flow through skeletal muscle; increased oxygen consumption; heart rate
Norepinephrine	Adrenal medulla; other chromaffn cells; adrenergic neurons	Adrenergic neurotransmitter; elevation of blood pressure; constricts arterioles and venules
Insulin	Pancreatic islets (β-cells)	Lowers blood glucose; increases utilization of glucose, and synthesis of protein and fat; decreases gluconeogenesis
Glucagon	Pancreatic islets (α-cells)	Increases blood glucose; stimulates catabolism of protein and fat
Androgens (e.g., testosterone)	Testis; adrenal cortex; ovary	Male sexual characteristics
Estrogens (e.g., estradiol)	Ovary; placenta; testis; adrenal cortex	Female sexual characteristics
Progestogens (e.g., progesterone)	Ovary; placenta; adrenal cortex	Maintenance of pregnancy; inhibition of reproductive cycles
Relaxin	Ovary; uterus; placenta	Enlargement of birth canal by relaxation of uterine cervix and pelvic ligaments
Glucocorticoids (e.g., cortisol, corticosterone)	Adrenal cortex	Promote synthesis of carbohydrate; protein breakdown; anti-inflammatory and antiallergic actions
Mineralocorticoids (e.g., aldosterone)	Adrenal cortex	Sodium retention and potassium loss through kidneys
Melatonin	Pineal gland	May mediate systemic responses to environmental lighting; effects on pigment cells
Human chorionic gonadotrophin (HCG)	Placenta	Various effects on gonads; some actions similar to pituitary LH
Pregnant mare serum gonadotrophin (PMSG)	Placenta	Ovulation in immature rats; various effects on gonads
Placental lactogen	Placenta	Simulates activities of pituitary growth hormone and prolactin
Gastrin	Stomach	Secretion of gastric juice
Secretin	Small intestine	Secretion of fluid by acinar pancreas
Cholecystokinin	Small intestine	Contraction of gallbladder; enzyme secretion by pancreas
1,25-$(OH)_2$-cholecalciferol	Kidney	Elevates serum calcium; promotes intestinal absorption of calcium and mobilizes bone calcium

hypophysial principles exert their actions upon blood vessels, kidneys, mammary glands, and uterus. Certain endocrine organs, such as the gastrointestinal mucosa, pancreatic islets, parathyroid glands, and adrenal medulla, seem to function with little, if any, dependence upon pituitary hormones. Table 2–2 provides a list of the best known hormones derived from vertebrate endocrine glands other than the pituitary. All of these exert multiple and sometimes very complex actions; only a few representative effects are listed in the table.

PROBLEMS AND CONCEPTS

The brief presentation of the organization of the vertebrate endocrine system does not do justice to the tremendous amount of research work that has been done to accumulate this wealth of information. Neither does it describe adequately the many interesting techniques used to obtain this knowledge, nor does it emphasize the many problems and concepts that provide the basis for current and future endocrinological investigations. Many of these problems and concepts are of a general nature and apply not only to particular glands but to the entire endocrine system. In other words, such problems as how hormones are made and released, how they are transported, how they recognize their targets or *vice versa,* and how they bring about their effects are common to the study of every endocrine gland. In the forthcoming sections we shall consider some of these problems in a general way, and later, when the various glands and hormones are discussed individually, the peculiarities of the particular hormone in question will be attended to.

Methods of Study

Ablation by Surgery or Disease

Removal of a gland would deprive the organism of its normal source of hormone, so that measurable abnormalities should appear in the individual during its life history. Varying degrees of hypofunction may be produced by subtotal ablations.

Because many, if not all, processes are regulated by multiple hormones working in unison, defects resulting from the extirpation of one kind of gland may be due to the unopposed action of secretions from another gland. Experiments involving multiple ablations may be performed to assess the relative significance of several glands in a particular process. For example, removal of the pancreas elevates the blood sugar and produces other symptoms of diabetes mellitus; if the pituitary is removed from the same animal, the diabetic symptoms are ameliorated (Houssay preparations). Long and Lukens discovered that removal of the adrenals has a similar effect in clearing up some of the impairments resulting from ablation of the pancreas.

Permissive actions may be determined by removing the gland in question and maintaining the animal in a responsive state by a constant intake of hormones from that gland while another hormone is being tested. Large doses of estrogen increase the liver glycogen of intact fasting rats, but do not exert this effect after the adrenals are removed. However, if adrenalectomized rats are maintained on minimal amounts of adrenal cortical extracts, estrogen raises the liver glycogen; this effect could not have been mediated by the adrenal cortex. The cortical hormones in the extract are said to have a "permissive" role, inasmuch as they normalize the functions of organs and thereby condition the animal's capacity to adapt and respond to the estrogen.

Through disease, accident, or defective heredity, Nature sometimes produces glandular abnormalities that would be difficult to simulate experimentally. Hereditary diabetes insipidus has been found in rats of the Brattleboro strain; the neurohypophysis cannot synthesize the antidiuretic principle (vasopressin); consequently, these rats consume much water and excrete copious amounts of dilute urine.[47] The hereditary nephrogenic diabetes insipidus in the mouse, on the other hand, is characterized by abnormally small kidneys having a reduced number of nephrons.[8] This hereditary condition is the consequence of a kidney defect, and there is no deficiency of pituitary or hypothalamic secretions. An inherited form of pseudohermaphroditism in the male rat has been extensively studied; androgen production by the adult testis is deficient, and the onset of this defect was probably during fetal life.[3] Many hereditary lesions such as these have been analyzed with profit.

Chemical Ablation or Impairment

Antiandrogens such as cyproterone acetate compete with androgenic steroids (*e.g.,* testosterone) for binding sites in target organs and thus block their actions. These agents, by preventing the response of androgen targets, provide a convenient method of producing physiologic states that are equivalent to those following bilateral orchiectomy. The development of mammary gland primordia in male fetuses is normally suppressed by testicular androgens; following the exposure of rat fetuses to cyproterone, the mammary anlagen of males differentiate as fully as those of normal females.[13] The same effects upon the nipple primordia of rats may result from the administration of agents which selectively inhibit certain enzyme systems that are essential for androgen biosynthesis by the testis. There is abundant evidence that feminine organogenesis ensues in mammalian fetuses deprived of androgen, and this general problem can be elucidated by using antiandrogens on fetuses in whom surgical removal of the testes is difficult.[34] From these examples, it is apparent that chemical procedures may be employed to prevent the synthesis of androgens by the testis, or to block the androgens at the level of the targets, and the end results will be the same.

When radioactive iodine is administered, it collects principally in the thyroid. The ionization within the thyroid destroys the organ partially or completely, without appreciably damaging other parts of the body. This method of radiothyroidectomy is especially advantageous in fishes, in which the follicles are so widely scattered that surgical ablation would be impossible. A large number of chemical agents may be used to block the production of thyroid hormones by interfering at some level with their biosynthesis in the gland. Animals receiving adequate treatment with the antithyroid agents (e.g., thiouracil) cannot manufacture thyroid hormones and hence are counterparts of thyroidectomized subjects.

Alloxan is a compound that selectively destroys the B-cells of the pancreatic islets. Since these cells are the source of insulin, alloxan provides a convenient method of reducing the output of insulin sufficiently to produce diabetes mellitus. Neutral red is a useful tool in selectively impairing the A-cells of the pancreas, thus inducing a deficiency of glucagon.[35]

Many organic compounds are capable of suppressing the formation of germ cells by the testis without any apparent effect on endocrine functions. Such agents include nitrofurans, dinitropyrroles and thiophenes. Hexamethylphosphoramide is a potent antispermatogenic agent; it has been employed to sterilize male houseflies and is known to induce prolonged sterility with aspermia in several laboratory mammals.[22]

There are a number of organic preparations (e.g., Metopirone, SU 4885) that inhibit particular enzymes involved in the biosynthesis of steroids by the adrenal cortex. As the adrenocortical hormones in the circulation diminish, the anterior pituitary responds by accelerating its release of ACTH, and this induces adrenocortical hyperplasia. Such compounds may be used by clinicians to test the competence of the anterior pituitary to respond to an adrenocortical deficiency. Metopirone has been found useful in elucidating pituitary-adrenal functions in fishes, in which the steroideogenic tissue of the adrenal is dispersed in the lymphoid kidney and cardinal veins, and hence is not amenable to surgical removal.[36]

Many substances may be administered to endocrine cells to impair basic cellular function. Metabolic inhibitors, such as iodoacetamide, dinitrophenol, and cyanide, are especially striking in this regard and have been shown to inhibit the secretion of MSH.[15] The secretory process for some hormones is said to involve the action of subcellular organelles, microtubules and microfilaments.[29] Administration of the microtubule inhibitors, vinblastine and vincristine, and cytochalasin B, a substance that disrupts microfilaments, profoundly affects the secretory process.

With improved techniques in immunochemistry and the availability of purified protein and polypeptide hormones, it has been demonstrated that mammalian species may form antibodies (antihormones) which neutralize heterologous hormones, whether exogenously injected or endogenously secreted. This antigen-antibody reaction can be employed to elucidate the action of many highly purified hormones on their target organs. For example, if purified interstitial cell-stimulating hormone (ICSH, or luteinizing hormone [LH]) derived from the sheep is injected into the rabbit, an antibody develops in the serum that specifically acts against this hormone. When the rabbit antiserum is given to young rats, the testes shrink in size, sperm formation ceases, and insufficient androgen is produced to maintain the accessory sex glands, such as prostates and seminal vesicles.[19] In female rats, this antiserum stops the estrous cycles and produces striking atrophy of the ovaries and female accessories. Normal rabbit serum, injected in equivalent amounts, produces no demonstrable effect upon the genital organs of rats. The rabbit antiserum acts to negate the intrinsic ICSH of the rats, and the gonadal effects are quite comparable to those resulting from surgical removal of the pituitary; the gonadal effects, however, are reversible in both sexes if the treatments are discontinued.

Chemical Extraction and Cellular Sources

It should be possible to extract a hormone from the particular gland that produces it and also from the blood stream, which conveys it. This has been accomplished in many instances. The urine sometimes is a better source of hormones than is the blood, but the excreted metabolites may be quite different chemically and physiologically from the compounds obtained directly from glandular tissues. Many of the hormones within the circulation are bound to serum proteins and hence do not filter through the renal glomeruli. Consequently, the urine generally contains only traces of the hormone in its original form. In certain diseases of the adrenal cortex, the abnormal metabolites of the steroid hormones appearing in the urine reflect enzymatic blocks in the biosynthetic pathway within the adrenal itself.

Isotopic and immunologic methods are of value in extracting, purifying, and assaying antigenic hormones present in crude tissue extracts. There are strong indications that the primate placenta secretes a protein hormone that has properties similar to pituitary growth hormone and pituitary prolactin. It is called human (or simian) placental lactogen, and was first identified in crude placental extracts by its cross reaction with antiserum to human growth hormone.[25]

It is often of great value to know the cellular sources of the hormones being studied, and there are many histochemical methods for determining this. The fluorescent antibody technique has been used to advantage in some instances.[18] Frozen or paraffin sections of the fresh tissue are exposed to labeled antibodies that a heterologous species produced against the particular hormone (antigen) whose location is being determined. The antiserum gamma globulin (antibody) is labeled with a fluorescent dye (fluorescein isothiocyanate), and the staining of particular cells depends upon their content of hormone, which forms a stable complex with the labeled antibody. Adjacent sections of the tissue may be stained by conventional methods in order to check the identification of cell types. Using fluorescent antibodies to sheep prolactin, the type of cell in the rat's pituitary that secretes this hormone has been identified. As another example, the cellular source of placental lactogen has been determined: anti-GH and anti-placental lactogen sera, labeled with the fluorescent dye, became localized within the syncytiotrophoblast, an epithelial covering of the chorionic villi.[41]

Ultrastructurally, these cells have a highly developed endoplasmic reticulum and probably participate in many of the steroid hormone transformations that occur in the placenta.

Isotopic Tracer Methods[4]

Isotopes are of two general kinds: *stable* and *radioactive.* The stable isotopes differ from ordinary atoms only in their mass and may be prepared by fractionation from natural sources. The radioactive isotopes, besides differing in mass, possess unstable nuclei and undergo spontaneous decomposition with the emission of radiation. Most of the radioactive isotopes that are used in biochemistry do not occur in nature but are prepared by bombardment in the cyclotron. The reacting uranium pile, used for the production of atomic instruments, is the best source of neutrons for the preparation of isotopes. The stable isotopes, not being radioactive, are identified by means of a mass spectrometer. The radioactive ones are assayed by instruments such as the Geiger-Müller radiation counter and various types of scintillation counters. Since the analytical methods for the measurement of radioactive isotopes are extremely sensitive, they are used more commonly in biochemical studies than are the stable isotopes. The rate of decomposition of radioactive isotopes is commonly expressed as their *half-life;* this is the time required for the isotope in any given sample to diminish to half its original value. The half-life of I^{131} is 8.1 days, whereas that of C^{14} is 5760 years.

The isotopic method makes it possible to label an element or compound and to follow the fate of the substance *in vivo* under conditions that cause a minimum of physiologic disturbance to the experimental organism. For example, if we administered elemental iodine (I) to an organism, it would become mixed with like atoms already in the "metabolic pool"; hence, it would be impossible to trace its metabolic pathway within the body. On the other hand, when we administer the radioactive isotope of iodine (I^{131}), these atoms can be distinguished from those already in the body. Their uptake by the different tissues, their incorporation into compounds, and the breakdown of the compounds can be followed. Even in those cases in which there is no net increase, or in which there is an actual decrease, in the concentration of the product, isotopic labeling provides a method for proving the transformation of one compound into another. Special procedures make it possible to demonstrate unstable metabolic intermediates that cannot be isolated by ordinary methods. Competitive protein-binding methods are widely used in the assay of hormones, and these procedures require an isotopic form of the hormone being tested.

There is abundant evidence that hormones are selectively concentrated by particular receptor tissues; for example, estrogens are promptly taken up by the uterus. It is not difficult to determine in what cells and tissues labeled hormones have become localized. This can be shown by taking two adjacent microtome sections, staining one in the usual way, and leaving the other in contact with a photographic plate or film for an appropriate time and developing the image. The areas of high isotopic concentration can be determined by comparing the stained section with the "autoradiograph." Labeled compounds on paper chromatograms may also be located by this method.

It is thought that a number of steroid hormones produce their effects by acting directly upon certain genes and, if this is the case, one would expect to find hormone binding sites in the nuclei of target cells. In several instances, these intracellular proteins that serve as binding sites for steroid hormones have been located by using isotopically labeled hormones as tracers. Aldosterone is an adrenal steroid that promotes sodium transport, and nuclear receptor sites for it have been located in the mucosal cells of the toad bladder and in the kidney cells of the rat.[2] Much progress in modern endocrinology is due to the availability of pure hormones labeled with radioisotopes.

The use of labeled elements and compounds, supplemented by other techniques, is the most important procedure yet devised for the study of metabolic pathways and the rates of turnover of substances in the organism. Today the isotopes not only are used in laboratory experimentation but have found an important role in clinical diagnosis and treatment.

In Vitro Techniques

The perfusion of whole organs, such as adrenals, testes, and ovaries, has been a useful procedure in determining biosynthetic pathways of the steroid hormones. The endocrine gland is carefully removed and placed in a closed system that allows it to be perfused either with the animal's own blood or with a physiologic solution of approximately the same electrolyte content as that of the blood. The excised organs survive for a considerable time; hence isotopically labeled materials may be introduced and samples of the perfusate withdrawn for analysis. One advantage of this method is that metabolic products may be removed as they are formed, instead of accumulating and interfering with the speed of chemical reactions. An extension of this method involves the culture of two or more organs or tissues. Thus, it is possible to culture an endocrine gland in close proximity to a target gland or tissue, and to assess the effects of one upon the other.

In some types of studies, very thin slices of living organs are suspended in appropriate physiologic solutions and kept alive for hours or days. Various test materials may be added to the suspension fluid and the transformations determined by analytical procedures. Rapid progress has been made in the refinement of tissue culture techniques and it is now possible to culture individual endocrine cells for many weeks. In some exciting experiments, clonal strains of functional pituitary cells have been grown in culture and have been used in the study of the regulation of growth hormone and prolactin production.[21]

Tissue minces and homogenates are often used in studying enzymatic transformations. In such preparations, the cellular organization is disturbed, and many or all of the individual cells are destroyed. A cell-free homogenate actually consists of a liquid in which the soluble components of protoplasm have been dissolved, and suspended in this liquid are the solid components of cells such as microsomes, mitochondria, nucleoli, etc. The insoluble components of homogenates may be separated from the suspension medium by centrifugation. It appears that many of the important cellular enzymes are bound to the organelles found in homogenates; extracts containing only the soluble constituents may carry some of the enzymes in solution, but their natural relationships in the intact cell have been completely destroyed. Until there is absolute proof, it should not be assumed that the results of *in vitro* procedures are identical with those that normally operate within the whole organism.

It is obvious that no single method of study is uniquely sufficient for the elucidation of every aspect of endocrine function. All of the techniques mentioned have contributed importantly to our understanding, and data obtained by different techniques often reinforce one another and thus become increasingly significant.

The Assay of Hormones

Progress in endocrinology depends upon the development of techniques which enable the investigator to know what hormone he is dealing with and to determine how much of the hormone is present in the material being considered. Until a hormone becomes available in pure form, its assay must depend upon some relatively unique biologic alteration that it produces. To mention only a few examples, insulin lowers the level of blood sugar, thyrocalcitonin lowers plasma calcium and phosphate, androgens promote growth of the capon's comb, estrogens cornify the vaginal epithelium of rodents, MSH peptides cause dispersion of melanin granules in the melanophores of the frog's skin, gonadotrophins induce specific alterations in the gonads, and thyrotrophin brings about structural and functional changes in the thyroid gland. The most valid bioassays are based upon changes which are produced exclusively by a particular hormone under rigidly controlled conditions. Elevation of the blood sugar, for example, is not a specific indicator of epinephrine action because pancreatic glucagon, pituitary ACTH, and adrenocortical steroids produce the same end result by acting in different ways.

Perhaps all hormones produce a multitude of responses within the body and different responses among different species. In view of such divergent actions, selection of the best biologic indicator must depend upon the degree of objectivity, accuracy, sensitivity, specificity, reproducibility, and convenience afforded by the test.

It is always desirable to base assay techniques upon structural and functional changes that can be measured objectively by instruments, instead of relying upon subjective estimations. Body configuration and hair distribution are reliable indicators of gonadal steroids in human beings, but both parameters are difficult to standardize and measure objectively. Hormones within the organism are typically effective in minute amounts, and indicators that are sensitive enough to respond to physiologic quantities of the hormone are most preferable. If sensitivity is lacking, and tremendous amounts of hormone are required, the response is likely to be pharmacologic rather than physiologic. The response must be reproducible, and a dose-response relationship should be evident.

Many factors may alter responses to hormones and thus influence bioassays. Important variables are the route of administration, the vehicle in which the hormone is dissolved or suspended, the species and strain of animal, sex, age, and general health. Since most of the natural hormones are not effective orally, they are generally given parenterally, *i.e.,* subcutaneously or intramuscularly. The intravenous route is employed only when a prompt response is desired, or when it is advantageous to have high, but transient, titers present in the blood. Steroid hormones are generally not given intravenously. Hormones in oil vehicles are absorbed more slowly than are those in aqueous ones, thus giving relatively constant and prolonged effects. Modifications of the hormone molecule may alter its rate of absorption, degradation, or excretion, without changing its characteristic type of action. On the other hand, even slight changes in chemistry of the molecule may render it ineffective or may alter its effect within the organism.

Once the structure of a hormone molecule is known, physical and chemical procedures may be developed for its detection and quantitative determination. Highly sensitive and specific physicochemical methods are available for the assay of steroid hormones in the blood and urine. Since it is desirable to assay occasionally on the basis of a biologic indicator to make sure that the molecule is active, it is not likely that the physicochemical or immunologic procedures will entirely replace the bioassays. The immunologic methods may not be absolutely valid unless the antigenic site and the active center of the protein molecule coincide. When antigenicity and activity are located at different levels in the molecule, the immunologic information must be verified by some bioassay procedure. This is especially important if the hormone being assayed for is not homogeneous. Heterogeneity of the peptide hormone being assayed can lead to differences between results obtained by immunologic methods and those obtained by bioassay.

It is well known that smaller molecules (ligands) characteristically bind to larger protein molecules, and some of these associations are highly specific, as, for example, those between antigens and antibodies, between enzymes and substrates, and between the neurohypophysial octapeptides and a protein (neurophysin) present in the pars nervosa of the pituitary. It is now recognized that protein and polypeptide hormones generally elicit the formation of "antihormones" when injected into heterologous species. The availability of highly purified hormones and improved immunologic methods has provided the basis for the development of highly sophisticated methods of *radioimmunoassay* (RIA), the use of which has become widespread because of its high degree of sensitivity, wide range of application, quickness, and adaptability to automation. In present usage, radioimmunoassay is a general term that includes not only RIA, but saturation analysis, radioligand binding assay, and competitive protein binding. All of these techniques involve immunochemical reactions in which labeled and unlabeled antigens compete for sites on a limited amount of antibody or other receptor.[43]

Nonantigenic hormones such as adrenocortical and gonadal steroids and thyroxine spontaneously associate and dissociate with specific proteins in the blood, and this makes it possible to assay them by the competitive protein-binding technique. This method is extremely sensitive and is used to assay hormones present in the body fluids. The principle employed is essentially the same as that of radioimmunoassay: Both require a binding protein of high specificity and an isotopic form of the hormone to be measured. In one case, the binding protein is an antibody; in the other, the binding protein is normally present in the plasma or within cells as hormone receptor sites.

The reactions occurring in competitive protein-binding assays follow the law of mass action, and the principle can be illustrated as follows: If a binding protein is mixed with tracer and nontracer ligands, and the two ligands exceed the number of binding sites on the protein, they will compete with each other for binding sites in proportion to their concentrations. The amounts of binding protein and tracer ligand are kept constant as more nontracer ligand is added. This displaces increasing numbers of tracer molecules and the amount of tracer ligand bound to the protein falls rapidly. The final step is separation of the protein-bound ligand from the unbound ligand in order to determine the distribution of radioactivity. This may be accomplished by electrophoresis, dialysis, protein precipitation, gel filtration, or by adsorption of the unbound fraction onto various kinds of insoluble particles. The percentage of bound tracer ligand may be plotted against the amount of nontracer ligand added.[33]

It is possible to induce the formation of antibodies against hormonal steroids and other small molecules by using them as haptens. Since antibodies are stable and highly specific, this is advantageous in cases in which specific binding proteins are not naturally present in the body fluids. After obtaining suitable antibodies against such hormone-protein conjugates, the assay may be performed by standard radioimmunologic procedures.

Hormone Synthesis, Release, and Transport

Ultrastructure of Synthesis and Release

During the last two decades, electron microscopic and biochemical studies have provided substantial information on the manner in which the various cell organelles participate in the secretory process.[9] In addition, the contributions of molecular biology have been applied to endocrine cells. Thus, through the processes of transcription and translation, the endocrine cell synthesizes structural proteins, enzymes necessary for various functions including the formation of non-peptide hormones, and peptide or protein hormones. There is now much interest in the possibility that some hormones may activate specific genes (DNA), thus promoting the transcrip-

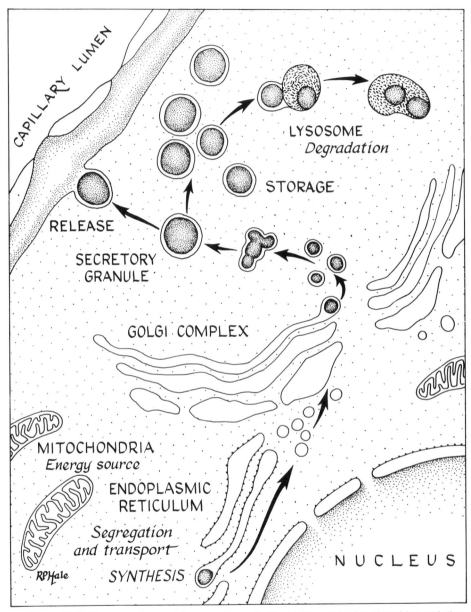

Figure 2–3. Diagram of a protein-secreting cell, illustrating some functional interrelationships of the organelles. The protein synthesized on the ribosomes is transported through the lumen of the endoplasmic reticulum, and is concentrated and packaged in the Golgi complex; the secretion is released from the granules after the fusion of their membranes with the cell membrane. Excess secretory granules are degraded by lysosomes.

tion of new kinds of messenger RNA (m-RNA), which then code for the synthesis of specific proteins at the ribosomal level.[27]

Under the electron microscope, pores are visible in the nuclear membrane, and m-RNA molecules are assumed to move through them into the cytoplasm. The endoplasmic reticulum (ER) in protein-secreting cells is highly developed and of the granular or rough type. Varying numbers of ribosomes become associated with each m-RNA molecule to form the polysomes, which are oriented along the outer surface of the ER. In the translation process, transfer RNA brings amino acids to the ribosomes, where they are assembled as dictated by the codons of the m-RNA molecule attached to the ribosomes. The protein molecules move through the ER to the Golgi complex, where they are concentrated and formed into membrane-bound droplets or granules. In such cells, probably the most common method of discharge is for the membrane of the granule to adhere to the cell membrane, thus permitting the egress of the secretion without leaving a rupture in the cell membrane (Fig. 2–3). At present much attention is being given to the mechanism of insulin release from the B-cells of the pancreas.[29] The actions of microtubules and microfilaments have been implicated in the secretory process. It has been suggested that granules of the hormone are released by emiocytosis, a process which involves the fusion of the granule limiting membrane with the plasma membrane and the subsequent escape of the granule contents through a small pore of transitory existence.

Lysosomes appear to be important organelles for clearing the cells of accumulated secretions, excessive membranes, and ribosomes, when the need for the secreted product diminishes. Such unnecessary materials are accumulated in autophagic vacuoles and are broken down by enzymes contained in the lysosomes. Following thyroid stimulation by pituitary TSH, lysosomes appear in the luminal ends of the epithelial cells lining the follicle. It is probable that these cells take in colloid (thyroglobulin) from the lumen of the follicle by pinocytosis, and that hydrolytic enzymes of the lysosomes degrade the protein to liberate thyroxine and triiodothyronine.[14] These hormones are then released from the basal end of the cell into the parafollicular capillaries.

Endocrine cells that synthesize steroid hormones present certain ultrastructural features that distinguish them from cells specialized for the production of protein or polypeptide secretions. Steroid-secreting cells such as those of the gonads and adrenal cortices contain a very extensive agranular (smooth) ER, which is frequently arranged into whorls, and the granular (rough) ER is much less conspicuous than in protein-secreting cells. Lipid droplets accumulate in the cytoplasm, but membrane-bound granules are absent. The Golgi complex is typically very prominent. Lysosomes may be numerous, and there is frequently some accumulation of lipochrome pigment. Mitochondria represent energy sources and are always present in gland cells; their internal structure is sometimes very complex.[9] Lipid droplets appear to be extremely important in the secretion of steroid hormones. In the adrenal cortex, lipid droplets originating either from Golgi elements or from the smooth ER enlarge, and ultimately outer elements of the droplet membrane fuse with the plasma membrane. Finally, the lipid droplets, presumably containing adrenocorticosteroid hormones, are discharged from the cell surface by a process that has been termed endoplasmocrine secretion.[40]

Transport

The endocrine glands are among the most highly vascularized organs of the body, and their secretions are typically distributed by the circulation. There are increasing indications, however, that certain hormones may diffuse through tissues and thus give rise to local field effects. Ultrastructural and biochemical studies have shown that the sustentacular cells of Sertoli, within the seminiferous tubules, synthesize cholesterol and various androgenic steroids, but it is probable that these are largely retained within the testis tubule where they exert a local effect on spermatogenesis.[5] By contrast, the interstitial cells of the testis are richly vascularized and promptly deliver their androgens to the circulation for the maintenance of distant targets. Certain androgens are known to be present in mammalian semen and it is probable that these derive, in part at least, from the seminiferous tubules or the epithelial lining of certain accessory sex ducts, rather than from the circulation. It has been shown that cells lining the epididymis and ductus deferens can synthesize cholesterol from acetate, or even produce compounds beyond cholesterol, such as androgens (dehydroepiandrosterone).[17] This activity of accessory ducts is testis-dependent, and it is probable that the secretions are added to the epididymal fluid instead of being released into the circulation. Such cells might qualify as exocrine glands; even though they must possess some of the same enzyme systems as the gonads and adrenal cortices, they could not properly be regarded as endocrine in nature. Integradations are often encountered in biology, and the distinctions between exocrine and endocrine glands may not be as sharp as once was supposed.

Hormones in the circulation are frequently bound to specific carrier proteins, and are present in very minute amounts. The amounts of androgen (testosterone) in the blood of normal men is about 0.6 μgm per 100 milliliters. Hormones may persist for only short periods in the blood, particularly if they are not bound to proteins. They are continuously subjected to enzymatic inactivation or destruction in such organs as the liver and kidneys. All chemical messengers are released in response to specific stimuli, arising externally or internally, and these may fluctuate from time to time. Since the adrenal medulla is under neural control, its catecholamines can be quickly released in response to sudden requirements of the body.

It was discovered many years ago that the neurohypophysial octapeptides stored within the pars nervosa were bound to a protein (neurophysin) with a molecular weight of about 30,000. As is pointed out in Chapter 6, it seems that both the neurohypophysial peptides and neurophysin are synthesized in the hypothalamus and that the peptides are bound to the protein. Subsequently, they reach the neurohypophysis by axonal transport mechanisms and are stored in this bound form. Some evidence suggests that they are released into the circulation in this bound form and that they are conveyed by the blood in this manner. The plasma contains specific carrier proteins for thyroxine and many of the steroid hormones. Thyroxine-binding globulin (TBG) is highly specific for thyroxine, but it binds triiodothyronine to a lesser extent. Thyroxine also binds to some degree to plasma prealbumin and albumin. Human corticosteroid-binding globulin (CBG), or *transcortin,* binds strongly with progesterone and adrenocortical steroids such as cortisol and corticosterone; the affinity of CBG for various steroids varies with the species. The sex hormone-binding globulin (SHBG) appears to be the only high-affinity binding site for testosterone and estradiol in human plasma.

This reversible association between hormones and carrier proteins appears to be much more than a convenient transport mechanism; it may serve as a storage and buffer system as well. The binding regulates the levels of hormones reaching the targets and the amounts metabolized, and it may protect the organism against excessive concentrations. It is probable that the large carrier proteins do not readily cross the blood-brain and placental barriers, whereas the smaller steroid molecules are known to do so. A striking increase in serum thyroxine occurs during human pregnancy, but the basal metabolic rate remains normal since most of the thyroxine is bound and does not reach the tissues. A testosterone-binding protein becomes markedly elevated during pregnancy in certain mammals. The increased binding of certain steroids during pregnancy may prevent the wrong hormones from acting on the sensitive genital and nervous tissues of the mother and the developing young *in utero.*[7] There are strong indications that the high levels of progesterone during pregnancy may serve to protect the fetus against excessive androgens.

Receptor Mechanisms

It is obvious that organismal responses to hormones depend upon the capacity of target tissues and organs to respond to them. This is illustrated by a rare congenital anomaly called "feminizing testes" that results from an inability of target organs to respond to androgenic hormones. This androgen unresponsiveness begins before birth and continues throughout life. The patients appear feminine, but they are genetic males with normal XY chromosomes. The testes produce amounts of testosterone equal to those of normal males, and also amounts of estrogen within the normal female range. The administration of tremendous amounts of androgen is ineffective since the target cannot respond. Analogous genital defects may be produced in male rats by treating them prenatally with antiandrogens.

Since labeled hormones became available for experimental use, it has been amply demonstrated that particular hormones are selectively concentrated by specific target cells and tissues; for example, estrogens by the uterus, androgens by the male accessory glands, and FSH and LH by the gonads. In general, the tissues that respond most profoundly show the highest uptake of the hormone and retain it longest. The mechanism of ac-

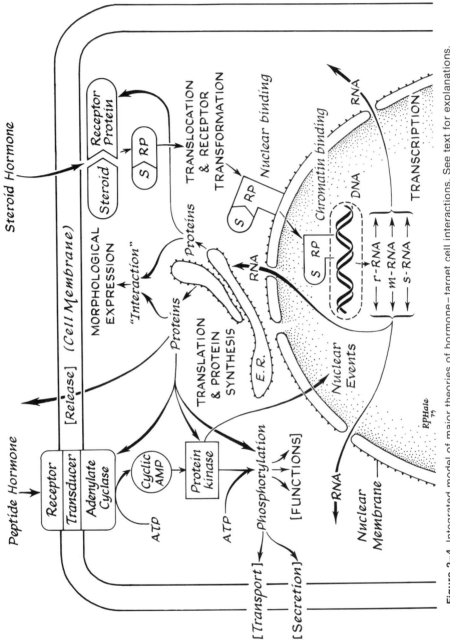

Figure 2–4. Integrated model of major theories of hormone–target cell interactions. See text for explanations.

tion of a hormone involves its interaction with *receptor sites* of the target cells and the ensuing chain of intracellular events that eventually leads to the organismal adjustments generally regarded as the effects of the hormone. The receptor hypothesis is that every target cell has specific sites that bind particular hormones, and some progress has been made in identifying and characterizing the macromolecules which serve the cells in this capacity. There seem to be two major hormone receptor sites: those on the cell surface associated with the plasma membrane, and others within the cell, either as part of the internal membrane structure or present in the cytosol itself (Fig. 2–4). Much attention has focused on each of these receptor sites, and it has been found in many cases that the receptor is or involves a protein. Since the results of most hormone activity ultimately involve intracellular events such as protein synthesis or enzyme activation, it becomes important to understand how the interaction of a hormone with a surface receptor can bring about an appropriate internal effect. An adequate explanation is derived from the first-messenger-second messenger concept developed by Sutherland and his colleagues.[44, 45] This subject will be taken up in more detail in the following section; however, in essence the concept considers that a hormone is a first messenger which, following its interaction at the cell surface, leads to the elaboration of an intracellular second messenger that has been identified as cyclic AMP. A sequence of events involving the latter ultimately evokes the appropriate endocrine response.

While the use of isotopic techniques has contributed much to our recent knowledge about receptor mechanisms, classical pharmacological methods had already established the concept that the response of some cells to catecholamines such as epinephrine or norepinephrine occurs through the stimulation of adrenergic receptors. These receptors are considered to be of two types, *alpha* or *beta,* and each is thought to control responses that are opposite to the other.[1] Thus, stimulation of the alpha receptors of vertebrate smooth muscle usually evokes contraction, while stimulation of beta receptors on these cells causes relaxation. Often cells contain both types of receptors; however, when alpha receptors are present, they usually dominate over beta receptors. The presence of beta receptors under these circumstances can be shown by the preferential blocking of alpha receptors with specific blocking agents. Several pharmacological agents, such as dibenamine, phentolamine, and ergotamine, block the alpha adrenergic receptor and prevent the expected response to catecholamine stimulation. If such blocked effector cells also contain beta adrenergic receptors, stimulation by catecholamines will bring about the opposite response, or "epinephrine reversal."[6] The presence or absence of alpha and beta adrenergic receptors on given effector cells is variable between species or races. For example, epinephrine or norepinephrine can cause an aggregation of pigment in melanophores of northern races of the leopard frog through stimulation of alpha adrenergic receptors on these cells; however, when this experiment is repeated on southern races, dispersion of pigment occurs because alpha receptors are lacking and the remaining beta adrenergic receptors respond with pigment dispersion.[16] Adrenergic receptors are not limited to effectors that respond in a mechanical way, such as with pigment migration or muscle responses, but have been shown to play a role in such metabolic responses as the release of glucose from the liver and of fatty acids from adipose tissue. There is strong evidence that adrenergic receptors may be implicated with cyclic AMP, for it has been reported that stimulation of beta adrenergic receptors in many tissues leads to an increase in tissue levels of cyclic AMP, while alpha stimulation decreases cyclic AMP levels.[46]

The actions of many peptide or protein hormones, such as insulin, glucagon, ACTH, prolactin, and calcitonin, are thought to result from an interaction with the cell surface, and in the case of insulin, specific proteins have been implicated as binding sites.[10] With various steroid hormones it appears that the hormone enters the cell and binds to a specific receptor protein found outside the nucleus. In a series of interesting studies by Jensen and his colleagues, it was shown that in the uterus, estradiol first associates with an extranuclear receptor protein.[24] This estradiol-receptor complex is then translocated to the nucleus, and in the process the receptor protein changes its physical characteristics, a process called "receptor transformation." The transformed receptor protein-estradiol complex has now acquired the ability to bind to uterine nuclei and to initiate nuclear events that the original untransformed complex could not induce. It appears that by its binding to the cytosol receptor protein, estradiol has induced the formation of a new biochemically functional form. It is interesting that, in the uterus, the reaction and transformation are highly specific for estradiol; however, there is evidence that in other steroid target organs similar steroid-receptor protein complexes undergo a similar transformation.

Application of the receptor concept should not be limited to the interaction of hormones with target cells, for the endocrine cell producing a given hormone generally does so in response to a stimulus. In such cases this response probably results from the stimulation of receptors possessed by the endocrine cell. The secretion of insulin by B-cells in response to the presence of glucose seems to be one of the best examples of this concept. It seems that the initial release of insulin occurs following recognition of glucose by a glucose receptor, and it is also likely that such receptor stimulation leads to synthesis of the hormone. These physiological responses to glucose are accompanied by prominent structural changes in the plasma membrane which are apparently manifestations of insulin secretion.

Target cell competence depends upon many factors, such as the species of animal, sex, pregnancy, nutrition, photoperiods, refractory states, temperature, age, other hormones in the system, etc. All of the hormones that are necessary for milk secretion are present during pregnancy, but they are not normally effective until after parturition. In vitro experiments have shown that prolactin increases the respiratory activity of mammary slices from lactating rats, but slices of the glands from pregnant rats do not respond.[42] Wild and domesticated species may respond differently to the same hormone.[32] Certain hormones produce little or no response if the body protein stores are exhausted and labile proteins are unavailable.[30] Immature organs (e.g., leg discs or ovaries of Drosophila) are unable to metamorphose when subjected prematurely to large quantities of hormones

that normally elicit developmental changes. In both insects and vertebrates the competence of target organs may be dependent upon a certain
degree of maturation. On the other hand, some hormones produce their
characteristic actions only during critical periods of embryonic, fetal, or
neonatal development.

Mechanisms of Hormone Action

Although some progress has been made during the past decade in determining how hormones act at the cellular level, the problems are exceedingly complex and unifying concepts, applicable to all hormones, have only
begun to emerge. Since natural hormone molecules come in many sizes
and shapes, ranging in complexity from modified amino acids through steroids to complex proteins, and since different hormone types utilize different
receptor systems, it is not likely that all would employ the same mechanisms in evoking their actions. Some hormones exert a multitude of different effects in various species and must employ a variety of targets; for example, thyroxine influences amphibian metamorphosis, the metabolic rate
in homoiotherms, maze-learning ability in rats, deposition of guanine in fish
scales and of melanin in bird feathers, eruption of teeth in young mammals,
schooling behavior in fishes, growth of antlers in deer, the rate of glucose
absorption in mammals, and water diuresis in mammals. It would be difficult to visualize all of these widespread effects of thyroxine as resulting
from a single, uniform mode of action. On the other hand, since the character of all of these events must ultimately be accounted for by the genetic
constitution of the organism, it is reasonable to consider that all hormone
action could occur at the level of gene transcription, following the model of
Jacob and Monod.[23] Thus, appropriate protein synthesis could occur and,
depending upon which proteins are formed, all the events listed above
could ultimately be accounted for. Obviously, the actions of some genes are
not achieved by the immediate action of the hormone at the transcriptional
level. We know this for a number of reasons, not the least of which is the
fact that the action of some hormones is not blocked by inhibitors of gene
transcription or translation. It can be said, then, that while some hormonal
activities occur at the level of the nucleus, others involve the use of elements
already available. In any event, these activities are expressed by the target
cell following the stimulation of hormone receptors, be they found at the cell
surface or within the cell.

The Second Messenger Hypothesis

As was pointed out earlier, many hormones, including peptides, proteins, and catecholamines, act as first messengers and interact with receptors on the cell surface. It is considered that, with many such hormones,
their actions are mediated by an intracellular second messenger, which is
elaborated in the cell following receptor stimulation by the hormone or first

messenger. Sutherland and his colleagues have shown the second messenger to be 3′, 5′ cyclic adenosine monophosphate (cyclic AMP).[44, 45] Through the action of adenylate cyclase, ATP is converted to cyclic AMP, which then acts within the effector cell to produce the appropriate hormonal response. Cyclic AMP is destroyed by the enzyme cyclic nucleotide phosphodiesterase. As would be predicted, specific hormonal events can be mimicked in the effector system by the application of cyclic AMP or its more permeable dibutyryl derivative. Such responses can also be duplicated by methylxanthines such as caffeine and theophylline, that are known to elevate cellular cyclic AMP levels by inhibiting phosphodiesterase. Cyclic AMP has been established as a second messenger that mediates some of the effects of quite a number of hormones: parathyroid hormone on bone and kidney, ACTH on the adrenal cortex, TSH on the thyroid, vasopressin on the kidney, epinephrine and glucagon on the liver, MSH on pigment cells, LH on bovine corpus luteum, ICSH on the testis, and others. In all of these instances, the hormones increase the intracellular content of cyclic AMP, and it is noteworthy that this molecule produces a variety of strikingly different general effects including transport, synthesis, and secretion (Fig. 2–4). It is thought that cyclic AMP mediates these effects by first activating a class of enzymes called protein kinases and that these, in turn, bring about the phosphorylation of other proteins, finally leading to the circumscribed hormonal effects. The fact that the same small molecule, operating on different target cells, mediates such diverse responses in organisms as widely separated as mammals and slime molds is fascinating and underlines the important position that cyclic AMP holds in nature. It is important to note that hormones whose actions have been ascribed to second messenger mediation are for the most part peptide or protein hormones that are usually considered to act on the surface of the effector cell. In keeping with this view it is held that adenylate cyclase is somehow related to the hormone receptor at the cell surface. It has been suggested that adenylate cyclase may be an actual part of the receptor or that it is connected to the receptor in some way, possibly by a "transducer." The nature of the transducer is unknown; however, the prostaglandins are among the candidates. Some of these interesting prostanoic acid derivatives (see Chapter 16) have been shown to bind to extracted receptor protein preparations and to stimulate cyclic AMP accumulations. Resolution of the problem of how hormone-receptor interaction is translated into intracellular augmentation of cyclic AMP levels is still in the realm of speculation.

Among the present considerations of the second messenger hypothesis is the fact that some of the events mediated by the action of cyclic AMP are bidirectionally controlled. For instance, glycogen breakdown attributable to epinephrine and glucagon is associated with increased levels of cyclic AMP. On the other hand, glycogen synthesis mediated by insulin does not involve an alteration in cyclic AMP levels and implies the existence of another mediator. It has been proposed that another cyclic nucleotide, 3′,5′ cyclic guanosine monophosphate (cyclic GMP), is the mediator of this response and of others which seem to be bidirectionally controlled and in which cyclic AMP is implicated. In other words, it appears that the opposing effects of cyclic AMP and cyclic GMP regulate the activities of bidirectionally controlled systems.[12] This hypothesis, which has been referred to as the "Yin-Yang hypothesis," is still in its infancy. However, it must be given serious consideration. It should be noted that cyclic GMP has been found in all living systems that have been looked at, albeit at concentrations much lower than those of cyclic AMP. This has made studies of its regulatory activities rather difficult.

The Nucleus and Hormone Action

Some hormones, notably steroids, may produce their effects directly by activating or suppressing particular genes. By acting either at the transcriptional or translational level, hormones could alter the rate of synthesis of new enzyme molecules. Such agents as actinomycin, puromycin, and cycloheximide have been employed in many of the experiments in order to block the synthesis of RNA in the nucleus or of protein in the cytoplasm.

This hypothesis is an outgrowth of studies on insect development, particularly the effect of ecdysone upon the giant chromosomes of the salivary glands.[26] Ecdysone is a steroid hormone that stimulates growth and differentiation in insects and crustaceans; it was shown that minute amounts of this steroid (as little as 10^{-5} μgm) lead to a characteristic "puffing" pattern in the giant or polytene chromosomes of the midge *Chironomus.* In this insect, as in most Diptera, the daughter chromatids fail to separate following replication, and line up side by side to form a chromosome consisting of hundreds of fine threads. The threads are aligned gene for gene and this gives the chromosomes a banded appearance; segments rich in DNA alternate with areas containing much less DNA. The puffs result from a loosening of the bundles of threads at specific gene loci, and represent the main sites of RNA synthesis on the chromosomes. These puffs induced by ecdysone are not artifacts; characteristic patterns of puffing are found normally during different developmental stages and in specific tissues. Much experimental evidence supports the concept that ecdysone activates specific genes; this leads to the synthesis of specific m-RNA, evidenced by the chromosomal puffs, and to the synthesis of specific proteins (*e.g.,* enzymes) required in the developmental process. There is a very short lapse of time between the injection of ecdysone and the appearance of the first chromosomal puffs, and, if actinomycin (DNA inhibiter) is given in conjunction with the hormone, the puffs do not appear. These facts support the belief that the hormone affects the genes *directly.* Similar conclusions have been drawn about the mode of action of vertebrate hormones, and although it has not been restricted to steroid hormones, the most convincing and most conclusive experimentation has been done on the mode of action of estrogen and progesterone on the chick oviduct.

While the studies described above concerning the mechanism of action of ecdysone demonstrate the synthesis of RNA, they do not constitute direct proof of action in the transcription of specific structural genes. Such proof is difficult to obtain in the absence of a specific and quantifiable end product of specific gene activation. However, as a result of the important experiments of O'Malley and his colleagues, this proof is now available. The chick oviduct, which they utilized in their studies, is unique in that estrogen and progesterone each initiate synthesis of specific proteins, ovalbumin and avidin, respectively, which can be readily extracted in quantities sufficient for accurate measurements.[38] Through the appropriate techniques of cellular dissection, experiments involving chemically defined cell-free systems have provided evidence that estrogen and progesterone activate specific genes, permitting the transcription of new species of m-RNA which code for these proteins. As striking as these experiments are, it must be remembered that they provide data only for the induction of one or two specific proteins. It is obvious that the synthesis of other proteins is also induced by these hormones in order to produce the appropriate growth and differentiation effects which occur during hormone mediation. How these synthetic events are coordinated is not yet known. In any event, we now have some understanding of the sequence of events that occurs in the mechanism of steroid hormone action. The sequence probably includes the formation of the steroid-receptor protein complex in the cytoplasm, transport of the complex to the nucleus and transformation of the receptor protein, binding of the now active complex to specific sites on the genome, activation of the transcription mechanism leading to the production of specific m-RNA's, transport of the induced RNA's to the cytoplasm leading to the synthesis of new protein species on the ribosomes, and the interaction of these proteins with other cellular elements to produce responses characteristic of that target cell.

HORMONAL INTERRELATIONS

The endocrine system is a highly integrated affair, and excesses or deficiencies in one gland may alter the rate of production of hormones by others. Almost every physiologic adjustment with which the endocrinologist deals is effected by a balance between hormones acting together or in sequence. Complete and normal functioning of the mammary glands, for example, requires estrogens, progesterone, insulin, prolactin, oxytocin, adrenal steroids, pituitary gonadotrophins, thyroid hormones, and perhaps others. The estrous and menstrual cycles are complicated phenomena and a multitude of hormones act in concert to produce the observed changes.[20] Since hormones in the body form interlocking complexes, a variety of secondary effects may be mediated by other hormones. Hormones in the body fluids never act alone, and one may be modified (potentiated or limited) by others that are present with it. For example, there is evidence that progesterone, emanating from the placenta, prevents premature expulsion of the fetus by blocking the response of the uterine musculature to other hormones. Progesterone augments the action of estrogen on female mating behavior in birds and mammals, although it has little or no effect alone.

Several hormones, acting in proper sequence, may be required for many adjustments. Complete development of the rabbit's uterus requires the sequential action of both estrogen and progesterone, neither hormone acting alone can produce the type of uterus (endometrium) required for the implantation of blastocysts. As was pointed out in the previous section, the white of the chicken's egg contains several proteins which are secreted by the magnum of the oviduct: ovalbumin and lysozyme are secreted in response to estrogen, whereas the production of avidin is specifically induced by progesterone when it acts upon an estrogen-primed oviduct.[37]

Synergisms have received a great deal of attention by experimental endocrinologists. Some hormones increase the effectiveness of others that are present with them in low concentrations. Although pituitary somatotrophin (STH) dramatically affects the skeleton, it also influences a wide spectrum of metabolic processes.[28] It enhances the effectiveness of a large number of other hormones; it appears to do this by producing in target tissues the kind of environment that is essential for other hormones to exert their fullest activities. Without mentioning more specific examples at this time, it may be stated that STH alone has little effect on some of the pituitary targets (*e.g.,* thyroid, gonads, adrenal cortex), but it markedly enhances the effectiveness of the hormones that are specific for these targets when administered together with them.

PERSPECTIVES

After having discussed the major problems and concepts of modern endocrinology and after having reviewed the current methodology in this actively growing field, we are in a position to assess some of the directions that future endocrinological research might take. It is obvious that some of the themes we have considered, notably receptor mechanisms and mechanisms of hormone action, are dynamic ones that command the interest of investigators in diverse fields including pharmacology, biochemistry, and genetics. Ongoing research into the ultrastructure of endocrine target cells will continue on a high plane and provide much information about the synthesis and release of both hormones and products resulting from hormonal stimulation. Surely, many of these ultrastructural observations will have important bearing on studies concerning receptors and mechanisms of hormone action.

Among the older themes that have always played an important role in our understanding of endocrinology is that of evolution. An understanding of evolutionary principles has been a great unifier and has allowed us to bring together seemingly unrelated characteristics found in different organisms, species, and phyla. Thus, the many endocrine homologies and analogies that exist can be better understood. When the role of evolution is viewed together with findings in various fields such as developmental biology and physiology, surprising revelations occur; and often they lead to the formulation of unifying hypotheses that have important ramifications in current and future endocrinological investigations. One such hypothesis, advanced by Pearse, considers that endocrine polypeptide cells are derived from the neural crest.[39] He specifically refers to cells that are endowed with cytochemical characteristics described as APUD (*Amine Precursor Uptake and Decarboxylation*). Some 16 cell types belong to the APUD series, including ACTH- and MSH-secreting cells of the pituitary, adrenal medullary cells, melanophores, some cells of the ultimobranchial bodies and of the carotid body, and various endocrine cell types of the gastrointestinal tract including all the endocrine cells of the pancreas. While all of the endocrine polypeptide cells he refers to have in common the APUD characteristics, there is little definitive proof that all of these types are of neural crest origin. The best support for the hypothesis comes from the unequivocal observation that the calcitonin-secreting cells of the avian ultimobranchial body are derived from the neural crest (see Chapter 8). Some ancillary support for the concept is derived from other experiments; however, definitive substantiation is wanting. There are many reasons to believe that the concept is too inclusive, that an attempt to unify the polypeptide-secreting cells into one group is presumptuous and invalid. Nevertheless, the concept is reasonable, interesting, and thought-provoking, and it is such hypotheses which stimulate experimentation, ultimately leading to the acquisition of new knowledge.

REFERENCES

1. Ahlquist, R. P.: A study of adrenergic receptors. Am. J. Physiol. *153*:586–600, 1948.
2. Ausiello, D. A., and Sharp, G. W. G.: Localization of physiological receptor sites for aldosterone in the bladder of the toad, *Bufo marinus*. Endocrinology 82:1163, 1968.
3. Bardin, C. W., Allison, J. E., Stanley, A. J., and Gumbreck, L. G.: Secretion of testosterone by the pseudohermaphrodite rat. Endocrinology 84:435, 1969.
4. Chase, G. D., and Rabinowitz, J. L.: Principles of Radioisotope Methodology. Minneapolis, Burgess Publishing Co., 1962.
5. Christensen, A. K., and Mason, N. R.: Comparative ability of seminiferous tubules and interstitial tissue of rat to synthesize androgens from progesterone-4-^{14}C *in vitro*. Endocrinology 76:646, 1965.
6. Dale, H. A.: On some physiological actions of ergot. J. Physiol. (London) *34*:163–206, 1906.
7. Diamond, M., Rust, N., and Westphal, U.: High-affinity binding of progesterone, testosterone and cortisol in normal and androgen-treated guinea pigs during various reproductive stages: Relationship to masculinization. Endocrinology 84:1143, 1969.
8. Falconer, D. S., Latyszewski, M., and Isaacson, J. H.: Diabetes insipidus associated with oligosyndactyly in the mouse. Genet. Res. 5:473, 1964.
9. Fawcett, D. W., Long, J. A., and Jones, A. L.: The ultrastructure of endocrine glands. Rec. Progr. Horm. Res. 25:315, 1969.
10. Freychet, P., Brandenburg, D., and Wollmer, A.: Receptor-binding assay of chemically modified insulins: Comparison with *in vitro* and *in vivo* bioassays. Diabetologia 10:1, 1974.
11. Fuxe, K., and Hökfelt, T.: The influence of central catecholamine neurons on the hormone secretion from the anterior and posterior pituitary. *In* F. Stutinsky (ed.): Neurosecretion. New York, Springer-Verlag, 1967, p. 165.
12. Goldberg, N. D.: Cyclic nucleotides and cell function. Practice 9:69, 1974.
13. Goldman, A. S., and Neumann, F.: Differentiation of the mammary gland in experimental adrenal hyperplasia due to inhibition of Δ^5, 3 β-hydroxysteroid dehydrogenase in rats. Proc. Soc. Exp. Biol. Med. *132*:237, 1969.
14. Greer, M. A., Grimm, Y., and Inoue, K.: Fate of iodide derived from intrathyroidal hydrolysis of thyroglobulin. Endocrinology 85:837, 1969.
15. Hadley, M. E., Bower, A., and Hruby, V.: Cellular mechanisms controlling melanophore stimulating hormone (MSH) release. Gen. Comp. Endocr. 26:24, 1975.

16. Hadley, M. E., and Goldman, J. M.: Adrenergic receptors and geographic variation in *Rana pipiens* chromatophore response. Am. J. Physiol. *219*:72, 1970.

17. Hamilton, D. W., Jones, A. L., and Fawcett, D. W.: Cholesterol biosynthesis in the mouse epididymis and ductus deferens: A biochemical and morphological study. Biol. Reproduction *1*:167, 1969.

18. Hayashida, T.: Immunological reactions of pituitary hormones. *In* G. W. Harris and B. T. Donovan (eds.): The Pituitary Gland, Vol. 2. Berkeley, University of California Press, 1966, p. 613.

19. Hayashida, T.: Inhibition of spermiogenesis, prostate and seminal vesicle development in normal animals with antigonadotrophic hormone serum. J. Endocr. *26*:75, 1963.

20. Hisaw, F. L., Velardo, J. T., and Goolsby, C. M.: Interactions of estrogens on uterine growth. J. Clin. Endocr. *14*:1134, 1954.

21. Ivey, J. L., and Tashjian, A. H., Jr.: Regulation of prolactin and growth hormone production by clonal strains of functional pituitary cells in culture. Amer. Zool. *15*:249, 1975.

22. Jackson, H.: Antispermatogenic agents. Brit. Med. Bull. *26*:79, 1970.

23. Jacob, F., and Monod, J.: Genetic regulatory mechanisms in the synthesis of proteins. J. Mol. Biol. *3*:318, 1961.

24. Jensen, E. V., and DeSombre, E. R.: Estrogen-receptor interaction. Science *182*:126, 1973.

25. Josimovich, J. B., and MacLaren, J. A.: Presence in the human placenta and term serum of a highly lactogenic substance immunologically related to pituitary growth hormone. Endocrinology *71*:209, 1962.

26. Karlson, P.: Biochemical studies of ecdysone control of chromosomal activity. J. Cell. Comp. Physiol. *66*(Suppl. 1):69, 1965.

27. Karlson, P.: New concepts on the mode of action of hormones. Perspect. Biol. Med. *6*:203, 1963.

28. Knobil, E.: The pituitary growth hormone: Some physiological considerations. *In* M. X. Zarrow (ed.): Growth in Living Systems. New York, Basic Books, 1961, p. 353.

29. Lacey, P. E., and Malaisse, W. J.: Mictrotubules and beta cell secretion. Rec. Progr. Horm. Res. *29*:199, 1973.

30. Leathem, J. H.: Hormones and protein metabolism. Rec. Progr. Horm. Res. *14*:141, 1958.

31. Li, C. H.: Pituitary growth hormone as a metabolic hormone. Science *123*:617, 1956.

32. Mosier, H. D., and Richter, C. P.: Response of the glomerulosa layer of the adrenal gland of wild and domesticated Norway rats on low and high salt diets. Endocrinology *62*:268, 1958.

33. Murphy, B. E. P.: Protein binding and the assay of nonantigenic hormones. Rec. Progr. Horm. Res. *25*:563, 1969.

34. Neumann, F., and Elger, W.: Physiological and physical intersexuality of male rats by early treatment with an antiandrogenic agent (1,2α-methylene-6-chloro-Δ⁶-hydroxyprogesterone acetate). Acta Endocr. (Kobenhavn), Suppl., *100*:174, 1965.

35. Okuda, T., and Grollman, A.: Action of neutral red on the secretion of glucagon and glucose metabolism in the rat. Endocrinology *78*:195, 1966.

36. Olivereau, M.: Action de la métopirone chez l'anguille normale et hypophysectomisée, en particulier sur le systeme hypophyso-corticosurréjalien. Gen. Comp. Endocr. *5*:109, 1965.

37. O'Malley, B. W., McGuire, W. L., Kohler, P. O., and Korenman, S. G.: Studies on the mechanism of steroid hormone regulation of synthesis of specific proteins. Rec. Progr. Horm. Res. *25*:105, 1969.

38. O'Malley, B. W., Woo, S. L., Harris, S. E., Rosen, J. M., Comstock, J. P., Chan, L., Bordelon, C. B., Holder, J. W., Sperry, P., and Means, A. R.: Steroid hormone action in animal cells. Amer. Zool. *15*(Suppl. 1):215, 1975.

39. Pearse, A. G. E.: The cytochemistry and ultrastructure of polypeptide hormone producing cells of the APUD series and the embryologic, physiologic, and pathologic implications of the concept. J. Histochem. Cytochem. *17*:303, 1969.

40. Rhodin, J. A. G.: The ultrastructure of the adrenal cortex of the rat under normal and experimental conditions. J. Ultrastruct. Res. *34*:23, 1971.

41. Sciarra, J. J., Kaplan, S. L., and Grumbach, M. M.: Localization of anti-human growth hormone serum within the human placenta: Evidence for a human chorionic "growth hormone-prolactin." Nature *199*:1005, 1963.

42. Sgouris, J. T., and Meites, J.: Differential inactivation of prolactin by mammary tissue from pregnant and parturient rats. Am. J. Physiol. *175*:319, 1953.

43. Skelley, D. S., Brown, L. P., and Besch, P. K.: Radioimmunoassay. Clin. Chem. *19*:146, 1973.

44. Sutherland, E. W.: Studies on the mechanism of hormone action. Science *177*:401, 1972.

45. Sutherland, E. W., Robison, G. A., and Butcher, R. W.: Some aspects of the biological role of adenosine 3′,5′ monophosphate (cyclic AMP). Circulation *37*:279–306, 1968.

46. Turtle, J. R., and Kipnis, D. M.: An adrenergic receptor mechanism for the control of cyclic 3′,5′ adenosine monophosphate synthesis in tissues. Biochem. Biophys. Res. Commun. 28:797–802, 1967.

47. Valtin, H.: Hereditary hypothalamic diabetes insipidus in rats (Brattleboro strain). Am. J. Med. 42:814, 1967.

CHAPTER 3

Neuroendocrinology

Neurology and endocrinology developed as separate disciplines, but the line of demarcation between them is not as sharp as formerly supposed. During recent decades it has been established that the nervous and endocrine systems are reciprocally interrelated and work together in many ways. Survival of the organism often depends upon the ability to adjust to a wide variety of stimuli, arising from within and without the body, and this involves the exchange of information between the nervous and endocrine systems. Perhaps the time is near at hand when it will be more instructive and correct to think in terms of one coordinatory system (neuroendocrine) rather than viewing the two components as separate entities, operating in distinctive manners to facilitate integration of the individual. The discovery of neurosecretory cells (gland-like neurons) added a new dimension to regulatory biology and resulted in establishment of the rapidly expanding science of neuroendocrinology.[16, 31, 32]

All definitions proposed for hormones seem to be either too expansive or too restrictive. Regardless of the definition one prefers, it must be recognized that chemical messengers are not all the same, and the differences may be very important under certain circumstances. The classic definition of Starling emphasized their dissemination via the bloodstream. Much confusion has resulted from the discovery that many regulatory agents confine their activities to localized tissues and do not attain effective concentrations in the blood. It should be appreciated, however, that the intercellular fluid originates from the blood plasma and is returned from the tissues to the general circulation via the capillaries and lymphatic vessels. This relatively slow circulation of *tissue fluids* permits many biologically active substances to exert localized effects.

There is merit to the point of view that hormones act essentially to integrate the organism by transferring information from one set of cells to another.[13, 26] To define hormones as information-transferring molecules has several broadening effects: (1) it would obliterate the distinction between neurotransmitters and neurohormones, and emphasize the similarities rather than the differences between the nervous and endocrine systems; (2) it puts less emphasis on the mode of transmission within the organism than is allowed by the classic definition, and (3) it should help to delimit hormones from vitamins and other agents primarily functioning in energy metabolism.

THE CONCEPT OF NEUROSECRETION

Exteroceptive stimuli may be perceived through any sensory modality (auditory, visual, olfactory, thermal, tactile, and so forth); interoceptive stimuli include many chemical changes in the body fluids, such as pH, temperature, hormones, water, glucose, salt, and oxygen. Emotional states clearly influence certain endocrine glands, but little can be said of these except that they are mediated by the higher brain centers. Cues that have been received and integrated by the central nervous system are passed by neurons to neurosecretory cells, which respond by releasing neurohormones in the vicinity of effector cells or into vascular pathways for more remote action. The neurosecretory cells, being of dual nature, perform the important function of tying together the nervous and endocrine systems. They constitute a final common path for the conversion of nerve impulses into endocrine messengers.

With neurosecretory cells serving as "go-betweens," the central nervous system is able to control the functional activities of many endocrine glands and adjust their activities in accordance with the requirements of varying internal environments. It is not surprising that neuroendocrine mechanisms participate in such organismal adjustments as growth, reproductive development and sexual behavior, molting, diapause, regeneration, water balance, color change, migration, and blood chemistry. The reverse relationship, whereby hormones affect the nervous system, is equally important. The concept that the nervous and endocrine systems are reciprocally interrelated is well documented and generally accepted.

The Nature of Neurosecretory Cells

Neuroscretory cells are neurons which have differentiated in the direction of glands, the elaboration and discharge of secretions being of prime importance. In terms of phylogeny, they are the oldest hormone-secreting cells in the animal kingdom. Though functioning as glands, they are morphologically similar to conventional neurons, with dendrites, axons, Nissl bodies, neurofibrillae, neurotubules, and Golgi complexes. Dendrites may be absent from these cells in the invertebrates. It is certain that at least some neurosecretory cells can conduct impulses,[14] and it is possible that this is concerned in some manner with the release of secretions. In the best established instances, the neurosecretory products are proteinaceous, which is consistent with the ultrastructure of the cells.

The proteinaceous neurosecretion is synthesized on ribosomes associated with the endoplasmic reticulum, and is passed to the Golgi apparatus for packaging into the elementary granules. These are electron-dense spheres which range in size from 1000 to 3000 Å in diameter, and are bounded by membranes. This synthesis is presumed to occur largely in the perikarya, but it is possible that synthesis or reorganization of the secretion may occur to some extent in the axons. The protein that is produced by some neurosecretory cells, called *neurophysin,* is regarded as a carrier of the ac-

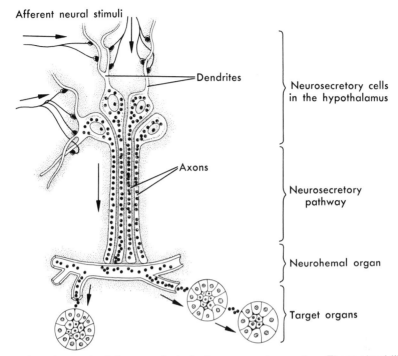

Figure 3–1. Generalized diagram of a typical neurosecretory system. These gland-like neurons synthesize neurohormones which are freed from the axonic terminals, often within storage and release centers called neurohemal organs. The secretions typically enter the circulation and affect distant targets. The neurosecretory cells receive nervous impulses from many sources, as indicated by arrows and synapses. Such neurosecretory systems form important links between the nervous and endocrine organs of both invertebrates and vertebrates. (From Frye, B. E.[10] after Scharrer, E., and Scharrer, B.[31])

tual neurohormone. The granules are thought to be transported by axoplasmic flow from the perikaryon to the axon terminals, from whence they are discharged. The granules often collect in bulbous enlargements of the axons prior to release (Fig. 3–1). Small electron-lucent vesicles are also present in axon terminals of neurosecretory cells. These measure 200 to 500 Å and appear quite similar to the synaptic vesicles of cholinergic terminals. The significance of these small vesicles has not been established, though some studies suggest that they may play a role in the release of neurosecretory material from the membrane-bound granules, or aid in its passage through the axon membrane.[3]

The perikarya of neurosecretory cells are often clumped in the central nervous system, but their axon terminals typically extend outside the nervous system and end in close association with blood vessels or hemocoels. These may form *neurohemal organs* for the storage, or possibly modification, of the neurohormones. The best known neurohemal organs are the posterior lobe (pars nervosa) of the pituitary, the median eminence and its equivalent structures in certain vertebrates, the caudal neurosecretory system (urophysis) of fishes, the sinus gland of crustaceans, and the corpus cardiacum of insects. The perikarya of these cells are surprisingly constant in number and location within the central nervous system.

To a greater extent than in vertebrates, it appears that the invertebrates depend heavily on axonal transport for the dissemination of their neurosecretions; the elongated axons often extend through intricate systems of commissures and connectives before reaching their targets. In some instances, at least, the secretion is discharged at the target, without relying on blood transport. Neurosecretory cells of invertebrates are widely distributed within the nervous system, but there is a tendency in vertebrates for such cells to become aggregated in the diencephalic portion of the brain.

It must be clearly understood that no unique granule, vesicle, or other structural feature can be employed to distinguish all neurosecretory cells from conventional neurons. In most instances electron-microscopic, cytochemical, and physiologic information is required to make this decision. Many types of confirmatory evidence depend upon knowing the actions and chemical identity of the secretion.

The Neurohypophysial Neurohormones

The first and clearest instance of neurosecretion among vertebrates was proof that the neurohormones stored in the posterior lobe are the products of neurosecretory neurons whose perikarya are located in hypothalamic nuclei. Since these hormones are transported in conjunction with carrier proteins (neurophysins), the secretion could be selectively stained and followed throughout the neuron to its point of discharge and storage in the pars nervosa. These cells are clearly distinct from conventional neurons since they synthesize and discharge peptidergic secretions close to blood vessels, and do not function in synaptic transmission. Conventional neurons from many areas of the brain establish synaptic connections with the neurosecretory neurons.

The Median Eminence-Adenohypophysial Relationship

In 1930, attention was directed to a system of portal veins extending along the pituitary stalk and connecting a capillary plexus in the median eminence with another in the adenohypophysis. It was apparent that this arrangement must have great physiologic significance, but it took nearly a decade to convince all concerned that the direction of blood flow is from the brain to the pituitary. It follows that nearly all of the blood reaching the adenohypophysis has first traversed the capillary plexus located in the median eminence region of the hypothalamus.[25, 36]

Many neurosecretory neurons terminate on the capillary loops of the median eminence, and these resemble those of the neurohypophysis except for the fact that they do not contain granules that take the Gomori stain. Various physiologic and chemical experiments make it reasonably certain that these neurons are peptidergic and that they synthesize at least nine hypophysiotrophic neurohormones (releasing and inhibiting factors) and discharge them into the median eminence. They are then transported by the portal circulation to control secretion by the multiple kinds of adenohypo-physial cells. In this manner, the small peptide neurohormones serve as the main functional link between the brain and the adenohypophysis. There are indications that some of the releasing factors may be transported by epen-dymal tanycytes from the third ventricle to the median eminence.

The neurosecretory cells which produce the hypophysiotrophic pep-tides are themselves subject to regulation by neurons of a more conven-tional type emanating from different parts of the brain. These particular neurons employ monoamines as synaptic transmitters and appear to be re-stricted in their distribution. The three transmitters, collectively referred to as monoamines, are dopamine, norepinephrine, and serotonin. Monoami-nergic endings may be identified by fluorescence techniques or through the use of radioactive transmitter compounds which are specifically bound by the nerve terminals.

Some New Dimensions to Neurosecretion

Electron-microscopic studies and refined biochemical techniques have provided information that may require modulation of current concepts and definitions. It appears that ordinary neurons and neurosecretory cells over-lap to a greater degree than was formerly supposed, and it is becoming in-creasingly difficult to support the conventional distinction usually drawn between neurotransmitters and neurohormones. Distinctions have usually been made on such criteria as how the secretion is transported (range of action), chemistry of the secretion, and how the secretion is used. Perhaps it is a matter of deciding how gland-like a neuron must become before it is properly called a neurosecretory cell.

Depending upon the chemistry of the neurohormone, neurosecretory cells have been classed as "peptidergic" or "aminergic."[15] Convincing evidence from both invertebrates and vertebrates indicates that neurosecre-tory cells may release amines as well as proteins or polypeptides into the body fluids. For example, amine-secreting neurons have been identified by fluorescence microscopy in the central nervous systems of annelids. These secretions appear to be released from the perikarya, rather than from the axons, and are probably taken up by the capillary circulation.[4]

The following special situations deserve further study:[30]

(1) With exception of the adrenal medulla, it has generally been be-lieved that the endocrine organs are only sparsely innervated, if at all, and hence depend almost exclusively on blood-borne messengers. Some of the nerve terminals found in endocrine glands abut upon blood vessels and probably have some effect on blood flow through the gland. Recent elec-tron-microscopic studies have revealed that endocrine cells themselves receive signals via conventional neurons to an extent not appreciated pre-viously. Such secretomotor endings have been found in the adenohypo-physis, the pancreatic islets, and several other glands. This indicates that these endocrine cells are capable of responding to neural signals, instead

of being wholly dependent upon circulating neurohormones, but the significance of this has not been evaluated.

(2) It is known that some neurosecretory cells, having their perikarya in hypothalamic nuclei and releasing peptidergic secretions from their axons, may bypass the hypophysial portal veins and terminate directly on or between adenohypophysial cells. These may form special secretomotor junctions, but the nerve cell and endocrine cell may be no further apart than are neurons at conventional synaptic junctions. An analogous situation has been observed in the corpus allatum of insects. By depositing the peptide messenger near the target cell, prompt delivery is assured and dilution of the messenger by blood is prevented. Fluorescence and labeling techniques have shown that in some instances aminergic messengers, instead of peptidergic ones, may be delivered in this manner by neurons presumed to be neurosecretory. Very little is known about the special circumstances that call for this type of regulation.

(3) It has been found in both vertebrates and invertebrates that non-endocrine targets such as muscle fibers and exocrine glands may be supplied by pepetidergic neurosecretory cells. The axons, with perikarya in the central nervous system, discharge peptides in very close proximity to the effector cells, thus avoiding the circulatory system. This is reminiscent of a primitive condition in which neurosecretory cells were the only sources of hormones, as is still the case with coelenterates and other invertebrate groups. Except for the method of transport, these neurosecretory cells are very comparable to those of the neurohypophysis which secrete oxytocin and vasopressin, neurosecretions delivered by the blood to non-endocrine targets such as the kidney and uterus.

It is important to recognize borderline situations of this kind and to modulate current concepts when the evidence becomes sufficient. On the other hand, they may represent intermediate gradations which do not carry enough physiologic significance to warrant radical changes of concepts and definitions.[29]

The Evolution of Regulatory Mechanisms

Plants are devoid of nervous systems and glands of internal secretion and, from this, it may be assumed that integrations within multicellular plants are accomplished largely through the dispersal of chemical messengers, these perhaps being formed and released by all living cells of the plant body. Each cell has its own system of homeostatic controls, and this is supplemented by auxins and other phytohormones which make intercellular communication possible.

Neural and endocrine controls represent innovations that evolved in multicellular animals as they began to differentiate tissues and organs for the performance of particular functions. The chemical messengers operating to integrate the organism may be considered as evolutionary extensions of the autoregulatory devices functioning at the cellular level. Hormones and related substances must be geared to these intracellular regulating systems. Considerable evidence could be amassed to support the view that the following progressive changes occurred during evolution: intracellular messengers → nerve cells (neurohumors) → neurosecretory cells (neurohormones) → endocrine glands (hormones).

Among invertebrates, the neurosecretory cells tend to be widely scattered throughout the nervous system; in the vertebrates, particularly in mammals, neurosecretory centers tend to concentrate in one small area of the diencephalon, namely the *hypothalamus*. Ductless glands are not present in the lower invertebrates and most, if not all, of the major functions such as metabolism, reproduction, regeneration, and behavior are directly conditioned by neurosecretions. It is inferred from this that the neurosecretory system antedated the circumscribed endocrine glands. When ductless glands did appear, most of them came under the regulatory control of neurosecretory cells. This arrangement makes it possible for various kinds of external and internal stimuli impinging upon the nervous system to act via neurosecretory cells and endocrine glands. In this manner, the effects within the organism are amplified and prolonged.

While endocrine glands are present in some of the invertebrates, they are few in number and much less specialized than in the vertebrates. From the standpoint of comparative anatomy, the endocrine glands have not undergone any very striking structural changes in the various vertebrate classes, but there have been important phylogenetic changes in the chemistry and actions of the hormones within the body.

CONTROL OF THE ENDOCRINE SYSTEM

General Nature of Hormonal Actions

The endocrine glands function to a large extent in maintaining relatively constant states (homeostasis) in the internal fluid environment of the body. They generally cooperate with the nervous system in effecting responses to a large variety of exteroceptive and interoceptive stimuli, and in order to do so they must be subject to complex control systems which regulate their output of secretions. Since endocrine tissues maintained in tissue culture or used in perfusion experiments retain some slight capacity to secrete their characteristic hormones, provided that necessary precursors are supplied, it is apparent that extrinsic controls are not essential for minimal activity. In the normal organism, however, controls are essential to increase or decrease the hormonal output in accordance with current or anticipated needs. Reproductive cycles, for example, depend upon profound fluctuations in the titers of the multiple hormones that bring about the structural and functional changes.

Since hormones are transported by the vascular system, the blood at all times contains small quantities of all hormones that are being actively secreted. The form of the circulating hormone may not be identical with that liberated by the gland. Some of the hormones in the blood are bound to carrier proteins, and many of them have to undergo enzymatic transformations at the level of target tissues before they can be utilized. Prohormonal compounds may undergo transformations in several organs before the active form of the hormone is released. Since the secretion of hormones is precisely controlled, it is obviously essential that those in the circulation be inactivated and excreted rather promptly. Enzymatic breakdown occurs principally in the liver and kidneys, the end products being eliminated via the bile or urine.

The actions of a hormone are entirely dependent upon the ability of target tissues to respond. The hormone does not create in the target cell any new potentiality; it merely triggers the metabolic machinery already possessed. If the receptor sites (proteins or lipoproteins) on target cells are absent or already occupied, the hormone produces no effect. An organ may respond to a hormone produced by one of its tissues, but endocrine cells are typically unable to respond directly to their own secretions, possibly because they lack the necessary receptor macromolecules. For example, the Leydig cells of the testis are the main source of androgens, and these steroids are required for proper functioning of the germinal epithelium that lines the testis tubules. The Leydig cells themselves do not respond to androgens but do respond to luteinizing hormone from the anterior pituitary. Growth hormone, prolactin, and insulin are examples of hormones that employ a great variety of effector cells; thyrotrophin and other trophic hormones from the anterior pituitary employ a more restricted range of targets.

In many instances, multiple hormones must act upon a target tissue in correct sequence in order to elicit maximal responses. Growth hormone, for example, is limited in its actions if thyroxine is deficient or lacking. Thyroxine is said to perform a *permissive function,* and many hormones act in that manner. The uterus and many other tissues respond more fully to progesterone if they have been subjected first to estrogens.

There are numerous instances of hormones acting with others to produce opposing effects. Insulin, for example, has the overall effect of reducing the levels of blood sugar, whereas glucagon has the reverse action. Post-embryonic development in insects is controlled largely through the interactions of two hormones: juvenile hormone encourages the retention of larval characters, whereas ecdysone promotes the differentiation of adult characters. Some of the anterior pituitary cells are controlled by dual hypophysiotrophic hormones of the median eminence, one promoting release of the secretion and the other inhibiting it.

Feedback Control Systems

The adrenal medulla is one of the few endocrine glands whose secretions (catecholamines) are released in response to direct nervous stimulation. Impulses arising in various brain centers are relayed over the sympathetic system and reach the medulla via preganglionic (cholinergic) fibers contained in the splanchnic nerves. The embryonic cells (neuroblasts) that form the medulla are of neural crest origin, and it is interesting that this gland retains its intimate association with the nervous system. Being under nervous control, the medullary hormones can be released quickly; they produce widespread systemic actions, some of which (such as rising blood pressure and elevated plasma glucose) act back via central nervous pathways to reduce the output of hormones.

Most endocrine glands are components of homeostatic feedback loops whereby the resultant of target-cell activity (controlled variable) acts back to accelerate or retard hormone production by the controlling gland. *Negative feedback* systems are the simplest and most prevalent type; here the output, consequent upon target-cell responses, retards the control action (Fig. 3–2). In the case of *positive feedback* the output accelerates the control action. Some kind of "sensing" mechanism must be present in all feedback systems to evaluate the concentration of the controlled variable. One may conceive of mineral homeostasis and such processes as involving the operation of multiple feedback loops. It must be recognized, however, that many modifying factors enter at all levels and no simple engineering scheme accurately depicts all that occurs within the living organism.

By reference to Figure 3–2 we may illustrate how insulin, a hormone from the B-cells of the pancreatic islets, helps control the levels of blood glucose. In the first place, it has to be assumed that the B-cells possess some kind of sensory mechanism which enables them to monitor the level of glucose in the blood (controlled variable). When blood sugar begins to rise, the B-cells increase their release of insulin, which stimulates liver cells and other targets to remove sugar from the blood for storage or utilization. The gland diminishes its secretion of insulin as blood sugar levels fall. Glucagon, a hormone of the pancreatic A-cells, functions in the opposite manner. This kind of control is possible when the controlled variable is an alteration in chemistry of the body fluids which serves as a secretory stimulus.

Insulin secretion is a much more complex activity than might be inferred from this brief discussion. Increasing attention is being given to the manner in which islet functions are affected by autonomic nerves, as well as by the gastrointestinal hormones. Various hormones from the anterior pituitary and adrenals are indirectly involved. There are receptors in the intestinal wall that monitor glucose concentrations there and employ both neural and hormonal signals to alert the B-cells to augment the insulin output in

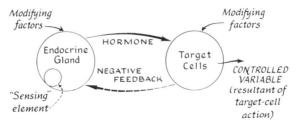

Figure 3–2. A simple negative feedback. A hormone from an endocrine gland acts on target cells to produce a change (controlled variable) which acts back on the gland to decrease the rate of hormone release. This general type of control exists between insulin and blood sugar, glucagon and blood sugar, parathyroid hormone and blood calcium, and calcitonin and blood calcium.

anticipation of a glucose load. This is a kind of feedback control having positive features.

A more complex arrangement is illustrated in Figure 3–3; precursor compounds undergo successive enzymatic transformations in multiple organs before the most effective form of the hormone is released. Vitamin D_3 (cholecalciferol) may be synthesized in the skin, under the influence of ultraviolet light, or consumed as a dietary constitutent. Cholecalciferol undergoes successive hydroxylations in the liver and kidneys to form 1,25-dihydroxycholecalciferol, which functions as a steroid hormone in helping to regulate serum calcium levels. Several of the intermediate compounds possess slight biological activity, and production of the final hormone may require considerable time.[24]

Neuroendocrine integrations involving the brain and pituitary gland are far more complex than the arrangements just mentioned (Fig. 3–4). All components of the pituitary are closely associated with the central nervous system, and this subjects the many pituitary targets to a wide variety of influences arising from changes in the external and internal environments. A *neuroendocrine reflex* is an arrangement whereby sensory impulses from the nervous system are converted into hormonal signals and eventually into a physiologic response. The neurosecretory cell is the key that makes such pathways possible; it is able to receive impulses from nerve cells that are widely dispersed in the nervous system and, being able to secrete chemical messengers, translates the neural signals into hormonal signals which can be received by endocrine glands that are not richly innervated. In this manner, the neurosecretory cells constitute a final common pathway over which environmental stimuli can exert powerful effects on processes that depend upon endocrine controls.

Three levels of complexity in the neuroendocrine system are usually recognized (Fig. 3–4). In *first order* arrangements, neurosecretory products (neurohormones) act upon non-endocrine target tissues or organs. This is illustrated by the neurohypophysial peptides (vasopressin and oxytocin), which affect such targets as the uterus, kidneys, and mammary glands. In a *second order* process, a neurohormone from the hypothalamus (hypophysiotrophic peptide) acts on an endocrine gland (anterior pituitary), which then

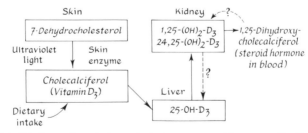

Figure 3–3. In this type of control, a substrate compound is enzymatically altered by multiple organs before the final hormone is attained. As an example, cholecalciferol (vitamin D_3) may be synthesized in the human skin or consumed in the diet; it then is metabolically transformed in the liver and kidney, and dihydroxycholecalciferol is released into the blood where it functions as a steroid hormone. Its overall effect is to increase the levels of plasma calcium.

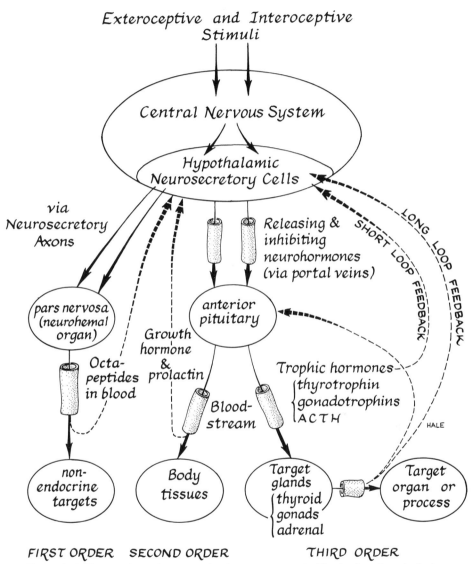

Figure 3–4. Three orders of neuroendocrine arrangements. The broken lines indicate negative feedback; the action may be directly upon the anterior pituitary, more indirectly upon the neurosecretory cells in the periventricular brain, or upon both.

secretes a hormone that acts on a final set of targets. Anterior pituitary growth hormone and prolactin are examples. *Third order* neuroendocrine controls are the most complex; they include hypothalamic neurohormones, anterior pituitary trophic hormones, and target glands (thyroid, adrenals, gonads) and their respective targets.

Hormonal feedback loops become very complex in the neuroendocrine arrangement, and there is not perfect agreement among investigators. Two types of hormonal feedback have been described with respect to the length of the loop: (1) *long-loop feedback,* in which the blood concentrations of hormones from pituitary target glands act back upon the hypothalamus or other parts of the brain to affect anterior pituitary functions, and (2) a *short-loop* system, whereby the trophic hormones of the anterior pituitary may themselves act back on the hypothalamus or other brain areas (Fig. 3–4).

Endocrine glands such as the testes, ovaries, thyroid, and adrenal cortices depend to a large extent upon the circulating levels of pituitary trophic hormones and have, at best, only limited powers of autonomous regulation. By feedback mechanisms, target gland hormones in the blood increase or decrease the production of the pituitary trophic hormones. When the titers of gonadal steroids in the blood are high, some chemoreceptive mechanism in the hypothalamus acts to reduce the release of pituitary gonadotrophins, and, consequently, the output of steroids by the gonad is diminished. It is well known that the excessive administration of gonadal steroids may result in severe impairment of testicular and ovarian functions. Low titers of gonadal steroids in the circulation affect the feedback mechanism in the reverse manner. In the female, ovarian steroids (estradiol and progesterone) condition the reproductive cycles, and these may act through both negative and positive feedbacks to coordinate the sequential release of neurohormones from the median eminence and of hormones from the anterior pituitary. The regulation of thyroid activity by TSH and of the adrenal cortex by ACTH are other examples of long-loop feedback (Fig. 3–4).

Examples of Neuroendocrine Reflex Arcs

Afferent pathways derive information about the external and internal environment through organs of special sense and transmit neural signals to neurosecretory cells in the brain; these gland-like neurons release blood-borne chemical signals (neurohormones) that activate non-endocrine or endocrine targets. This kind of a circuit is called a *neuroendocrine reflex,* and these vary greatly in the degree of complexity (Fig. 3–4). The afferent portion of the arc is usually neural, but in some cases it may be hormonal. Only a few examples, illustrating slightly different situations, can be mentioned here.

Responses Related to Reproduction

In certain birds (*e.g.,* junco finches) and mammals (*e.g.,* ferrets), exposure to increasing periods of illumination during the winter months, when the day length is naturally decreasing, stimulates the gonads and brings the animals prematurely into breeding conditions. In birds, at least, the photoreceptors may be ocular (retinal) or encephalic (within the brain).[22] In some animals, such as sheep and goats, which normally breed during the autumn, exposure to light has the reverse effect: breeding activity may be stimulated prematurely by exposing the animals artificially to diminishing periods of light during the early summer, when the days are naturally lengthening. Impulses from the photoreceptors are channeled through the brain to centers that control the release of gonadotrophins from the anterior pituitary; the latter hormones stimulate the gonads to proliferate gametes and to secrete steroid hormones, which in turn promote development of the accessory sex organs and secondary sex characters and condition breeding behavior. Sexual activity and quiescence appear to be regulated by an inherent rhythm, but the timing of these events can be modified in certain species by light.

Ovulation in the rabbit occurs 10 hours after copulation, and this timing is remarkably constant. Stimulation of the cervix by the penis, coupled with the act of mating, sets up impulses that reach the spinal cord and travel up the cord to the hypothalamic portion of the brain lying above the pituitary gland. Neurosecretory neurons discharge hypophysiotrophic peptides (release factors) which are carried to the anterior pituitary via a system of portal veins. These stimulate the pituitary to discharge the necessary gonadotrophins into the systemic circulation. The latter hormones stimulate ovarian changes and make the release of eggs (ovulation) possible.

Copulation in rabbits and rats produces a reflexive release of pituitary luteinizing hormone (LH) in both sexes. The LH stimulates the cells of Leydig in the testis and leads to large increases in the amount of testosterone in peripheral plasma. The act of coitus is not essential for this effect in male rabbits; merely placing them with females is sufficient to elevate testosterone levels.[27]

Egg laying in many birds ceases after a customary number of eggs has accumulated. The house sparrow generally lays four or five eggs, but if the eggs are removed, oviposition may be continued until the ovaries are exhausted and as many as 50 eggs have been laid in succession. Female pigeons do not lay if they are kept in complete isolation, but laying is induced by the presence of males or other females. Ovulation will eventually occur if the isolated female is permitted to observe herself in a mirror. Brooding behavior in pigeons is normally associated with the presence of at least one egg in the nest. Medway found that denervation of that part of the pigeon's breast which covers the eggs does not terminate broodiness.[21] This suggests that the maintenance of broodiness does not depend upon tactile stimuli alone; multiple sensory receptors apparently are involved. Social factors, operating through neuroendocrine pathways, are extremely important in the reproduction of many invertebrates and vertebrates.

It has been known for years that in many mammals (cow, goat, rabbit, dog, human, and others) the first half minute of milking or suckling yields little milk, but at the end of this period, milk begins to flow suddenly and freely. This is known as the "let down" or "draught," and the mechanism involved is now understood. It is a neuroendocrine reflex, the afferent limb of the arc being formed by sensory nerves and pathways and the efferent limb by the release of oxytocin from the neurohypophysis into the circulating blood. This hormone acts specifically to cause contraction of the myoepithelial cells surrounding the mammary alveoli, squeezing out the milk that is contained in the alveolar cells. Many sensory modalities other than tactile stimulation of the teats may induce the milk-ejection reaction. In cattle, the sound of milking equipment, sight of the calf, various odors, manipulation of the external genitalia, the presence of a male, the act of copulation, the arrival of the scheduled time for milking, and many other situations may initiate this neuroendocrine chain of events.

Afferent pathways may be hormonal instead of nervous. For example, in certain crustaceans a male sex hormone is secreted by special *androgenic glands* that are spatially separate from the testes. Male sex behavior is abolished by surgical removal of these glands or is induced in females by transplanting the glands into them. The hormone apparently influences behavior through its action on the nervous system.[6]

A comparable situation exists in the mouse, where aggressive behavior is conditioned by testicular hormone (androgen). Orchiectomy of the adult reduces fighting; androgen treatments restore this behavior in such males and induce the behavior in ovariectomized females. Aggressive behavior can even be induced by androgen when it is given to adult males that had been orchiectomized at birth. It is clear from this that the nervous components mediating aggressive behavior can still be altered in adulthood by the presence or absence of androgen. On the other hand, the neural substrates that determine the cyclic release of pituitary gonadotrophins are irrevocably determined during a critical period of fetal life or a short period following birth. Unless androgens act on the brain during the critical period, the release of gonadotrophins is cyclic as in normal females and, unlike aggressive behavior, cannot be reversed later in life by hormonal manipulation.[1]

Metabolic Adjustments

Exposure of rats to low environmental temperatures increases the output of thyroid-stimulating hormone from the anterior pituitary; this augments the synthesis of thyroid hormones, which act to enable the body to oxidize more food and maintain the body temperature. This effect is mediated by neurosecretory centers in the brain. Profound metabolic changes occur in organisms preparing for molt, migration, hibernation, estivation, and diapause; all of these involve complex neuroendocrine mechanisms.

In mammals, an excessive loss of water (dehydration) increases the osmotic pressure of the blood. As the blood circulates through the capillaries of the brain, certain osmoreceptors in the hypothalamus are stimulated and the neurohypophysis releases increasing amounts of vasopressin (antidiuretic principle). This neurohormone, a product of neurosecretory cells, acts directly upon the kidney tubules to promote the return of water to the circulation. Consequently, the organism eliminates a smaller amount of urine than it otherwise would. Excessive hydration decreases the osmotic pressure of the blood and has the opposite effect.

Growth and Development

Growth in arthropods occurs during the periods when the hard exoskeletons are lost. It is well known that nymphal molting in the hemipteran *Rhodnius* is dependent upon the consumption of a heavy meal of blood. Stretching the abdominal wall causes impulses to be relayed to the brain over afferent pathways, and these elicit the secretion of hormones that are essential for molting.

In the rat and other mammals that come into estrus and copulate shortly after delivering a litter, the young embryos (blastocysts) are often held in the uterine lumen, in a state of developmental arrest (facultative diapause), until lactation subsides and the brain-pituitary-gonadal axis can readjust to prepare the type of uterus in which nidation is possible. In such mammals as the mink *(Mustela vison)* and European badger *(Meles meles),* delayed implantation is prolonged and occurs regularly as a part of the pregnancy cycle (obligate diapause). The spotted skunk *(Spilogale putorius latifrons)* has an extremely long gestation period of 230 to 250 days, but the unimplanted blastocysts are held in a state of arrested development for 200 to 220 days. Progesterone levels in the plasma are low during the long preimplantation period, but are elevated markedly a few days prior to nidation. Very little is known about the neuroendocrine mechanisms that operate during this type of pregnancy.[20]

Adjustments Related to Stress

Fertility in male and female rats is greatly reduced by auditory stimuli (ringing bell) applied at frequent intervals during the day and night. Under these conditions, females may develop persistent estrus; during early pregnancy the implantation of blastocysts is frequently prevented and pregnancy is terminated. This kind of pregnancy block is comparable to that produced in female mice by a pheromone from a strange male (Fig. 1–1). These auditory-gonadal effects are mediated by the neurosecretory cells of the brain that regulate the secretion of pituitary gonadotrophins.[38]

It is common knowledge that many wild animals kept in captivity fail to reproduce even though they are well cared for and appear in good health. Under captive conditions, reproduction probably fails because environmental conditions are stressful; the stimuli derived from the physical environment or from social contacts with other individuals of the same species do not duplicate those normally met in the wild.

The adrenal glands of socially subordinate mice, repeatedly defeated in combat, are heavier than those of dominant members of the group. It is known that exposure of mice to trained fighters results in hyperactivity of the adrenal cortices of the untrained, attacked subjects. Mice that suffered previous defeats show a much greater adrenal response to the fighter's presence than animals that never before experienced this social stress. In situations of this type, cues derived from the external environment are received and integrated by the central nervous system; this leads to an augmented output of ACTH from the pituitary and this hormone acts to increase the release of adrenal steroids into the blood. There is evidence that the growth of mammalian populations may be regulated to an appreciable degree by social pressures operating through neuroendocrine mechanisms. At the human level, clinicians are aware that emotional stimuli of many sorts may produce dramatic changes in endocrine glands and their target organs.[5, 7]

Pheromones are of great importance in the induction of migratory behavior in locusts, and these act via neurosecretory cells and the endocrine glands dependent on them.[12, 19] Solitary and gregarious (swarming) phases of the desert locust *(Schistocerca gregaria)* differ in many ways and can be distinguished quickly on the basis of body color and behavior. The pheromone is produced by the epidermis of mature males, and it promptly stimulates both male and female recipients; it apparently acts through the central nervous system, since it brings about an immediate behavioral response — twitching of the mouthparts and kicking movements of the legs. In male recipients, the pheromone triggers the release of a brain neurohormone which stimulates an endocrine gland (corpus allatum); this gland secretes a hormone that induces pheromone production by the integument, stimulates the accessory sex organs, and changes the color of the body from gray to yellow (morphologic color change). In females, the pheromone stimulates the brain to activate the corpus allatum — a hormone from this gland acts with a gonadotrophin of neural origin to promote the maturation of eggs. These are examples of second order neuroendocrine reflexes (Fig. 3 – 4).

Acting in these ways, the pheromone accelerates sexual maturation of other males as well as of females. The synchronization of reproductive development of all members of the group, and a consequent over-crowding, are important features of migratory behavior in this species. Animal migrations, whether in fishes, amphibians, birds, mammals, or insects, often enable the group to cope with one kind of stress or another.

HORMONAL ACTIONS ON THE BRAIN

The foregoing examples illustrate how indispensable the central nervous system is in effecting endocrine adjustments to a great variety of exteroceptive and interoceptive stimuli. Of equal importance is the fact that many circulating hormones act back upon the brain to regulate pituitary secretions, to influence brain development in fetal and neonatal animals and, in adults, to condition the psychologic and behavioral characteristics of the species. There can no longer be any doubt that the relationship between the nervous and endocrine systems is one of reciprocity. The modern point of view is that the brain is not only an endocrine organ, but also a hormone target.[34]

The Concept of Hypophysiotrophic Neurohormones

The adenohypophysis is the source of multiple hormones, whose concentrations in the peripheral circulation are highly variable. The functions of this gland are regulated largely by chemical messengers in the blood rather than by direct neural signals. Feedback mechanisms are known to be of great importance in regulating the output of pituitary trophic hormones; the titers of target gland hormones act upon the pituitary itself or upon brain neurons to accelerate or retard the release of specific trophic hormones. Feedback mechanisms are interrupted by surgical excision of target glands (gonads, adrenal cortices, thyroid) and the titers of the respective pituitary hormones in the blood are increased. The administration of excessive target gland hormone has the reverse effect (Fig. 3–4).

Much experimental evidence supports the belief that adenohypophysial secretions are adjusted largely by messengers (hypophysiotrophic neurohormones) that derive from neurosecretory cells in the brain and reach the pituitary by means of the hypophysial portal veins. Support has been derived from many kinds of experiments: (1) transplantation of the pituitary to many ectopic sites, (2) electrical stimulation of brain areas, (3) surgical interruptions of pathways within the brain, (4) sectioning of the pituitary stalk, (5) the actions of various pharmacologic agents on the brain, (6) the accurate placements of electrolytic lesions, (7) studies on feedback controls and sex behavior, (8) the implantation of crystalline hormones into particular brain regions, (9) the nuclear retention of tritiated steroid hormones by brain neurons, (10) the isolation and chemical identification of hypophysiotrophic neurohormones from extracts of the median eminence, and (11) the preparation and testing of analogues. The chemistry and actions of these factors are treated more fully in Chapter 4.

Target Neurons Within the Brain

The hypophysiotrophic neurohormones are conceptualized as the products of specific neurosecretory cells within the brain, but the identity of these cells has remained unknown or at best conjectural. Since the brain is clearly involved in various feedback adjustments, it appeared that secretory neurons would respond to hormones in the same manner as do non-neural targets—that is, by binding the hormone. Promising results have been obtained in the rat with the dry-mount autoradiographic technique.[33] This has made it possible to identify hormone target cells in the pituitary and to map the distribution of steroid hormone-sensitive neurons in the brain. The nuclear concentration of tritium-labeled estradiol, testosterone, and cortisol by certain anterior pituitary cells supports the generally held view that these hormones may exert feedback effects at the pituitary level.

[3]H-estradiol is retained by the nuclei of neurons located in defined areas of the phylogenetically old periventricular brain, in both male and female animals. Such neurons therefore are not confined to the hypothalamus. Steroid hormones, labeled by tritium, are not taken up by cells in such brain structures as the neopallium and cerebellar cortex. A distinct labeling pattern is also observed following the administration of ^{3}H-testosterone, and there is considerable overlap of the anatomical sites where estrogen-sensitive and androgen-sensitive neurons are found.[28] In some brain areas there is a high labeling index for both estrogen and androgen, and

this suggests the possibility that some neurons may be addressed by both kinds of steroids to influence the secretion of hypophysiotrophic neurohormones or to affect sex behavior. The neurosecretory cells serving as targets for gonadal and adrenal hormones seem to be associated with certain nerve fiber tracts within different regions of the periventricular brain. The view that neurosecretory cells are present only in the hypothalamus appears not to be valid.[34]

Gonadal Hormones and Brain Differentiation

There are great variations in the patterns of breeding activity among different species. Vertebrate reproductive cycles are controlled by a complex interplay of neural and endocrine factors. The production of pituitary and gonadal hormones, and hence the rhythmic alternation of sexual receptivity and nonreceptivity, is set by some inherent "biologic clock," which assures a relatively constant pattern of activity for any one species. With the onset of the breeding period, the circulating hormones act not only on the reproductive organs to induce their full anatomic development, but also upon the nervous system to assure a behavioral repertoire commensurate with the fully developed genital organs. The behavior of the rat in estrus, for example, is strikingly different from that of the same animal during diestrus or following ovariectomy. These behavioral differences are explainable on the basis of the types of hormones that act back upon the brain. [8]

In female mammals, the hypothalamus exerts rhythmic influences upon the anterior pituitary, by means of the hypophysiotrophic neurohormones, so that there is a rhythmic discharge of gonadotrophins. In the male, on the other hand, the hypothalamus is relatively arrhythmic, which accounts for the continuous production of gonadotrophins and the steady-state pattern of male activity.[35] Studies on fetal and neonatal mammals indicate that circulating gonadal hormones have an organizing action upon certain brain neurons, particularly those in the periventricular region. There are critical periods in development during which the immature brain is especially sensitive to gonadal hormones. In rats and mice, this critical period extends from shortly before birth to about the tenth day of postnatal life; in mammals with a longer gestation period, such as the guinea pig and monkey, the sensitive period occurs entirely before birth. Whether the brain causes the anterior pituitary of the adult to produce gonadotrophins rhythmically (female type brain) or continuously (male type brain) depends upon the kind of gonadal hormone to which the central nervous system is exposed during early life. The important factor in differentiation of the mammalian brain seems to be the presence or absence of testicular hormone.[8, 17]

When the ovaries or testes are surgically removed before the brain is fully differentiated, it matures as a female type organ in both genetic males and genetic females. Two criteria have been used in assessing brain functions: (1) whether it stimulates the pituitary to release follicle-stimulating hormone (FSH) and luteinizing hormone (LH) rhythmically or arrhythmically; and (2) the type of sexual behavior that the animal displays after attaining adulthood. Genetic female rats, given a small dose of testosterone shortly after birth (androgen-sterilized female), show marked masculine behavioral patterns when they become adults, instead of normal female behavior.[2, 11] When the ovaries or testes are removed from newborn rats, they both grow up to display female behavior. If genetic male rats are exposed to a potent antiandrogen (e.g., cyproterone) during the last part of intrauterine life and for several weeks postnatally, they develop vaginae and behave as females.[23]

It has been suggested that androgen, acting at this early critical period, might interfere with the development of estrogen receptor proteins on the brain neurons that normally trap estrogen.[9] This defect could render the estrogen-sensitive neurons incapable of mediating negative and positive feedbacks on the pituitary cells that secrete gonadotrophins. Since the pituitary is non-cyclic, ovulation fails and corpora lutea do not form in the ovaries. The overall effect is permanent sterility.

Observations on guinea pigs and monkeys indicate that the pattern of gonadotrophic secretion and the pattern of adult sexual behavior depend upon whether or not the brain differentiates under the influence of testicular androgen. Since human fetuses cannot be used for such experimental purposes, it is not known to what extent these principles apply to human beings. At the human level, however, there is no doubt that abnormal hormone levels during embryonic life are responsible for a variety of genitourinary deformities, and some of these may not become apparent until after puberty. Neither is there doubt that sexual orientation of human individuals is frequently at variance with their genetic sex. Many subtle aspects of human sexual behavior remain totally obscure, and these need to be studied with scientific objectivity.[37]

REFERENCES

1. Barkley, M. S., and Goldman, B. D.: Effects of castration and silastic implants of testosterone on aggression and gonadal activity in mice. Abstract, 57th Ann. Meeting Endocrine Society (U.S.A.), p. 181, 1975.
2. Barraclough, C. A.: Modifications in reproductive function after exposure to hormones during the prenatal and early postnatal period. In L. Martini, and W. F. Ganong (eds.): Neuroendocrinology, Vol. 2. New York, Academic Press, 1967, p. 61.
3. Bern, H. A., and Knowles, F. G. W.: Neurosecretion. In L. Martini and W. F. Ganong (eds.): Neuroendocrinology, Vol. 1. New York, Academic Press, 1966, p. 139.
4. Bianchi, S.: The amine secreting neurons in the central nervous system of the earthworm (Octolasium complanatum) and their possible neurosecretory role. Gen. Comp. Endocr. 9:343, 1967.
5. Bronson, F. H., and Eleftheriou, B. E.: Adrenal responses to fighting in mice: Separation of physical and psychological causes. Science 147:627, 1965.
6. Charniaux-Cotton, H.: Androgenic gland of crustaceans. Gen. Comp. Endocr. (Suppl.) 1: 241, 1962.
7. Christian, J. J., and Davis, D. E.: Endocrines, behavior and population. Science 146:1550, 1964.
8. Davidson, J. M., and Bloch, G. J.: Neuroendocrine aspects of male reproduction. Biol. Reprod. (Suppl.)1:67, 1969.
9. Flerko, B.: Steroid hormones and the differentiation of the central nervous system. In L. Martini and V. H. T. James (eds.): Current Topics in Experimental Endocrinology, Vol. 1. New York, Academic Press, 1971, p. 41.

10. Frye, B. E.: Hormonal Control in Vertebrates. New York, The Macmillan Co., 1967.
11. Gorski, R. A.: Gonadal hormones and the perinatal development of neuroendocrine function. *In* L. Martini and W. F. Ganong (eds.): Frontiers in Neuroendocrinology. Oxford University Press, 1971.
12. Highnam, K. C., and Lusis, O.: The effect of mature males on the neurosecretory control of ovarian development in the desert locust. Quart. J. Microscop. Sci. *103*:73, 1962.
13. Huxley, J. S.: Chemical regulation and the hormone concept. Biol. Rev. *10*:427, 1935.
14. Ishibashi, T.: Electrical activity of the caudal neurosecretory cells in the eel, *Anguilla japonica,* with special reference to synaptic transmission. Gen. Comp. Endocr. 2:415, 1962.
15. Knowles, F.: Neuroendocrine correleations at the level of ultrastructure. Arch. Anat. Microscop. *54*:343, 1965.
16. Kopec, S.: Studies on the necessity of the brain for the inception of insect metamorphosis. Biol. Bull. *42*:323, 1922.
17. Levine, S., and Mullins, R. F., Jr.: Hormonal influences on brain organization in infant rats. Science *152*:1585, 1966.
18. Lisk, R. D., and Barfield, M. A.: Sites and mechanisms of steroid effects on behavior. *In* Stumpf, W. E., and Grant, L. D. (eds.): Anatomical Neuroendocrinology. Basel, Karger, 1975.
19. Loher, W.: The chemical acceleration of the maturation process and its control in the male of the desert locust. Proc. Roy. Soc. (B) *153*:380, 1960.
20. Mead, R. A.: Effects of hypophysectomy on blastocyst survival, progesterone secretion and nidation in the spotted skunk. Biol. Reprod. *12*:526, 1975.
21. Medway, L.: Domestic pigeons; the stimulus provided by the egg in the nest. J. Endocr. *23*: 9, 1961.
22. Menaker, M., Roberts, R., Elliott, J., and Underwood, H.: Extraretinal light perception in the sparrow: The eyes do not participate in photoperiodic photoreception. Proc. Nat. Acad. Sci. (U.S.A.) *67*:320, 1970.
23. Neumann, F., and Elger, W.: Physiological and psychical intersexuality of male rats by early treatment with an antiandrogenic agent (1,2α-methylene-6-chloro-Δ⁶-hydroxyprogesterone acetate). Acta Endocr. (Kobenhaven), Suppl., *100*:174, 1965.
24. Norman, A. W., and Henry, H.: 1,25-Dihydroxycholecalciferol — a hormonally active form of vitamin D_3. Rec. Prog. Horm. Res. *30*:431, 1974.
25. Popa, G. T., and Fielding, U.: A portal circulation from the pituitary to the hypothalamic region. J. Anat. (London) *65*:88, 1930.
26. Robison, G. A., Butcher, R. W., and Sutherland, E. W.: Cyclic AMP. New York, Academic Press, 1971, p. 19.
27. Saginor, M., and Horton, R.: Reflex release of gonadotropin and increased plasma testosterone concentration in male rabbits during copulation. Endocrinology *82*:627, 1968.
28. Sar, M., and Stumpf, W. E.: Autoradiographic localization of radioactivity in the rat brain after the injection of 1,2-³H-testosterone. Endocrinology *92*:251, 1973.
29. Scharrer, B.: The role of neurons in endocrine regulation: a comparative overview. Amer. Zool., *15*(Suppl. 1):7, 1975.
30. Scharrer, B.: The spectrum of neuroendocrine communication. In K. Lederis and K. E. Cooper (eds.): Recent Studies of Hypothalamic Function, Symposium, Calgary, Alberta, May, 1973. Basel, Karger, 1974, p. 8.
31. Scharrer, E., and Scharrer, B.: Neuroendocrinology. New York, Columbia University Press, 1963.
32. Speidel, C. C.: Gland-cells of internal secretion in the spinal cord of the skates. Carnegie Inst. Wash. Pub. No. 13, pp. 1–31, 1919.
33. Stumpf, W. E.: Autoradiographic techniques and the localization of estrogen, androgen, and glucocorticoid in the pituitary and brain. Amer. Zool. *11*:725, 1971.
34. Stumpf, W. E.: The brain: an endocrine organ and hormone target. *In* Stumpf, W. E., and Grant, L. D. (eds.): Anatomical Neuroendocrinology. Basel, Karger, 1975.
35. Takewaki, K.: Some experiments on the control of hypophyseal-gonadal system in the rat. Gen. Comp. Endocr., Suppl. 1:309, 1962.
36. Wislocki, G. B., and King, L. S.: The permeability of the hypophysis and hypothalamus to vital dyes, with a study of the hypophyseal vascular supply. Amer. J. Anat. *58*:421, 1936.
37. Young, W. C., Goy, R. W., and Phoenix, C. H.: Hormones and sexual behavior. Science *143*: 212, 1964.
38. Zondek, B., and Tamari, I.: Auditory stimulation and fertility. Amer. J. Obstet. & Gynecol. *80*: 1041, 1960.

CHAPTER 4

Pituitary Gland:
Anatomy; Secretions of
the Adenohypophysis

Although the human pituitary gland, or hypophysis, is a relatively small organ, weighing about 600 mg. in adult men and slightly more in women, no part of the body is exempt from its influences. It is concerned with a multiplicity of vital processes, and at least nine protein or polypeptide hormones have been isolated from it. The *trophic* hormones of the pars distalis stimulate specific endocrine glands, but probably do not limit their actions to these targets. A reciprocal relationship exists between the hypophysis and other endocrine glands, as well as between the hypophysis and the central nervous system.

The pituitary is closely applied to the floor of the brain and remains attached to it by means of a delicate stalk. This relationship is not fortuitous since the functional capacity of the entire pituitary depends upon its neural and vascular connections with the hypothalamus. These anatomic connections make it possible for the organ to adjust its output of hormones in response to stimuli arising from the exterior as well as from within the organism. The pituitary gland is an essential link in the neuroendocrine system, but it has little capacity to function independently. Since it is subservient to the nervous system and to some of the other endocrine glands, it is misleading to refer to it as the "master" gland of the body.

ANATOMY

Gross Anatomy

The pituitary is a compound gland of internal secretion located in the sella turcica, a concavity in the sphenoid bone (Fig. 4–1). Topographically, it is one of the best protected and most inaccessible organs of the body. The gland is encapsulated by the dura mater; a shelflike fold of this membrane forms the diaphragma sellae and extends around the infundibular stalk. The pituitary enlarges during pregnancy and in certain other conditions, and, since it is situated immediately behind the optic chiasm, visual

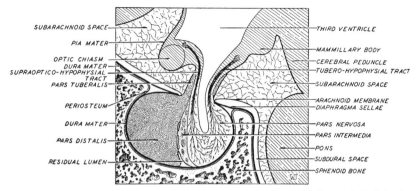

Figure 4–1. A diagrammatic sagittal section through the hypophysis cerebri of the human being, showing the relationships of this gland to adjacent structures.

symptoms may result when the enlarged organ presses upon the optic tracts.

A variety of anatomical designations have been applied to the pituitary, but the most widely used terminology is that provided below. It is based upon the fact that the pituitary is derived from both epithelial and neural components.

Adenohypophysis { lobus glandularis { pars distalis } anterior lobe
pars tuberalis
pars intermedia

posterior lobe

Neurohypophysis {
lobus nervosus { processus
(pars nervosa) infundibuli

infundibulum { infundibular stem
(neural stalk) median eminence of
tuber cinereum

The pars tuberalis, a constituent of the adenohypophysis, is a thin epithelial plate of cells that is formed by the fusion of two outgrowths from the embryonic pars distalis. The pars tuberalis of the adult may surround the infundibular stalk and extend some distance below the tuber cinereum. When the pituitary gland is removed surgically (hypophysectomy), it is practically impossible to ablate all of the pars tuberalis without some injury to the hypothalamus. Although the tuberalis is the most vascular region of the hypophysis and receives many sympathetic fibers it is not known to have any definite endocrine function. During the hypophysectomy of laboratory mammals, the delicate stalk usually breaks at the level of the diaphragma sellae.

In young human beings and in the majority of other vertebrates, a narrow band of tissue, the pars intermedia, is demonstrable between the pars distalis and the neural lobe. The pars intermedia is conspicuous in most human infants, but in adults it merges with the neural lobe and tends to become obscure. This lobe is absent in birds and in certain mammals, such as the whale, Indian elephant, and armadillo.

The vascular supply of the pituitary varies with the species and from one individual to another, but the same general pattern is found in all of the mammalian species that have been studied. A pair of posterior hypophysial arteries, originating from the internal carotid arteries, supplies blood chiefly to the neural lobe. A series of anterior hypophysial arteries originates from the internal carotids and from the posterior communicating arteries of the circle of Willis. Some of these vessels supply the pars distalis directly, whereas others pass into the pars tuberalis and break up into a primary plexus in the median eminence. Venules, forming the hypophysial portal system, convey blood from the capillary meshwork of the median eminence to the sinusoids of the pars distalis. It thus appears that the arterial supply to the adenohypophysis, particularly to the pars distalis, is largely independent of that of the neurohypophysis. The whole organ is drained by means of short veins that empty into sinuses in the dura mater or in the basisphenoid bone (Fig. 2–2).

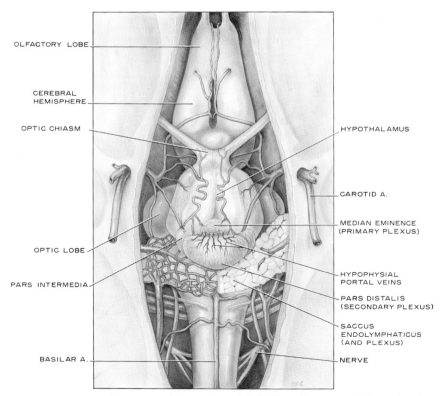

OLFACTORY LOBE

CEREBRAL HEMISPHERE

OPTIC CHIASM

OPTIC LOBE

PARS INTERMEDIA

BASILAR A.

HYPOTHALAMUS

CAROTID A.

MEDIAN EMINENCE (PRIMARY PLEXUS)

HYPOPHYSIAL PORTAL VEINS

PARS DISTALIS (SECONDARY PLEXUS)

SACCUS ENDOLYMPHATICUS (AND PLEXUS)

NERVE

Figure 4–2. Ventral view of the brain of an adult bullfrog *Rana catesbeiana,* showing the pituitary gland and hypothalamus. The hypophysial portal veins, extending from the median eminence to the pars distalis, are clearly seen. (From a dissection by Mr. Hsien-Sung Lin.)

The nerve supply of the hypophysis consists of sympathetic fibers from the surrounding perivascular plexuses, parasympathetic fibers from the petrosal nerves, and the hypothalamo-hypophysial tract. A comprehensive study of pituitaries from 75 species of vertebrates from cyclostomes to man revealed the presence of sympathetic fibers in the pars tuberalis but none in the pars distalis. Very few workers still hold that the bulk of the anterior lobe cells receive any direct innervation. Since the pars tuberalis is not known to secrete hormones, the nerve fibers that end there are probably vasomotor rather than secretomotor. The weight of evidence indicates that if the main secreting mass of the pars distalis receives any nerve endings at all, they are very few; if any are present, it remains to be shown whether they are secretomotor or vasomotor. There is no convincing evidence that the sympathetic and parasympathetic innervations play any important role in regulating the secretory functions of the pars distalis.[47]

A conspicuous feature of the pars nervosa is the large number of secretory axons that terminate there. The perikarya of these axons are located in certain hypothalamic nuclei. The fibers sweep down the pituitary stalk and are grouped into supraoptico- and tubero-hypophysial tracts. Some of these fibers are known to terminate in the median eminence and in the pars intermedia, but it is doubtful that any of them enter the pars distalis (Fig. 2–2).

Amphibians have been used extensively in experiments involving the pituitary gland. Figure 4–2 is a drawing of a ventral dissection of the frog's brain, showing the pituitary gland and adjacent structures.

Developmental Anatomy

The entire pituitary is ectodermal, but this tissue arises from two different sources (Fig. 4–3). The neurohypophysis originates from the infundibulum of the brain, an outpocketing of the hypothalamus. The stalk permanently connects the neural lobe with the hypothalamus. The anterior and intermediate lobes differentiate from Rathke's pouch, an outgrowth from the roof of the mouth. This pouch promptly meets the infundibulum and loses its connection with the buccal epithelium. The cavity of Rathke's pouch becomes the residual lumen of the hypophysis. This lumen may persist between the anterior and intermediate lobes, or it may be obliterated entirely in certain species. The pars intermedia differentiates from the wall of Rathke's pouch, which comes into contact with the infundibulum. The remainder of the pouch thickens greatly and becomes the pars distalis. Paired lateral extensions differentiate from this anlage and eventually fuse to produce a thin plate of tissue, the pars tuberalis, which grows around the infundibular stalk and spreads out below the hypothalamus.

A body of typical anterior lobe tissue, the pharyngeal hypophysis, is commonly found in the vault of the human nasopharynx. This structure apparently differentiates from a fragment of Rathke's pouch which is left behind.[11]

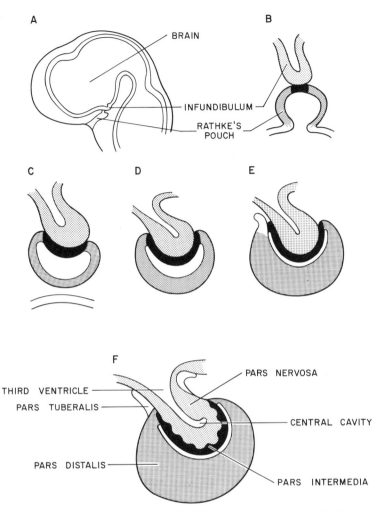

Figure 4–3. Diagrams showing progressive stages in the embryonic development of the pituitary gland. Rathke's pouch becomes detached from the oral epithelium at stage *C*. (Stage *A* is from Villee, C. A., Walker, W. F. Jr., and Smith, F. E.: General Zoology, 2nd ed. Philadelphia, W. B. Saunders Co., 1963.)

In amphibians, the hypophysial primordium is found outside the mouth as a wedge of tissue immediately in front of the prospective stomadeum and just beneath the forebrain. This placode is completely homologous to Rathke's pouch and provides a convenient approach for experimental manipulation of the prospective pituitary. It was therefore possible to show that in amphibians such as *Hyla regilla,* a pars intermedia fails to differentiate unless the adenohypophysial anlage comes into contact with the infundibulum; the pars distalis, on the other hand, does develop.[27]

It is possible to remove surgically the posterior hypothalamic primordium (hypothalectomy) in the open neurula stages of *Rana pipiens.*[18, 50]

Such animals fail to develop a neurohypophysis and a pars intermedia, but a pars distalis develops without any anatomical connections with the brain. This is taken as evidence that in normal development, the infundibular region of the hypothalamus induces the development of the pars intermedia from the innermost portion of the hypophysial placode.

Microscopic Anatomy

Pars Distalis

This part of the gland is composed of irregular masses and cords of epithelial cells separated by sinusoids and supported by a loose framework of connective tissue. Routine staining of the adenohypophysis with such stains as hematoxylin and eosin, or with Mallory aniline blue or azan, reveals two major varieties of gland cells: The *chromophils* contain characteristic cytoplasmic granules and are generally considered to be secretory, whereas the *chromophobes* do not possess conspicuous secretory granules and are thought to be inactive in this respect. Most cytologists have interpreted the chromophobes as being progenitors of the other cell types or as degranulated, resting stages of the chromophils. Chromophils are further divided into *acidophils* and *basophils* on the basis of their tinctorial responses. This terminology is very inadequate, since cytoplasmic granules often respond to both acid and basic stains, but it cannot be easily discarded until it becomes possible to redefine the cells confidently on the basis of the specific hormones they secrete.

In recent years, a more specific scheme for designating hormone-secreting cells of the pars distalis has evolved (Table 4–1). This scheme was established from data obtained largely from experiments on the rat, but it is probable that these same designations can apply to other mammals, including humans.

Table 4–1 HORMONE-SECRETING CELLS IN THE ANTERIOR PITUITARY OF THE RAT. THE FSH GONADOTROPHS ARE LOCATED IN THE PERIPHERY OF THE GLAND, WHEREAS THE LH GONADOTROPHS ARE UNIFORMLY DISTRIBUTED.*

CELL TYPE	HORMONE SECRETED	STAINING REACTIONS			GRANULE SIZE (mμ DIAMETER)
		General	*Orange G*	*PAS†*	
Somatotrophs	Growth hormone	Acidophil	+	−	350
Lactotrophs (mammotrophs)	Prolactin	Acidophil	+	−	600
Corticotrophs	ACTH	Chromophobe	−	−	100
FSH gonadotrophs	FSH	Basophil	−	+	200
LH gonadotrophs	LH	Basophil	−	+	200
Thyrotrophs	TSH	Basophil	−	+	140

*Modified from Ganong, W. S.: Review of Medical Physiology. New York, Springer Verlag, 1969.
†PAS, periodic acid-Schiff reaction.

Since six protein or polypeptide hormones can be extracted from the pars distalis, it is pertinent to know whether there is a cell type specialized for the secretion of each hormone or whether a single pituitary cell can secrete several hormones. If the latter is the case, we should like to know whether the multiple hormones are elaborated simultaneously or alternately by a given pituitary cell. Although considerable progress has been made in cytochemical techniques, and there is some measure of agreement regarding the source of several anterior lobe hormones, it is still premature to conclude that any available stain unmistakably identifies a pituitary hormone with its cell of origin. The relative proportions of the cells may vary markedly during physiologic states; they may also undergo changes, such as granulation, degranulation, hyalinization, and vacuolation. While the significance of such fluctuations is not always certain, it is felt that some of these changes are associated with synthesis, release, and resorption of secretory granules. Studies of the pituitary with the electron microscope indicate that the intracellular biosynthesis of hormones is not unlike that of proteins in other organs. Using the example of prolactin[131] (Fig. 2–3), it can be considered that the hormone is probably synthesized on ribosomes of the rough endoplasmic reticulum and is transported to the Golgi complex, where it is concentrated into granules. In the Golgi cisternae, these small granules are aggregated to form the mature secretory granule. In response to cues for hormone release, the secretory granules fuse with the cell membrane and are discharged. In the absence of hormone release, excess secretory granules are taken up into lysosomes and degraded. Since mitotic figures are extremely sparse in the pituitary gland, it has seemed apparent that cells are transformed from one variety to another, and the literature abounds with proposals for cell lineages based upon supposed transition stages.

Mammals. Pituitary cytology has been most intensively studied in the rat and in other laboratory mammals. The periodic acid-Schiff technique and Gomori's aldehyde fuchsin have proved valuable in studying the cell types of the adenohypophysis. Electron microscopy has been of great help in identifying cell types on the basis of differences in cytoplasmic granules, endoplasmic reticulum, mitochondria, Golgi apparatus, nuclear structure, cell size and shape, etc.[4, 36] The cytochemical procedures, coupled with electron microscopy, have yielded important information when applied to animals known to be in various physiologic states, such as those produced by gonadectomy, adrenalectomy, thyroidectomy, pregnancy, lactation, and stress. Structural and functional changes in the pituitary may be detected following the administration of such agents as metyrapone (adrenocortical inhibitor) and thiourea (thyroid inhibitor).

Three of the anterior lobe hormones, viz., follicle-stimulating hormone, luteinizing hormone, and thyroid-stimulating hormone, in contrast to the other hormones of this gland, are glycoproteins. The periodic acid-Schiff method (PAS stain) is used for the identification of mucopolysaccharides and mucoproteins, and its application to the adenohypophysis has been informative. A positive PAS reaction is interpreted as resulting from the presence within the cells of a carbohydrate-containing pituitary hormone.

The Pearse PAS trichrome stain and other modifications have been useful in making differential cell counts.

On the basis of electron microscopy and various tinctorial methods, it is generally agreed that the rat's pars distalis contains two kinds of acidophils and four kinds of basophils. The somatotrophic acidophils (somatotrophs) secrete growth hormone (STH) and are distinct from lactotrophic acidophils (lactotrophs), which are the source of prolactin. The basophils are gonadotrophic cells (FSH gonadotrophs and LH gonadotrophs), thyrotrophic cells (TSH thyrotrophs), and corticotrophic cells (ACTH corticotrophs). Electron micrographs show that the chromophobes are not devoid of cytoplasmic granules, but that they merely have fewer than the chromophils.[34, 35, 60, 115, 129]

It has been suspected for many years that the acidophils were concerned with the secretion of somatotrophin. Pituitary dwarfism in man and in other mammals correlates with a deficiency of acidophils, whereas in acromegaly and gigantism, characterized by excessive growth of the skeleton, there is typically a striking increase in the number of acidophils. In genetic dwarf mice, the acidophils are sparse and bioassays indicate that the pituitaries of such animals are deficient in STH.[71, 100]

Cytologic observations on the rat's pituitary from birth to maturity indicate that the gonadotrophic cells undergo degranulation at puberty, perhaps indicating an increased release of gonad-stimulating hormones at this time. Thyrotrophic cells, staining with aldehyde-fuchsin, are present in the rat's pituitary from birth onward.[108, 128]

Castration of various laboratory mammals results in a striking alteration of the gonadotrophic cells. Many of them become enlarged and degranulated, and eventually develop large cytoplasmic vacuoles that compress the nucleus against the cell membrane. The castration cells (signet-ring cells) appear after removal of either the testes or ovaries and persist indefinitely unless the animal is treated with gonadal steroids. Though not so extreme as in the rat, comparable cells appear in the human hypophysis after gonadectomy and are also seen in the glands of aged persons.[53]

In thyroidectomized rats and mice, as in certain other species, the thyrotrophic cells undergo degranulation and increase in size and number, forming the so-called thyroidectomy cells. The thyrotrophic cells of the rat's anterior lobe become almost completely degranulated within two days following thyroid ablation and, by the sixth day, they have enlarged sufficiently to be recognized as thyroidectomy cells.

The term *amphophil* was originally used to refer to the thyroidectomy cells of the mouse. After the thyroid glands of the mouse are destroyed by appropriate treatment with ^{131}I, the thyroidectomy cells in the pars distalis first increase in numbers, then form focal hyperplasias, and finally give rise to adenomatous nodules. The modified thyrotrophic cells, composing the tumors, contain PAS-positive granules, but by varying the fixatives and stains, the granules can be made to appear either basophilic or acidophilic. The amphoteric nature of cytoplasmic granules in these cells suggested the name "amphophils." Such cells are commonly found in the pituitaries of human subjects suffering from thyroid deficiency.[14, 40]

In the rat, at least, it appears that the six cell types, responsible for the six hormones secreted by the pars distalis, can be identified. A similar situation may prevail in many other mammals, but it would be premature to conclude that the same cell types are present in non-mammalian species; the pituitaries of different vertebrates show considerable variation in cytochemical patterns.[7]

Birds. The avian pituitary lacks a pars intermedia, and the anterior lobe is histologically divisible into caudal and cephalic regions. The cytology of the pars distalis is generally similar to that of mammals, but the functional roles performed by the different cell types have not been established with certainty. Two types of acidophils (Payne's A_1 and A_2 cells) can be delineated; these differ slightly in staining reactions and occur in different regions of the gland. The acidophils are conspicuous at the time of hatching and are more numerous in pullets than in cockerels. According to Yasuda, prolactin is secreted by one of the acidophil types.[144]

Assay of gonad-stimulating potencies of pituitaries from normal and caponized birds, as well as correlated changes in the basophils during development, indicates that the large basophils are the source of one or more gonadotrophins. Degranulation of basophils, suggesting a discharge of hormone, can be induced by exposure to light. A similar degranulation of basophils occurs in the mallard at the height of sexual activity.[58] Castration causes an increase in the number of basophils, but these do not transform into signet-ring cells as they do in mammals.

Acidophilic granules have been observed in the basophils of laying hens, but appear to be entirely absent from the basophils of cocks and non-laying hens. Since ovulation-inducing hormone (OIH) is freed from the hen's pituitary between 6 and 4 hours before the release of an egg from the ovary, it may be that the acidophilic granules in these basophils are related in some manner to the formation of OIH.

As in mammals, thyroidectomy or treatment with antithyroid agents produces characteristic alterations in pituitary cytology. Thyroidectomy cells (Payne's T cells) appear during thyroid deficiency. While these cells may be markedly basophilic, Payne found that they differed from basophils in nuclear structure and in site of origin within the gland, and hence regarded them as neither basophils nor acidophils.[104]

A striking alteration in the pars distalis of the domestic hen occurs at the onset of broodiness. The ordinary basophils and acidophils almost disappear and *broody cells* dominate the picture (Fig. 4–4). Although the latter cells may contain acidophilic granules, differences in size, nuclear configuration, and position in the gland suggest that they are distinguishable from both acidophils and basophils. Strangely, maximum development of the broody cells has been observed in the White Leghorn hen, which seldom exhibits broody behavior. While Payne was of the opinion that the broody cells might be the source of prolactin, Yasuda regarded them as chromophobes and hence not connected with such a role.[12, 105, 106, 144]

Amphibians and Fishes. Seasonal alterations in the cytology of the pituitary have been observed in a variety of reptiles, amphibians, and fishes. The pars distalis generally enlarges and undergoes structural changes in

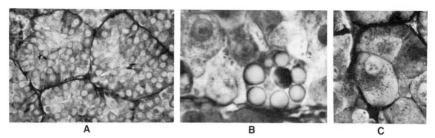

Figure 4–4. Pituitary cytology in the domestic fowl. *A,* Broody cells; *B,* aging change in a basophil of an old cock; *C,* a thyroidectomy cell (T cell). (Courtesy of Fernandus Payne.)

connection with the annual breeding periods.[89] Several tinctorial types are present in the pars distalis of some amphibians including *Rana, Notophthalmus (Diemictylus),* and *Xenopus,* but it appears too early to assign functional roles to them. A closely related group of cells appears to be present in the frog pituitary, and the identification of transitional stages suggests that one type may transform into another.[101] A study using both light and electron microscopes has indicated that certain glycoprotein-contain-

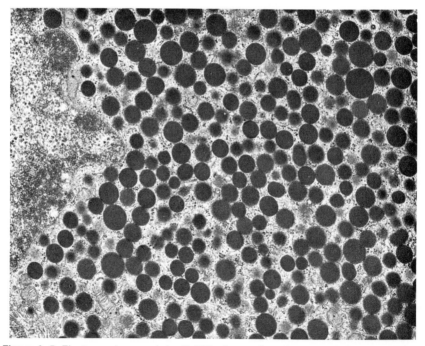

Figure 4–5. Electron micrograph (× 18,000) of a portion of an orange G acidophil from the pituitary gland of the salamander *Notophthalmus viridescens.* These cells are believed to contain and secrete somatotrophin, which appears to be stored in the dark spherical granules. It is thought that the hormones are synthesized in the rough endoplasmic reticulum and transported to the Golgi complex, where they are condensed into protein granules. These lie in the cytoplasm until the cell is stimulated to release its hormone. The granules are then discharged into the pericapillary space and diffuse into the capillary lumen. The nucleus is to the left. (Courtesy of Robert R. Cardell, Jr.)

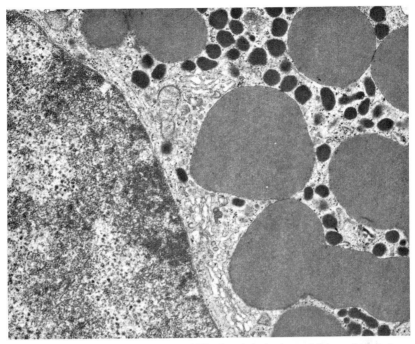

Figure 4–6. Electron micrograph (× 18,000) of a globular basophil from the pituitary gland of *Notophthalmus viridescens*. A significant feature of this cell type is that it contains two distinct types of cytoplasmic granules, the large globules and the smaller, irregularly shaped granules. This cell probably secretes two distinct hormones. The large globules are probably related to gonadotrophins; it is not known what the smaller granules contain. The nucleus is to the left. (Courtesy of Robert R. Cardell, Jr.)

ing cells of *Xenopus* bear a close resemblance to the thyroidectomy cells of the rat and they are considered, therefore, to be thyrotrophs.[139] Earlier studies made on the ultrastructure of amphibian pituitary glands have revealed that various cell types can be distinguished on the basis of specific granular size (Figs. 4–5 and 4–6),[16, 24, 25, 26, 63] and strides are now being made toward the elucidation of their functional activities.[26] In some cyto-immunochemical studies of the hypophysial cells of several amphibian species, the distribution of specific cell types was shown. Antisera were made against several purified mammalian polypeptide and protein hormones and were applied to thin sections of various amphibian pituitaries. The localization of the antisera, detected by fluorescence methods, revealed that every antiserum marked a special cell type. While specific results were obtained with this technique, it is still premature to make any fast generalization about the designation of function to specific cell types of the amphibian pituitary. However, in general it appears that corticotrophic cells are rostral in distribution, while prolactin cells are more anterior and ventral. Somatotrophic and gonadotrophic cells are more irregular in distribution, and thyrotrophic cells are found in a more median position.

The adenohypophysis of teleost fishes is characterized by a zonation that is a reflection of the regional distribution of specific cell types (Fig. 4–

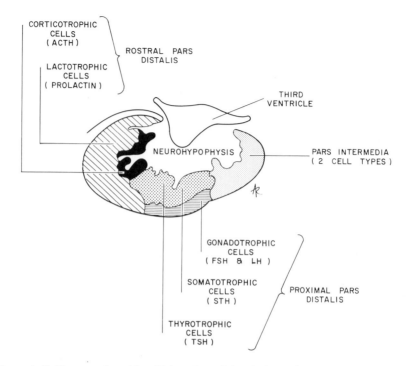

Figure 4–7. Diagram of a midsagittal section of the pituitary gland of a bony fish *(Poecilia)*, showing localization of cell types in the adenohypophysis. (Modified from Olivereau, M., and Ball, J. N.: Gen. Comp. Endocr. *4:*523, 1964.)

7).[37, 126] This is especially true of the rostral pars distalis, whose predominant cell type is the source of prolactin. These cells contain large granules that stain heavily with azocarmine, acid fuchsin, and erythrosin. It has been observed that under conditions favoring prolactin release, the presumed prolactin cells of the rostral pars distalis of salmonids, cyprinodonts, eel, and mullet undergo numerous cytologic changes. These include an enhancement of endoplasmic reticulum, RNA increase, nucleolar hypertrophy, increased number of Golgi bodies, decreased number of granules, and increased mitotic activity.[37, 98, 126] That these cells elaborate prolactin has been confirmed by immunofluorescence techniques. In the internal zone of the rostral region are cells thought to be corticotrophs. This function has been assigned to these cells by means of various methods of stimulation or inhibition of corticotrophic activity.

The proximal region of the pars distalis of some teleosts, including *Poecilia,* contains thyrotrophic cells. However, such cells, characterized by their glycoprotein granulations and by periodic acid-Schiff (PAS) staining, are sometimes seen in the rostral lobe bordering the proximal zone. This seems to be the case in some salmonids and anguillids.[37] The thyrotrophic nature of such cells in the carp has been confirmed by immunological methods. Also present in the proximal zone are non-glycoprotein, orangeophilic cells that contain large granules. Both because of their staining reactions and because of various physiological correlations, these cells are thought to be somatotrophs. In the salmon, *Oncorhynchus nerka,* these cells are said to concentrate anti-STH ovine antibodies. Gonadotrophic cells are localized in the proximal zone, and while they are often caudal in distribution, they may, in some species, invade the rostral zone. Several different cell types have been identified as gonadotrophs, a complication due in part to a variation in staining characteristics depending upon the stage in the reproductive cycle. Various anti-gonadotrophin antisera are known to react with various gonadotrophs, but the situation is obfuscated by the possibility that only one gonadotrophin, serving both FSH and LH functions, is present in some teleosts.

While much more is known about the functional roles of specific cell types in the teleost pars distalis, knowledge is beginning to accumulate about the functional cytology of the pituitary of more primitive fishes.[37] Elasmobranchs have been studied most effectively; by the use of appropriate staining reactions in correlation with various physiological tests, it has been indicated that cells having prolactin and corticotrophic activity are found in the rostral lobe and that gonadotrophic and thyrotrophic cells are found in the ventral lobe.

Pars Intermedia

The intermediate lobe is composed of polygonal cells that take basic dyes and in which secretory granules have been described. Vesicles containing colloid are present in certain species. Although the colloid contains small amounts of iodine, it has not been shown to have any functional significance. Cytological alterations occur in the intermediate lobes of frogs and salamanders during various physiological conditions, such as adaptation to black and white backgrounds or following transplantation of the hypophysis. At the ultrastructural level, MSH synthesis and release are reflected in an increased activity of the endoplasmic reticulum and in the presence of dense, membrane-bound granules in association with the Golgi region (Fig. 5–10).[86, 124] Only few secretory granules are observed, while in the non-secreting gland the pars intermedia cells contain many such granules.

In addition to glandular cells, at least two types of nerve endings have been found in the pars intermedia of both frogs and elasmobranchs. Each type, found in synaptic connection with secretory cells, can be distinguished on the basis of differences in the size of granules it contains. These observations support the results of fluorescence microscopy, which indicate the presence of monoamines in the amphibian pars intermedia.[29] By contrast, no nerve endings of any kind have been found in the pars intermedia of at least two species of lizards.[102, 116]

Neural Lobe

This portion of the neurohypophysis consists of branching cells, called pituicytes, and thick networks of fine unmyelinated nerve fibers that are the terminations of the hypothalamo-hypophysial tract. These fibers form plexuses in the vicinity of blood vessels and appear not to form synapses with the pituicytes. Most workers feel that the hormones of the neurohypophysis are not secreted by the pituicytes, but that they are products formed by certain neurosecretory cells of the hypothalamic nuclei. The neurosecretory material is thought to move along the axons of the hypothalamo-hypophysial tract into the neural lobe, where it is discharged, stored, possibly modified, and released into the general circulation as needed. It follows that the neural lobe *per se* is a depot for the storage of hormones.

Comparative Anatomy

The anatomic constituents of the vertebrate pituitary gland are remarkably constant. The most conspicuous phylogenetic changes have been the appearance of a consolidated neurohypophysis, the development of a system of portal vessels passing from the median eminence to the adenohypophysis, and the lack of a pars intermedia in birds and a few mammals.

The adenohypophysis of the cyclostome is an elongated structure, divided by connective tissue septa into three regions, for which the noncommittal names pro-, meso-, and meta-adenohypophysis were proposed by Pickford and Atz.[109] The most posterior component is the pars intermedia, and the two anterior components are the rostral pars distalis and the proximal pars distalis (Fig. 4-8). The neurohypophysis is a slight thickening of the floor of the third ventricle, separated from the adenohypophysis by a thin layer of vascular tissue. Some of the hypothalamic neurosecretory axons, presumably conveying arginine vasotocin, terminate around blood vessels in the neurohypophysis, whereas others appear to liberate their secretions into the third ventricle.

The elasmobranchs and teleosts are specialized groups, and it is important to keep in mind that they are remote from the main line of vertebrate evolution (Fig. 4-8). The neurohypophysis of elasmobranchs is diffuse and intermingled with the pars intermedia, the two parts often being collectively referred to as the neurointermediate lobe. Neurosecretory axons from the preoptic nucleus and lateral hypothalamus terminate in the neurohypophysis, but these are absent from the anterior infundibular floor. A few such fibers terminate in the *saccus vasculosus,* a folded and highly vascularized structure lying posterior to the neurohypophysis. The function of the saccus has not been determined. The pars distalis lies below the infundibulum, and is divisible into proximal and rostral zones. The ventral lobe is a peculiar feature of the elasmobranch adenohypophysis; it varies greatly in size and shape among different species, and its function remains obscure. A primitive system of hypophysial portal veins, supplying both the distal and neurointermediate lobes, has been described. The presence of an anatomically differentiated median eminence is questionable.

In teleosts, the adenohypophysis consists of a pars intermedia and an anterior lobe which is sometimes divisible topographically into rostral and proximal regions. These regions of the pars distalis appear to contain all of

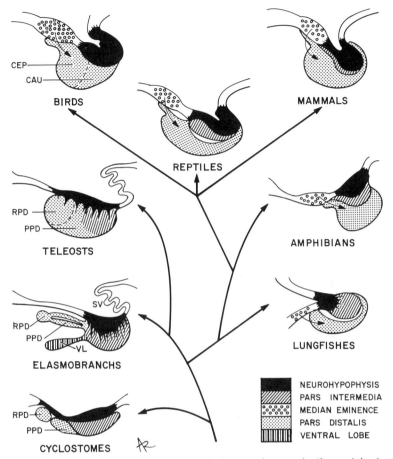

Figure 4–8. Schema showing probable evolutionary changes in the vertebrate pituitary gland. Arrows extending from the median eminence to the pars distalis represent the hypophysial portal system. CAU, caudal division of the avian anterior lobe; CEP, cephalic division of the avian anterior lobe; PPD, proximal pars distalis; RPD, rostral pars distalis; VL, ventral lobe of the elasmobranch pituitary; SV, saccus vasculosus.

the cell types characteristic of the mammalian anterior lobe. Some workers have homologized the rostral pars distalis of teleosts with the tetrapod pars tuberalis, but it is not certain that this is true. The neurohypophysis of teleosts, as in elasmobranchs, is diffuse and interdigitates with the cells of the pars intermedia and, to a lesser extent, with the cells of the pars distalis. Neurosecretory fibers from the preoptic nucleus and the lateral tuberal nucleus terminate in all parts of the neurohypophysis, but their secretions have also been found in both regions of the pars distalis. The saccus vasculosus is well developed in many teleosts, but it does not appear to be supplied by neurosecretory tracts. Whether equivalents of a median eminence and a portal system are present in teleosts remains a controversial point.[6]

Among lungfishes (Dipnoi), the neurohypophysis is separable from the pars intermedia, and a pars tuberalis is absent. A cleft is typically present between the pars distalis and the pars intermedia, and the saccus vasculosus does not develop. A primitive system of portal veins conveys blood from the median eminence to the pars distalis. Except for the absence of a pars tuberalis and the intermingling of nervous and pars intermedia tissue, the dipnoan pituitary is anatomically and histologically comparable to the pituitaries of tetrapod vertebrates[136] (Fig. 4–8).

The hypophysis of primitive urodeles is very similar to that of lungfishes; in anurans, the median eminence is more advanced and the portal system is conspicuous (Fig. 4–8). In some amphibians, a second distinct portal system supplies the pars intermedia and the pars nervosa.[23] The pars tuberalis is often lacking in reptiles, and a cleft is typically present between the pars intermedia and pars distalis. A pars intermedia is absent in birds, the neural and anterior lobes being separated by a connective tissue septum. The avian neurohypophysis is highly specialized and, in certain species, the zona externa of the median eminence, as well as the pars nervosa, serves as a storage site (neurohemal organ) for neurosecretory material from hypothalamic neurons.[97, 137] The portal blood vessels of the avian pituitary run to the anterior lobe via the pars tuberalis; not in direct apposition to the infundibular stalk, as in mammals. Thus, the portal vessels can be divided without injury to other parts of the gland.[58]

THE ADENOHYPOPHYSIS

Effects of Hypophysectomy

As early as 1886, clinicians had associated pituitary enlargement with the syndromes of acromegaly and gigantism and suspected that the organ had a great influence upon skeletal growth. Little progress was made in elucidating hypophysial functions until surgical methods were devised for removing the gland from laboratory animals without attendant injury to the brain. Around 1910, a transsphenoidal approach was employed for hypophysectomizing dogs, and a similar method was worked out in 1926 for the rat. A simple method of hypophysectomy for the rat, approaching the gland through the external auditory canal, has been used by some workers. Studies have now been made on many species of hypophysectomized vertebrates, ranging from fishes to man (Figs. 4–9 and 4–10). In most cases, the gland is removed from adult or young adult stages; however, in some cases it is possible to deprive an animal of its pituitary by removing the embryonic primordium of this gland. If this is accomplished before the organism develops its antigen recognition mechanism, the possibility is raised that at later stages it may be able to make antibodies against its own hormone kinds. Such an animal would be physiologically different from a sibling deprived of its hypophysis by removal of the fully differentiated gland. Because this possibility has never been studied and because the hypophysial primordium is accessible in so few species, no general problem is posed by this point. Nevertheless, the term "hypophysioprivic larva" is seen in the lit-

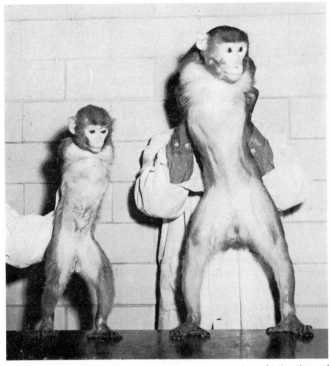

Figure 4–9. Hypophysectomy of the immature rhesus monkey. At the time of the operation, the experimental animal (left) weighed 2.7 kg. and the control (right) weighed 2.9 kg. After two years, when this photograph was taken, the hypophysectomized animal weighed 2.7 kg., whereas the control matured normally and weighed 8.4 kg. (From Knobil, E.: *In* Zarrow, M. X. (ed.): Growth in Living Systems. New York Basic Books, Inc., 1961.)

erature, in reference to amphibians which have been deprived of the hypophysial primordium.

Total hypophysectomy could not be performed for the treatment of malignant diseases in the human subject until it became possible to prevent death from hypopituitarism by an adequate replacement therapy. The operation is now employed rarely in cases of advanced metastatic cancer of the breast in an attempt to reduce the somatotrophin and steroid hormones of the body by one surgical intervention. Because of the surgical risks and the difficulties of postoperative care, hypophysectomy is generally employed only after other measures have failed to control the cancer or other condition. The physiologic disturbances in the hypophysectomized human being are quite the same as those that appear in other mammals.

The most striking alterations resulting from total hypophysectomy or from removal of the adenohypophysis alone may be summarized as follows:

1. Cessation of growth in young animals and the retention of juvenile hair coat and of other immature features (Fig. 4–10).[120] Very young hypophysectomized rats do not stop growing immediately, but growth does cease after they reach an age of about 1 month. When the pituitary is re-

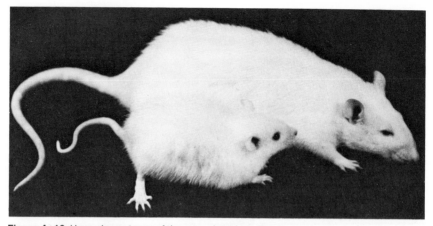

Figure 4–10. Hypophysectomy of the prepuberal rat. The two animals are littermate brothers. The smaller one (experimental) was hypophysectomized at 28 days of age, and each weighed 72 grams at that time. At the time of this photograph, the two animals were 10 months of age; the hypophysectomized animal weighed 81 grams and the control 465 grams. The hypophysectomized animal never developed adult pelage, and testicular descent failed to occur. The juvenile hair was lost rapidly, and bald areas frequently appeared on the back, particularly near the base of the tail. When rats are hypophysectomized as adults, the coarse adult hair is gradually replaced by the soft, fluffy hair characteristic of juveniles.

moved from rats at 6 days of age, they do not live to be more than 75 days of age. These deaths result from brain damage; the brain continues to grow to normal size, but the growth of the cranium is prematurely arrested and does not enlarge enough to accommodate the brain (Fig. 4–11). Failure of the cranium to increase in length and width is due to the cessation of endochondral osteogenesis in the basal region. The administration of somatotrophin to these young animals causes normal skull development, and they survive without showing any neural symptoms. In the absence of the pituitary there is no regeneration of bones removed from the top of the skull, whereas extensive replacement occurs in normal or hypophysectomized animals receiving somatotrophin.[1]

Nearly all primary and secondary centers of ossification are present in the skeleton of the 28 day female rat. The tibia of the rat or mouse is commonly used for the bioassay of STH since it normally retains an open epiphysial disc at its proximal end until late in life. After the pituitary gland is removed from the young animal, this disc promptly shows signs of inactivity. The disc diminishes in width and is far below normal width by two weeks after the operation. Thus, in the absence of the hypophysis and STH, long bone growth diminishes and skeletal dimensions are reduced.

2. Atrophy of the adrenal cortex and metabolic derangements resulting from a deficiency of adrenal steroid hormones occur. While some residual secretion of cortical hormones apparently can occur in the absence of the hypophysis, augmented production cannot be accomplished in response to stressful conditions. The adrenal medulla is thought to be independent of pituitary control and few if any changes seem to follow hypophysectomy.

3. The thyroid gland atrophies and becomes practically nonfunctional. This accounts for the low basal metabolic rate and other symptoms of hypothyroidism. Hypophysectomy of the rat leads to a profound reduction in all phases of thyroid iodine metabolism. The thyroglobulin content of the thyroid is greatly reduced: The meager amounts present contain low percentages of ^{131}I-thyroxine and other iodothyronines, but a normal percentage of ^{131}I-diiodotyrosine, and a greater than normal amount of ^{131}I-monoiodotyrosine. After the administration of ^{131}I to the hypophysectomized rat, no detectable amounts of ^{131}I-thyroxine appear in the blood. It is apparent that the synthesis of thyroid hormones is almost nihil in the absence of the pituitary gland.[134]

4. After hypophysectomy of the adult, the testes and ovaries become relatively nonfunctional and fail to produce mature germ cells or sufficient quantities of gonadal hormones to maintain the functional status of the accessory sex organs. After pituitary ablation in young animals, the gonads and sex accessories remain infantile and cyclic reproductive changes never occur. Although hypophysectomy may not terminate pregnancy, lactation fails to occur when the operation is performed during late pregnancy or post partum.

Hypophysectomy of the domestic cockerel is followed by a massive steatogenesis and formation of cholesterol in the seminiferous tubules of the testis. These degenerative changes appear to be identical to those that occur annually in wild birds at the end of the breeding season. As occurs normally in birds with seasonal cycles, the interstitial cells (Leydig cells) in the testes of hypophysectomized cockerels degenerate, and a new generation of Leydig cells begins to differentiate from connective tissue cells. In

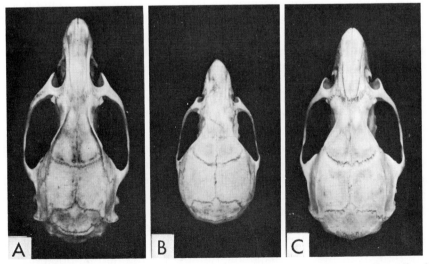

Figure 4–11. Effect of hypophysectomy and replacement therapy on the rat's skull. *A*, Normal rat 60 days of age; *B*, hypophysectomized at 6 days of age and killed at 60 days of age; *C*, hypophysectomized when 6 days of age and given growth hormone injections from 30 to 80 days of age. (From Asling, C. W., *et al.:* Anat. Rec. *114:*49, 1952.)

the absence of the pituitary, these presumptive Leydig cells become sudanophilic and cholesterol positive. This suggests an intrinsic rehabilitative mechanism within the gonad; however, there is no indication that the renewed interstitial tissue can secrete testicular steroids after removal of the adenohypophysis.[22]

5. Many disturbances occur in the metabolism of carbohydrates, lipids, and proteins in the hypophysectomized animal. In some species, such as the pig, the blood sugar drops to fatal levels if the appetite fails or if food is withheld for a moderate period. Glycogen stores in liver and muscle also fall much more rapidly than in intact fasting animals. Hypophysectomized individuals are much more sensitive than normal to the hypoglycemic action of insulin. Fasting ketonemia is more severe in hypophysectomized rats than in intact animals and becomes more marked with the lapse of time after the operation. Nitrogen is lost from the body at an excessive rate immediately after hypophysectomy but this rate is eventually reduced. There are indications that the incorporation of labeled amino acids into tissue proteins is diminished in the hypophysectomized rat. Hypophysectomy of the dog and certain other species causes a significant alteration in the pattern of proteins in the blood serum. The proliferation of red corpuscles is reduced in the hypophysectomized rat.

Since hypophysectomized animals are extremely sensitive to cold, infections, dietary deficiencies, and other stresses, they tend to live short lives unless given the very best attention. Chickens become very prone to hypoglycemia after removal of the pituitary. Nocturnal fasts and sudden temperature changes are often fatal.

6. In fishes, amphibians, and reptiles, ablation of the hypophysis causes a blanching of certain pigment cells in the skin and prevents the occurrence of usual color adaptations in these vertebrates. The immersion of yellow goldfish (*Carassius auratus* L.) in a 0.7 per cent solution of sodium chloride causes the appearance of pigment cells and the formation of melanin granules within them. This treatment does not elicit these changes after the pituitary has been removed.[19] The growth rate of tadpoles deprived of a pituitary gland is less than that of intact control animals, and the capacity of amphibians to carry out various types of regeneration is impaired by hypophysectomy. The importance of the pituitary in osmoregulation is underscored by the failure of hypophysectomized euryhaline teleost fish to survive in fresh water.

The hypothalamus and pituitary constitute a structural and functional unit, the components being bound together by nerves, neurosecretions, and blood vessels (Fig. 2–2). Because of this intimate and diffuse relationship, it is impossible to ablate the entire neural division surgically without injury to a vast number of contiguous structures. However, the physiology of the neurohypophysis has been clarified to some extent by using precision instruments that make it possible to induce small lesions accurately in different regions of the hypothalamus. Removal of the neural lobe only, other components of the neurohypophysis remaining *in situ,* does not have such far-reaching physiologic consequences as does total hypophysectomy or removal of the anterior lobe alone.

Hormones of the Adenohypophysis

At least seven hormones have been obtained from the adenohypophysis. These are: somatotrophin (STH, or growth hormone), corticotrophin (ACTH), thyrotrophin (TSH), prolactin (lactogenic hormone or luteotrophin, LTH), follicle-stimulating hormone (FSH), luteinizing hormone (LH, or interstitial cell-stimulating hormone, ICSH), and melanophore-stimulating hormone (MSH, or intermedin). Substantial evidence indicates that another hormone, β-lipotrophin (β-LPH), should be added to this list.[76] All these hormones are proteins or peptides and three of them (FSH, LH, and TSH) contain carbohydrate in addition to amino acids.

At one time or another, investigators have postulated the existence of additional diabetogenic, pancreatrophic, glycostatic, glycotrophic, and ketogenic hormones in anterior lobe extracts. Except for β-LPH, none of these factors has been convincingly established and nearly all workers feel that all these metabolic effects can be accounted for through the actions of the six or seven hormones already known to be produced by the pars distalis.

Hypophysial hormones are designated by their principal function. This is a gross oversimplification since hormone assay is rarely done on the species from which the hormone is derived. Moreover, as modern research points out, it now appears that activities that were once considered to be the result of hormone intercontamination are actually intrinsic functions of a given hormone. For example, while STH is usually thought of in terms of its capacity to stimulate skeletal growth, it has many other functions, including effects on metabolism and on the immune response.[77, 142] Even more striking is the fact that human somatotrophin exhibits a clear lactogenic effect and that it is chemically similar to a human placental lactogen. It is becoming increasingly more evident that certain groups of adenohypophysial hormones bear close physiological relationships to one another that are in turn based upon chemical similarities. The best example of such a relationship is a group of hormones composed of ACTH, α-MSH, β-MSH, and β-LPH. The question of whether these hormones are derived from common lines of evolution is currently the subject of investigation and speculation. Application of knowledge of the genetic code to questions concerning the origin of variations in the amino acid sequence of peptide and protein hormones provides interesting ground for speculation, which has been enhanced by new knowledge about the chemical structures of hormones of a variety of vertebrates.[41, 43]

Somatotrophin (STH)

Following recent studies on the comparative biochemistry of somatotrophins, it has become increasingly obvious from a comparison of molecular weight, amino acid composition, and partial amino acid sequence that the growth hormone molecules of various species are more similar than was once thought. Something is known of the nature of somatotrophin from the ox, the sheep, the horse, the pig, the whale, the dog, the rat, the rabbit, the

Table 4–2 AMINO ACID COMPOSITION OF EIGHT MAMMALIAN GROWTH HORMONES

AMINO ACID	HUMAN	BOVINE		OVINE	EQUINE		PORCINE	CANINE		RABBIT	RAT	
Lysine	9	11	12	13	8	11	11	11	12	10	10	10
Histidine	3	3	3	3	3	3	3	3	3	3	3	3
Arginine	11	13	13	13	11	13	12	13	12	12	11	8
Aspartic acid	20	16	16	16	14	14	15	17	18	14	13	16
Threonine	10	12	12	12	7	7	7	8	10	7	7	7
Serine	18	13	12	12	13	13	14	15	17	12	12	11
Glutamic acid	26	24	25	25	21	21	24	26	24	22	22	22
Proline	8	6	6	8	7	7	7	8	11	6	6	8
Glycine	8	10	10	10	9	9	8	8	10	9	7	10
Alanine	7	15	13	14	14	15	16	18	19	13	15	13
Half-cystine	4	4	4	4	4	2	4	4	4	3	3	2
Valine	7	6	6	7	7	7	8	8	7	6	4	8
Methionine	3	4	4	4	3	2	3	3	3	3	5	3
Isoleucine	8	7	7	7	6	5	6	6	6	4	6	7
Leucine	26	27	24	22	21	21	24	26	24	21	19	17
Tyrosine	8	6	6	6	6	5	7	7	7	6	6	5
Phenyl-alanine	13	13	13	13	9	9	12	13	12	10	10	8
Tryptophan	1	1	1	1		2	1			1	1	

Two sets of values are found in the literature for bovine, equine, canine and rat growth hormone. (Modified from Wilhelmi, A. E.: Chemistry of growth hormone. Handb. Physiol. Endocrinol. IV, Part 2:59, 1974.)

monkey, and man.[142] The average molecular weight of somatotrophins from all species studied is about 22,000; however, there is considerably more variation in isoelectric points, ranging from 4.9 for human STH to 6.8 for the sheep and the ox. Terminal amino acid residues are remarkably similar among these various somatotrophins. Immunochemical differences are highly variable and have no great correspondence with isoelectric point variation. In keeping with their similarities in molecular weight, the amino acid compositions of the various somatotrophins are quite similar. As is shown in Table 4–2, the profiles of amino acid distribution among the eight mammals indicated are remarkably alike.[141] The complete amino acid sequence is now known for somatotrophins of human, ovine, and bovine origin (Fig. 4–12), and partial sequences are known for porcine growth hormone. Many amino acid sequences among these molecules are similar to one another, and each possesses two disulfide bridges in approximately the same positions. These observations imply that there is a strong family resemblance among the growth hormones. A comparison of human and bovine STH's reveals that residues in 131 of 191 positions are alike. Bovine and ovine growth hormones are essentially identical. It is interesting that at position 127 in the bovine molecule, two allelic forms exist. At this position valine replaces leucine about 30 per cent of the time.

While this high degree of homology is seen between somatotrophins of different species, an even more striking similarity exists between the amino acid sequences of human STH and human placental lactogen (HPL), or

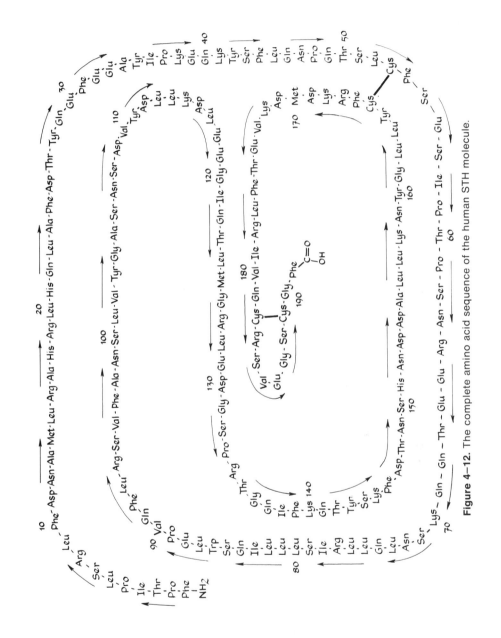

Figure 4–12. The complete amino acid sequence of the human STH molecule.

somatomammotrophin (HCS), as it is also called. Both hormones contain 191 residues, and 161 of these are identical in the two hormones. Most of the divergent positions can be accounted for by amino acid substitutions involving little change in the bases of the DNA template. These homologies in structure can be taken one step further by the inclusion of prolactin, whose amino acid composition and sequence very much resemble those of growth hormone and HPL. These observations strongly suggest that all three hormones have a common origin from an ancestral vertebrate molecule.

The chemical relatedness of somatotrophins from different species has important ramifications on the biological specificity of these hormones. For example, human beings and monkeys respond to primate growth hormones, but not to those from any other vertebrate. The guinea pig responds to no somatotrophin, not even to its own. Fishes respond to bovine STH, but fish STH is ineffective in the rat and in other mammalian species upon which it has been tested. Extracts of some teleost pituitaries, however, are known to be growth stimulating in the killifish. Bovine STH does not affect the growth of tadpoles of either *Rana pipiens* or *R. catesbeiana,* although ovine prolactin does exert a growth-promoting effect on these larvae. There is the possibility that antigenicity of the molecule may not coincide with the biologically effective "core" of somatotrophins. It is interesting that STH and prolactin preparations isolated from amphibian pituitaries showed a high cross-reactivity when tested in a rat STH radioimmunoassay system, implying that these amphibian hormones are structurally related to rat STH.[54] In this respect, it should be noted that the rat responds to somatotrophins from numerous species, including all mammals and a variety of other vertebrates. It is well known, however, that young hypophysectomized rats become resistant to repeated injections of primate STH and show no body weight gains after 10 or 12 days. In marked contrast, continuous body weight increases are evoked in such rats by the administration of bovine, ovine, porcine, and whale preparations. Ovine STH is highly antigenic in the guinea pig; when this hormone is given to recipients previously sensitized to the same preparation, 90 to 100 per cent of the animals die from anaphylactic shock.[64, 65]

Although growth is deficient in young birds deprived of their pituitary glands, a separate and distinct somatotrophin has not been demonstrated in avian species. Mammalian somatotrophins do not restore growth in hypophysectomized chickens, though sheep prolactin is effective in this respect.

The tibia test is most commonly employed for the bioassay of STH. After administration of the hormone, the increased width of the proximal epiphysial cartilage of the tibia of the hypophysectomized female rat or mouse is determined. STH produces continuous growth and widens the cartilages in proportion to the amount given. The tibia test is sensitive enough to detect STH in the blood of calves and young pigs and in humans with gigantism and acromegaly, but cannot detect STH in normal human plasma. The advantages of radioimmunoassay have made it a valuable tool in the assay of STH; however, since immunoreactivity and biological activity of this hormone are independent properties, the tibia test has continued to be important. It has a principal role in studies on the specificity of action of STH preparations, in which the activities of different hormones are measured on the same test system.

Biologic Actions. For many years, it was erroneously assumed that STH had only an effect on general body growth, particularly on the skeletal growth, and, when extracts rich in STH produced other actions, these effects were attributed to contaminating factors. It is known now that STH plays an important role in the metabolism of proteins, fats, and carbohydrates, and also serves as a synergist in enhancing the effects of other hormones.[44, 68] Human STH exerts a number of actions comparable to those generally attributed to prolactin, and this is consistent with the known chemical similarity between STH and prolactin. Highly purified human STH has about 20 per cent of the activity of highly purified ovine prolactin, both in pigeon crop gland stimulation and in luteotrophic activity in the mouse. It seems clear that human STH possesses intrinsic prolactin activity and that there is such a high concentration of growth hormone in the pituitary that a large amount of the prolactin activity of the gland could be attributed to growth hormone alone. Observations of this type have led some investigators to think that in the human, STH and prolactin may be the same molecule.[77, 78]

The fact that both STH and prolactin possess intrinsic activities of one another raises questions about the relatedness of active sites on the molecule.[78, 141] Some evidence concerning this problem is derived from experiments in which the biological activity of the molecule was tested after alterations in structural integrity. For example, it is known that partial digestion of STH's (15 to 25 per cent) from bovine, ovine, whale, and human sources can be carried out without serious impairment of growth-promoting activities. Similarly, with partial reduction of the disulfide bridges, in at least bovine and ovine growth hormones, there is little loss in activity. On the other hand, such treatment leads to about a 75 per cent loss in the growth-promoting action of human STH, but does not impair the prolactin activity of the molecule. A similar differential in the loss of biological activity of STH is seen following other chemical manipulations, and these observations suggest that these divergent biological activities involve different active sites on the molecule.

Hypophysectomy of the young animal results in attenuation of linear growth, due in large measure to impaired development of the skeleton. This results primarily from the loss of STH, which has a stimulatory effect on the formation of cartilage and bone. Changes resembling human acromegaly have been produced in various laboratory animals through the long-continued administration of STH. In the rat, for example, this increase in skeletal dimensions is accompanied by enlargement of visceral organs and hypertrophy of the musculature, the skin, connective tissues, and lymphoid organs. The nervous system seems to be exceptional inasmuch as it continues to grow in very young hypophysectomized animals, and its growth is not accelerated by the administration of exogenous STH. Some slight gain in weight may be observed in young animals following hypophysectomy, but this is due to the accumulation of fat rather than to the laying down of tissue protein. The carcasses of hypophysectomized animals, when compared with intact controls, are found to be deficient in protein and to contain proportionately too much fat. These parameters are reversed by the administration of STH.

Somatotrophin is a protein anabolic hormone which affects the growth of many tissues, not only of the skeletal system. It appears to retard the catabolism of amino acids and to encourage their incorporation into body proteins. The hormone induces a positive nitrogen balance and, in fasting animals, the levels of amino acids in the blood are diminished. A retardation in the rate of urea production is indicated by reduced concentrations in the blood and urine. The protein anabolic effect of STH is facilitated by normal amounts of pancreatic, adrenocortical, and thyroidal hormones acting in conjunction with it to stimulate the metabolism of fats and carbohydrates.[127] While there is insufficient evidence to establish definitely the mechanism of action of STH, one important aspect of its action is to promote the transfer of extracellular amino acids across cell membranes, particularly into muscle cells.[64]

The bulk of amino acids not utilized by the organism normally is converted to urea, which is eliminated through the urine. Somatotrophin, administered to the nephrectomized rat, retards the conversion of infused amino acids to urea. It thus appears that STH encourages the organism to retain amino acids, which are indispensable for the building of proteins. The increased body weight observed after hormone treatment is consequent upon an actual increase in tissue protein, water, and salts — not to an increased deposition of fat.

In view of its metabolic effects, STH has utility throughout the individual's life span, and studies have shown that the quantity of STH in the pituitary does not vary appreciably in the adult. It has been suggested that STH acts in a conservative capacity and enables the organism to retain its tissue supply of nitrogen, particularly when the exogenous supplies of protein and carbohydrate drop to low levels. If this is the case, STH may assist in effecting those metabolic adjustments that must be made when the lack of food becomes a threat to the economy of the organism.[119]

Hypophysectomy retards the mobilization of depot fat and tends to ameliorate the ketosis in diabetic subjects. Somatotrophin encourages the movement of unesterified fatty acids from fat reserves, consequently decreasing carcass fat and increasing the lipid content of the blood plasma and liver.[143] Certain adrenocortical steroids facilitate these effects of STH on lipid metabolism.

The discovery that the diabetic symptoms appearing in the dog after removal of the pancreas could be ameliorated by also removing the pituitary demonstrated convincingly that the hypophysis performs an important role in carbohydrate metabolism. The metabolism of carbohydrate is controlled by a well-regulated interplay of various hormones and other agents; in view of the many species differences and the complexity of the problem, no exhaustive treatment of the subject shall be attempted here. Several general statements may be made regarding the action of STH when administered to mammals: (1) The hormone tends to produce hyperglycemia, thus aggravating the diabetic state ("diabetogenic" effect); (2) it inhibits the action of insulin ("anti-insulin" effect); (3) it increases muscle glycogen when given to hypophysectomized subjects ("glycostatic" effect); and (4) it produces permanent diabetes mellitus in certain species when given over prolonged periods. The latter effect probably results from the eventual destruction of the β-cells of the pancreatic islets, which secrete insulin. The excessive blood sugar levels, evoked by STH, apparently overwork the β-cells, causing hypersecretion, hyperplasia, and eventually functional exhaustion and atrophy. It has been shown that rats receiving excessive carbohydrate by tube feeding develop temporary diabetes when given STH.

Some interesting studies have been made on the regulation of glycogen storage in the heart. Cardiac muscle, unlike skeletal muscles, must work continuously, and this muscle is known to maintain rather high levels of glycogen as an emergency substrate. When the heart works under anaerobic conditions, its glycogen is mobilized rapidly. Studies have shown that heart muscle incorporates C^{14}-glucose into cardiac glycogen to a greater extent than do ordinary skeletal muscles. It is also interesting to note that the glycogen content of the heart is increased during fasting, whereas the glycogen stores in other muscles tend to be depleted under these conditions. Hypophysectomy of the rat prevents the rapid increase in cardiac glycogen during fasting, but the administration of STH restores this capacity. When STH is given to normal subjects at the beginning of the fasting period, extremely high concentrations of glycogen accumulate in heart muscle. It has been suggested that the main role of STH in carbohydrate metabolism may be to promote the conservation of carbohydrate stores.[118]

Results of several investigations have demonstrated, both *in vivo* and *in vitro,* that somatotrophin stimulates the proliferation of thymic lymphocytes and of lymphoid cells in general. A recent study indicates that this action of STH is mediated by cyclic AMP.[85] The mitogenic capacity of bovine somatotrophin on rat thymocytes maintained *in vitro* is enhanced by caffeine, and cyclic AMP has the capacity to stimulate mitotic activity in the thymocyte populations. Thus, STH is one of a long list of hormones that use cyclic AMP as a "second messenger" in the mediation of specific responses.

STH as a Biologic Synergist. Four of the anterior lobe hormones (ACTH, TSH, FSH, and LH) are often referred to as "trophic" hormones because their principal actions are exerted upon specific target glands. Whereas STH alone has little effect on such target glands as the adrenal cortex, thyroid, and gonads, it markedly enhances the effectiveness of the trophic hormones specific for these organs when administered together with them. In the hypophysectomized mammal, the adrenal cortices become atrophic and incapable of secreting effective amounts of most of their steroid hormones. The cortices may be repaired by administering ACTH for a limited period after hypophysectomy, but the action of the latter hormone is enhanced by giving STH together with it.[72, 82]

In all vertebrates that have been studied, a full growth response requires both thyroid hormone and STH. The two hormones are complementary, although they differ in their specific manner of operation: Thyroid hormone encourages maturation but has little effect on growth; STH promotes growth without any effect on maturation.

The administration of STH to the hypophysectomized animal results in a modest improvement in the histologic appearance of several endocrine glands and of other tissues as well. The sex accessory organs of the hypophysectomized and castrated male rat are no exception. Furthermore, when the male sex hormone is given concurrently with STH, the two hormones function synergistically, and the male accessories are repaired rapidly and completely. Thus, STH enables the hypophysectomized animals to respond more effectively to other exogenous hormones.

There are reasons for believing that STH plays a supporting role in many biologic phenomena by producing in the tissues the type of environment that is necessary for certain hormones and other agents to express their functional potencies fully. Normal rats treated for long periods of time with STH often develop neoplastic growths, particularly in the lungs, adrenal medulla, and reproductive organs. Such neoplasms are seldom found in hypophysectomized animals similarly treated. Furthermore, removal of the hypophysis has been reported to suppress the response of the rat to carcinogenic agents such as 9,10-dimethyl-1,2-dibenzanthracene. Injecting purified STH into the hypophysectomized animals reinstates their usual capacity to respond to carcinogenic agents. While STH itself is not the cause of the tumors, it may create the type of biologic environment in which the carcinogen can manifest its actions speedily and completely.[90]

Prolactin (Lactogenic Hormone)[8]

The pituitary hormone that stimulates the crop glands of pigeons and doves is the same as that which elicits lactation in mammals. This hormone has gone by many names, including lactogenic hormone, mammotrophin, galactin, lactogen, and luteotrophin. The term "luteotrophin" was applied to this hormone after discovering that it is essential for activation of the corpora lutea in the rat. Since this ovarian effect has been demonstrated in only a few mammalian species, some workers feel that "luteotrophin" is not an appropriate name for the hormone. Indeed, in the light of an accumulating body of recent research findings, it appears that even "prolactin" is a questionable designation for this hormone. Prolactins have a myriad of effects among vertebrates, and one of their more striking actions is the ability of such preparations to stimulate growth in many forms, from amphibians to mammals. The importance of having both lactogenic activity and growth stimulating activity as functions of a single hormone called "prolactin" is underscored by the fact that it has not been possible to obtain a preparation from human pituitaries that is chemically unlike human somatotrophin and that possesses only lactogenic activity. As was pointed out earlier, the human pituitary contains such a high concentration of growth hormone that some prolactin functions can be accounted for by the intrinsic lactogenic properties of STH. Human STH preparations can bring about a spectrum of effects that are known to be properties of ovine or bovine prolactins. These include: (1) The stimulation of pigeon crop sac growth, (2) stimulation of the corpus luteum, (3) synergism with ovarian steroids in the stimulation of mammary gland development and growth, and (4) the induction of milk production in experimental animals and humans.

Highly purified preparations of prolactin have been secured from both ovine and bovine pituitary glands, and it is clear that they are very similar. Their biological potency, immunological spectra, and electrophoretic behavior seem identical, and they both have a molecular weight near 24,000.[78] That they are not completely identical is indicated by slight differences in solubility and in their content of tyrosine. A highly purified preparation of rat prolactin has also been obtained. It not only differs chemically from ovine prolactin, but is less active in the pigeon crop test. Whether common amino acid sequences exist in the prolactins of these two species is not known, for the amino acid sequence is known only for ovine prolactin. Comparison of the amino acid sequence of ovine prolactin with that of human STH reveals a strong similarity. Large segments of the molecules are homologous, and close examination reveals a common amino acid in about 50 per cent of the two chains. Ovine prolactin is composed of 198 amino acids and is slightly larger than human STH. It also has a third disulfide bridge involving a sequence non-homologous with that of STH. On the basis of many considerations, including chemical similarities, overlapping biological activities, and immunological relatedness, it would seem that the various vertebrate prolactins and somatotrophins have evolved from a common ancestral molecule or molecules.

Biologic Actions. Because of its broad spectrum of effects on vertebrates, prolactin is undoubtedly the most versatile of all adenohypophysial hormones.[8, 9] It would be advantageous to our understanding of the nature of the action of this hormone if this diversity of effects could be explained in terms of some general physiologic processes, but this does not seem to be possible, at least at present. Some prolactin effects are clearly metabolic, and others are distinctly morphologic or behavioral. Many of these effects involve integumental derivatives; however, it is not possible to associate exclusively these morphologic activities of prolactin with tissues of ectodermal origin because tissues of mesodermal origin are also known to be influenced by this hormone.

For the sake of dealing with such a large number of prolactin effects, the various actions are grouped into five categories and are listed in Tables 4–3 through 4–7. It is not possible to discuss each of these actions in detail, but certain of these occupy a special significance and deserve additional attention, which shall be given in this chapter and in Chapters 7 and 15.

The actions of prolactin on events associated with reproduction or parental care involve a diversity of animals, from teleost fishes to mammals. The most well-known amphibian effect concerns the phenomenon of water-drive. In certain geographic areas, the red eft stage of the spotted newt (*Notophthalmus viridescens*) metamorphoses and lives in terrestrial life for 3 or 4 years; it then returns to water, where it becomes sexually mature. Prolactin has been identified as the pituitary principle responsible for this migration to water. Hypophysectomized newts migrated to water from 4 to 10 days after being treated with mammalian prolactin, but they failed to acquire adult pigmentation and associated characteristics which presumably

Table 4–3   PROLACTIN ACTIONS RELATED TO REPRODUCTION AND
PARENTAL CARE*

1. Nest-building and fin-fanning [teleosts].
2. Skin mucus secretion (including secretion of discus milk) [teleosts].
3. Reduction of toxic effects of estrogen [teleosts].
4. Growth and secretion of seminal vesicles [teleosts].
5. Preparation for prespawning migration [teleosts].
6. Stimulation of eft water-drive (including skin changes) [amphibians].
7. Secretion of oviducal jelly [amphibians].
8. Spermatogenic and/or antispermatogenic (termination of cyclic male sexual activity) [amphibians].
9. Secretion of crop milk (columbids) [birds].
10. Formation of brood patch [birds].
11. Lipogenesis and deposition of fat (premigratory) [birds].
12. Antigonadal (antigonadotropic) [birds].
13. Premigratory restlessness (Zugunruhe) [birds].
14. Feeding of young (columbids) [birds].
15. Setting on eggs (domestic fowl) [birds].
16. Synergism with steroids on female reproductive tract [birds].
17. Stimulation of mammary gland development and lactation [mammals].
18. Synergism with androgen in male sex accessory growth [mammals].
19. Maintenance and secretion of corpus luteum in mouse, rat, ferret; possible synergism in other species [mammals].
20. Increased fertility of dwarf mice [mammals].
21. Retrieval of young by laboratory rats [mammals].
22. Decrease in copulatory activity in male rabbits [mammals].

*From Bern, H. A., and Nicoll, C. S.: The taxonomic specificity of prolactins. *In* M. Fontaine (ed.): La spécificité zoologique des hormones hypophysaires et de leurs activités. Paris, Centre National de la Recherche Scientifique, 1969, p. 193.

Table 4–4   PROLACTIN ACTIONS ON INTEGUMENT
AND DERIVATIVES*

1. Maintenance of hypophysectomized euryhaline fish in fresh water (gills) [teleosts].
2. Skin mucus secretion (including secretion of discus milk) [teleosts].
3. Melanogenesis and proliferation of melanocytes (synergist with MSH) [teleosts].
4. Stimulation of eft water-drive (including skin changes) [amphibians].
5. Proliferation of melanophores [amphibians].
6. Regulation of skin molting [reptiles].
7. Secretion of crop milk (columbids) (crop sac derived from ectoderm) [birds].
8. Formation of brood patch [birds].
9. Stimulation of feather growth [birds].
10. Stimulation of mammary gland development and lactation [mammals].
11. Sebaceous gland size and activity (including rat preputial gland) [mammal].
12. Hair maturation [mammals].

*From Bern, H. A., and Nicoll, C. S.: The taxonomic specificity of prolactins. *In* M. Fontaine (ed.): La spécificité zoologique des hormones hypophysaires et de leurs activités. Paris, Centre National de la Recherche Scientifique, 1969, p. 193.

Table 4–5 PROLACTIN ACTIONS RELATED TO
OSMOREGULATION (IONOREGULATION)*

1. Maintenance of hypophysectomized euryhaline fish in fresh water [teleosts].
2. Skin mucus secretion (including gill mucus-cell physiology) [teleosts].
3. Renal excretion [teleosts].
4. Preparation for prespawning migration (preadaptation to fresh water) [teleosts].
5. Stimulation of eft water-drive (including skin changes) [amphibians].
6. Renotropic [mammals].

*From Bern, H. A., and Nicoll, C. S.: The taxonomic specificity of pro-lactins. *In* M. Fontaine (ed.): La spécificité zoologique des hormones hypophysaires et de leurs activités. Paris, Centre National de la Recherche Scientifique, 1969, p. 193.

Table 4–6 PROLACTIN ACTIONS RELATED TO GROWTH*

1. Thyrotropin stimulation [teleosts].
2. Stimulation of eft water-drive (second metamorphosis) [amphibians].
3. Stimulation of larval growth and possible peripheral thyroxine antago-nism [amphibians].
4. Stimulation of limb regeneration [amphibians].
5. Goitrogenic [amphibians].
6. Stimulation of somatic growth [reptiles].
7. Stimulation of caudal regeneration [reptiles].
8. Hyperphagia [reptiles].
9. Stimulation of growth (splanchnomegaly) [birds].
10. Stimulation of growth (splanchnomegaly) [mammals].

*From Bern, H. A., and Nicoll, C. S.: The taxonomic specificity of prolac-tins. *In* M. Fontaine (ed.): La spécificité zoologique des hormones hypophy-saires et de leurs activités. Paris, Centre National de la Recherche Scientif-ique, 1969, p. 193.

Table 4–7 PROLACTIN ACTIONS RELATED TO
METABOLISM (FAT, CARBOHYDRATE)
AND ENERGETICS*

1. Thyrotropin stimulation [teleosts].
2. Lipid deposition [teleosts].
3. Resistance to high temperature stress [teleosts].
4. Hyperglycemic-diabetogenic [amphibians].
5. Goitrogenic [amphibians].
6. Reduction in lipid deposition [reptiles].
7. Hyperphagia [reptiles].
8. Lipogenesis and deposition of fat (premigratory) [birds].
9. Stimulation of growth (splanchnomegaly) [birds].
10. Hyperglycemic-diabetogenic [birds].
11. Hyperglycemic-diabetogenic [mammals].
12. Lipid deposition [mammals].
13. Stimulation of growth (splanchnomegaly) [mammals].
14. Erythropoietic [mammals].

*From Bern, H. A., and Nicoll, C. S.: The taxonomic specificity of prolactins. *In* M. Fontaine (ed.): La spécificité zoologique des hormones hypophysaires et de leurs activités. Paris, Centre National de la Recherche Scientifique, 1969, p. 193.

were dependent upon other pituitary hormones. Extracts and implants of fish pituitaries elicit the water-drive response in hypophysectomized newts, and this suggests that the fish pituitary contains prolactin or a related substance.[45]

In birds, prolactin seems to be involved in stimulation of the feather papillae to produce a new plumage. It acts synergistically with estrogen to produce brood patches in birds. These defeathered areas appear on the ventral surface of the body during incubation in one or both sexes, in species of many orders. After hypophysectomy, estrogen alone produces vascularization of these presumptive areas, but prolactin is required to produce edema and loss of feathers. Prolactin has no effect unless the area has first been vascularized by estrogen.[6]

In pigeons and doves, both parents participate in incubating the eggs and in feeding the young. "Crop milk" is a mass of desquamated cells from the epithelium of the crop sacs; this is regurgitated and given to the young. Under the influence of prolactin, these crop sac changes begin to occur during the second half of incubation and continue during the subsequent period of brooding and feeding the squabs (Fig. 4–13). There is some evidence that the pituitary increases its output of prolactin as a result of the stimulation provided by the experience of incubation. It is thought that prolactin elicits the regurgitation-feeding behavior by causing engorgement of the crop and suppression of sexual activities.[70]

There is substantial evidence that prolactin has antigonadal effects in both male and female birds. Whether these are direct effects on the gonads or are produced by suppressing the pituitary release of gonadotrophins is not known. Cooing in doves is suppressed by castration, and the administration of prolactin has the same effect. In avian species in which the male assists in feeding the young, the seminiferous tubules of the testes undergo fatty degeneration after the eggs are laid. This testicular collapse seems to correlate with the augmented secretion of prolactin by the pituitary. Similar testicular changes may be produced by hypophysectomy or by the administration of prolactin to intact animals.[80] Lipogenesis and the deposition of fat in migratory birds occur following injections of prolactin made at midday. Injections made earlier than this lead to a fat loss.

Prolactin functions in the rat and mouse to promote the secretion of progesterone by the corpora lutea—the so-called "luteotrophic" effect. When mammals are hypophysectomized during lactation, the production of milk ceases rapidly and completely, indicating that the pituitary hormones are essential for this process. After the mammary glands have been prepared anatomically, through the actions of ovarian hormones (estrogen and progesterone), the pituitary releases a hormone at the end of parturition to evoke milk secretion. This galactopoietic hormone of pituitary origin was formerly thought to be prolactin, but there are increasing indications that it may be growth hormone (STH). There is a high degree of functional overlap between these two protein hormones, and until there is more clarification of their chemical structures in different species, the problems are not likely to be resolved.

The actions of prolactin in osmoregulation have been studied mostly in fishes and are especially significant because they relate to the question of

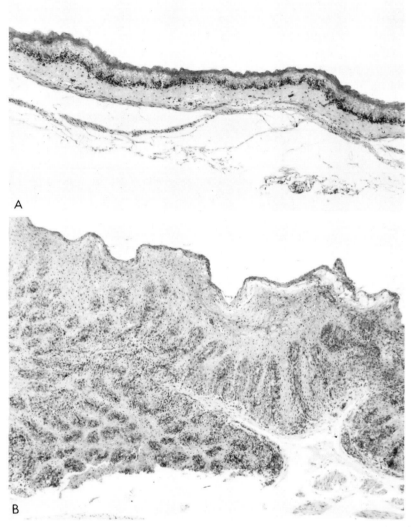

Figure 4–13. Histological sections of the crop-sac mucosa of untreated (A) and prolactin-injected (B) pigeons. Massive hypertrophy and hyperplasia of the mucosal cells are evident in the crop of the hormone-treated bird. (Courtesy of Charles S. Nicoll.)

the existence of a fish prolactin. It is clearly established that certain euryhaline fishes, but not all, require presence of the pituitary or injections of prolactin in order to survive in fresh water.[110] A variety of studies have implied that the ability of hypophysial extracts or prolactin to allow hypophysectomized fish to survive may be a complex phenomenon involving several sites of action. It seems that in euryhaline teleosts prolactin may act on several organs, including gill, gut, kidney, urinary bladder, and skin, to facilitate adaptation to a freshwater habitat. These specific organ effects have been ascertained from studies on numerous species, and it is not known that each organ is affected in each of the species tested. It seems probable that the effects on any one organ may be more important in one species than in another.

Evolution of Prolactin Function.   Because of the fact that something is known about prolactin activities of so many vertebrates, it is possible to make some generalizations about its functional evolution. These are summarized in the scheme indicated in Fig. 4–14. Of course, there are large gaps in our information because pituitaries of all the vertebrate classes have not been studied with respect to the many actions attributable to prolactin. Nevertheless, certain features stand out. One of these is the capacity to elicit various functions typical of animals of much more recent evolutionary origin. For example, pigeon crop stimulating activity seems to have emerged with the lungfishes, and mammary gland stimulating activity is already present in amphibians.[92, 93] This emergence of certain prolactin activities long before the targets of these actions have evolved is of special interest. Obviously, at the time that the prolactin molecule first acquired the capacity to stimulate crop epithelia or mammary glands, it could not be foreseen that these tissues were going to evolve. It follows, then, that the acquisition of these activities by the prolactin molecule was related to structural modifications imposed by pressures existing at that point in evolutionary time. These structural modifications were retained, were important features of the molecule when the crop epithelium or the mammary glands evolved, and were implicated in the mechanism of stimulation of these tissues.

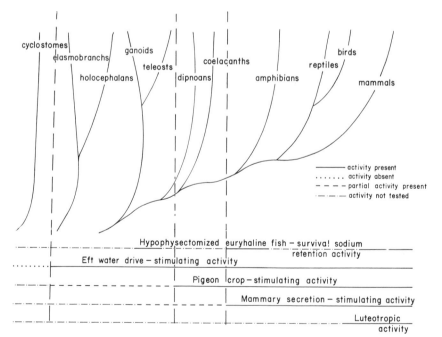

Figure 4–14. Distribution of some activities associated with prolactin among vertebrates. (Revised from Bern, H. Science *158*:455, 1967.)

Glycoprotein Hormones (FSH, LH, and TSH)

Three adenohypophysial hormones are glycoproteins: follicle-stimulating hormone (FSH), luteinizing hormone (LH), and thyrotrophin (thyroid-stimulating hormone, TSH). In addition to their carbohydrate content, the three molecules possess other chemical features in common.[38, 42, 111, 113, 122] They have a molecular weight of about 32,000, and all of them are composed of two chemically dissimilar subunits having a molecular weight of about 16,000. The subunits are non-covalently linked and thus can be readily dissociated by a variety of conditions. Only one of the subunits (beta) is endowed with structural characteristics that impart hormonal specificity. The alpha subunits of these three glycoprotein hormones are all similar to one another and are possibly identical. Recombination of alpha and beta subunits from the different hormones does not impair hormonal activity, but the activity of the hybrid molecule thus formed is always that pertaining to the beta subunit. The role of the alpha subunit is not known; however, it is functional, as is shown by the relative biological ineffectiveness demonstrated in the bioassay of the beta subunit alone. Following the development of more effective purification procedures, much has been learned about the amino acid composition of these glycoprotein hormones and considerable knowledge has been gained about the amino acid sequences found in the beta subunits of TSH and LH from ovine, bovine, and porcine sources. It appears that these various hormones have similar amino acid sequences, with as many as 50 per cent of the residues identical. Many other amino acid substitutions are simple ones that can be accounted for by single base modifications of the codon.

Additional evidence supporting the relationship of these three glycoprotein hormones is derived from immunologic investigations showing that antibodies can be developed that are common to human LH and TSH. In this respect, it should be pointed out that substances are present in the primate placenta that are functionally and immunologically similar to LH and TSH. Moreover, human chorionic gonadotrophin has been shown to be chemically similar to LH. Digestion of human LH by chymotrypsin leads to an almost complete loss of biologic activity, while loss of immunologic activity is less severe. It seems that biologic and immunologic activities involve different sites on the LH molecule. Human postmenopausal urinary luteinizing hormone is resistant to chymotryptic digestion, as is FSH from human, ovine, bovine, and porcine pituitaries. However, activity of FSH preparations from equine sources is destroyed by the action of this enzyme, indicating that FSH from the horse pituitary is different from that of other sources.[113]

An interesting and important discovery relative to the interrelationships of pituitary glycoprotein hormones concerns the heterothyrotrophic factors (HTF) of the teleost pituitary, which were studied extensively by Fontaine.[37] He has found these factors to be identical to gonadotrophic hormones of mammals. Accordingly, HTF, LH, and FSH all have the capacity to stimulate the thyroid gland of teleosts, but not that of mammals. These findings have fascinating evolutionary ramifications that have led Fontaine to suggest that the three glycoproteins of a species, having different activities, may be more closely related to one another than are hormones with the same functions isolated from more distantly related species. Resolution of problems of this type await the accumulation of more information about the chemistry of pituitary glycoprotein hormones of a variety of vertebrates. Nevertheless, it is an attractive speculation to consider that TSH, LH, FSH, and human chorionic gonadotrophin have evolved from a common ancestral molecule.

Bioassay and Biologic Actions of FSH.[21]   Since FSH activity is influenced by LH, it is essential to employ hypophysectomized animals in the bioassay of FSH. Two criteria have often been utilized in bioassay procedures: (1) increased ovarian weight and stimulation of young ovarian follicles in hypophysectomized rats, and (2) increased testicular weight, without stimulation of accessory sex organs, in hypophysectomized rats.

Because of their high degree of sensitivity, radioimmunoassay procedures have been used extensively in both qualitative and quantitative studies of all three hypophysial glycoprotein hormones.[117] The technique essentially involves the binding of an ^{131}I-labeled hormone such as FSH ^{131}I to an appropriate antiserum. The degree of radioactivity is used as a parameter of assay.

The main action of FSH in the female is to stimulate young ovarian follicles to develop multiple layers of granulosa and to form antra. When FSH acts alone in hypophysectomized females, LH being absent, these follicles do not reach full size, nor do they secrete estrogen. Under these conditions, the vagina, uterus, and oviducts remain infantile. FSH, acting alone in hypophysectomized male rats, stimulates the seminiferous tubules but does not activate the Leydig cells. The male accessories, therefore, remain atrophic. The principal function of FSH in the male concerns the process of spermatogenesis; while FSH was once considered to regulate the process, this function has now been assigned to LH.[132] Nevertheless, it is clear that FSH is essential for certain steps in spermatogenesis. FSH is known to concentrate specifically in Sertoli cells, and it may play a role in steroid biosynthesis attributed to these cells.

The same gonadotrophins are present in the pituitary glands of both sexes, but the hypothalamus is sexually dimorphic and this results in different patterns of pituitary release. The amount of prolactin in the pituitary glands of female rats not only varies with reproductive states, but has been shown to follow a circadian rhythm.[20]

That the gonadotrophins can act independently of other endocrine tissues is shown by the fact that the ovary of the mouse, maintained in an *in vitro* system, responds to such hormones as it ordinarily does under *in vivo* conditions.[81]

Gonad-stimulating hormones are known to be present in the pituitaries of fishes and other lower vertebrates, but they appear to be quite different from those of mammals. A purified factor from carp pituitaries was found to facilitate spermiation in the frog, to promote the uptake of ^{32}P by the testes of the eel, and to enlarge the testes of amphibian larvae. This factor was inactive in all mammalian tests.[15] Evidence is now beginning to accumulate about reptilian gonadotrophins. It is clear that both FSH and LH are present in reptiles such as chelonians and crocodilians, and that FSH from the snapping turtle has a wide spectrum of action.[79] The status of LH in snakes and lizards is uncertain, in that it has not been possible to show that the pituitary of these animals contains much of the hormone and it is not known how sensitive they are to its action.

Bioassay and Biologic Actions of LH. Ascorbic acid depletion from the luteinized ovary of the rat provides a highly sensitive and specific bioassay for LH. The method consists of administering the test solution intravenously to rats made pseudopregnant by treatment with pregnant mare serum followed by human chorionic gonadotrophin. The decrease in ovarian content of ascorbic acid is proportional to the amount of LH contained in the material being tested. Follicle-stimulating hormone has no effect on the content of ascorbic acid in the luteinized ovary.[39,103,123] A second assay method is based on the capacity of LH to increase hyperemia in the immature rat ovary. A method has been introduced for estimating the degree of hyperemia through the use of ^{131}I-labeled serum albumin.[28] This method is simple and rapid, but appears not to be valid if the material being tested contains an excess of FSH. Since LH acts upon the interstitial cells of the testis to induce androgen secretion, increased weights of male accessory sex organs (ventral prostate, etc.) of immature or hypophysectomized animals may be employed for assay purposes.

The weaver finch feather test is an interesting biologic reaction occasionally used for detecting the presence of LH activity. The weaver finch is a small bird, native to South Africa, but it has been imported into many countries and sold by bird dealers. With the onset of the breeding season, the male acquires a bright yellow and black plumage; at the close of the breeding season two or three months later, the animal molts and dons the hen-type plumage, like that worn by the female throughout the year. The hen plumage contains white feathers on the breast and lacks the black ones completely. Castrated males continue to don the nuptial plumage rhythmically, showing that the plumage change is not controlled by testicular hormones. The administration of anterior pituitary extracts to females or non-breeding males, castrate or intact, is followed by the appearance of dark feathers. The melanization of the feathers seems not to be a *direct* effect of LH.[112]

In testing an unknown preparation for LH, one plucks the breast feathers and waits until the white tips of the regenerating feathers become visible. The test material is then injected. If the material is positive for LH, a black band appears across the newly formed feathers; otherwise the pigmented band is absent.

The administration of purified LH to hypophysectomized rats repairs the involuted interstitial cells of the ovary; the uterus and vagina are not stimulated, and this indicates that the ovaries are failing to secrete estrogen. Luteinizing hormone acts synergistically with FSH to promote the secretion of estrogen by follicles undergoing maturation and to cause ovulation. It is also concerned with the formation of corpora lutea and, in the rat and mouse, works together with prolactin to stimulate the production of progesterone and estrogen by the corpora lutea.

Luteinizing hormone functions in the male to activate the interstitial cells of the testis (Leydig cells), with the consequent production of testicular androgen. Therefore, the extratesticular effects of LH are the same as those that result from the administration of male sex hormone.

The testes of adult hypophysectomized animals cease producing spermatozoa and the cells of Leydig do not secrete enough androgen to maintain the accessory sex organs. In certain mammals, the administration of androgen immediately after hypophysectomy prevents the loss of the spermatogenic function of the seminiferous tubules and may even reinstate spermatogenesis in atrophic tubules. From studies on the effects of impure FSH and LH preparations on the testes of hypophysectomized rats, the concept has developed that LH stimulates the cells of Leydig to produce testosterone, which in turn acts upon the accessory reproductive organs, whereas FSH promotes spermatogenesis by acting directly upon the seminiferous tubules. The action of LH on the Leydig cells has been confirmed, using an essentially pure preparation of the hormone, but there is doubt whether or not FSH is required to stimulate the seminiferous tubules. Sheep LH administered to hypophysectomized mice can reinvoke spermatogenic activity in the testes in the absence of FSH, even though the degeneration of the germ cells has progressed to the point where spermatozoa, spermatids, and secondary spermatocytes are no longer in evidence. When injections of LH were begun two weeks after hypophysectomy, degeneration and desquamation of the primary spermatocytes ceased, and, in about half of the injected animals, spermatozoa appeared in the epididymides. It thus appears that LH directly stimulates the Leydig cells to secrete androgen, and that the latter hormone affects the seminiferous tubules. Probably, the effects of FSH are essential for the last steps of spermatid maturation and for restoration of spermatogenic activity of the regressed germinal epithelium.[132]

Bioassay and Biologic Actions of TSH.   After ablation of the pituitary, the thyroid becomes atrophic and its secretory capacity is reduced to a minimum. The gland diminishes in size and appears less vascular than normal. Histologically, the secretory epithelium is flattened, and colloid is retained in the acini. The uptake of ^{131}I is reduced to very low levels. The thyroid of the hypophysectomized animal may be returned to normal by giving fresh pituitary implants, or by injecting purified preparations of TSH. Since TSH acts mainly on the thyroid, its administration is followed by the various metabolic changes that the thyroid hormones produce.

The most common methods of assay may be listed as follows: (1) procedures based on increased height of the secretory epithelium of the thyroid, (2) determination of the number of colloid droplets in the cells of the guinea pig thyroid after treatment with the test material, (3) iodine depletion in the thyroids of 1-day-old chicks, (4) the uptake of radioactive iodine by the thyroids of hypophysectomized rats, and (5) by radioimmunoassay of circulating TSH.

Corticotrophin (ACTH), Melanophore-Stimulating Hormone (MSH), and Lipotrophin (β-LPH)

The existence of adenohypophysial factors that stimulate the adrenal cortex and pigment cells has been known for more than 50 years. For a time it was felt that both these functions were attributable to the same factor; however, during the process of purification of pituitary extracts having these two activities, it was revealed that ACTH and MSH are separate hormones.

Highly purified ACTH has been isolated from beef, sheep, pig, and human pituitaries. In all four species, the hormone is a straight-chain polypeptide composed of 39 amino acid residues, with serine at the N-terminus and phenylalanine at the C-terminus. These natural hormones have molecular weights of about 4500. Though there are species differences in the structure of these hormones, it appears that they are equivalent in their abilities to stimulate the adrenal cortex. Furthermore, the species variations are confined to the amino acids that occupy positions 25 through 33, and this portion is not essential for biologic activity (Fig. 4–15). That portion of the molecule extending from position 25 to the C-terminus can be removed without impairing adrenal-stimulating activity. The active portion of the molecule (positions 1 through 24) is identical in all corticotrophins investigated.

Complete synthesis of the natural hormone has been accomplished, and much information has been obtained through the synthesis of fragments of the natural molecule. Peptides containing the first 20, 23, and 24 units of the peptide chain have been synthesized and they appear to possess full activity. A synthetic peptide, consisting of the first 19 units, has an activity of about 80 per cent of the natural product. Another synthetic fragment, consisting of the first 16 units, has very little ACTH potency. These studies indicate that the active core of the 39-amino acid chain consists of the first 20 or so NH_2-terminal residues.[55-57, 73-75]

During the search for the structure of ACTH, the compositions of three types of MSH were elucidated. These were: α-MSH, found in pituitaries of all mammals so far studied; "porcine" β-MSH (β-glutamyl MSH), also found in pituitaries of the sheep and the ox; and "bovine" β-MSH (β-arginyl MSH), also found in ovine and bovine pituitaries. With these revelations, it became apparent that the ability of ACTH to stimulate pigment cells is an intrinsic function of the hormone, based upon the fact that it is so similar to MSH. The amino acid sequence of α-MSH is identical to the 13 amino acids from the N-terminus of ACTH; the only difference is that in α-MSH, the α-amino group of the NH_2-terminal serine is acetylated, and the C-terminal residue is an amide. The elucidation of the two types of β-MSH from various mammalian sources reveals that, except for a few minor amino acid substitutions, this hormone is the same for most species. It is noteworthy that while macaque β-MSH is like other β-MSH's, that of the human has been reported to include four additional amino acids at the N-terminus (Fig. 4–15). Recent evidence indicates that this is an artifact of extraction due to the cleavage of β-LPH, and that human β-MSH does not exist *in vivo*. These observations are consistent with an interesting concept that has emerged concerning aspects of the evolution of ACTH and MSH.[83] In essence this theory considers that a similar cell type present in both the pars distalis and the pars intermedia has the capacity to synthesize both β-LPH and ACTH. Both of these hormones are secreted intact from the pars distalis; however, owing to the presence of certain enzymes in the pars intermedia, ACTH and β-LPH are cleaved and modified to the smaller peptides characteristic of

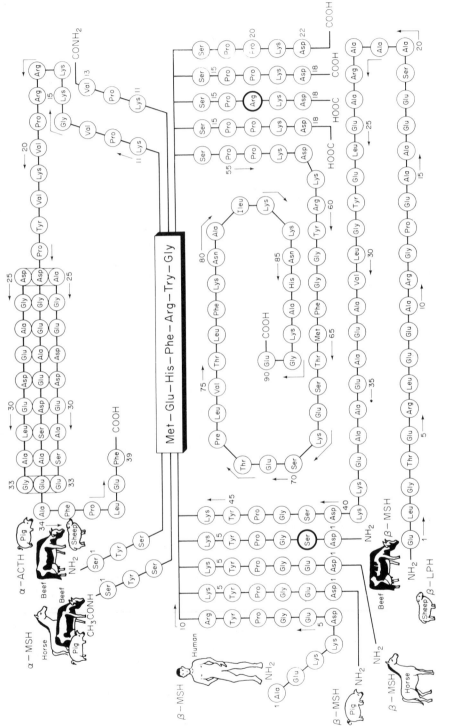

Figure 4–15. Structural comparison of pituitary ACTH, α-MSH, β-MSH, and β-LPH from various species. (After Li, C. H.[76] from Bagnara, J. T., and Hadley, M. E.: Chromatophores and Color Change: The Comparative Physiology of Animal Pigmentation. Englewood Cliffs, Prentice-Hall, Inc., 1973.)

pars intermedia secretion. Thus, β-LPH is modified to β-MSH and ACTH is cleaved into one peptide containing amino acids 1–17, and another corresponding to the 17–39 position of ACTH. The former is subsequently modified to α-MSH and the latter is unchanged, persisting as the corticotrophin-like intermediate lobe peptide (CLIP). There is good evidence to support this concept, not the least of which is the fact that, in species studied that lack a definitive pars intermedia, no MSH has been discovered. As was indicated above, the macaque, which has a pars intermedia, possesses α- and β-MSH's, whereas no MSH's are found in the human, which lacks a pars intermedia. Similarly, whales have no pars intermedia, and they also lack MSH.

Substantiation of this and other theories concerning the evolution of ACTH and MSH peptides can come only from an increase in knowledge about the existence of these hormones in a variety of other forms, including lower vertebrates. Gradually, such information is accumulating; the structures of ACTH, α-MSH, β-MSH, and CLIP are now known for the dogfish, *Squalus acanthias.*[17, 83] The structure of β-MSH from *Scyliorhinus canicula,* a related species, is also resolved. It is interesting to note that *Squalus* α-MSH is like that of the mammal; this is consistent with the fact that the first 19 amino acids of the N-terminal of ACTH of both *Squalus* and the mammal are virtually identical. Little is known about the structure of ACTH and MSH peptides from other vertebrates; however, the presence of ACTH and MSH activity in the pituitaries of most vertebrates strongly implies the existence of such molecules.

In the process of purifying ovine ACTH, a component was obtained that had distinctive properties quite different from those of ACTH.[76] Upon assay for its lipolytic activity, using the rabbit fat pad method, it proved to be as effective as ACTH. Because of its lipolytic activity, it was designated β-LPH, and subsequently similar substances were detected in porcine and bovine pituitary glands. Ultimately, when the structure of ovine β-LPH was revealed, it proved to resemble both ACTH and MSH and, as one would expect, it also possesses the ability to stimulate melanophores. It appears, therefore, that β-LPH is truly an adenohypophysial hormone having chemical and biologic properties that are between those of ACTH and β-MSH.

Two important features common to ACTH, MSH, and β-LPH underlie their close relationships. The first, a biologic one, is that all three have the ability to stimulate chromatophores, and the second, a chemical characteristic, is that all of these molecules have a similar composition. They all contain the heptapeptide, Met-Glu-His-Phe-Arg-Try-Gly, as well as other similar sequences of amino acids. One of many obvious questions asked by the close biologic and chemical relationship of these peptides concerns their evolution. This question has been discussed with increasing frequency.[41, 43, 83]

Bioassay and Biologic Actions.   The most common bioassay methods for ACTH are: (1) Measuring the loss of ascorbic acid from the adrenal cortex of the hypophysectomized rat after intravenous injection of the test substance. This appears to be a highly specific and sensitive test. The release of ascorbic acid from the cortex is not known to be accomplished by any agent other than this hormone. (2) Determining the reappearance of lipid in the atrophic cortices of the hypophysectomized rat after administering preparations that contain ACTH. (3) Determining the amount of ACTH-containing material that is necessary to maintain normal adrenal weights in rats when injected immediately after hypophysectomy. There are other techniques based upon the capacity of the adrenal cortical tissue, either *in vivo* or *in vitro,* to synthesize steroid hormones.

Activity of MSH is assayed on the basis of pigment cell changes induced in the integumentary chromatophores of amphibians *(e.g., Rana)* or reptiles *(e.g., Anolis).* This assessment may be derived from observations of changes in individual pigment cells (chromatophore index) or from alterations in the amount of light reflected from the surface of skin taken from the assay animals.

The adrenal cortex is the main target upon which ACTH acts, although a number of extra-adrenal functions have been described (Fig. 4–16). The hormone enlarges the adrenal cortices of normal animals and repairs the atrophic cortices of hypophysectomized subjects. It promotes the output of adrenocortical steroids, as is shown by the elevated titers of these hormones in adrenal venous blood after ACTH treatment. The metabolic changes resulting from ACTH are largely equivalent to those produced by specific steroids of the adrenal cortex.

It is now known that ACTH effects certain adjustments which are not mediated by its main target, the adrenal cortex. For example, when ACTH peptides are incubated with small pieces of epididymal fat tissue from rats, there is an increase in the concentration of nonesterified fatty acids in the

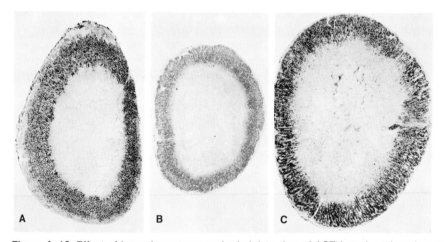

Figure 4–16. Effect of hypophysectomy and administration of ACTH on the adrenal cortex of the mouse. Frozen sections stained with Sudan black B stain. *A,* Adrenal of normal mouse, showing moderate amounts of lipid in the zona glomerulosa and abundant lipid in the zona fasciculata. *B,* Section showing marked shrinkage of the cortex 20 days after hypophysectomy. *C,* Adrenal of hypophysectomized mouse injected with α-corticotrophin for 7 days; the glomerulosa and fasciculata contain considerable lipid, and the cortical cells are large. (From Lostroh, A. J. and Woodward, P.: Endocrinology *62:*498, 1958.)

adipose tissue and in the medium. It is probable that ACTH produces this effect by activating a lipolytic enzyme in the tissue. Under these conditions, any possible mediation of the adrenal cortex is ruled out.[140] ACTH stimulates melanin synthesis in the xanthic goldfish through an extra-adrenal action. When pieces of caudal fin are grown in tissue culture by the roller tube method, the addition of ACTH stimulates melanogenesis in the dermal melanophores. Cortical steroids and, more surprisingly, MSH from various sources do not elicit this effect.[59] Melanophores in scales of the grey variety of goldfish are competent to respond to MSH, however.

It has been known for many years that the intermediate lobe of the pituitary gland is the source of hormones which act upon several kinds of chromatophores. The term "intermedin" was coined to designate the principle which affects the erythrophores of teleost fishes. While the term "melanophore-stimulating hormone" is misleading inasmuch as it implies that these agents employ only melanophores as their targets (see Chapter 5), it is currently used by so many researchers that it is now the preferred term.

HYPOTHALAMIC CONTROL OF ADENOHYPOPHYSIAL FUNCTIONS

Scientists and laymen alike have speculated for many years about the effects of the mind on the body and vice versa. There is no longer any doubt that "mind" or central nervous system, in response to exteroceptive and interoceptive stimuli, can bring about physiologic adjustments of many types. Emotional upsets, for example, prevailing for long periods of time without resolution, actually lead to physical sickness. At the human level, at least, much depends upon how the individual evaluates the stressful or threatening situation. There are at least two conceivable mechanisms whereby the brain and spinal cord could modulate bodily functions: The effects might be purely nervous, with impulses being relayed over chains of neurons directly to somatic and visceral targets; or the adjustments might be neuroendocrine in nature, with the nervous system activating glands of internal secretion which, in turn, affect various somatic and visceral targets. From many kinds of observations and experiments, it can now be stated with confidence that the nervous system does regulate and control certain endocrine glands, and that hormones in the blood act back upon the nervous system to condition the psychologic and behavioral characteristics of the organism.[51,62,69,91]

Environmental changes, often perceived through the organs of special sense, induce functional changes which are obviously mediated by the trophic hormones of the adenohypophysis. The sexual rhythms of many vertebrates are conditioned by environmental changes, such as photoperiods, temperature, food supply, nesting materials, and social contacts. It is common knowledge that ovulation in certain mammals (*e.g.,* rabbit, cat) is normally triggered by coitus, or by a comparable form of sexual excitement. Since reproductive functions are directly dependent upon gonadal hormones, and the functional capacity of the gonads is determined by gonadotrophic hormones of the pituitary, it is obvious that environmental effects on reproduction are mediated via the pituitary.

In man and in other vertebrates, an outpouring of adrenocortical steroids occurs in response to such emotional and sensory stimuli as intense light, sudden temperature changes, sound, restraint, handling, strange environments, and, in general, any situation resulting in anxiety, frustration, anger, or pain. The functional status of the adrenal cortex is regulated by adrenocorticotrophin (ACTH), and it is apparent that these environmental stimuli have affected the adenohypophysis. In agreement with these findings are clinical observations indicating that Graves' disease (exophthalmic goiter) is often preceded by emotional shock, and that the menstrual cycles can be altered by environmental changes and mental upsets. Since changes in the menstrual cycle involve both ovarian and pituitary hormones, the sequence of events may be: Emotional upset → central nervous system → adenohypophysis → ovary → uterus → clinical symptoms.

Observations such as these made it clear that environmental effects on the endocrine glands had to be mediated by the central nervous system, yet histologic studies of such endocrine glands as the adenohypophysis and adrenal cortices failed to reveal nerve terminals in close association with the secretory cells. The hypothalamus, in view of its close anatomic relationship with the pituitary gland, and its numerous afferent connections with the other parts of the brain, seemed to be a likely center for the integration of impulses which promote or suppress the release of adenohypophysial hormones. Since direct neural connections between the hypothalamus and adenohypophysis were found to be practically nonexistent, alternative pathways which might link the two structures were sought. Attention turned to the hypophysial portal veins, after it was established that the direction of blood flow is from the median eminence to the adenohypophysis, and the concept developed that the link is vascular rather than neural (Fig. 2–2). If adenohypophysial contact were indeed accomplished via vascular connections, the next problem would be to elucidate the source and identity of the blood-borne agents that transmit the information.

The Neurovascular Hypothesis

This working hypothesis was put forward in the 1940's to explain how a gland could be subject to nervous control without itself being supplied with secretomotor nerve terminals.[46] It is known that nerve fibers from the hypothalamus end in close association with capillaries of the primary plexus in the median eminence. These are presumably neurosecretory cells whose products enter the capillaries and are delivered to the adenohypophysis via the hypophysial portal veins. The first of these products to be described was associated with the release of ACTH and was designated "corticotropin-releasing factor" or CRF. Subsequently, other factors have been found to stimulate or retard the production or release of the various adenohypophysial hormones. The hypothalamic influence in mammals appears to be stimulatory with respect to FSH, LH, ACTH, TSH, and STH, but appears to be inhibitory with respect to prolactin.[32, 49, 92, 126]

The fundamental structure in this control mechanism is the median eminence. It has been the optimal source for the extraction of releasing factors and it has been much studied from the standpoint of ultrastructure. The belief that releasing factors are neurosecretions was strengthened by electron microscopic observations on the median eminence. Many axons in this region terminate along perivascular spaces that surround the capillaries. The terminals contain synaptic vesicles and opaque globules of neurosecretory material. The capillary endothelium is fenestrated, as is typically the case in areas where secretion and absorption are occurring.[52] Often structural alterations in the median eminence occur in correlation with the endocrine state of the organism. Kobayashi and Matsui[66] noted that after castration cytoplasmic organelles, including the Golgi apparatus, large vesicles of the rough endoplasmic recticulum, polyribosomes, glycogen granules, and other cellular inclusions, become more prominent in ependymal and hypendymal cells of the rat median eminence. Administration of estrogen to such animals did not restore the normal cytologic picture, but caused other changes, suggesting that the hormone stimulates ependymal secretion into the third ventricle. While these observations are difficult to interpret, they point out the importance of the median eminence in hypothalamic physiology. Reduced to its fundamental essence, it seems that the neurovascular hypophysis is composed of three connected features: hypothalamic nerve fibers → median eminence → hypophysial portal vessels. Coordinated control of pituitary function is achieved through a linkage of these structures.

It is now firmly established that the adenohypophysis is regulated by a feedback mechanism. According to the classic feedback system, controlling signals are hormones, produced by the peripheral glands, such as the gonads, adrenal cortex, and thyroid. Recently, the accumulation of a considerable body of evidence has led to the suggestion of a second mechanism, the "short loop" or automatic feedback hypothesis. This mechanism is an internal system in which specific adenohypophysial hormones themselves are the control signals (Fig. 3–4). It has been suggested that a short loop feedback system is involved in the control of all the hormones produced by the anterior and intermediate lobes of the pituitary gland. The suggestion has not yet been completely substantiated for all adenohypophysial hormones, but it seems likely that definitive proof will be forthcoming. There are indications that receptor sites for the classic "long loop" feedback systems are located in the brain, median eminence, or adenohypophysis. Receptors for signals from the short loop feedback system appear to be present in the brain, but have not been clearly demonstrated in the pituitary. The demonstration of the short loop system has been a welcome revelation because it may serve to explain the presence of adenohypophysial hormone-like activity in median eminence extracts. Of additional significance, it appears that the short loop system may be involved in controlling the secretion of prolactin, growth hormone, and MSH, hormones that do not have peripheral target glands. Regulation of the secretion of these hormones has been a question because their control would seem to be excluded from the classical long loop feedback systems.

The Nature of Hypothalamic Control

Various procedures have been employed to ascertain the extent and nature of the hypothalamic control of pituitary functions. Among these may be mentioned the induction of lesions in different areas of the hypothalamus, electrical stimulation of such areas, implantation of hormone pellets into the hypothalamus, sectioning of the pituitary stalk, transplantation of the adenohypophysis to ectopic sites, testing of extracts of the median eminence, *in vitro* techniques involving both pituitary and hypothalamic tissues, and surgical ablation of the hypothalamus in early amphibian embryos.

Ovulation in the rabbit depends upon copulation and normally occurs 10 hours thereafter. It is the consequence of a neuroendocrine reflex arc which results in the release of pituitary luteinizing hormone (LH). Electrical stimulation of certain areas of the hypothalamus was found to induce ovulation, in the absence of coitus, whereas direct stimulation of the adenohypophysis did not do so.

Sectioning of the pituitary stalk, including the portal vessels, generally produces only transient effects on pituitary functions because the blood vessels quickly revascularize the gland. If regeneration of the portal vessels is prevented by placing a sheet of metal foil between the pituitary and the hypothalamus, the release of pituitary hormones is seriously impaired.

When the pituitary gland of a female rat of reproductive age is removed from its normal position in the sella turcica and is autotransplanted below the kidney capsule, physiologic changes in the host reveal that the ectopic graft performs abnormally. Estrous cycles cease, functional corpora lutea persist in the ovaries for abnormally long periods, and the adrenal cortices and thyroid involute much as they do following hypophysectomy. The bulk of the pituitary graft consists of chromophobes and degranulated acidophils; all of the secretory cells are reduced in volume, and the gonadotrophs and thyrotrophs are less prevalent than in the normal gland. If the same graft is removed from the kidney and retransplanted to its normal position below the median eminence, it becomes vascularized by median eminence capillaries, undergoes cellular repair, and again produces its hormones normally. These experiments suggest that pituitaries, transplanted to ectopic sites, liberate reduced amounts of ACTH, TSH, FSH, and LH, but produce prolactin for abnormally long periods. It follows that the hypothalamic factor controlling prolactin secretion is inhibitory, whereas the others exert stimulatory influences. Ectopic pituitary grafts in the male rat function more completely than do similar grafts in females.[33, 96, 130]

The pituitary glands of rats may be maintained *in vitro,* and these are found to secrete much like the pituitary grafts that are removed from hypothalamic influences. The production of prolactin by the excised pituitary is inhibited by pieces of hypothalamic tissue cultured with it; the addition of small amounts of estrogen or thyroxine to the medium causes an accentuated release of prolactin.[88, 94, 95, 133]

There are numerous species differences in the extent to which adenohypophysial functions are dependent upon anatomic connections with the hypothalamus. In chickens, autotransplanted anterior lobes, persisting in the kidneys, fail to support testicular functions; however, they do have some capacity to maintain the adrenals, thus enabling the host to survive environmental stresses that would otherwise be fatal. While the kidney grafts do not produce gonadotrophins, they apparently can secrete some TSH and ACTH. The avian adrenal is somewhat more independent of pituitary support than that in mammals, and some workers believe that there may be an extrahypophysial source of ACTH. There is no evidence in birds that ectopic pituitary grafts liberate excessive prolactin.[84]

As was pointed out earlier (page 81), removal of the hypothalamic primordium from frog embryos does not prevent the development of the pars distalis, but the pars intermedia does not form. The hypothalectomized animals remain light in color, due to the absence of melanophore-stimulating hormones; they grow at about the same rate as unoperated controls and undergo delayed metamorphosis. It is apparent that the isolated pars distalis secretes "growth" hormone more or less normally and enough TSH to maintain thyroid secretion at levels sufficient for metamorphosis to be accomplished eventually. Production of TSH is probably subnormal since the thyroid glands show histologic indications of inactivity (Fig. 7-11).[18, 48]

The experiments of Etkin and Lehrer[30] on tadpoles of *Rana pipiens* gave different results. Tailbud embryos were hypophysectomized, and the adenohypophyses were autotransplanted to the tails. The animals carrying the ectopic grafts remained dark (hypermelanotic), and grew faster than the normal controls. The pars intermedia of the grafts was greatly hypertrophied, and the darkening of the skin indicated that this region was hyperactive in its output of MSH peptides. These workers suggested that, by analogy with the results obtained on rats, the ectopic pituitary grafts of the tadpoles might be releasing excessive prolactin, and that this hormone might serve as a "growth" hormone in these anurans. Since these ectopic grafts seem to liberate excessive amounts of MSH and "growth" hormone, it would be assumed that the hypothalamus normally exerts an inhibitory influence on the release of these particular secretions.[30, 31, 61, 138]

Pituitary glands of the fish *Poecilia* function abnormally after being separated from the hypothalamus. The ectopic pituitary grafts secrete TSH and prolactin in considerable amounts, moderate amounts of ACTH, very reduced amounts of STH, and no gonadotrophin.[5] The same type of results have been obtained with amphibians; however, variation is encountered. Ectopic transplantation of the pars distalis of *Xenopus* is accompanied by high levels of TSH release; however, such is not the case when *Rana* is used.

The studies on different species of vertebrates lead to the conclusion that the hypothalamus is an important terminus, which receives information channeled in from the external environment and other parts of the brain, and which translates this neural information into chemical messengers (neurohormones). These messengers, or release factors, are conveyed over the hypophysial portal system to the adenohypophysis, where they accelerate or suppress the output of particular homones. This is the essence of the neurovascular hypothesis, and it has turned out to be one of the most important conceptual formulations ever advanced in the field of endocrinology. Elevation of this scheme from the conceptual to the factual is beginning to occur, as more is learned about the nature of hypothalamic control factors.

The Nature of Hypothalamic Control Factors

It is now widely accepted that the release of most of the known adenohypophysial hormones is regulated by factors of hypothalamic origin. Because of their neural origin and because of their action on the adenohypophysis, these factors are generally thought of as hypophysiotrophic neurohormones.[125, 135] They are truly hormones because they are secreted into the hypophysial portal vessels and are thus transported to their target cells in the adenohypophysis. On this basis they are often referred to as releasing hormones, and are so designated in conjunction with the hypophysial hormone they regulate. Thus, the hypophysiotrophic hormone implicated in TSH release can be referred to as TSH-RH or TRH. Similar designations apply to other releasing hormones. Although these releasing substances are hormonal, they were originally referred to as releasing factors, and such terms as CRF or TRF have long been familiar terms in the literature. Because of their familiarity and because the use of the word "hormone" in the designation of these releasing substances might be confused with the adenohypophysial hormone that is actually being released, some workers have continued to use the term "releasing factor." Unfortunately, this has led to even more confusion because both designations are used in the literature and often are used interchangeably by authors in the same publication. In an attempt to clarify this terminology, the various designations are explained in Table 4–8. As was implied in the previous section, evidence indicates that the factors controlling the secretion of prolactin and MSH are

RELEASE OF PITUITARY HORMONES*

HYPOTHALAMIC HORMONE	ABBREVIATIONS
Corticotropin (ACTH) — releasing hormone	CRH, CRF
Thyrotropin (TSH) — releasing hormone	TRH, TRF
Luteinizing hormone (LH) — releasing hormone	LH-RH, LH-RF, LRH, LRF
Follicle-stimulating hormone (FSH) — releasing hormone	FSH-RH, FSH-RF, FRH, FRF
Growth hormone (GH) — releasing hormone	GH-RH, GH-RF, GRH, GRF
Growth hormone (GH) release-inhibiting hormone (Somatostatin)	GH-RIH, GIF (SRIF)
Prolactin release-inhibiting hormone	PRIH, PIF
Prolactin-releasing hormone	PRH, PRF
Melanocyte-stimulating hormone (MSH) release-inhibiting hormone	MRIH, MIF
Melanocyte-stimulating hormone (MSH) — releasing hormone	MRH, MRF

*From Schally, A. V., Arimura, A., and Kastin, A. J.: Hypothalamic regulatory hormones. Science *179:*341, 1973.

inhibitory and are thus designated as inhibiting factors: PIF for prolactin-inhibiting factor and MIF for MSH-inhibiting factor. On the basis of various experiments, some involving the placement of lesions in specific sites in the hypothalamus, followed by assay of the median eminence, it has become possible to suggest that certain locations in the hypothalamus synthesize specific releasing factors. The success of this type of experimentation is based upon the development and use of highly reliable assay procedures for the various hypothalamic releasing factors. Of great importance, the establishment of these assay methods has been instrumental in facilitating the purification of releasing factors from hypothalamic extracts. This has led to a fundamental accomplishment, the elucidation of the chemical structure and the synthesis of some of the hypophysiotrophic hormones. The significance of the identification of these releasing factors is profound, not only for their own sake, but also because it provides unequivocal support for the neurovascular hypothesis of adenohypophysial regulation.

The structure of porcine TRF is now known to be pyroGlu-His-Pro (NH_2)[10, 13] (Fig. 4–17). This substance was extracted from the hypothalamus and was shown to be biologically identical with the synthetic compound. It stimulates release of TSH from mouse or rat anterior pituitary glands both *in vivo* and *in vitro* and both responses are inhibited by triiodothyronine. Plasma TSH levels of rats and mice are elevated by this substance, and the same is true for hypophysectomized rats with pituitary transplants under the renal capsule. Ovine TRF appears to have an identical structure and it is likely that the relative lack of species specificity of this compound indicates that it is widely distributed among mammals. This viewpoint is supported by the fact that TRF is such a small molecule that there is little room for variation in composition. Substitution of an amino acid causes a drastic alteration in the molecule and is accompanied by a loss of biological activity. Many other analogs of TRF have been synthesized, and most of these have little or no activity. Attempts to identify TRF's of lower vertebrates have now begun. While there is reason to suggest that such factors exist in fishes and amphibians, mammalian TRF has proved inactive in those species so far tested.

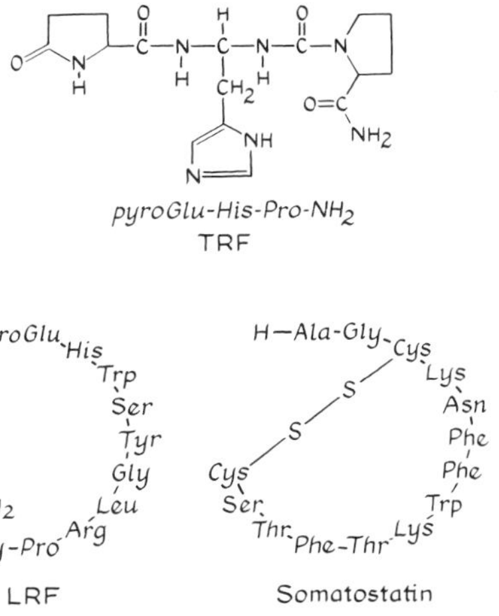

pyroGlu-His-Pro-NH₂
TRF

Figure 4–17. Chemical structures of three hypophysiotrophic hormones.

LRF

Somatostatin

The working out of TRF structure is surprising too from two stand-points—first because it is such a small molecule and second because its identification preceded that of CRF, which has been worked on for so long. The chemical nature of CRF is still unknown, despite the fact that it was thought to have been identified on several previous occasions. Following extractions of both pars nervosa and hypothalamus, at least two types of CRF were discovered. For a time, it was thought that a peptide closely related to α-MSH was α-CRF. It was also held, for a time, that vasopressin or a related peptide was CRF. At present, it appears that the CRF of the rat median eminence is a small compound of a peptide nature and probably containing a disulfide group. It appears to be relatively unstable, a feature which has made its identification difficult.

The only other hypophysiotrophic hormone whose chemical nature is understood is LRF (Fig. 4–17).[121, 135] It is a decapeptide whose biological identity is proved by the fact that antibodies made against it can block ovulation and can inhibit release of gonadotrophins. Its amino acid sequence was first determined from extracts of porcine hypothalamus, and soon after its structure was established, the molecule was synthesized. It has proved active in all mammalian species tested. The fact that LRF can stimulate the release of both LH and FSH has led to the suggestion that it may really be a "gonadotrophin releasing factor." Such suggestions are supported by the failure, thus far, to obtain a definitive FSH releasing factor. On the other hand, it is known that FSH and LH are not always secreted together, for example, in the female rabbit after copulation. In all probability, future investigation will disclose the identity of a separate FRF. The remaining gonadotrophin, prolactin, seems to be mediated by a substance that inhibits release. Such seems to be the case for most vertebrates, including poikilotherms; however, there is also some evidence for the existence of factors stimulating prolactin release. This seems to be especially true in birds. In any event, little is known about the chemistry of either PIF or PRF.[121, 135]

The status of a GRF controlling the release of somatotrophic hormone is still unclear. Various peptides have been isolated that have been claimed to have GRF activity; however, the purest of these fail to cause STH release *in vivo* as detected by radioimmunoassay. Apparently, the use of this assay has detected measurable release following the administration of more crude preparations, but the identity of the active components of these preparations is unknown. On the other hand, a peptide inhibiting the release of STH has been purified and synthesized.[67] This tridecapeptide has been designated "somatostatin," and it is quite unusual in containing a disulfide bridge that gives the molecule a cyclic configuration (Fig. 4–17).

The status of hypophysiotrophic hormones that control the release of MSH is highly questionable (see Chapter 5). However, the literature contains indications of the existence of both MIF's and MRF's. In particular, claims that the tripeptide tail of oxytocin is an MIF have received most attention. Results are controversial in this area; at present it seems most likely that MSH release does not involve hypophysiotrophic hormones, but is mediated directly by inhibiting neurons from the hypothalamus.

As is true following most research efforts, the acquisition of new information signals a step forward in the hierarchy of knowledge. Studies on the hypophysiotrophic hormones have revealed that, indeed, these are active substances that represent definitive points in the chain of events by which the nervous system ultimately regulates adenohypophysial function. However, these revelations lead to the next question: By what means is the release of the hypophysiotrophic hormones controlled? Already, answers to these questions are being sought and some have been obtained. For instance, there are now adequate data to support the view that the catecholaminergic control of gonadotrophin release occurs through the regulation of release of LRF and FRF.[87, 114] The same may be true for the hypothalamic release of TRF. Similarly, it has been suggested that gamma-aminobutyric acid (GABA) plays a role in the discharge of LRF.[99] It seems, then, that while much work is being done on the nature of the releasing hormones, a new frontier concerns the mediation of their release.

Among the many interesting discoveries made during the course of investigation on the hypophysiotrophic hormones is the fact that some of these agents exert unexpected effects. For example, LRF has direct effects on mating reactions that are independent of its involvement in gonadotrophin release. Injections of LRF can cause lordosis behavior in hypophysectomized ovariectomized female rats.[107] Somatostatin also has activity beyond the inhibition of STH release. It has a well-documented inhibitory action on the release of insulin which appears to occur directly at the level of the endocrine pancreas. It is possible that TRF may function as a PRF. No PRF has as yet been isolated, but it has been clearly shown that, in addition to its action in TSH release, TRF can bring about prolactin release in humans.

At present, the mechanisms by which the hypothalamus regulates the secretion of adenohypophysial hormones constitute one of the major areas of endocrinologic research. In the course of a few years, many of the points covered in this section will seem elementary, indeed. Most of the true releasing factors will be elucidated and contributions from neurochemistry will allow us to properly assess the biologic role of various compounds, such as biogenic amines, on hypophysial function.

REFERENCES

1. Asling, C. W., Walker, D. G., Simpson, M. E., Li, C. H., and Evans, H. M.: Death in rats submitted to hypophysectomy at an extremely early age and the survival effected by growth hormone. Anat. Rec. *114*:49, 1952.
2. Atz, E. H.: Experimental differentiation of basophil cell types in the transitional lobe of the pituitary of a teleost fish, *Astyanax mexicanus.* Bull. Bingham Oceanogr. Coll. *14*:94, 1953.
3. Bailey, R. E.: The incubation patch of passerine birds. Condor *54*:121, 1952.
4. Baker, B. L.: Functional cytology of the hypophysial pars distalis and pars intermedia. Handb. Physiol. Endocrinol. IV, Part 1:45, 1974.
5. Ball, J. N., Olivereau, M., Slicher, A. M., and Kallman, K. D.: Funçtional capacity of ectopic pituitary transplants in the teleost *Poecilia formosa,* with a comparative discussion of the transplanted pituitary. Phil. Trans. Roy. Soc. London, B. *249*:69, 1965.
6. Belsare, D. K.: Vascular supply of the pituitary gland in *Channa punctatus* Bloch. Nature *206*(4980):211, 1965.
7. Benoit, J., and DaLage, C. (eds.): Cytologie de l'adénohypophyse. Colloq. Intern. Centre Natl. Rech. Sci. (Paris), No. 128, 1963.

8. Bern, H. A., and Nicoll, C. S.: The comparative endocrinology of prolactin. Rec. Progr. Horm. Res. *24*:681, 1968.

9. Bern, H. A., and Nicoll, C. S.: The taxonomic specificity of prolactins. *In* M. Fontaine (ed.) La spécificité zoologique des hormones hypophysaires et de leurs activités. Paris. Centre National de la Recherche Scientifique, 1969, p. 193.

10. Bowers, C. Y., Schally, A. V., Enzmann, F., Bøler, J., and Folkers, K.: Porcine thyrotropin releasing hormone is (Pyro) Glu-His-Pro(NH$_2$). Endocr. *86*:1143, 1970.

11. Boyd, J. D.: Observations on the human pharyngeal hypophysis. J. Endocr. *14*:66, 1956.

12. Breneman, W. R.: Reproduction in birds: the female. Mem. Soc. Endocr., No. 4, 94, 1955.

13. Burgus, R., Dunn, T. F., Desiderio, D., Ward, D. N., Vale, W., and Guillemin, R.: Characterization of ovine hypothalamic hypophysiotropic TSH-releasing factor. Nature *226*:321, 1970.

14. Burt, A. S., Landing, B. H., and Sommers, S. C.: Amphophil tumors of the hypophysis induced in mice by [131]I. Cancer Res. *14*:497, 1954.

15. Burzawa-Gerard, E., and Fontaine, Y. A.: Activités biologiques d'un facteur hypophysaire gonadotrope purifié de poisson téléostéen. Gen. Comp. Endocr. *5*:87, 1965.

16. Cardell, R. R., Jr.: Observations on the cell types of the salamander pituitary gland: An electron microscopic study. J. Ultrastr. Res. *10*:317 (515), 1964.

17. Chadwick, A., and Lowry, P. J.: The purification and analysis of MSH from the pituitary gland of the dogfish, *Squalus acanthias.* Gen. Comp. Endocr. *13*:497, 1969.

18. Chang, C. Y.: Hypothalectomy in *Rana pipiens* neurulae. Anat. Rec., *128*:531, 1957.

19. Chavin, W.: Pituitary-adrenal control of melanization in xanthic goldfish, *Carassius auratus* L. J. Exp. Zool. *133*:1, 1956.

20. Clark, R. H., and Baker, B. L.: Circadian periodicity in the concentration of prolactin in the rat hypophysis. Science *143*:375, 1964.

21. Cole, H. H. (ed.): Gonadotropins: Their Chemical and Biological Properties and Secretory Control. San Francisco, W. H., Freeman & Co., 1964.

22. Coombs, C. J. F., and Marshall, A. J.: The effects of hypophysectomy on the internal testis rhythm in birds and mammals. J. Endocr. *13*:107, 1956.

23. Cruz, A. R.: Sur l'existence d'un système porte dans la neuro-hypophyse des amphibiens anoures. Acta Anat. *36*:153, 1959.

24. Dent, J. N.: Cytological response of the newt pituitary gland to thyroidal depression. Gen. Comp. Endocr. *1*:218, 1961.

25. Dent, J. N., and Gupta, B. L.: Ultrastructural observations on the development cytology of the pituitary gland in the spotted newt. Gen. Comp. Endocr. *8*:273, 1967.

26. Doerr-Schott, J.: Cyto-immunochemical study of the hypophysial cells of amphibians by light- and electron-microscopy. Fortsch. Zool. *22*:245–267, 1973.

27. Eakin, R. M., and Bush, F. E.: Development of the amphibian pituitary with special reference to the neural lobe. Anat. Rec. *129*:279, 1957.

28. Ellis, S.: Bioassay of luteinizing hormone. Endocrinology *68*:334, 1961.

29. Enemar, A., Falck, B., and Iturriza, F. C.: Adrenergic nerves in the pars intermedia of the pituitary in the toad, *Bufo arenarum.* Z. Zellforsch. *77*:325, 1967.

30. Etkin, W., and Lehrer, R.: Excess growth in tadpoles after transplantation of the adenohypophysis. Endocrinology *67*:457, 1960.

31. Etkin, W., and Sussman, W.: Hypothalamo-pituitary relations in metamorphosis of *Ambystoma.* Gen. Comp. Endocr. *1*:70, 1961.

32. Everett, J. W.: Central neural control of reproductive functions of the adenohypophysis. Physiol. Rev. *44*:373, 1964.

33. Everett, J. W., and Nikitovitch-Winer, M.: Physiology of the pituitary gland as affected by transplantation or stalk section. *In* A. V. Nalbandov (ed.): Advances in Neuroendocrinology. Urbana, University of Illinois Press, 1963, p. 289.

34. Farquhar, M. G., and Rinehart, J. F.: Cytologic alterations in the anterior pituitary gland following thyroidectomy: An electron microscope study. Endocrinology *55*:857, 1954.

35. Farquhar, M. G., and Rinehart, J. F.: Electron microscopic studies on the anterior pituitary gland of castrate rats. Endocrinology *54*:516, 1954.

36. Fawcett, D. W., Long, J. A., and Jones, A. L.: The Ultrastructure of Endocrine Glands. Rec. Progr. Horm. Res. *25*:315, 1969.

37. Fontaine, M., and Olivereau, M.: Aspects of the organization and evolution of the vertebrate pituitary. Amer. Zool. *15* (Suppl. 1):61–79, 1975.

38. Fontaine, Y. A.: Studies on the heterothyrotropic activity of preparations of mammalian gonadotropins of teleost fish. Gen. Comp. Endocr., Suppl. 2, 417, 1969.

39. Foreman, D.: Effects of gonadotrophic hormones on the concentration of ascorbic acid of the rat ovary. Endocrinology *72*:693, 1963.

40. Furth, J., and Burnett, W. T., Jr.: Pituitary adenomas in ^{131}I thyroidectomized mice. Proc. Soc. Exp. Biol. Med. *78*:222, 1951.

41. Geschwind, I. I.: Molecular evolution of peptide and protein hormones. Amer. Zool. 7:89, 1967.
42. Geschwind, I. I.: Comparative biochemistry of pituitary gonadotropins. Gen. Comp. Endocr., Suppl. 2, 180, 1969.
43. Geschwind, I. I.: The main lines of evolution of the pituitary hormones. *In* M. Fontaine (ed.): La spécificité zoologique des hormones hypophysaires et de leurs activités. Paris, Centre National de la Recherche Scientifique, 1969, p. 385.
44. Goodman, H. M., and Schwartz, J.: Growth hormone and lipid metabolism. Handb. Physiol. Endocrinol. IV, Part 2:211, 1974.
45. Grant, W. C., Jr., and Grant, J. A.: Water drive studies on hypophysectomized efts of *Diemyctylus viridescens:* The role of the lactogenic hormone. Biol. Bull. *114*:1, 1958.
46. Green, J. D., and Harris, G. W.: The neurovascular link between the neurohypophysis and adenohypophysis. J. Endocr. *5*:136, 1947.
47. Green, J. D., and Maxwell, D. S.: Comparative anatomy of the hypophysis and observations on the mechanism of neurosecretion. *In* A. Gorbman (ed.): New York, John Wiley & Sons, 1959, p. 368.
48. Guardabassi, A.: The hypophysis of *Xenopus laevis* Daudin larvae after removal of the anterior hypothalamus. Gen. Comp. Endocr. *1*:348, 1961.
49. Guillemin, R., and Schally, A. V.: Recent advances in the chemistry of neuroendocrine mediators originating in the central nervous system. *In* A. V. Nalbandov (ed.): Advances in Neuroendocrinology. Urbana, University of Illinois Press, 1963, p. 314.
50. Hanoaka, Y.: The effect of hypothalectomy at open neurula embryos in *Rana pipiens.* Amer. Zool. *3*:509, 1963.
51. Hansel, W.: The hypothalamus and pituitary function in mammals. Int. J. Fertil. *6*:241, 1961.
52. Harris, G. W.: The central nervous system and the endocrine glands. Triangle 6:242, 1964.
53. Hartley, M. W., McShan, W. H., and Ris, H.: Isolation of cytoplasmic pituitary granules with gonadotropic activity. J. Biophys. Biochem. Cytol. 7:209, 1960.
54. Hayashida, T., Licht, P., and Nicoll, C. S.: Amphibian pituitary growth hormone and prolactin: Immunochemical relatedness to rat growth hormone. Science *182*:169, 1973.
55. Hofmann, K.: Chemistry and function of polypeptide hormones. Ann. Rev. Biochem. *31*:213, 1962.
56. Hofmann, K., and Yajima, H.: Synthetic pituitary hormones. Rec. Progr. Horm. Res. *18*:41, 1962.
57. Hofmann, K., Yajima, H., Yanaihara, N., Liu, T., and Lande, S.: The synthesis of a tricosapeptide possessing essentially the full biological activity of natural ACTH. J. Amer. Chem. Soc. *83*:487, 1961.
58. Höhn, E. O.: Endocrine glands, thymus and pineal body. *In* A. J. Marshall (ed.): Biology and Comparative Physiology of Birds, Vol. 2. New York, Academic Press, 1961, p. 87.
59. Hu, F., and Chavin, W.: Induction of melanogenesis *in vitro* (Abst.). Anat. Rec. *125*:600, 1956.
60. Hymer, W. C., McShan, W. H., and Christiansen, R. G.: Electron microscopic studies of anterior pituitary glands from lactating and estrogen-treated rats. Endocrinology 69:81, 1961.
61. Jörgensen, C. B., and Larsen, L. O.: Nature of the nervous control of pars intermedia function in amphibians: rate of functional recovery after denervation. Gen. Comp. Endocr. *3*: 468, 1963.
62. Kanematsu, S., and Sawyer, C. H.: Blockade of ovulation in rabbits by hypothalamic implants of norethindrone. Endocrinology 76:691, 1965.
63. Kerr, T.: Histology of the distal lobe of *Xenopus laevis* Daudin. Gen. Comp. Endocr. *5*:232, 1965.
64. Knobil, E.: The pituitary growth hormone: Some physiological considerations. *In* M. X. Zarrow (ed.): Growth in Living Systems. New York, Basic Books, Inc., 1961, p. 353.
65. Knobil, E., and Sandler, R.: The physiology of the adenohypophyseal hormones. *In* U. S. von Euler and H. Heller (eds.): Comparative Endocrinology, Vol. 1. New York, Academic Press, 1963, p. 447.
66. Kobayashi, H., and Matsui, T.: Fine structure of the median eminence and its functional significance. *In* W. F. Ganong and L. Martini (eds.): Frontiers in Neuroendocrinology. New York, Oxford University Press, 1969, p. 3.
67. Koerker, D. J., Ruch, W., Chideckel, E., Palmer, J., Goodner, C. J., Ensinck, J., and Gale, C. C.: Somatostatin: Hypothalamic inhibitor of the endocrine pancreas. Science *184*:482, 1974.
68. Kostyo, J. L., and Nutting, D. F.: Growth hormone and protein metabolism. Handb. Physiol. Endocrinol. IV, Part 2:187, 1974.
69. Kuroshima, A., Ishida, Y., Bowers, C. Y., and Schally, A. V.: Stimulation of release of folli-

cle-stimulating hormone by hypothalamic extracts *in vitro* and *in vivo*. Endocrinology *76*:614, 1965.
70. Lehrman, D. S.: The physiological basis of parental feeding behavior in the ring dove (*Streptopelia risoria*). Behavior *7*:16, 1955.
71. Lewis, U. J., Cheever, E. V., and VanderLaan, W. P.: Studies on the growth hormone of normal and dwarf mice. Endocrinology *76*:210, 1965.
72. Li, C. H.: Pituitary growth hormone as a metabolic hormone. Science *123*:617, 1956.
73. Li, C. H.: Synthesis and biological properties of ACTH peptides. Rec. Progr. Horm. Res. *18*:1, 1962.
74. Li, C. H.: Perspectives in the biochemical endocrinology of adenohypophyseal hormones. Bull. N.Y. Acad. Med. *39*:141, 1963.
75. Li, C. H.: The ACTH molecule. Sci. Amer. *209*:46, July, 1963.
76. Li, C. H.: β-Lipotropin, a new pituitary hormone. *In* M. Fontaine (ed.): La spécificité zoologique des hormones hypophysaires et de leurs activités. Paris, Centre National de la Recherche Scientifique, 1969, p. 93.
77. Li, C. H.: Recent studies on the chemistry of human growth hormone. *In* M. Fontaine (ed.): La spécificité zoologique des hormones hypophysaires et de leurs activités. Paris, Centre National de la Recherche Scientifique, 1969, p. 175.
78. Li, C. H.: Chemistry of ovine prolactin. Handb. Physiol. Endocrinol. IV, Part 2: 103, 1974.
79. Licht, P., and Crews, D. P.: Stimulation of ovarian and oviducal growth and ovulation in female lizards by reptilian (turtle) gonadotropins. Gen. Comp. Endocr. *25*:467, 1975.
80. Lofts, B., and Marshall, A. J.: The effects of prolactin administration on the internal rhythm of reproduction in male birds. J. Endocr. *13*:101, 1956.
81. Lostroh, A. J.: The response of ovarian explants from post-natal mice to gonoadotrophins. Endocrinology *65*:124, 1959.
82. Lostroh, A. J., and Woodward, P.: Changes in the adrenal of the hypophysectomized C3H mouse with α-corticotropin and growth hormone. Endocrinology *62*:498, 1958.
83. Lowry, P. J., and Scott, A. P.: The evolution of vertebrate corticotrophin and melanocyte stimulating hormone. Gen. Comp. Endocr. *26*:16, 1975.
84. Ma, R. C. S., and Nalbandov, A. V.: *In* A. V. Nalbandov (ed.): Advances in Neuroendocrinology. Urbana, University of Illinois Press, 1963, p. 306.
85. MacManus, J. P., and Whitfield, J. F.: Mediation of the mitogenic action of growth hormone by adenosine 3′,5′-monophosphate (cyclic AMP). Proc. Soc. Exp. Biol. Med. *132*:409, 1969.
86. Masur, S. K.: Fine structure of the autotransplanted pituitary in the red eft, *Notophthalmus viridescens*. Gen. Comp. Endocr. *12*:12, 1969.
87. McCann, S. M., and Moss, R. L.: Putative neurotransmitters involved in discharging gonadotropin-releasing neurohormones and the action of LH-releasing hormone on the CNS. Life Sci. *16*:833, 1975.
88. Meites, J., Nicoll, C. S., and Talwalker, P. K.: The central nervous system and the secretion and release of prolactin. *In* A. V. Nalbandov (ed.): Advances in Neuroendocrinology. Urbana, University of Illinois Press, 1963, p. 238.
89. Miller, M. R., and Robbins, M. E.: Cyclic changes in the pituitary gland of the urodele amphibian *Taricha torosa (Triturus torosus)*. Anat. Rec. *122*:105, 1955.
90. Moon, H. D., Li, C. H., and Simpson, M. E.: Effect of pituitary hormones on carcinogenesis with 9,10-dimethyl-1,2-dibenzanthracene in hypophysectomized rats. Cancer Res. *16*:111. 1956.
91. Nalbandov, A. V. (ed.): Advances in Neuroendocrinology. Urbana, University of Illinois Press, 1963.
92. Nicoll, C. S.: Physiological actions of prolactin. Handb. Physiol. Endocrinol. IV, Part 2:253, 1974.
93. Nicoll, C. S., Bern, H. A., and Brown, D.: Occurrence of mammotrophic activity (prolactin) in the vertebrate adenohypophysis. J. Endocr. *34*:343, 1966.
94. Nicoll, C. S., and Meites, J.: Estrogen stimulation of prolactin production by rat adenohypophysis *in vitro*. Endocrinology *70*:272, 1962.
95. Nicoll, C. S., and Meites, J.: Prolactin secretion *in vitro*: effects of thyroid hormones and insulin. Endocrinology *72*:544, 1963.
96. Nikitovitch-Winer, M., and Everett, J. W.: Functional restitution of pituitary grafts re-transplanted from kidney to median eminence. Endocrinology *63*:916, 1958.
97. Oksche, A., Wilson, W. O., and Farmer, D. S.: The hypothalamic neurosecretory system of *Coturnix Cotournix Japonica*. Z. Zellforsch. *61*:688, 1964.
98. Olivereau, M.: Functional cytology of prolactin-secreting cells. Gen. Comp. Endocr., Suppl. 2, 32, 1969.
99. Ondo, J. G.: Gamma-aminobutyric acid effects on pituitary gonadotropin secretion. Science *186*:738, 1974.

100. Ortman, R.: A study of some cytochemical reactions and of the hormone content of the adenohypophysis in normal and genetic dwarf mice. J. Morph. *99*:417, 1956.
101. Ortman, R.: Anterior lobe of pituitary of *Rana pipiens.* A cytological and cytochemical study. Gen. Comp. Endocr. *1*:306, 1961.
102. Pandalai, K. R., and Sheela, R.: Hypothalamic control of the pars intermedia of the pituitary gland in the garden lizard, *Calotes versicolor.* Gen. Comp. Endocr., Suppl. 2, 477, 1969.
103. Parlow, A. F.: *In* A. Albert (ed.): Human Pituitary Gonadotropins. Springfield, Ill., Charles C Thomas, 1961, p. 300.
104. Payne, F.: Anterior pituitary-thyroid relationships in the fowl. Anat. Rec. *88*:337, 1944.
105. Payne, F.: Effects of gonad removal on the anterior pituitary of the fowl from 10 days to 6 years. Anat. Rec. *97*:507, 1947.
106. Payne, F.: Some observations on the anterior pituitary of the domestic fowl with the aid of the electron microscope. J. Morph. *117*:185, 1965.
107. Pfaff, D. W.: Luteinizing hormone-releasing factor potentiates lordosis behavior in hypophysectomized ovariectomized female rats. Science *182*:1148, 1973.
108. Phillips, J. B., and Piip, L. K.: A cytochemical study of pituitary glands of 1- to 15-day-old rats utilizing the aldehyde-fuchsin staining technique. Anat. Rec. *129*:415, 1957.
109. Pickford, G. E., and Atz J. W.: The Physiology of the Pituitary Gland of Fishes. New York, New York Zoological Society, 1957.
110. Pickford, G. E., Robertson, E. E., and Sawyer, W. H.: Hypophysectomy, replacement therapy, and the tolerance of the euryhaline killifish *Fundulus heteroclitus,* to hypotonic media. Gen. Comp. Endocr. *5*:160, 1965.
111. Pierce, J. G.: Chemistry of thyroid-stimulating hormone. Handb. Physiol. Endocrinol. IV, Part 2: 79, 1974.
112. Ralph, C. L., Hall, P. F., and Grinwich, D. L.: Failure to demonstrate a direct action of luteinizing hormone (LH or ICSH) on regenerating feathers in African weaver birds. Amer. Zool. *5*:212, 1965.
113. Reichert, L. E.: New data on the comparative biochemistry of mammalian gonadotropins. *In* M. Fontaine (ed.): La spécificité zoologique des hormones hypophysaires et de leurs activités. Paris, Centre National de la Recherche Scientifique, 1969, p. 315.
114. Reichlin, S., Jackson, I. M. D., Seyler, L. E., Jr., and Grimm-Jorgenson, Y.: Regulation of the secretion of thyrotropin releasing hormone (TRH) and luteinizing hormone releasing hormone (LRH). *In* P. Seeman and G. M. Brown (eds.): Frontiers in Neurology and Neuroscience Research 1974. University of Toronto, 1974, p. 48.
115. Rennels, E. G.: An electron microscope study of pituitary autograft cells in the rat. Endocrinology *71*:713, 1962.
116. Rodriguez, E. M., and LaPointe, J.: Light and electron microscopic study of the pars intermedia of the lizard, *Klauberina riversiana.* Z. Zellforsch. *104*:1, 1970.
117. Rosselin, G., Dolais, J., and Freychet, P.: Etude de la spécificité des hormones gonadotropes et thyréotrope par la methode radioimmunologique. *In* M. Fontaine (ed.): La spécificité zoologique des hormones hypophysaires et de leurs activités. Paris, Centre National de la Recherche Scientifique, 1969, p. 321.
118. Russell, J. A.: Hormonal control of glycogen in the heart and other tissues in rats. Endocrinology *58*:83, 1956.
119. Russell, J. A.: Effects of growth hormone on protein and carbohydrate metabolism. Amer. J. Clin. Nutr. *5*:404, 1957.
120. Rust, C. C.: Hormonal control of pelage cycles in the short tailed weasel *(Mustela erminea bangsi).* Gen Comp. Endocr. *5*:222, 1965.
121. Saffran, M.: Chemistry of hypothalamic hypophysiotropic factors. Handb. Physiol. Endocrinol. IV, Part 2: 563, 1974.
122. Sairam, M. R., and Papkoff, H.: Chemistry of pituitary gonadotrophins. Handb. Physiol. Endocrinol. IV, Part 2: 111, 1974.
123. Sakiz, E., and Guillemin, R.: On the method of ovarian ascorbic acid depletion as a test for luteinizing hormone (LH). Endocrinology *72*:804, 1963.
124. Saland, L. C.: Ultrastructure of the frog pars intermedia in relation to hypothalamic control of hormone release. Neuroendocrinology 3:72, 1968.
125. Schally, A. V., Arimura, A., and Kastin, A. J.: Hypothalamic regulatory hormones. Science *179*:341, 1973.
126. Schreibman, M. P., Leatherland, J. F., and McKeown, B. A.: Functional morphology of the teleost pituitary gland. Amer. Zool. *13*:719–742, 1973.
127. Scow, R. O., Wagner, E. M., and Ronov, E.: Effect of growth hormone and insulin on body weight and nitrogen retention in pancreatectomized rats. Endocrinology *62*:593, 1958.
128. Siperstein, E., Nichols, C. W., Griesbach, W. E., and Chaikoff, I. L.: Cytological changes in the rat anterior pituitary from birth to maturity. Anat. Rec., *118*:593, 1954.

129. Siperstein, E. R., and Allison, V. F.: Fine structure of the cells responsible for secretion of adrenocorticotrophin in the adrenalectomized rat. Endocrinology 76:70, 1965.
130. Smith, P. E.: Postponed pituitary homotransplants into the region of the hypophysial portal circulation in hypophysectomized female rats. Endocrinology 73:793, 1963.
131. Smith, R. E., and Farquhar, M. G.: Lysosome function in the regulation of the secretory process in cells of the anterior pituitary gland. J. Cell Biol. 31:319, 1966.
132. Steinberger, E., and Steinberger, A.: Hormonal control of testicular function in mammals. Handb. Physiol. Endocrinol IV, Part 2:325, 1974.
133. Talwalker, P. K., Ratner, A., and Meites, J.: The in vitro inhibition of pituitary prolactin synthesis and release by hypothalamic extract. Amer. J. Physiol. 205:213, 1963.
134. Taurog, A., Tong, W., and Chaikoff, I. L.: Thyroid ^{131}I metabolism in the absence of the pituitary: The untreated hypophysectomized rat. Endocrinology 62:646, 1958.
135. Vale, W., Grant, G., and Guillemin, R.: Chemistry of the hypothalamic releasing factors — Studies on structure-function relationships. In W. F. Ganong and L. Martini (eds.): Frontiers in Neuroendocrinology, 1973. New York, Oxford University Press, 1973, p. 375.
136. van Oordt, P. G. W. J., and Kerr, T.: Comparative morphology of the pituitary in the lungfish, Protopterus aethiopicus. J. Endocr. 37:8, 1966.
137. Vitums, A., Mikami, S., Oksche, A., and Farner, D. S.: Vascularization of the hypothalamo-hypophysial complex in the white-crowned sparrow, Zonotrichia leucophrys gambelii. Z. Zellforsch. 64:541, 1964.
138. Voitkevich, A. A.: On the relation of neurosecretion to growth and cell differentiation in the amphibian adenohypophysis. Gen. Comp. Endocr. 3:554, 1963.
139. Watanabe, Y. G.: The acidophilic granules (AG) in the thyrotrophs and their relation to thyroid hyperplasia among laboratory-reared Xenopus. J. Fac. Sci., Hokkaido Univ., Series VI, 16:339, 1968.
140. White, J. E., and Engel, F. L.: Fat mobilization by purified corticotropin in the mouse. Proc. Soc. Exp. Biol. Med. 102:272, 1959.
141. Wilhelmi, A. E.: Chemistry of growth hormone. Handb. Physiol. Endocrinol. IV, Part 2:59, 1974.
142. Wilhelmi, A. E., and Mills, J. B.: The chemistry of the growth hormone of several species. In M. Fontaine (ed.): La spécificité zoologique des hormones hypophysaires et de leurs activités. Paris, Centre National de la Recherche Scientifique, 1969, p. 165.
143. Wislocki, N. I., and Szego, C. M.: Acute reduction of plasma nonesterified fatty acid by growth hormone in hypophysectomized and Houssay rats. Endocrinology 76:665, 1965.
144. Yasuda, M.: Cytological studies of the anterior pituitary in the broody fowl. Proc. Japan Acad. 29:586, 1953.
1:00

CHAPTER 5

Pars Intermedia: Chromatophore Regulation Among Vertebrates

Most vertebrates, especially the poikilotherms, possess integumentary pigment cells which function as chromatic effectors. These special cells, called chromatophores, enable the organism to change color in response to many environmental stimuli. Color changes may serve several functions: (1) The animal may be rendered inconspicuous by imitating the color pattern of the environment, as in background adaptation, or the animal may be made more conspicuous, as in warning coloration; (2) colors "signal" to other individuals a state of sexual readiness; (3) the body tissues can be protected against excessive radiation. Since dark surfaces absorb heat and light surfaces reflect it, integumentary pigments may be important in thermoregulation in certain species of amphibians and reptiles.

At least three general types of chromatophores exist among vertebrates[9]: (1) Melanophores (black, brown, or red chromatophores) are the most well known; (2) iridophores (guanophores, leucophores, xantho-leucophores) function to reflect or scatter light; and (3) xanthophores and erythrophores (yellow, orange, or red chromatophores), found exclusively in poikilotherms. The chromatophores of all vertebrates differentiate from cells that migrate out of the neural crest.[20, 35] These cells, referred to as "chromatoblasts," have the capacity to migrate over long distances and ultimately to differentiate in response to given developmental cues. These cues may be part of the immediate environment of the chromatoblast, or they may be more general in nature, such as the titer of circulating chromatophore-stimulating hormones.[10] Chromatophores are found mainly in the integument, but they may be found in other tissues such as the peritoneal and meningeal membranes and the walls of blood vessels.

Color changes occur in response to a variety of environmental conditions, such as light, temperature, humidity, psychic stimuli, and inherent rhythms. Usually these environmental factors do not affect the pigment cells directly. However, there are examples of direct chromatophore effects of environmental stimuli. One of the best demonstrations of this occurs in the tail fin of tadpoles of the African clawed toad, *Xenopus*.[2] Melanophores of this region respond directly to light; in fact, localized paling of darkened tails can be brought about by the use of fine beams of light focused on portions of single melanophores.[66] For the most part, various environmental stimuli that bring about color changes do so through the action of hormones. Melanophore-stimulating hormone (MSH) from the pituitary is the major hormonal element affecting pigment cells; however, various other humoral agents, including indoles (*e.g.,* melatonin) and catecholamines (*e.g.,* norepinephrine), are implicated in normal pigment cell responses.[10] The role of the nervous system should not be discounted, for it has been shown clearly that chromatophores of certain, but not all, fishes and reptiles are innervated. Thus far, it has not been demonstrated conclusively that chromatophores of any of the amphibians are under direct nervous control.

The responses of chromatophores are of two basic types[49] — the physiologic and the morphologic response. Physiologic color change is a rapid response of the chromatophore, in which pigments within the cell aggregate or disperse. This response is typical of poikilotherms. The morphologic response or morphologic color change is a relatively slow event characterized by pigment synthesis. It may be expressed by an increase in the total amount of pigment found in the chromatophore, by the cytocrine deposition of pigment by chromatophores, or by an increase in the number of chromatophores in a given area.[10] Prolonged physiologic color change is usually accompanied by the morphologic response, but the nature of their connection is not yet understood.

THE NATURE OF PIGMENTATION

Melanophores have been studied to a greater extent than any other type of pigment cell and information gained from such investigations has led to a better understanding of other pigment cells. Many concepts established from observations on melanophores have been extended to other types of pigment cells. For example, it has been shown clearly that in the response of a melanophore to an appropriate stimulus, pigments migrate into or out of static processes of the cells (Fig. 5–1). This phenomenon has not been demonstrated unequivocally in other chromatophore types, although we assume it holds for these cells as well. While the various chromatophore types possess many characteristics in common, they are also quite distinctive with respect to their function and composition.

Types of Chromatophores

Melanophores.   Basically, two types of melanophores exist among vertebrates. These are categorized separately as "dermal melanophores" or "epidermal melanophores," not only because of their specific locations in the dermis and epidermis, respectively, but also because of their specific characteristics. Rapid color changes of poikilotherms usually involve the participation of dermal melanophores, which generally are larger than epidermal melanophores. Dermal melanophores often exist in a flattened form

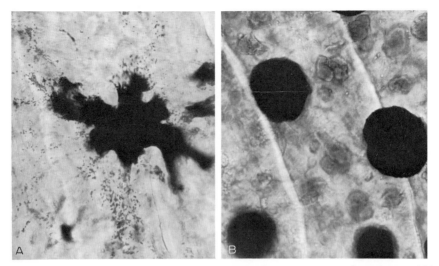

Figure 5–1. The effect of hypophysectomy on the integumentary melanophores of black goldfish. *A,* The beginning or perinuclear migration of melanin granules in a macromelanophore 3 hours after hypophysectomy. Many granules are still present in the cell dendrites. *B,* Complete perinuclear aggregation of melanin granules in macromelanophores 24 hours after hypophysectomy. The pigment cells eventually degenerate after loss of the pituitary gland. (Courtesy of Walter Chavin, Wayne State University.)

and have radially directed processes that allow a relatively large portion of the integumental surface to be covered when the chromatophore is in a dispersed state. In adult amphibians and reptiles, processes of dermal melanophores often extend upward from the plane of the cell to present a basket-like appearance.

A fundamental characteristic of all melanophores is that they deposit their pigment, melanin, on subcellular organelles called melanosomes[46, 61] (Fig. 5–2). Melanins are complex polymers of tyrosine derivatives and proteins that are categorized into eumelanins (brown or black) and phaeomelanins (yellow, orange, or red).[55] In addition to differences in color, phaeomelanins differ from eumelanins by the incorporation of cysteine into the melanin molecule. The formation of melanin is catalyzed by tyrosinase, which is found in formative stages of the melanosomes, called premelanosomes. Only after melanin deposition is completed is the organelle designated a melanosome. Most studies on melanosome formation have been made on epidermal melanophores, although the processes are probably the same in both melanophore types.

Epidermal melanophores are the most widely distributed of all vertebrate chromatophores and, in all classes, both their form and their function are remarkably consistent. They are long and thin and include dendritic processes that extend outward from the poles of the cell (Fig. 5–3). Epidermal melanophores are primarily agents of morphologic color change, which is accomplished through an association with adjacent epidermal cells. During prolonged exposure to stimuli that cause darkening of the animal, such

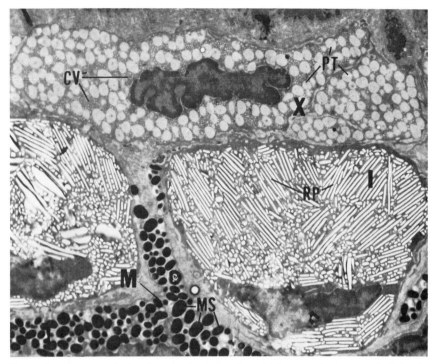

Figure 5–2. Electronphotomicrograph of the dorsal integument of an adult *Hyla cinerea* showing pigmentary organelles. Reflecting platelets (RP) are oriented in stacks in the iridophore (I). Melanophores (M) containing melanosomes (MS) are obvious. Xanthophores (X) containing pterinosomes (PT) and carotenoid vesicles (CV) are above iridophores. (From Bagnara, J. T., and Hadley, M. E.: Amer. Zool. 9:465, 1969.)

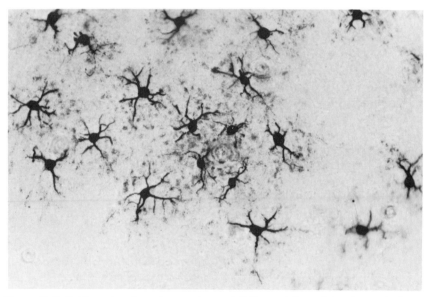

Figure 5–3. Epidermal melanophores of an adult *Rana pipiens*. Cytocrine melanin can be seen in epidermal cells near the thin dendritic processes. (Courtesy of M. E. Hadley, University of Arizona.)

as dark backgrounds, low temperature, or increased radiation, melanin synthesis occurs within the melanophore and epidermal melanophores respond by depositing excess melanin into adjacent epidermal cells.[25, 32] This takes place through the prominent cytocrine activity of melanophore dendrites that terminate in epidermal cells. Through this process, epidermal cells donate cytocrine melanin to the epidermis of all classes, to the hair of mammals, and to the bills and feathers of birds. It is considered that epidermal melanophores of man and other homoiotherms are homologous to those of lower vertebrates.

Iridophores. Iridescent pigment cells that function primarily through the reflection of light are called iridophores.[9] Their pigmentary organelles are called reflecting platelets (Fig. 5–2) and are composed of crystalline deposits of purines, notably guanine and hypoxanthine. Reflecting platelets are often arranged in stacks and the orientation and size of these organelles are the basis for the chromatic function of iridophores.[63] Iridophores are characteristic of poikilotherms; however, they have also been found in irises of birds.[24]

Xanthophores and Erythrophores. The bright-colored yellow, orange, or red chromatophores of lower vertebrates are called xanthophores or erythrophores.[9] Because the pigments of some of these cells are carotenoids that are soluble in lipid solvents, these chromatophores have been called "lipophores." It appears that pteridines are more prevalent xanthophore pigments which, unlike carotenoids, are synthesized by the xanthophores or erythrophores. Pteridines are found in pterinosomes,[44] organelles that are composed of a series of concentric lamellae, while carotenoids are contained in vesicles of various sizes (Fig. 5–2). Often pteridines and carotenoids are found in the same xanthophore or erythrophore.

INTEGRATED FUNCTION OF DERMAL
CHROMATOPHORES IN COLOR CHANGE

The primary function of dermal chromatophores in amphibians and reptiles is the regulation of rapid color changes. This is accomplished by the rapid mobilization of the pigment-containing organelles of the various chromatophores during physiologic color change. These color changes are brought about by coordinated responses of the three basic chromatophore types, which are so situated that they comprise an integral, functional unit, which has been designated the "dermal chromatophore unit"[12] (Fig. 5–4). Uppermost in the unit, just below the basement membrane, xanthophores are present, and immediately beneath this layer of yellow pigment are found iridophores. In frogs, the iridophore layer that forms the reflecting component of the unit consists of a single layer of cells. In lizards, it consists of many layers.[64, 69] The basal component of the unit is composed of a layer of melanophores that have dendrites extending upward. In frogs, these dendrites terminate in finger-like processes on the surface of the iridophore, just beneath the xanthophore layer. During adaptation to dark-colored backgrounds, melanosomes fill these processes, thus obscuring the reflect-

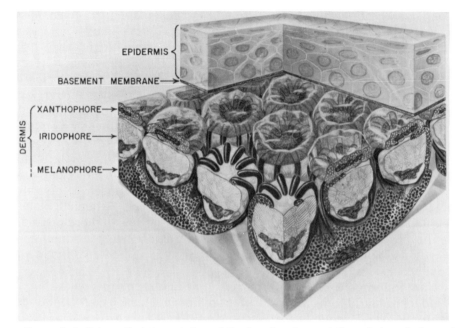

Figure 5–4. Schematic interpretation of the functional association of dermal chromatophores ("dermal chromatophore unit") from several anurans. Adaptation to a dark background is represented. (From Bagnara, J. T., Hadley, M. E., and Taylor, J. D.: Gen. Comp. Endocr., Suppl. 2, 1969.)

ing surface of the iridophore and leading to consequent darkening of the animal. When the animal lightens, melanosomes move from the terminal processes and occupy a perinuclear position. As a result, their dermal melanophores are almost completely obscured by overlying xanthophore and iridophore layers, and the animal appears light in color. The pigmentary role of the xanthophore layer relates to the establishment of the green color of many forms. In such animals, light waves leaving the iridophore surface appear blue because of tyndall scattering, and as the light waves pass through overlying yellow pigment cells, the shortest wavelengths are absorbed, so that finally the animal appears green.

THE ROLE OF THE PITUITARY

The fundamental role of the pituitary in controlling pigmentation was first revealed from experiments on frogs, during which the hypophysial primordium was removed from embryos at the early tailbud stage.[62] Light-colored or "silvery tadpoles" were derived from such embryos (Fig. 5–5), and it was found they could be darkened by being fed mammalian pituitaries. Examination of the skins of these silvery tadpoles indicated that iridophores were expanded (reflecting platelets dispersed) and melanophores were contracted (melanosomes aggregated), while dark tadpoles exhibited punctate

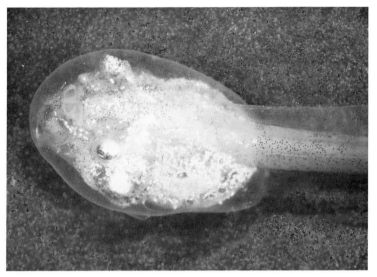

Figure 5–5. A larva of *Hyla regilla* developing from a gastrula which was treated with a 10 per cent solution of sucrose. The light coloration is due to a deficiency of the melanophore-stimulating hormone of the pars intermedia; the melanophores are punctate whereas the iridophores are expanded. The left eye is poorly developed and the external nares are fused. (From Eakin, R. M.: Science *111*, 1950.)

iridophores and melanophores in the dispersed state (Fig. 5–6). It was concluded that the pituitary contained a chromatophore-stimulating principle. Ultimately it was demonstrated that the source of this hormone is the pars intermedia, and following studies on teleost pituitaries, the substance was designated "intermedin."[72] Subsequently, during the process of purifying

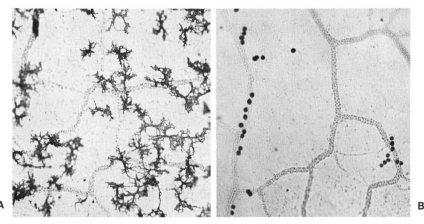

Figure 5–6. Integumentary melanophores of the frog *Hyla regilla*. *A*, Normal animal showing expanded melanophores; *B*, a similar mount from a sugar-treated embryo, showing hypoplasia and contracted state of the melanophores resulting from developmental failure of the pars intermedia. (From Driscoll, W. T. and Eakin, R. M.: J. Exp. Zool. *129*, 1955.)

this chromatophorotrophic substance it was referred to as MSH (melano-phore-stimulating hormone), and this designation has become more popular, although the term "intermedin" appears in the literature frequently.

For a time, the existence of a true MSH, separate from ACTH, was questioned. Because of contamination with MSH, ACTH preparations often had as much melanophore-stimulating activity as did MSH preparations. Definitive proof for the existence of MSH came with the availability of highly purified MSH and ACTH preparations and with the ultimate elucidation of the structures of these two hormones. Of course, as was discussed in Chapter 4, it is now known that the chromatophore-stimulating capacity of ACTH preparations is, in at least some measure, based upon the fact that the first 13 amino acids of the ACTH molecule comprise an amino acid sequence identical to that of the entire α-MSH molecule. It is nevertheless possible that ACTH plays a pigment-stimulating role in some vertebrates. In the goldfish, it seems that melanogenesis is a function of ACTH rather than of MSH[17]; however, in another teleost, *Fundulus,* ACTH has no melanogenic effect, but prolactin does.[53] In many species (*e.g.,* humans, the deer mouse, the weasel), both ACTH and MSH affect melanophores.[16, 40, 58] Resolution of the question of whether MSH or ACTH is the true chromatophorotrophin in these various examples is difficult because the structure of MSH has been revealed for only a few species, and none of these are normally used for studies on chromatophore stimulation. In any case, there can be no doubt that the pituitary plays a definitive role in chromatophore stimulation of vertebrates, as has been shown for many mammals, including man; for many fishes, including cyclostomes,[71] elasmobranchs, and teleosts (Fig. 5–1); for amphibians (Fig. 5–5); and for reptiles, such as the lizards *Anolis, Chameleo,* and *Phrynosoma,* and the rattlesnake.[30] In the weasel, MSH appears to play a role in the normal regulation of color pelage cycles.[58] The white winter coat results from the presence of low titers of MSH in the circulation during hair growth, while the brown summer coat results from MSH stimulation of melanophores in the hair follicles. Even in species such as the laboratory mouse, in whom the pituitary seems to play no pigmentary role, mutants exist which are sensitive to MSH[26] (Fig. 5–7).

Functions of MSH

Melanophore Stimulation.   The best known activity of MSH is to stimulate the dispersion of melanosomes within melanophores. In the absence of MSH, melanophores assume a punctate configuration, wherein melanosomes are aggregated in the perinuclear area of the cell. During stimulation by MSH, melanosomes are dispersed to peripheral regions of the chromatophore. Both dermal and epidermal melanophores respond to stimulation by MSH; a short period of stimulation leads to physiologic color change, while a prolonged exposure to the hormone is conducive to morphologic color change.

Iridophore Stimulation.   During the early experiments on tadpoles deprived of the pituitary gland (hypophysioprivic tadpoles), it was discov-

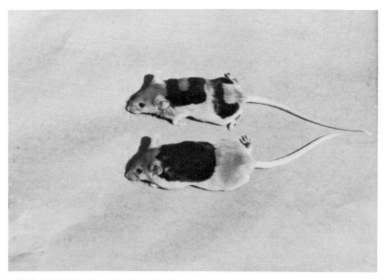

Figure 5–7. Melanization of pelage in A^y mice induced by alpha-MSH injection. Their coats were plucked in the patterns visible, and during MSH administration melanin was deposited in the growing hairs. (Courtesy of I. I. Geschwind, University of California at Davis.)

ered that the expanded iridophores of hypophysioprivic larvae could be made to aggregate by administration of pituitary extracts. Subsequently, it was demonstrated that iridophore contraction was brought about through the action of MSH.[3] Thus, administration of MSH darkened tadpoles and adult frogs by causing opposite responses of two different pigment cells: concentration of pigment in the iridophores and dispersion of pigment in melanophores. It was surprising to learn that both of these events require the same site on the MSH molecule.[7] This was demonstrated by making use of the facts that the entire MSH molecule is not essential for melanophore-stimulating activity and that some melanophore response can be produced by the centrally located amino acid sequence, His-Phe-Arg-Try-Gly. Injection of this and longer MSH peptides into hypophysioprivic larvae induced iridophore contraction and, in every case, the iridophore response was always paralleled by melanophore expansion.

The role of iridophores in physiologic color change is pronounced, and the morphologic responses of iridophores to MSH administration are also exceedingly prominent. Hypophysioprivic tadpoles injected with high concentrations of MSH may lose most of their purine pigments.[3] At the ultrastructural level, this loss is demonstrated by a diminution in the size and thickness of the reflecting platelets.[63]

Xanthophore Stimulation. The participation of xanthophores in physiologic color change is most obvious in fishes.[54] For the most part, in elasmobranchs and teleosts maintained on light backgrounds, xanthophores are punctate. Hypophysectomy has the same effect, while hypophysial extracts bring about dispersal of xanthophore pigments, as does exposure to dark backgrounds. In some species, xanthophores are unresponsive to

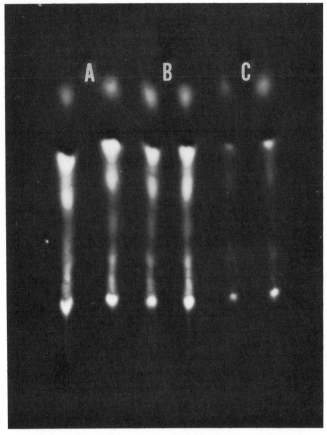

Figure 5–8. Chromatogram of skin squashes of *Pleurodeles waltlii* larvae showing separated pteridine pigments, which appear as fluorescent spots under ultraviolet illumination. *A,* Normal; *B,* partially hypophysioprivic; *C,* hypophysioprivic. The normal larvae have much more fluorescence than do the hypophysioprivic ones. (From Bagnara, J. T.: Responses of pigment cells of amphibians to intermedin. *In* M. Fontaine [ed.]: La spécificité zoologique des hormones hypophysaires et de leurs activitiés. Paris, Centre National de la Recherche Scientifique, 1969, p. 153.)

MSH, but do respond to the administration of prolactin.[60] Xanthophore responses in physiologic color change of other poikilotherms are not prominent; however, at least one example occurs in amphibians, in whom it has been shown that punctate xanthophores can be caused to disperse their pigments under the influence of MSH.[10]

The endocrine control of xanthophore expression in morphologic color change is best known from studies on amphibian larvae (Fig. 5–8). Larvae of both frogs and salamanders that have been deprived of their pituitary gland contain much smaller amounts of pteridine pigments in their xanthophores than do intact animals.[5] Administration of MSH to these hypophysioprivic larvae constitutes an effective replacement therapy, for it elevates pteridine levels to essentially normal values. This is especially significant considering the fact that the effect is just the opposite of that which occurs with respect to purines in the reflecting platelets or iridophores. Because pteridines and purines are chemically related and have a common synthetic pathway,[9] it appears that the MSH level in the circulation determines which of these pigment classes is to be synthesized. The morphologic effect of MSH on xanthophores is manifested in the appearance of the xanthophore. Thus, xanthophores of hypophysioprivic salamander larvae contain thin, delicate processes that stand out individually, while those of normal larvae have broad "arms" that spread out over a large surface area. Thus far, it has not been demonstrated at the ultrastructural level that pterinosomes are affected by either the removal of the hypophysis or the administration of MSH.

Hypothalamic Control of the Pars Intermedia

Because of its profound chromatophore stimulating activities, MSH has long been considered to be the major hormone used in vertebrate color adaptation, and it has provided the basis for the unihormonal theory of chromatophore control.[49] In essence, this theory proclaims that during adaptation to white backgrounds, little or no MSH is released from the pars intermedia, leading to a decrease in circulating MSH levels and a conse-

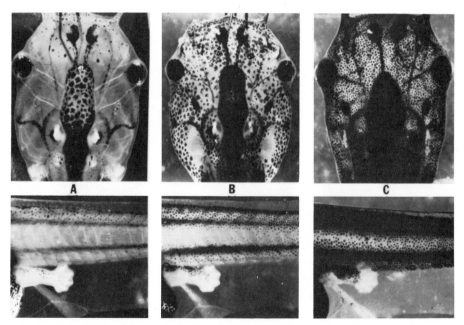

Figure 5–9. Head and base of tail of *Xenopus* larvae at stage 55. *A,* On a white background since stage 20. *B,* Normal control. *C,* Separation of the hypothalamus from the hypophysis by section of the prosencephalon at stage 29. Secretion of MSH is minimal in *A,* leading to a reduction in melanophore response and number. In *C,* MSH secretion is uninhibited, leading to an augmentation of melanophore response and number. (From Pehlemann, F. W.: Zool. Anz., Suppl. 29, 1967.)

quent lack of chromatophore stimulation (Fig. 5–9). Thus, melanophores become punctate and iridophores expand. Adaptation to black backgrounds leads to MSH release; consequently, melanophore pigments disperse and iridophore pigments aggregate.

In order to adapt to alterations in background, it is necessary that the animal perceive these background changes. It is generally agreed that the lateral eyes are involved, but it is not really understood how the retina discriminates among background differences. Ultimately, perception of background is expressed in terms of the release of MSH from the pars intermedia, and the vehicle for this expression is the hypothalamus. Unlike its relationship to other adenohypophysial hormones, the hypothalamus is believed to control MSH release by a mechanism of inhibition. Accordingly, MSH is released from the pars intermedia spontaneously until its release is suppressed by the hypothalamus. In this way, in animals on a black background, MSH is being released freely, but in those on a white background, release is being inhibited by the hypothalamus.

During adaptation to a dark-colored background, pars intermedia cells are characterized by an increase in the rough endoplasmic reticulum with a dilation of its cisternae, and by a decrease in the number of secretory granules present (Fig. 5–10). On light-colored backgrounds such cells show a reduction in the amount of rough endoplasmic reticulum, and their cyto-

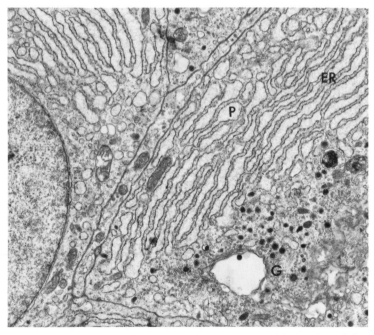

Figure 5–10. Pars intermedia secretory cells from 14 day black-adapted *Rana pipiens.* Cells show an increase in the stacks of rER with a filamentous precipitate in the dilated cisternae; electron dense secretory granules and possible junctional vesicles are around the Golgi complex. ×14,182. (Courtesy of E. K. Perryman.)

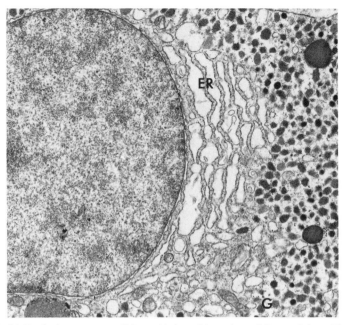

Figure 5–11. Typical secretory cell from 14 day white-adapted *Rana pipiens.* The cytoplasm is filled with granules, the rER is reduced in amount, and the filamentous precipitate is absent. ×14,746. (Courtesy of E. K. Perryman.)

plasm is filled with granules (Fig. 5–11). Presumably, the latter are a reflection of a stored hormone product and are present in reduced numbers in cells on dark-background adapted animals because of a rapid release of MSH. That the granule-containing cells of the pars intermedia contain MSH has been suggested from cyto-immunological experiments in which anti-alpha and anti-beta MSH antibodies interact specifically with the secretory granules present in pars intermedia cells.[19] Moreover, such granules have been isolated by differential centrifugation and have been shown by bioassay to contain MSH-like activity.[38]

This mechanism of hypothalamic control of pars intermedia function can be used to explain ontogenetic changes in the adaptive response of tadpoles. It is known that during the development of larvae there is a distinct point, for each species, at which the ability to adapt to background is acquired.[10] Before this point, the larvae are referred to as being in a primary stage in which they cannot respond to alterations in background. It is considered that they have not yet acquired the capacity to inhibit MSH release and thus remain darkly pigmented whether they are on dark or light backgrounds. Older larvae that are able to adapt to background changes are considered to be in a secondary stage that is based upon the maturation of the mechanism whereby MSH release can be inhibited.

The concept that MSH release is under inhibitory control is derived from a number of experiments involving the isolation of the pituitary either by hypophysial transplantation or by hypophysial stalk section[23, 51] (Fig. 5–

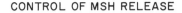

CONTROL OF MSH RELEASE

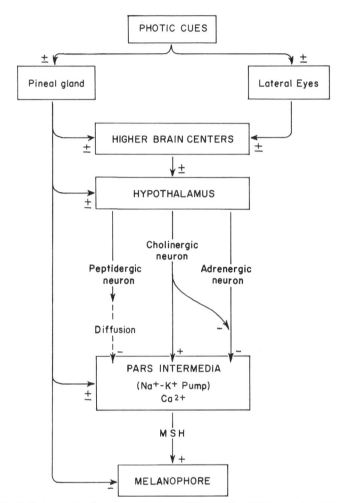

Figure 5–12. Scheme for the control of pars intermedia MSH secretion. Both stimulatory (+) and inhibitory (−) inputs to MSH release are indicated. (From Hadley and Bagnara, 1975)

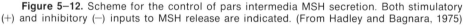

11). Hypophysioprivic tadpoles containing transplants of the whole adeno-hypophysis or of the pars intermedia alone become intensely dark. The same is true for tadpoles or adults suffering hypothalamic damage.

    The nature of the hypothalamic inhibitory action on the pars intermedia is not yet resolved; however, this has been a subject of much investigation and many concepts have emerged.[10, 29] The integration of some of these concepts is presented in the scheme shown in Figure 5–12. It has been thought that a neurosecretory mechanism is involved or that normal nerves mediate the response. Studies with the electron microscope have demonstrated the presence of nerve endings in the pars intermedia, and it has been suggested that their synaptic vesicles contain norepinephrine.[36] These observations, taken together with the demonstration, by the flourescence technique, that catecholamine-containing nerve endings are present in the pars intermedia of adult amphibians,[22] lend strong support to the concept that hypothalamic control of the pars intermedia is mediated by monoamines released from adrenergic neurons terminating in the pars intermedia.[37] The viewpoint that catecholamines inhibit MSH release has been supported by a variety of studies and possibly explains why the administration of epinephrine and norepinephrine to intact amphibians causes blanching, while immersion of skins from these animals in solutions of these catecholamines has little effect on their pigment cells.[28]

While the view of adrenergic inhibition of MSH release is attractive, the matter is much more complicated. For example, there is evidence that acetylcholine can cause MSH release; and on this basis a cholinergic pathway may somehow be involved in the hypothalamic control of the pars intermedia. Even more perplexing, it has been shown clearly that the pars intermedia of some lizards is not innervated.[57] In such forms it is possible that peptidergic neurons might mediate pars intermedia activity through the release of a diffusible inhibitory neurosecretion.

Many studies on the control of MSH release have involved *in vitro* incubation of the pars intermedia.[33] From such experiments it was revealed that the Ca^{2+} ion is required for MSH release, and subsequent investigation disclosed the existence of a Na^+-K^+ pump. Thus, it has been revealed that the release of MSH from the pars intermedia utilizes an active transport mechanism.

Some interesting studies have been made on *Rana pipiens* after surgically removing the primordium of the posterior hypothalamus at the open neurula stage (stage 13 – 14). Tadpoles resulting from the operated neurulae lack a pars intermedia, infundibulum, median eminence, and pars nervosa. The pars distalis, on the other hand, differentiates independently and lies below the brain, without connecting to any part of it. The operated animals grew at about the normal rate, suggesting that the adenohypophysis produced "growth" substance at a normal rate, notwithstanding the lack of normal connections with the hypothalamus. As might be expected, the hypothalectomized tadpoles were light in color since they lacked a pars intermedia as a source of MSH. Observations on the thyroid indicated that the hypothalectomized animals secreted subnormal amounts of thyroid-stimulating hormone[34] (Fig. 7 – 12).

ADAPTATION TO DARKNESS

Larval stages, but not adults, of most amphibians undergo a marked blanching when maintained in darkness. A similar response is displayed by many fishes. It is likely that blanching is due in some measure to a decrease in MSH release in darkness, but for the most part it is believed that the principal effect results from the release of melatonin (N-acetyl-5-methoxytryptamine) from the pineal. This hypothetical scheme, advanced by Bagnara[4, 6] and supported by others,[15] suggests that under conditions of darkness, the pineal is stimulated to release melatonin, presumably a pineal hormone, into the general circulation. Melatonin exerts a profound contracting effect on dermal melanophores leading to rapid blanching. The involvement of the pineal in this response relates to two aspects of its physiology, light reception and endocrine function. Morphologic and electrophysiologic studies have clearly established that the pineal can function as a photoreceptor,[21] but its role as an endocrine organ is more obscure, despite the fact that circumstantial evidence strongly indicates that this is the case.

The first evidence indicating that the pineal contains a humoral agent comes from the classic experiments of McCord and Allen,[41] who made the important discovery that tadpoles underwent a profound blanching when they were fed mammalian pineals. Because prevailing thought at that time excluded the possibility that the pineal was involved in pigmentary changes, they dismissed their data as being purely of pharmacologic significance. The presence of a melanophore-stimulating agent in the pineal was not forgotten, however, and over the years others extracted mammalian pineal glands until finally Lerner and his colleagues isolated a potent melanosome-aggregating agent from beef pineal glands, which they identified as melatonin.[39] Subsequently, this indole has been found in the pineals of other mammals (*e.g.,* monkey, cow, rat, birds, and amphibians). Of great interest is the fact that relatively large amounts are found in the lateral eyes.[56] For example, the first reports of the discovery of melatonin in extracts of *Xenopus*[67] were followed by the observation that this substance was located largely in the lateral eyes.[13] The lateral eyes as well as the pineals contain all the substrates and enzymes essential for the synthesis of melatonin. Chemically, melatonin consists of an indole nucleus, an N-acetylated side chain, and a methoxy group (Fig. 5–13). Melatonin is synthesized from serotonin (5-hydroxytryptamine) in the following manner: (1) An N-acetylating enzyme converts serotonin to N-acetylserotonin; (2) the latter compound is O-methylated through the action of hydroxyindole-O-methyltransferase (HIOMT). Serotonin is metabolized to 5-hydroxyindole acetaldehyde by the enzyme monoamine oxidase (MAO). The activity of this enzyme in the destruction of serotonin and that of HIOMT in the O-methylation of N-

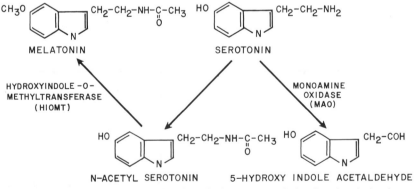

Figure 5–13. The synthesis of melatonin from serotonin by the pineal gland.

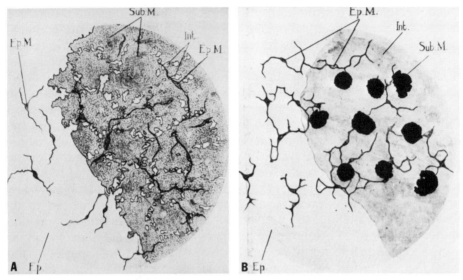

Figure 5–14. Whole mount preparations from dorsal skin of *Rana pipiens* tadpoles. *A,* Normal tadpole: The epidermal melanophores (Ep.M.) of the epidermis (Ep.) are expanded, as are the subepidermal (dermal) melanophores (Sub.M.) of the integument (Int.). *B,* The feeding of pineal extracts to tadpoles causes a rapid blanching of the skin, which results from dermal melanophore contraction. The epidermal melanophores are unresponsive and remain expanded. (From McCord, C. P., and Allen, F. P.: J. Exp. Zool. *23*:207, 1917.)

acetylserotonin provide convenient vehicles for controlling the amount of melatonin present in an organism at any one time.

The concept that the body-blanching reaction is under pineal control is based on the fact that the reaction occurs in blinded tadpoles, but is abolished by "pinealectomy." Temporal events in the onset of and recovery from the reaction are consistent with an endocrine mediation of the response. Most important of all is the fact that pigmentary changes induced by the action of melatonin duplicate the response that occurs in darkness.[11] For example, in darkness, only the dermal melanophores of primary stage tadpoles respond; the epidermal melanophores and iridophores remain essentially unchanged. Since it is known that dermal melanophores, but not epidermal melanophores and iridophores, are affected by melatonin, it seems reasonable to attribute the blanching induced by darkness to melatonin (Fig. 5–14). This argument is strengthened by the fact that such primary stage larvae have not yet acquired the capacity to inhibit MSH release from the pituitary. The persistence of dendritic epidermal melanophores and punctate iridophores during the body-blanching reaction of these primary stage tadpoles indicates that circulating levels of MSH are still high.

The body blanching that ensues when secondary stage tadpoles are placed in darkness is attributable both to the release of melatonin and to the "turning off" of MSH release. The latter is witnessed by the fact that body-blanched, secondary-stage larvae may exhibit partially dendritic iridophores and partially contracted epidermal melanophores. It is not known which mechanism, that through the pineal or that through the pituitary, is most "important" in regulating the body-blanching reaction of secondary stage tadpoles; however, it is certain that the reaction can occur in the absence of the pituitary. This was demonstrated in experiments in which hypophysioprivic larvae, darkened by immersion in MSH, showed a definite body blanching when placed in the dark.[8] Probably this blanching resulted from the release of melatonin in a quantity sufficient to overcome the effects of MSH. These observations on hypophysioprivic larvae are strong arguments against the view that the amphibian body-blanching reaction results from a pineal inhibition of MSH release. Any inhibition of MSH release that occurs when larvae are placed in darkness appears to be a function of the lateral eyes. This is shown by the fact that MSH levels of blinded secondary-stage larvae do not change under conditions of darkness, as witnessed by the absence of any alteration in the state of epidermal melanophores or iridophores. Only dermal melanophores of these larvae contract; presumably this is in response to the release of melatonin. At present, the possibility that melatonin "turns off" MSH release cannot be completely discounted, for this may be the case in some mammals.[59] It has been shown that the implantation of melatonin into male weasels, who should be acquiring a brown coat following the spring molt, results instead in the growth of a white coat. Similar melatonin-implanted animals with pituitary autografts under the kidney capsule grow a brown coat, suggesting that melatonin does not act at the level of the pituitary. It has been suggested from these experiments that melatonin acts on the hypothalamus, causing the release of an MSH-inhibiting factor, which prevents the elaboration of MSH and thus leads to the growth of a white coat.

In the light of all the available data, the hypothesis that the body-blanching reaction of amphibian larvae is mediated by the pineal seems rather convincing. However, it must be emphasized that this mechanism is restricted to larvae and does not persist into adulthood. Melanophores of adult fishes and amphibians are generally unresponsive to melatonin,[28] and the same seems to be true of *Anolis,* the only lizard so far tested in this regard.[30] Moreover, adult amphibians generally do not blanch in darkness. These observations preclude the suggestion that melatonin might mediate adaptation to white backgrounds. This conclusion is reinforced by the observation that hypophysectomized adult frogs retain the ability to adapt to a white background.

MECHANISMS OF HORMONE ACTION ON PIGMENT CELLS

While it appears certain that MSH is the major hormonal agent controlling pigment cells, our knowledge of the mechanism of its action is much less certain. The same can be said for other hormones that exert pigmentary effects, especially those such as catecholamines, which may induce one response in one species and another in a different species. Fortunately, because of the advancement of the two important concepts mentioned in

Chapter 2 (the first messenger–second messenger hypothesis and the adrenergic receptor scheme), we are now in a better position to understand mechanisms of hormone action on pigment cells.

The First Messenger–Second Messenger Hypothesis of MSH Action

According to this hypothesis, hormones such as MSH are thought to act as first messengers, bringing about their effects by promoting an intracellular increase of a second messenger, cyclic AMP, which in turn is re-

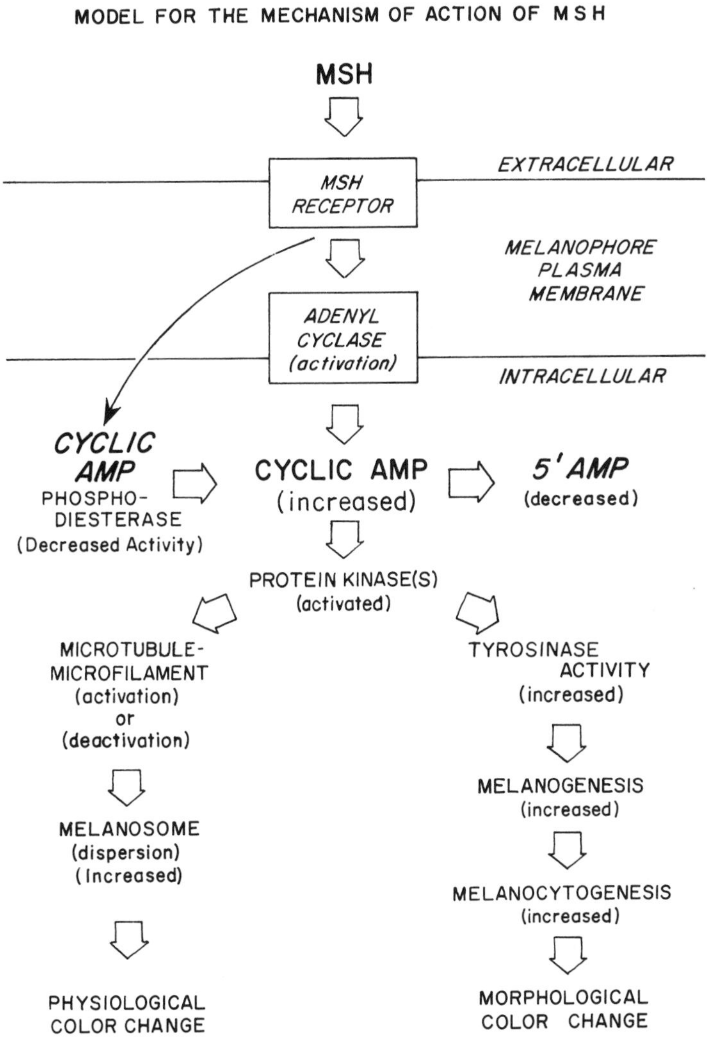

MODEL FOR THE MECHANISM OF ACTION OF M S H

Figure 5–15. Model for the mechanism of action of MSH on vertebrate melanophores. (Hadley and Bagnara, 1975)

sponsible for the particular response of the effector cell (Fig. 5–15). Thus, experimental administration of cyclic AMP or its more permeable dibutyryl derivative to the system should lead to a response that mimics that of the first messenger. In accordance with this scheme, it is known that cyclic AMP or the dibutyryl compound mimics the action of MSH by bringing about the dispersion of melanosomes in melanophores and the aggregation of reflecting platelets in iridophores.[10] These two responses, different as they may be, occur in a parallel way following stimulation by MSH peptides. This parallelism, which has always seemed a little mysterious, can now be explained adequately through the function of the second messenger. Probably both iridophores and melanophores contain similar or identical MSH receptor sites. This could account for the fact that both iridophores and melanophores can be stimulated in a parallel way. The specificity of the response, namely aggregation of reflecting platelets and dispersion of melanosomes, could then be explained in terms of the specific interaction between the second messenger and the specific functional elements of the particular chromatophore that are responsible for the movements of reflecting platelets or melanosomes.

If the intracellular level of the second messenger, cyclic AMP, is indeed responsible for evoking the responses of both iridophores and melanophores, it should be possible to effect these chromatophore responses by altering the activity of enzymes involved in the synthesis or breakdown of cyclic AMP. This is the case, for it is known that methylxanthines such as caffeine or theophylline, which are known inhibitors of phosphodiesterase

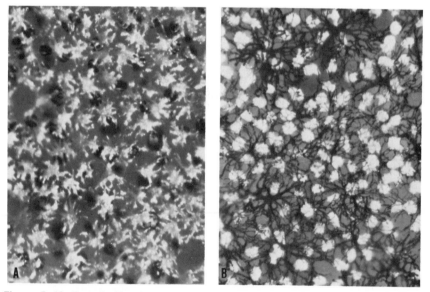

Figure 5–16. Dorsal skins from adult *Rana pipiens* photographed with reflected light. *A,* Control maintained in Ringer solution. Iridophores, which appear silvery, are expanded; dermal melanophores are punctate. *B,* Experimental skin in Ringer solution containing caffeine. Iridophores are contracted to the punctate state, melanophores are well expanded.

(the enzyme that breaks down cyclic AMP), can cause iridophore contraction and melanophore expansion[10] (Fig. 5–16). Presumably, the action of these methylxanthines leads to an increase in the intracellular levels of cyclic AMP, which in turn brings about these specific chromatophore effects.[1]

The Role of Adrenergic Receptors

Although it is clearly established that MSH is the major humoral factor regulating vertebrate chromatophores, other hormones also play important roles. Especially significant are the catecholamines, epinephrine and norepinephrine, that are important in bringing about the rapidly occurring chromatophore events that form the basis of "excitement pallor" and "excitement darkening."

Catecholamines are considered to mediate their effects through two types of receptors, *alpha* and *beta,* each of which evokes responses that are antagonistic to the other. Thus, the response of an adrenergic system is based upon the relative amounts of the two receptor types present. A responsive tissue may contain only one type or the other, it may contain both alpha and beta receptors, or both receptors may be present in different quantities. Recently, it has been demonstrated that both alpha and beta receptors are present on amphibian chromatophores and that there is a wide variation in the receptor pattern in the chromatophores of any one species or race.[31] The emergence of the receptor concept has made it possible to elucidate some previously unexplained effects that were indeed paradoxical. For example, while both epinephrine and norepinephrine lighten the skins of adult *R. pipiens* these catecholamines darken the skins of *Xenopus* and the spade-foot toad, *Scaphiopus.*[27] These different responses to the same compounds are thought to be due to the presence of alpha receptors in *R. pipiens* and the predominance of beta receptors in *Xenopus* and *Scaphiopus.* Stimulation of alpha adrenergic receptors leads to paling, while stimulation of beta adrenergic receptors causes darkening.

The total color change following receptor stimulation includes the participation of both iridophores and melanophores; thus, it would seem that the adrenergic receptor patterns of these chromatophore types should complement one another. This seems to be the case in *R. pipiens,* wherein catecholamine-induced paling results from stimulation of alpha receptors on melanophores that mediate melanosome aggregation and of alpha receptors on iridophores that mediate reflecting-platelet dispersion. In *Scaphiopus,* in whom darkening ensues after adrenergic stimulation, it seems that beta receptors are present on only the melanophores, for iridophores remain unchanged.[27] This is reminiscent of the paling response induced in *Anolis* by catecholamines, wherein stimulation of alpha adrenergic receptors on melanophores causes melanosome aggregation, while iridophores remain unaffected.[30] In assessing the role of adrenergic receptors on poikilotherm color changes, it seems obvious that the system is complicated by variations in the pattern of distribution of receptors on the various chromatophores. It is even more difficult to understand *in vivo* responses because of additional participation of the catecholamines in the control of MSH release.

The concept of receptor stimulation and pigment cell response should not be confined to alpha and beta receptors, for it is evident that MSH reacts with a receptor to initiate the chain of events ultimately leading to the buildup of intracellular concentrations of cyclic AMP. Moreover, it is possible that a relationship may exist between adrenergic receptors and cyclic AMP. During melanosome aggregation following alpha receptor stimulation, it has been shown that intracellular levels of cyclic AMP decline.[1] In addition, in many other tissues it is known that beta receptor stimulation is accompanied by an elevation of cyclic AMP concentrations, and the same is probably true for melanophores. There is evidence that receptors for MSH and beta receptors are both components of the plasma membrane; however, the structural and functional relationships of these receptors are not yet understood.[50] Possibly, prostaglandins are involved.[68] These substances are known to disperse melanophores, and they may act in a position intermediary between the first messenger and adenylate cyclase (Fig. 5–15).

Intracellular Movement of Pigment Granules

Whatever the mechanism of chromatophore stimulation (*e.g.,* hormonal, nervous, direct action of light), the ultimate expression of color change is based upon the aggregation or dispersion of pigment-containing organelles within the chromatophore. So far, the mechanism or mechanisms of how this is accomplished has escaped elucidation. However, there are some theories which may prove helpful in the resolution of the problem.

One of the older theories entertains the possibility that melanosome movements are related to sol-gel changes in the chromatophore cytoplasm.[43] In support of this contention, it has been observed that increases in hydrostatic pressure cause melanosome dispersion in fish melanophores, while factors that stabilize the gelated state counterbalance this effect. Colchicine, which has been shown to cause melanosome dispersion in frog melanophores[70] is well-known for its action in disrupting the mitotic spindle apparatus. Possibly the melanosome dispersing effects of colchicine relate to its ability to cause solation of the melanophore cytoplasm.[42] It is possible that sol-gel changes in the chromatophore cytoplasm are related to the role of microtubules. It has been demonstrated that in the melanophores of *Fundulus,* arrays of microtubules are oriented in the dendritic processes in a manner parallel to the movement of melanosomes. On this basis, it has been suggested that they play a role in the intracellular migration of pigmentary organelles.[14]

Microfilaments have also been considered to play a role in melanosome mobilization, especially in the process of dispersion. In part, this concept is based upon the fact that cytochalasin B, a substance known to interfere selectively with microfilament function, inhibits melanosome dispersion in response to either MSH or cyclic AMP. Investigations of the incidence and the localization of both microfilaments and microtubules have revealed a wide variation between species, and it has not been possible to demonstrate a general relationship among poikilotherms between melanosome movements and the presence or absence of either microtubules or microfilaments.[45]

A considerable body of additional data relating to the intracellular migration of pigments is available, but much of this evidence is difficult to place in proper perspective. So many different species have been used that generalizations are difficult to make. Two particular areas of investigation that hold promise of providing important new information relate to (1) the role of sulfhydryl agents in chromatophore responses, and (2) the energy requirements necessary for these chromatophore events to occur.

In considering the action of MSH on chromatophores, most studies have dealt with physiologic color changes, those events involving the intracellular migration of pigment granules. In addition, it is known that pigment synthesis is also greatly affected by the action of this hormone, for events involving pigment synthesis *in vivo* are related to prolonged aggregation or dispersion of pigment-containing organelles. It is possible that this is a fortuitous connection really based on separate manifestations of MSH stimulation (Fig. 5–15). For example, it has been shown *in vitro* that tyrosinase activity and subsequent melanin synthesis can be stimulated in mouse melanoma cells, a system that does not involve melanosome dispersion.

EXTRAPIGMENTARY EFFECTS OF MSH

While the evidence seems to show that the principal role of MSH concerns the control of chromatophore responses, the possibility arises that MSH may have other functions. In this regard, it is most interesting to note that while the majority of pigmentary effects ascribed to MSH relate to poikilotherms, these effects are induced experimentally by the employment of MSH extracted from homoiotherms. While mammalian melanophores respond to MSH in some degree, the response is neither general nor is it pronounced. On these grounds it seems likely that MSH may play roles which have hitherto escaped attention. There are several reports alluding to extrapigmentary functions of MSH;[48] notably, thyrotrophic action, steroidogenic action, lipolytic action, antigonadal action, interactions with sex steroids, induction of menstrual bleeding, natriuretic action, hypocalcemic action, aqueous flare response, positive chronotrophic action, action on monosynaptic potentials, induction of stretching and yawning, action on knifefish electrical discharge, hypersensitivity in mice, actions on conditioned reflexes, and electroencephalographic actions. Among the most thoroughly studied of these are the behavioral actions of MSH and ACTH peptides.[18] Such studies have revealed that amino acids 4–7, common sequences in the MSH and ACTH molecules, are important in the acquisition and extinction of conditioned behavior.

REFERENCES

1. Abe, K., Butcher, R. W., Nicholson, W. E., Baird, C. E., Liddle, R. A., and Liddle, G. W.: Adenosine 3',5'-monophosphate (cyclic AMP) as the mediator of the actions of melanocyte stimulating hormone (MSH) and norepinephrine on the frog skin. Endocrinology 84:362, 1969.
2. Bagnara, J. T.: Hypophysectomy and the tail-darkening reaction in *Xenopus*. Proc. Soc. Exp. Biol. Med. 94:572, 1957.
3. Bagnara, J. T.: Hypophyseal control of guanophores in anuran larvae. J. Exp. Zool. 137:265, 1958.
4. Bagnara, J. T.: Pineal regulation of the body lightening reaction in amphibian larvae. Science 132:1481, 1960.
5. Bagnara, J. T.: Chromatotropic hormone pteridines and amphibian pigmentation. Gen. Comp. Endocr. 1:124, 1961.
6. Bagnara, J. T.: The pineal and the body lightening reaction of larval amphibians. Gen. Comp. Endocr. 3:86, 1963.
7. Bagnara, J. T.: Stimulation of melanophores and guanophores by melanophore-stimulating hormone peptides. Gen. Comp. Endocr. 4:290, 1964a.
8. Bagnara, J. T.: Independent actions of pineal and hypophysis in the regulation of chromatophores of anuran larvae. Gen. Comp. Endocr. 4:299, 1964b.
9. Bagnara, J. T.: Cytology and cytophysiology of non-melanophore pigment cells. Int. Rev. Cytol. 20: 173, 1966.
10. Bagnara, J. T., and Hadley, M. E.: Chromatophores and Color Change: The Comparative Physiology of Animal Pigmentation. Englewood Cliffs, N. J., Prentice-Hall, Inc., 1973.
11. Bagnara, J. T., and Hadley, M. E.: Endocrinology of the amphibian pineal. Amer. Zool. 10: 201, 1970.
12. Bagnara, J. T., Taylor, J. D., and Hadley, M. E.: The dermal chromatophore unit. J. Cell Biol. 38:67, 1968.
13. Baker, P. C.: Melatonin levels in developing *Xenopus laevis*. Comp. Biochem. Physiol. 28: 1387, 1969.
14. Bikle, D., Tilney, L. G., and Porter, K. R.: Microtubules and pigment migration in melanophores of *Fundulus heteroclitus* L. Protoplasma 61:322, 1966.
15. Bogenschütz, H.: Extraokulare Steuerung des Farbwechsels bei Qualquappen. Experientia 21:451, 1965.
16. Bronson, F. H., and Clarke, S. H.: Adrenalectomy and coat color in deer mice. Science 154:1349, 1966.
17. Chavin, W.: Pituitary hormones in melanogenesis. *In* M. Gordon (ed.): Pigment Cell Biology. New York, Academic Press, 1959, p. 63.
18. DeWied, D.: Pituitary-adrenal system hormones and behavior. *In* F. O. Schmitt and F. G. Worden (eds.): The Neurosciences Third Study Program. Cambridge, Mass., MIT Press, 1974, p. 653.
19. Doerr-Schott, J.: Cyto-immunochemical study of the hypophysial cells of amphibians by light- and electron-microscopy. Fortschr. Zool. 22:245, 1974.
20. DuShane, G. P.: An experimental study of the origin of pigment cells in Amphibia. J. Exp. Zool. 72:1, 1935.
21. Eakin, R. M.: Photoreceptors in the amphibian frontal organ. Proc. Nat. Acad. Sci. 47:1084, 1961.
22. Enemar, A., and Falck, B.: On the presence of adrenergic nerves in the pars intermedia of the frog, *Rana temporaria*. Gen. Comp. Endocr. 5:577, 1965.
23. Etkin, W.: Hypothalamic inhibition of the pars intermedia activity in the frog. Gen. Comp. Endocr., Suppl. 1, 70, 1962.
24. Ferris, W. R., and Bagnara, J. T.: Iridophores in the iris of doves. J. Invest Derm. 54:86, 1970.
25. Fitzpatrick, T. B., and Breathnach, A. S.: Das epidermale Melanin-Einheit-System. Derm. Wschr. 147:481, 1963.
26. Geschwind, I. I.: Change in hair color in mice induced by injection of alpha-MSH. Endocrinology 79:1165, 1966.
27. Goldman, J. M., and Hadley, M. E.: The beta adrenergic receptor and cyclic 3',5'-adenosine monophosphate: Possible roles in the regulation of melanophore responses of the spadefoot toad, *Scaphiopus couchi*. Gen. Comp. Endocr. 13:151, 1969.
28. Hadley, M. E., and Bagnara, J. T.: Integrated nature of chromatophore responses in the *in vitro* frog skin bioassay. Endocrinology 84:69, 1969.
29. Hadley, M. E., and Bagnara, J. T.: Regulation of release and mechanism of action of MSH. Amer. Zool. 15 (Suppl. 1):81, 1975.

30. Hadley, M. E., and Goldman, J. M.: Physiological color changes in reptiles. Amer. Zool. 9: 489, 1969.
31. Hadley, M. E., and Goldman, J. M.: Adrenergic receptors and geographical variation in Rana pipiens chromatophore responses. Am. J. Physiol. 219:72, 1970.
32. Hadley, M. E., and Quevedo, W. C., Jr.: The role of epidermal melanocytes in adaptive color changes in amphibians. Advan. Biol. Skin 8:337, 1967.
33. Hadley, M. E., Bower, Sr. A., and Hruby, V. J.: Regulation of melanophore-stimulating hormone (MSH) release. Yale J. Biol. Med. 46:602, 1973.
34. Hanaoka, Y.: The effect of hypothalectomy at open neurula embryos in Rana pipiens. Amer. Zool. 3:509, 1963.
35. Horstadius, S.: The neural crest. London, Oxford Univ. Press, 1950.
36. Iturriza, F. C.: Electron-microscopic study of the pars intermedia of the pituitary of the toad, Bufo arenarum. Gen. Comp. Endocr. 4:494, 1964.
37. Iturriza, F. C.: Monoamines and control of pars intermedia in the toad pituitary. Gen. Comp. Endocr. 6:19, 1966.
38. Kikuyama, S., and Yasumasu, I.: Separation of granules containing melanophore stimulating hormone from the frog (Rana catesbeiana) pars intermedia. Endocr. Jap. 19:549, 1972.
39. Lerner, A. B., Case, J. D., Takahashi, Y., Lee, T. H., and Mori, W.: Isolation of melatonin; the pineal gland factor that lightens melanocytes. J. Amer. Chem. Soc. 80:2587, 1958.
40. Lerner, A. B., and McGuire, J. S.: Melanocyte stimulating hormone and adrenocorticotrophic hormone. New Eng. J. Med. 270:539, 1964.
41. McCord, C. P., and Allen, F. P.: Evidences associating pineal gland function with alterations in pigmentation. J. Exp. Zool. 23:207, 1917.
42. Malawista, S. E.: On the action of colchicine. J. Exp. Med. 122:361, 1965.
43. Marsland, D. A.: Mechanism of pigment displacement in unicellular chromatophores. Biol. Bull. 87:252, 1944.
44. Matsumoto, J.: Studies of fine structure and cytochemical properties of erythrophores in swordtail, Xiphophorus helleri, with special reference to their pigment granules. J. Cell Biol. 27:493, 1965.
45. Moellman, G., McGuire, J., and Lerner, A. B.: Intracellular dynamics and the fine structure of melanocytes. Yale J. Biol. Med. 46:337, 1973.
46. Moyer, F. H.: Genetic effects on melanosome fine structure and ontogeny in normal and malignant cells. Ann. N. Y. Acad. Sci. 100:584, 1963.
47. Murphy, D. B., and Tilney, L. G.: The role of microtubules in the movement of pigment granules in teleost melanophores. J. Cell Biol. 61:757, 1974.
48. Novales, R. R.: Actions of melanocyte-stimulating hormone. In R. O. Greep and E. B. Astwood (eds.): Handbook of Physiology, Section 7, Endocrinology, Volume IV, Part 2. Baltimore, Williams & Wilkins Co., 1974, p. 347.
49. Parker, G. H.: Animal colour changes and their neurohumours. London, Cambridge Univ. Press, 1948.
50. Pawelek, J., Wong, G., Sansone, M., and Morowitz, J.: Molecular controls in mammalian pigmentation. Yale J. Biol. Med. 46:430, 1973.
51. Pehlemann, F. W.: Experimentelle Beeinflussung der Melanophorenverteilung von Xenopus-laevis larven. Zool. Anz., Suppl., 29:571, 1967.
52. Perryman, E. K.: Fine structure of the secretory activity of the pars intermedia of Rana pipiens. Gen. Comp. Endocr. 23:94, 1974.
53. Pickford, G. E.: Melanogenesis in Fundulus heteroclitus. Anat. Rec. 125:603, 1956.
54. Pickford, G. E., and Atz, J. W.: The physiology of the pituitary gland of fishes. New York, New York Zoological Society, 1957.
55. Prota, G., and Nicolaus, R. A.: On the biogenesis of phaeomelanins. Advan. Biol. Skin 8: 323, 1967.
56. Quay, W. B.: Indole derivatives of pineal and related neural and retinal tissues. Pharmacol. Rev. 17(3):321, 1965.
57. Rodriquez, E. M., and La Pointe, J.: Light and electron microscopic study of the pars intermedia of the lizard, Klauberina riversiana. Z. Zellforsch. 104:1, 1970.
58. Rust, C. C.: Hormonal control of pelage cycles in the short-tailed weasel (Mustela erminea bangsi). Gen Comp. Endocr. 5:222, 1965.
59. Rust, C. C., and Meyer, R. K.: Hair color, molt, and testis size in male, short-tailed weasels treated with melatonin. Science 165:921, 1969.
60. Sage, M.: Control of prolactin release and its role in color change in the teleost Gillichthys mirabilis. J. Exp. Zool. 173:121, 1970.
61. Seiji, M., Shimao, K., Birbeck, M. S. C., and Fitzpatrick, T. B.: Subcellular localization of melanin biosynthesis. Ann. N. Y. Acad. Sci. 100:497, 1963.

62. Smith, P. E.: The pigmentary growth and endocrine disturbances induced in the anuran tadpole by the early ablation of the pars buccalis of the hypophysis. Amer. Anat. Mem., No. 11, 1920.

63. Taylor, J. D.: The effects of intermedin on the ultrastructure of amphibian iridophores. Gen. Comp. Endocr. *12*:405, 1969.

64. Taylor, J. D., and Hadley, M. E.: Chromatophores and color change in the lizard, *Anolis carolinensis*. Z. Zellforsch. *104*:282, 1970.

65. Taylor, J. D., and Bagnara, J. T.: Dermal chromatophores. Amer. Zool. *12*:43, 1972.

66. Van der Lek, G.: Photosensitive melanophores [Ph.D. thesis]. Utrecht, Netherlands, Univ. of Utrecht, 1967.

67. Van de Veerdonk, F. C. G.: Demonstration of melatonin in amphibia. Cur. Mod. Biol. *1*:175, 1967.

68. Van der Veerdonk, F. C. G., and Brouwer, E.: Role of calcium and prostaglandin (PGE₁) in the MSH-induced activation of adenylate cyclase in *Xenopus laevis*. Biochem. Biophys. Res. Commun. *52*:130, 1973.

69. Von Geldern, C. E.: Color changes and structure of the skin of *Anolis carolinensis*. Proc. Calif. Acad. Sci. *10*:77, 1921.

70. Wright, P. A.: Physiological responses of frog melanophores *in vitro*. Physiol. Zool. *28*:204, 1955.

71. Young, J. Z.:The photoreceptors of lampreys. II. The functions of the pineal complex. J. Exp. Biol. *12*:254, 1935.

72. Zondek, B., and Krohn, H.: Ein Hormon der Hypophyse. Zwischenlappenhormon (Intermedin). Naturwissenschaften, *20*:134, 1932.

CHAPTER 6

Neurohypophysis: Neurohormonal Peptides

The oxytocins and vasopressins are neurosecretory products of the neurohypophysis, and a large body of information is available on their chemical structures, physiologic and pharmacologic actions, and their phyletic distribution among the vertebrates. The extremely rapid progress made in the elucidation of these peptides since 1953 stems largely from the fact that their molecular structures are known and their natural secretions, as well as many analogues not found in nature, may be prepared synthetically. Information is accumulating on relationships between chemical structure and biologic effectiveness, and on possible mechanisms whereby they may act at the cellular level.

A variety of functions have been ascribed to these neurohormones, including: (1) contraction of the smooth muscle of the uterus (oxytocic effect), (2) contraction of the myoepithelial cells which surround the mammary alveoli (milk ejection), (3) actions upon the kidney to prevent excessive loss of water (antidiuretic effect), and (4) contraction of the smooth muscle in the walls of blood vessels (vasopressor effect). An examination of these actions reveals that the effectors employed are contractile elements and semipermeable membranes, such as the kidney tubules, and, in anuran amphibians, the skin and urinary bladder. The action on the kidney promotes the reabsorption of water from the glomerular filtrate, thus resulting in the excretion of a concentrated urine. The effect in amphibians is not only upon the kidney, but also upon the skin, to increase its permeability and allow water from the environment to pass into the body. The mammalian vasopressins are often referred to as antidiuretic hormones (ADH) since their main action is to conserve water. Although vasopressin elevates the blood pressure of mammals, and has the reverse effect in birds, there is no satisfactory evidence that it normally plays any role in the regulation of vascular tone or blood pressure. The effect may be pharmacologic rather than physiologic since the dose required is seemingly in excess of the amounts normally released by the intact neurohypophysis.

CHEMISTRY AND PHYLETIC DISTRIBUTION

Chemistry

All of the neural lobe secretions are octapeptides; that is, they consist of eight different amino acids, the two sulfur-linked cysteine molecules generally being counted as one cystine molecule (Fig. 6–1). Three of the amino acids are present in the form of amides. The sulfur linkage forms a pentapeptide ring (five amino acids), to which is attached a side chain composed of three amino acids. All of the neurohypophysial principles whose structures are known show this pattern. Substitutions occur in the natural secretions at positions 3, 4, and 8, producing peptides with different biologic potencies. The nine naturally occurring principles known at present are oxytocin, arginine vasopressin, lysine vasopressin, vasotocin, mesotocin, isotocin, glumitocin, valitocin, and aspartocin (Fig. 6–2).

The secretions that are stored in the mammalian pars nervosa are oxytocin and vasopressin. Oxytocin is very potent in causing uterine contractions, in lowering the blood pressure of birds, and in promoting milk ejection. One milligram of pure oxytocin contains about 500 USP units; the three types of activity per unit weight are found in a constant proportion (Table 6–1). Vasopressin also produces all of these effects, to a much slighter degree. On the other hand, vasopressin is unquestionably the main pressor and antidiuretic principle; oxytocin produces the same effects, but only to about 1 per cent and 0.5 per cent, respectively, of the activity possessed by vasopressin. These overlapping biological activities of oxytocin and vasopressin are a reflection of basic similarities in the structure of the two hormones; as is demonstrated in Table 6–1, even synthetic analogs of these principles may also elicit all three types of action.[9] By appropriate amino acid substitutions, organic chemists are synthesizing a variety of peptides, some of which have even higher specific physiologic activities than the naturally occurring peptides. Other synthetic peptides have highly restricted specific action, possessing only one of the neurohypophysial hormone activities and none of the overlapping activities.

Oxytocin was first identified in extracts prepared from the pituitary glands of cattle and swine, and was synthesized in 1953 by du Vigneaud and his colleagues. Shortly thereafter, the molecular structures of the vaso-

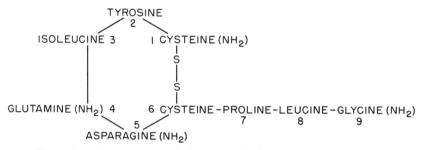

Figure 6–1. The arrangement of amino acids in a molecule of oxytocin.

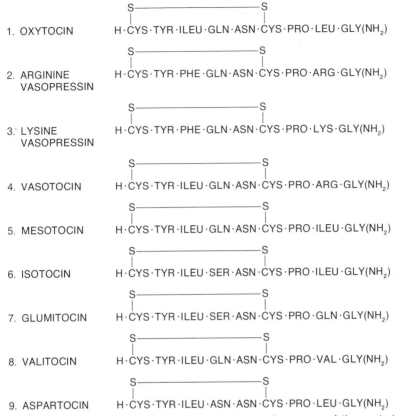

Figure 6–2. Amino acid sequences in the natural neurohormones of the posterior lobe (neurohypophysis).

pressins were determined and duplicated synthetically. These were brilliant chemical achievements since these were the first peptides to be synthesized. The mammalian neurohypophysis is the source of three principles: oxytocin, arginine vasopressin, and lysine vasopressin. By referring to Figure 6–2, we may see that oxytocin has isoleucine at position 3 and leucine at position 8; the vasopressins have phenylalanine at position 3, and either arginine or lysine at position 8. While these differences in molecular structure might seem to be slight, they have profound effects upon biologic potencies.

Arginine vasotocin was first identified in the chicken. It has isoleucine at position 3 (like oxytocin) and arginine at position 8 (like arginine vasopressin). This analogue had been synthesized and named "arginine vasotocin" before it was found to be present in the pituitaries of a large variety of nonmammalian vertebrates.[20] An analogue of oxytocin, called *ichthyotocin* or *isotocin,* has been obtained from the pituitary glands of holostean and teleostean fishes. This peptide is the same as oxytocin, except for serine at position 4 and isoleucine at position 8. Chemically, the compound is 4-ser-

Table 6–1   MOLECULAR ACTIVITIES (INTERNATIONAL UNITS PER MG)
OF SOME SUBSTITUTED ANALOGS OF OXYTOCIN*

TRIVIAL NAMES	RAT OXYTOCIC ACTIVITY	CHICKEN DEPRESSOR ACTIVITY	RAT PRESSOR ACTIVITY
Oxytocin	450 ± 30	450 ± 30	5 ± 1
[4-Serine] Oxytocin	190 ± 30	220 ± 20	<0.1
Isotocin	145 ± 12	310 ± 15	0.6 ± 0.01
Glumitocin	7.8 ± 0.6	–	0.4 ± 0.1
Arginine Vasotocin	120 ± 16	300 ± 42	255 ± 16
[4-Serine] Arginine Vasotocin	66 ± 15	311 ± 28	20.2 ± 3.4
Lysine Vasotocin	80 ± 10	215 ± 3	133 ± 13
Arginine Vasopressin	17 ± 4	62 ± 6	412 ± 41
Lysine Vasopressin	5 ± 0.5	42 ± 5	285 ± 21
[4-Serine] Lysine Vasopressin	0.9 ± 0.2	10 ± 0.7	3.3 ± 0.5

*Modified from Chauvet, J., Chauvet, M. T., and Acher, R.: Experientia *28*:1493, 1972.

ine, 8-isoleucine oxytocin. A peptide extracted in relative abundance from rays has been isolated and purified.[2] This peptide, called *glumitocin,* differs from isotocin only in the replacement of isoleucine by glutamine at position 8. Another oxytocin-like principle, *mesotocin,* (8-isoleucine oxytocin) has been identified in the pituitaries of the primitive ray-finned fish *Polypterus,* lungfishes, and several species of amphibians.[16, 28] Two hormones, valitocin and aspartocin, extracted from shark pituitary glands are the most recent of the neurohypophysial hormones to be identified.[4] Valitocin contains valine instead of leucine in the 8-position; in aspartocin, asparagine replaces glutamine in position 4.

Phyletic Distribution

Neurohypophysial octapeptides are found in all classes of vertebrates, but they have undergone changes in amino acid composition which make them pharmacologically different. The natural peptides vary in potency, when tested in the same or in different species, and this suggests that the receptor sites have also changed during the course of evolution.

Arginine vasotocin is the most widely distributed neurohormone (Fig. 6–3). It is the only principle present in cyclostomes, the most primitive of all living vertebrates. Even though it is not known to occur among adult mammals, it must be regarded as a very ancient molecule. This concept is supported by the interesting discovery of the transitory presence of arginine vasotocin in fetal mammalian pituitaries.[37] Its absence in the adult suggests that this is a kind of molecular recapitulation. Arginine vasotocin is present in the four major lines of evolution that led respectively to cyclostomes, the chondrichthyes (shark-like fishes), the actinopterygians (ray-finned fishes), and the tetrapods. Arginine vasotocin, together with isotocin, has been identified in the pituitaries of teleostean fishes. Mesotocin and arginine vasotocin are fundamental neurohypophysial hormones of amphibians, reptiles, and birds. It appears that no fundamental variation in neurohypo-

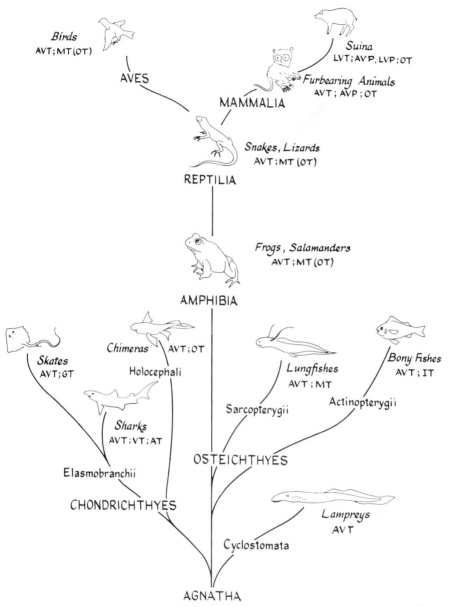

Figure 6–3. The family tree of vertebrate classes and the phylogenetic distribution of neuro-hypophysial peptides. Classes in capital letters; subclasses, orders, or suborders in capitals and lower case letters; AVT, arginine vasotocin; AVP, arginine vasopressin; LVP, lysine vasopressin; OT, oxytocin; MT, mesotocin; GT, glumitocin; IT, isotocin; VT, valitocin; AT, aspartocin. Hormones separated by semicolons are assumed to be determined by different gene loci; those representing established polymorphisms are separated by commas. A hormone enclosed in parentheses represents an uncertain situation that may be either mistaken identity or polymorphism. AVT of furbearing animals was extracted from fetal pituitary glands and adult pineal glands. LVT of suina was extracted from adult pineal glands. (From Valtin, Stewart and Sokol, Chapter 7. *In* R. O. Greep and E. B. Astwood (eds.): Handbook of Physiology, Section 7, Endocrinology, Vol. IV, Part I, p. 156. Baltimore, Williams & Wilkins Co., 1974.)

physial hormones occurred during the evolutionary transition from amphibians to reptiles.[1]

Two vasopressins are found among mammals, the arginine variety being most widely distributed. Arginine vasopressin has been identified in marsupials and also in *Echidna,* an egg-laying monotreme, and this suggests that it appeared very early in the evolution of mammals.[29] Lysine vasopressin has only been identified in the neural lobes of surviving Suiformes, a suborder of the Artiodactyla or even-toed ungulates. Lysine vasopressin alone occurs in the domestic pig, whereas both kinds of vasopressin are found in certain wart hogs, peccaries, and the hippopotamus.[12] Thus a genetic polymorphism with respect to these two vasopressins has been disclosed for all three families of the Suiformes. The absence of arginine vasopressin from the domestic pig may well have resulted from domestication. It is possible that arginine vasopressin is present in other strains of domesticated pigs which have not been tested. Arginine vasopressin could have evolved from arginine vasotocin, present in the reptilian ancestors of mammals, by a single mutation causing isoleucine at position 3 to be replaced by phenylalanine. Lysine vasopressin could have arisen from arginine vasopressin through other mutations causing arginine in position 8 to be replaced by lysine.

While the evolution of the pressor principles seems straightforward, the origin of oxytocin-like molecules is more confusing. Such compounds must be very ancient molecules, and oxytocin itself is present in the holocephalian elasmobranch *Hydrolagus collei.*[25] Similarly, valitocin and aspartocin are molecules that appeared early in neurohypophysial peptide evolution. They have so far been discovered only in sharks.[35] Of the later appearing peptides, isotocin seems to be restricted to the teleosts, while mesotocin has persisted in the main lines of tetrapod evolution.

As our knowledge of the chemistry and phylogenetic distribution of neurohypophysial hormones has increased, several schemes for the evolution of these hormones have appeared.[15, 35] A summary of these, presented in Figure 6–4, illustrates the proposed sequence of evolutionary steps that possibly took place. Except for the scheme of Acher, who proposes the existence of a precursor molecule with as yet undetermined amino acids in positions 3, 4, and 8, the other proposals have in common the suggestion that arginine vasotocin is the ancestral molecule of Agnatha that gave rise, by various amino acid substitutions, to the other neurohypophysial petides. This is an attractive hypothesis that is supported by the almost universal occurrence of arginine vasotocin among lower invertebrates, its presence in fetal mammals, and the fact that mesotocin, oxytocin, and arginine vasopressin can all arise from it by single amino acid substitutions. It becomes obvious from the amino acid composition of these peptides that some transitions require replacement in two different positions. Thus, an evolution of isotocin or glumitocin from arginine vasotocin would require substitution of two amino acids, at positions 4 and 8 (Fig. 6–2). Depending upon the specific amino acid substitutions that take place, several intermediates could possibly exist between arginine vasotocin and glumitocin as this postulated evolutionary transition occurs. Constraints imposed by the genetic code

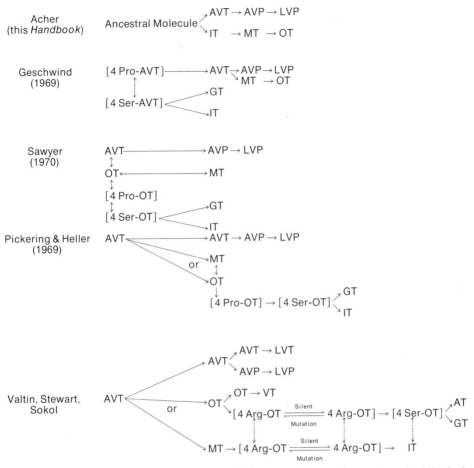

Figure 6–4. Proposed schemes for the evolutionary pathways of neurohypophysial principles. With the exception of the first example, each arrow denotes an amino acid substitution that
could be accomplished by a single nucleotide base substitution; compounds in brackets are
hypothetical molecules. The models by Geshwind and Sawyer were constructed to accomodate
the minimum number of mutations. (From Valtin, Stewart and Sokol, Chapter 7. *In* R. O. Greep
and E. B. Astwood (eds.): Handbook of Physiology, Section 7, Endocrinology, Vol. IV, Part I,
p. 156. Baltimore, Williams & Wilkins Co., 1974.)

must also be taken into account in the evaluation of evolutionary steps. For
example, while the transition between isotocin and mesotocin involves the
replacement of a single amino acid, the genetic code requires that two
steps take place, because the amino acids involved are serine and glutamine at position 4 (Fig. 6–2). The codons for these amino acids are so different that two base changes are necessary for this transition to occur. In
the light of all these considerations, it is impossible to indicate, with any
assurance, a clear pathway for the evolution of neurohypophysial principles. Such will only become possible following the acquisition of new
knowledge about the distribution, pharmacology, and biochemistry of
known neurohypophysial peptides and of others that may yet be discovered.
     It is apparent from the above discussion that the octapeptide neurohor-

mones are very similar in chemical structure. Thus, as indicated in Table 6-1, there is considerable overlapping of pharmacologic properties, though relative potencies may be strikingly different in the various bioassays. Arginine and lysine vasopressins are antidiuretic principles in mammals, but arginine vasotocin performs this function in amphibians, reptiles, and birds. Antidiuresis is an adaptation to terrestrial life, and it is therefore not surprising to find that the neurohypophysial principles have no effect on water conservation in fishes, though they may promote the loss of sodium through the kidneys. Oxytocin is known to regulate milk ejection, and probably facilitates parturition and sperm transport in the female reproductive tract of mammals; its function in male mammals, if it has any, is unknown. Arginine vasotocin acts in birds to stimulate contractions of the oviduct and to promote oviposition, effects that are essentially oxytocic. When administered to mammals, vasotocin has potent oxytocic and milk-ejecting actions, whereas the vasopressins are less active. It appears that during evolution vasotocin was discarded in mammals, and a clear separation appeared between octapeptides promoting water conservation (vasopressins) and the octapeptide controlling uterine contractility and milk ejection (oxytocin). The functions of neurohypophysial principles in aquatic vertebrates remain largely undetermined. However, the mere presence of these peptides in the pituitaries of the lowest vertebrates does not mean that they have to function as systemic hormones in these groups.

FORMATION, STORAGE, RELEASE, AND TRANSPORT

Oliver and Schäfer demonstrated in 1895 that whole pituitary extracts, administered intravenously to the dog, induced vasoconstriction and elevated the blood pressure. Other workers promptly showed that this effect was attributable to the pars nervosa, and not to any other component of the pituitary. Since this part of the pituitary does not show cytologic characteristics of a gland, the source of the active principle became a problem. Some investigators postulated that the active material might be secreted by the adenohypophysis and passed to the pars nervosa for storage; others thought that it might be produced in situ by the pituicytes, even though these cells did not appear to be glandular. Kamm and his co-workers (1928) succeeded in separating two active fractions from neural lobe extracts, one being especially potent in elevating the blood pressure of mammals and the other acting principally to induce uterine contractions. Evidence contributed by many other workers made it clear that blood-borne hormones were present in neural lobe tissue, but it remained hard to believe that they could originate in such a nonglandular structure. The problem was finally clarified by the Scharrers and Bargmann and their co-workers in the early 1950's. They established the concept that oxytocin and vasopressin are neurosecretory products which arise in the neurons of certain hypothalamic nuclei. The paired supraoptic and paraventricular nuclei are the most important ones for the production of these neurohormones. The neurohormones are actually synthesized by these glandular neurons, moved along the axons of the hypothalamo-hypophysial tract, and discharged around blood vessels in the pars nervosa (a neurohemal organ). The pituicytes are neuroglia and are no longer regarded as the source of these secretions; there is still the possibility, however, that the pituicytes may be involved in either the release mechanism or in the separation of the active peptides from the carrier substance.[6, 7, 30]

In birds, in whom a septum separates the two lobes of the pituitary, it is possible to remove the pars nervosa without disturbing the adenohypophysis. Ablation of the posterior lobe of the laying hen results in a prompt and permanent diuresis, but impairs neither ovulation nor oviposition. The consumption of water increases rapidly, and birds weighing 1000 to 2000 grams may drink as much as 1000 grams of water daily. The diabetes insipidus in the operated birds may be controlled by the administration of neurohypophysial principles. The posterior lobe principles are known to facilitate oviposition in birds but, in the absence of the posterior lobe, enough oxytocin is apparently released from the hypothalamic neurons to take care of this need.[23]

Totally hypophysectomized mammals seldom show any serious disturbances in water metabolism. In the hypophysectomized rat, neurosecretory material accumulates at the broken end of the pituitary stalk, the latter undergoing reorganization to form a normal but miniature neural lobe. On the other hand, if the hypothalamo-hypophysial tracts are severed near the supraoptic nuclei, the cell bodies of the latter deteriorate, and the organism is practically deprived of oxytocin and vasopressin. Under these conditions, a permanent diabetes insipidus results, the animals consuming large quantities of water and eliminating it through the kidneys.

The factors involved in the release of neurohypophysial secretion have not been completely elucidated. The release of antidiuretic hormone (ADH; synonymous with vasopressin) may be altered by changes in osmotic pressure and volume of the blood, certain sensory reflexes, and action occurring within the central nervous system itself. In snakes, as in other amniotes, intraperitoneal injections of sodium chloride, or the withholding of water, cause neurosecretory material in the hypothalamic nuclei and pars nervosa to be rapidly depleted. The osmoreceptors in dogs are thought to be located in some area of the prosencephalon, which is supplied by the internal carotid artery. If hypertonic solutions of sugar or salt are injected into the carotid artery of normal animals during water diuresis, a prompt fall in urine output occurs. Changes in blood volume and electrolyte concentration of the plasma can bring about striking increases in ADH. Various emotions, as well as coitus and pain, reflex stimulation (as in suckling and milking), changes in environmental temperatures, etc., are known to promote the release of such neurohormones.[26]

Certain drugs, probably acting on hypothalamic nuclei, are known to reduce the flow of urine by increasing the release of ADH. Among these may be mentioned morphine, nicotine, ether, and various barbiturates. Since the main nervous connection between the hypothalamus and pars nervosa is the hypothalamo-hypophysial tract, one wonders whether the neurons that elaborate neurosecretions can also conduct nervous impulses. There is some evidence that they do both.

Various staining techniques have been employed in order to identify neurosecretory cells in different components of the neurohypophysial complex. It is possible that these techniques stain a protein "carrier substance," to which the peptide principles are adsorbed or attached.[36] Van Dyke and his colleagues isolated a protein from neurohypophysial extracts which has vasopressor and oxytocic activities in the ratio of 1:1. These activities could be separated from the protein by treatment with acid. The van Dyke protein has been named "neurophysin," and has been obtained from a number of mammalian species. Bovine and porcine neurophysins are best known, and it has been shown that they contain several hormone-binding proteins. Two major bovine neurophysins have been distinguished from those of the pig; however, there is evidence that other protein components of both bovine and porcine origin have very similar or identical properties.[19]

Probably, all of the bovine neurophysins and porcine neurophysins I and III are monomeric polypeptide chains having molecular weights of about 10,000. Evidently, these monomers associate readily to form dimers and oligomers, thus accounting for higher molecular weights such as that of 30,000 originally assigned to the van Dyke protein. The complete amino acid sequences have been reported for bovine neurophysins I and II and porcine neurophysin I, and obviously large sections of these molecules are identical. Preliminary observations on a human neurophysin indicate that its composition resembles those of porcine and bovine origin.[13] Neurophysins are so specific in their binding of neurohypophysial principles that they can be used to separate these principles from other peptides which are present in pituitary extracts. Indeed, the specificity is such that individual peptides may have preferential affinities for the various neurophysins. Thus, it has been suggested that in supraoptic and paraventricular regions of the bovine hypothalamus, oxytocin binds specifically to neurophysin I and vasopressin to neurophysin II.[38] It appears that both the neurohypophysial peptides and the neurophysins are synthesized together in these regions of the hypothalamus and that they are transported to the pars nervosa, where they are stored and then released together.[19] The association of neurohypophysial peptides and neurophysins in secretory granules and their release in parallel can be readily accomplished by the process of exocytosis described by Douglas.[10] The process involves the fusion of the granule membrane with the plasma membrane and results in the extrusion of the entire granule contents. Whether the neurophysins released in this manner play an additional physiological role is currently under investigation.

BIOLOGIC ACTIONS OF NEUROHYPOPHYSIAL PRINCIPLES

It appears that the principles of the neurohypophysis may not be indispensable for life. Although vasopressin has strong pharmacologic actions on the circulation, there is no proof that it performs such a physiologic role. Oxytocin has been assigned a role in promoting uterine contractility in mammals during coitus and at the time of delivery, but individuals of some species seem to deliver young quite well after the supply has been eliminated, or reduced, by hypothalamic lesions. Most mammals could not rear their young without ejecting milk, but the individual could live without doing so. Even in the absence of the antidiuretic principle, mammalian organisms may rely upon other homeostatic mechanisms for the regulation of body water. To what extent desert animals conserve water through the release of ADH is not known. When the laboratory rat is deprived of water, it not only increases the output of ADH but also diminishes the consumption of food, thus reducing the loss of water through the feces.

Antidiuretic Effects

Even before the chemical identification of neurohypophysial principles, physiologists had demonstrated that they act upon the kidney to reduce the volume of urine. If a dog's kidney is isolated and perfused with blood from the trunk of another dog, it produces a large volume of dilute urine. The addition of small amounts of pituitary extract to the perfusate causes the kidney to excrete a smaller volume of more concentrated urine. Inclusion of the dog's head in the perfusion circuit causes the excised kidney to diminish its output of urine, but this effect of the head is abolished by removing the pituitary gland.

There can be no doubt that ADH (vasopressin) is of physiologic utility in the regulation of water balance in mammals. By acting upon the epithelial cells of the distal portion of the renal tubule, it encourages the reabsorption of water. Diabetes insipidus (excretion of a large volume of dilute urine) can be produced in mammals, such as the cat, dog, and monkey, by hypothalamic lesions that destroy the supraoptico-hypophysial tracts. Approximately 90 per cent of the fibers in these tracts must be severed before any profound disturbances occur in water metabolism. Such diabetic animals consume large quantities of water (polydipsia) and eliminate a large volume of urine (diuresis); the excessive water loss may be corrected by the administration of vasopressin. The essential effect of the peptide on the distal segment of the nephron is to increase the permeability of the epithelial surface to water.

Hereditary diabetes insipidus has been described, exemplifying clearly that the condition can result either from the lack of vasopressin or from the lack of a vasopressor effect on the renal tubules. Rats homozygous for hypothalamic diabetes insipidus (Brattleboro strain) are apparently unable to synthesize arginine vasopressin and thus consume copious amounts of water (80 per cent of body weight) and excrete large volumes of urine (70 per cent of body weight).[33, 34] These manifestations are reflected in a lack of neurosecretory material in the hypothalamo-neurohypophysial system. Rats heterozygous for this condition possess features between those that are normal and those that are homozygous. In the mouse, diabetes insipidus is associated with oligosyndactyly caused by the dominant gene Os.[11] Because these animals possess small kidneys with fewer nephrons and are resistant to exogenous vasopressin, it is concluded that the condition is probably of renal origin.

Members of most mammalian species die when 20 per cent of the body water is lost, but the camel can survive after losing more than 40 per cent of its body water. Hibernating mammals, such as the hedgehog and certain desert rodents, have remarkable abilities to economize on water. The Mongolian gerbil and similar desert species can survive for years without drinking water, living on a diet of dry grain without weight loss. The kangaroo rat (Dipodomys) obtains water through the oxidation of its food, but it does not store an excess of water in the tissues and has no especial resistance to dehydration. When excess water is administered by stomach tube, it is excreted with great difficulty, and the animals are likely to show symptoms of "water intoxication." The urine volume is about half that of the laboratory rat and is much more concentrated. The neural lobe of the kangaroo rat is relatively larger than that of the laboratory rat and contains more vasopressin per microgram of tissue. This suggestion that vasopressin may have special importance in the water metabolism of the kangaroo rat is supported from studies of neurohypophysial ultrastructure.[31] Electron microscopic observations have revealed the presence of rich stores of osmiophilic neurosecretory material in the neural lobes of normal, unstressed *Dipodomys merriami* (Fig. 6–5). The neural lobes of rats dehydrated by the injection of hypertonic sodium chloride contain large, clear vesicles which have been depleted of their osmiophilic secretion as a result of the injection (Fig. 6–6).

Striking antidiuretic actions have been demonstrated in birds, reptiles, and certain amphibians. Most anurans, maintained in water and injected with neurohypophysial peptides, increase in weight. This is known as the "Brunn" or "water balance" effect. This weight increase results from a composite effect of the neurohormones; water loss through the kidneys is diminished, water uptake through the skin is increased, and water is absorbed from the urinary bladder and returned to the blood. Pieces of frog skin *in vitro* respond to ADH by accelerating the movement of water from the outside to the inside, but only if the inside is hypertonic to the outside as it normally is *in vivo*. The urinary bladder of toads and frogs may also be used in *in vitro* experiments; it responds to ADH by increasing water absorption from the luminal surface. Of the three neurohypophysial peptides that have been obtained from amphibians, vasotocin is far more active than either oxytocin or mesotocin when tested *in vitro* or *in vivo* on the water and sodium metabolism of *Bufo marinus*.[8] Following injection of vasotocin into other amphibian species, differences are found in the amount of water that is retained. Probably this is due to species and individual variation in the peptide receptors found on the three effectors: kidney, skin, and urinary bladder. Among anurans, all three effectors participate. In urodeles, on the other hand, only the kidney responds, although *Salamandra maculosa* is an exception in that its bladder also is affected. In many urodele amphibians that never leave the water (e.g., Necturus), antidiuresis either cannot be produced by these peptides, or the required dose is so high that it is obviously

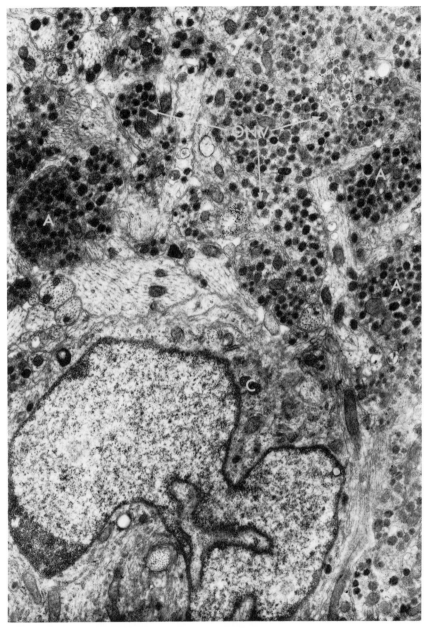

Figure 6–5. Relatively high magnification micrograph from the neural lobe of a normal kangaroo rat. In addition to the rich stores of osmiophilic neurosecretion (ONV) in the axons (A) of the field, the other noteworthy feature is the presence of a cell (C). This type of cell is commonly observed in both normal and acutely dehydrated kangaroo rats. (From Scott, D. E.: Neuroendocrinology 4:347, 1969.)

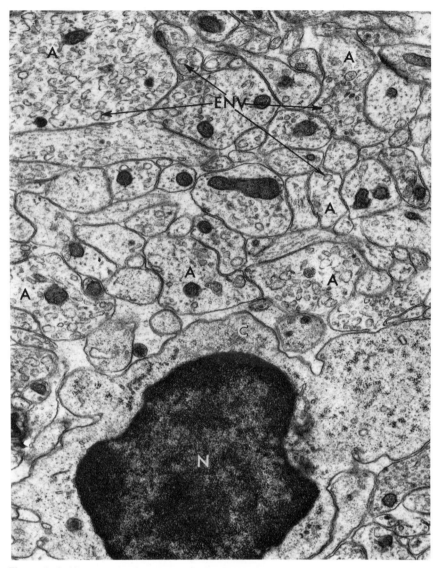

Figure 6–6. Micrograph of a section from the neural lobe of a kangaroo rat sacrificed 30 minutes after acute dehydration. Note the abundance of electron-lucent neurosecretory vesicles (ENV) in the axis cylinders of transient fibers (A). A prominent cell (C) with a distinct nucleus (N) can also be observed. (From Scott, D. E.: Neuroendocrinology *4*:347, 1969.)

of unphysiologic proportions. Sodium transport across the skin of anurans is augmented by vasotocin, and in at least one urodele *(Notophthalmus),* the same is true. Posterior lobe principles have not been demonstrated to exert antidiuretic effects in fishes, though they may be important in these vertebrates in promoting a renal vascular action that in some teleosts and in *Protopterus* leads to an increase in urine volume. The administration of vasotocin to the teleost *Carassius auratus* causes sodium to be lost through the kidneys and promotes the intake of sodium, perhaps by an effect on the gills.[17, 22] The role of the gills of marine teleost fishes in electrolyte exchange is quite prominent in comparison with other avenues, such as the kidneys or gut. An exchange of sodium across the gills of such species can be stimulated by the injection of strong doses of oxytocin and vasotocin.

Amphibian skin and bladder are useful tissues since they may be observed *in vitro* after the application of neurohypophysial principles. Evidence has been adduced that ADH acts upon amphibian membranes by dilating the pores. Isotopically labeled thiourea penetrates the toad's skin at a slower rate than water, presumably because of the larger molecules. Antidiuretic hormone increases the rate of flux of the thiourea molecules. On the basis of the *pore theory,* this is explained by assuming that the pores of the skin are normally just large enough to admit water molecules, but ADH dilates them sufficiently for thiourea molecules to pass through. It has been suggested that the pore theory may be applied to account for the actions of ADH on the kidney.[5, 14, 21, 27]

The question of how ADH mediates its effect has been studied extensively, and while several other theories have appeared, the most attractive hypothesis maintains that the permeability changes brought about by vasopressin occur through the action of the second messenger, cyclic AMP.[24] The experiments performed to test this hypothesis are classic, and the evidence obtained leaves little doubt that cyclic AMP is an intracellular intermediate in the action of ADH (Fig. 6–7). The majority of experiments have been performed on the isolated toad bladder, but results obtained from studies on the kidney are in agreement. The hypothesis was based initially upon the fact that cyclic AMP mimics the vasopressin reaction with respect to all characteristics. Subsequently, it was learned that the reaction could be duplicated by administration of theophylline, which leads to an increase in cellular levels of cyclic AMP through the inhibition of phosphodiesterase, an enzyme which catalyzes the breakdown of cyclic 3', 5'-AMP to 5'-AMP. Additional convincing evidence derives from the fact that both

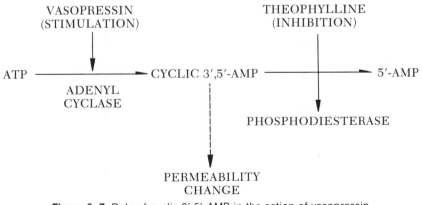

Figure 6–7. Role of cyclic 3',5'-AMP in the action of vasopressin.

ADH and theophylline can elevate the concentration of cyclic AMP in both the kidney and the toad bladder. It should be noted that in the toad bladder only 15 per cent of the mucosal cells are responsive to neurohypophysial peptides.[32] In *in vito* studies, oxytocin caused a 235 per cent increase in the amount of cyclic AMP in these mitochondria-rich responsive cells, but had no effect on granular cells which are another major constituent of the bladder mucosa. While the evidence that cyclic AMP is the second messenger for ADH action is most convincing, the important question of how it affects permeability changes remains unsolved.

Much of the early experimentation on the mode of action of ADH centered on the fact that it contains a disulfide linkage which appears essential for its activity. It was considered that the sulfhydryl groups of the hormone might bind to the active membrane through the formation of disulfide linkages. This concept was supported by experiments showing that sulfhydryl agents such as N-ethylmaleimide and parachloromercuribenzoate interfere with the binding and the action of ADH. While these data are extremely convincing, they do not at the same time contradict the second-messenger hypothesis. In all probability, the sulfhydryl involvement in ADH action resides at the level of the ADH receptor on the cell surface, while the cyclic AMP effect is an internal one that follows the interaction of vasopressin and its receptor.

Oxytocic Effects

Two main functions have been ascribed to oxytocin in the promotion of uterine contractility: (1) to facilitate the ascent of spermatozoa in the female tract after intromission, and (2) to expel the fetus from the female tract at parturition. Owing to the intermittent nature of these events, it has been difficult to obtain quantitative information. Many workers have felt that in many species the spermatozoa reach the fallopian tubes too rapidly to be accounted for by the flagellate motility of the spermatozoa themselves. Moreover, nonmotile spermatozoa are known to ascend the female tract as quickly as do motile ones. Oxytocin has been observed to increase the speed of ascent of spermatozoa and of various fluids introduced into the bovine uterus maintained *in vitro*.

Increased contractility of the uterus has been demonstrated in domestic animals after natural mating, tactile stimulation of the external genitalia, and mechanical stimulation of the uterus. In cows, the content of oxytocin in external jugular blood was found to be increased after rectal palpation of the uterus and cervix. Milk ejection may accompany natural mating in several species, suggesting that there is an augmented release of oxytocin at this time.

Extracts containing oxytocin have been used clinically for many years to induce uterine contractions and facilitate delivery of the fetus. The neural lobes of rats and dogs contain very little oxytocin for several hours after labor, suggesting that the stored peptides have been used to support the process. The fact that parturition may occur normally in the absence of the pituitary gland does not prove that oxytocin is unimportant in parturition; sufficient quantities of neurohormone may continue to be produced by the hypothalamus. It is generally agreed that the sensitivity of the uterine muscle to oxytocin varies in accordance with the sex hormones that act upon it. Furthermore, there are differences in the reactivity of different regions of the same uterus. While the evidence is suggestive, no final conclusions can be made concerning the physiologic role of oxytocin in parturition.

There are indications that posterior lobe peptides may be important in the reproductive physiology of birds and reptiles. They effect oviposition in the hen by inducing contraction of the shell gland and of the vagina. Vasopressin stimulates contractions of the oviducts of the painted turtle, *Chrysemis picta*. Assay studies have shown that the oxytocic activity of the hen's neural lobe is practically depleted prior to oviposition.

Neural lobe secretions appear to influence reproductive behavior in certain fishes. It has been reported that synthetic oxytocin induces the spawning reflex in *Fundulus.*

Milk Ejection

One of the best-established functions of oxytocin is its role in stimulating milk ejection. The milk-ejection reflex manifests itself by a sudden rise in milk pressure within the glands and, as with other reflexes, it can be conditioned. The lactating female becomes conditioned to a variety of tactile, visual, and auditory stimuli associated with suckling or milking. In this manner, the lactating mother unconsciously participates and makes it possible for the nursing young to obtain a full supply of milk. This reflex arc is a neurohormonal one, the efferent component being a neurohormone that is, in all probability, oxytocin. This principle is released from the neurohypophysis and causes contraction of the branching myoepithelial cells around the mammary alveoli.

The development of the mammary glands and milk secretion require a large number of hormones. There are indications that all of the anterior pituitary hormones may be involved in normal mammary functions. It has been proposed that an important effect of oxytocin is to prevent involution of the lactating mammary gland. Oxytocin, reflexively discharged, is thought to reach the anterior pituitary and cause it to release prolactin. The latter hormone then maintains the functional integrity of the mammary alveolar tissue. Factors involved in lactation are discussed more fully in Chapter 15.

REFERENCES

1. Archer, R. : Chemistry of the neurohypophysial hormones: an example of molecular evolution. *In* R. O. Greep and E. B. Astwood (eds.): Handbook of Physiology, Section 7, Endocrinology, Vol. IV, Part 1, pp. 119–130. Baltimore, Williams & Wilkins Co., 1974.
2. Archer, R., Chauvet, J., Chauvet, M. T., and Crepy, D.: Phylogénie des peptides neurohypo-

physaires: Isolement d'une nouvelle hormone, la glumitocine (Ser$_4$-Gln$_8$-ocytocine) présente chez un poisson cartilagineux, la raie *(Raia clavata)*. Biochem. Biophys. Acta *107*: 393, 1965.

3. Acher, R., Chauvet, J., Chauvet, M. T., and Crepy, D.: Phylogeny of vertebrate neurohypophysial hormones. Gen. Comp. Endocr. *5*:662, 1965.
4. Acher, R., Chauvet, J., and Chauvet, M. T.: Identification de deux nouvelles hormones neurohypophysaires, la Valitocine (Val^8-oxytocine) et l'Aspartocine (Asn^4-oxytocine) chez un poisson sélacien, l'Aiguillat *(Squalus acanthias)*. Compt. Rend. *274*:313, 1972.
5. Anderson, B., and Ussing, H. H.: Solvent drag on non-electrolytes during osmotic flow through isolated toad skin. Acta Physiol. Scand. *39*:228, 1957.
6. Bargmann, W.: The neurosecretory system of the diencephalon. Endeavour *19*:125, 1960.
7. Bargmann, W., and Scharrer, E.: The site of origin of the hormones of the posterior pituitary. Amer. Sci. *39*:255, 1961.
8. Bentley, P. J.: Comparison of actions of neurohypophysial hormones in amphibia. *In* M. Fontaine (ed.): La spécificité zoologique des hormones hypophysaires et de leurs activités. Paris, Centre National de la Recherche Scientifique, 1969, p. 57.
9. Chauvet, J., Chauvet, M. T., and Acher, R.: Biological properties of synthetic Ser^4-Arg^8-oxytocin (Ile^3-Ser^4-arginine vasopressin): Role of the residue No. 4 in the hormone-pressor receptor interaction. Experientia *28*:1493, 1972.
10. Douglas, W. W.: Mechanism of release of neurohypophysial hormones: Stimulus-secretion coupling. *In* R. O. Greep and E. B. Astwood (eds.): Handbook of Physiology, Section 7, Endocrinology, Vol. IV, Part 1, pp. 191–224. Baltimore, Williams & Wilkins Co., 1974.
11. Falconer, D. S., Latyszewski, M., and Isaacson, J. H.: Diabetes insipidus associated with oligosyndactyly in the mouse. Genet. Res. *5*:473, 1964.
12. Ferguson, D. R., and Pickering, B. T.: Arginine and lysine vasopressins in the hippopotamus neurohypophysis. Gen. Comp. Edocr. *13*:425, 1969.
13. Foss, I., Sletten, K., and Trygstad, O.: Studies on the primary structure and biological activity of a human neurophysin. FEBS Letters *30*:151, 1973.
14. Frazier, H. S., Dempsey, E. F., and Leaf, A.: Movement of sodium across the mucosal surface of the isolated toad bladder and its modification by vasopressin. J. Gen. Physiol. *45*: 529, 1962.
15. Geschwind, I. I.: The main lines of evolution of the pituitary hormones. *In* M. Fontaine (ed.): La spécificité zoologique des hormones hypophysaires et de leurs activités. Paris, Centre National de la Recherche Scientifique, 1969, p. 385.
16. Heller, H.: Neurohypophyseal hormones. *In* U. S. von Euler and H. Heller (eds.): Comparative Endocrinology, Vol. 1. New York, Academic Press, 1963, p. 25.
17. Heller, H., and Bentley, P. J.: Phylogenetic distribution of the effects of neurohypophysial hormones on water and sodium metabolism. Gen. Comp. Endocr. *5*:96, 1965.
18. Heller, H., and Spickett, S. G.: The polymorphism of the neurohypophysial hormones. Mem. Soc. Endocr. *15*:89, 1967.
19. Hope, D. B., and Pickup, J. C.: Neurophysins. *In* R. O. Greep and E. B. Astwood (eds.): Handbook of Physiology, Section 7, Endocrinology, Vol. IV, Part 1, pp. 173–189. Baltimore, Williams & Wilkins Co., 1974.
20. Katsoyannis, P. G., and du Vigneaud, V.: Arginine-vasotocin, a synthetic analogue of the posterior pituitary hormones containing the ring of oxytocin and the side chain of vasopressin. J. Biol. Chem. *233*:1352, 1958.
21. Leaf, A., and Hays, R. M: The effects of neurohypophyseal hormone on permeability and transport in a living membrane. Rec. Progr. Horm. Res. *17*:647, 1961.
22. Maetz, J., Bourguet, J., Lahlough, B., and Hourdry, J.: Peptides neurohypophysaires et osmoregulation chez *Carassius auratus*. Gen. Comp. Endocr. *4*:508, 1964.
23. Nalbandov, A. V.: Reproductive Physiology, 2nd ed. San Francisco, W. H. Freeman and Company, 1964, p. 107.
24. Orloff, J., and Handler, J. S.: Cellular mode of action of antidiuretic hormone, J. Clin. Path. *18*:533, 1965.
25. Pickering, B. T., and Heller, H.: Oxytocin as a neurohypophysial hormone in the holocephalian elasmobranch fish, *Hydrolagus collei*. J. Endocr. *45*:597, 1969.
26. Pickford, M.: Factors affecting milk release in the dog and the quantity of oxytocin liberated by suckling. J. Physiol. *152*:515, 1960.
27. Ridley, A.: Effects of osmotic stress and hypophysectomy on ion distribution in bullfrogs. Gen. Comp. Endocr. *4*:481, 1964.
28. Sawyer, W. H.: Evolution of neurohypophysial principles. Arch. Anat. Micr. Morph. Exp. *54*: 295, 1965.
29. Sawyer, W. H., Munsick, R. A., and van Dyke, H. B.: Pharmacological characteristics of neurohypophysial hormones from a marsupial *(Didelphis virginiana)* and a monotreme *(Tachyglossus [Echidna] aculeatus)*. Endocrinology *67*:137, 1960.

30. Scharrer, E., and Scharrer, B.: Hormones produced by neurosecretory cells. Rec. Progr. Horm. Res. *10*:183, 1954.
31. Scott, D. E.: Ultrastructural changes in the neural lobe of the hypophysis of the kangaroo rat (*Dipodomys merriami*) following intraperitoneal injection of hypertonic sodium chloride. Neuroendocrinology *4*:347, 1969.
32. Scott, W. N., Sapirstein, V. S., and Yoder, M. J.: Partition of tissue functions in epithelia: Localization of enzymes in "mitochondria-rich" cells of toad urinary bladder. Science *184*:797, 1974.
33. Sokol, H. W., and Valtin, H.: Morphology of the neurosecretory system in rats homozygous and heterozygous for hypothalamic diabetes insipidus (Brattleboro strain). Endocrinology *77*:692, 1965.
34. Valtin, H.: Hereditary hypothalamic diabetes insipidus in rats (Brattleboro strain). Amer. J. Med. *42*:814, 1967.
35. Valtin, H., Stewart, J., and Sokol, H. W.: Genetic control of the production of posterior pituitary principles. *In* R. O. Greep and E. B. Astwood (eds.): Handbook of Physiology, Section 7, Endocrinology, Vol. IV, Part 1, pp. 131–171. Baltimore, Williams & Wilkins Co., 1974.
36. van Dyke, H. B., Chow, B. F., Greep, R. O., and Rothen, A.: The isolation of a protein from the pars neuralis of the ox pituitary with constant oxytocic, pressor and diuresis-inhibiting effects. J. Pharmacol. *74*:190, 1942.
37. Vizsolyi, E., and Perks, A. M.: New neurohypophysial principle in foetal mammals. Nature *223*:1169, 1969.
38. Zimmerman, E. A., Robinson, A. G., Husain, M. K., Acosta, M., Frantz, A. G., and Sawyer, W. H.: Neurohypophysial peptides in the bovine hypothalamus: The relationship of neurophysin I to oxytocin, and neurophysin II to vasopressin in supraoptic and paraventricular regions. Endocrinology *95*:931, 1974.

CHAPTER 7

The Thyroid Gland

The human thyroid consists of two lobes that lie on either side of the trachea and are usually connected by a thin isthmus extending over the anterior surface of the trachea. Thyroids are present in all vertebrates, but they are quite variable in shape and anatomic position. In some of the lower vertebrates, thyroid follicles are present, but they are not organized into a compact, encapsulated gland. The thyroid follicles of lampreys and bony fishes tend to be dispersed along the ventral aorta and are frequently found along the branchial arteries of the gills. The thyroid tissue of certain teleosts is extremely mobile and may disperse from the pharyngeal region to distant areas, such as the eye, brain, spleen, and kidney. The function of the thyroid is to elaborate, store, and discharge secretions that are concerned principally with the regulation of metabolic rate. However, that the thyroid secretions of adult, cold-blooded vertebrates perform similar metabolic functions remains to be demonstrated convincingly.

The hormonal variants that derive from the thyroid gland will be referred to by the term *thyroid hormone,* which, unless otherwise stated, will designate thyroxine, 3,5,3'-triiodothyronine, and any other active compounds that may be produced from these in the body.

ANATOMIC FEATURES

Gross Anatomy

The human thyroid is encapsulated by two layers of connective tissue; the outer layer is continuous with the cervical fascia and is loosely connected to the inner capsule that adheres intimately to the surface of the gland. The normal thyroid of the adult weighs 25 to 40 gm, but it is one of the most labile organs of the body, and its size fluctuates with age, reproductive states, habitation, and diet. The vascular supply to the thyroid is exceptionally rich (Fig. 7 – 1). It is probable that more blood flows through this gland, in proportion to its size, than through any other organ of the body, with the possible exception of the adrenal gland. The most outstanding feature of the thyroid is its ability to concentrate large amounts of iodine; the amount of iodine within the gland may be 50 to several hundred times that of the blood plasma.

Postganglionic sympathetic fibers from the superior and inferior cervical ganglia and vagal fibers from the superior and inferior laryngeal nerves

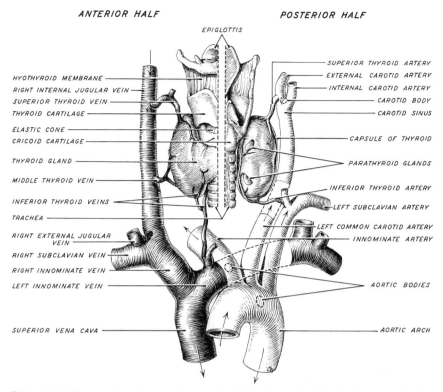

ANTERIOR HALF   *POSTERIOR HALF*

EPIGLOTTIS

SUPERIOR THYROID ARTERY
EXTERNAL CAROTID ARTERY
HYOTHYROID MEMBRANE
INTERNAL CAROTID ARTERY
RIGHT INTERNAL JUGULAR VEIN
SUPERIOR THYROID VEIN
CAROTID BODY
THYROID CARTILAGE
CAROTID SINUS
ELASTIC CONE
CRICOID CARTILAGE
CAPSULE OF THYROID
THYROID GLAND
PARATHYROID GLANDS
MIDDLE THYROID VEIN
INFERIOR THYROID ARTERY
INFERIOR THYROID VEINS
LEFT SUBCLAVIAN ARTERY
TRACHEA
LEFT COMMON CAROTID ARTERY
RIGHT EXTERNAL JUGULAR VEIN
INNOMINATE ARTERY
RIGHT SUBCLAVIAN VEIN
RIGHT INNOMINATE VEIN
LEFT INNOMINATE VEIN
AORTIC BODIES
SUPERIOR VENA CAVA
AORTIC ARCH

Figure 7–1. Diagram showing the human thyroid and parathyroid glands and their relationships to adjacent structures. The anterior surfaces of the thyroid, larynx, and trachea are shown in the left half of the figure; the posterior surfaces are shown in the right half.

enter the gland along with the blood vessels. The fact that the thyroid secretes when its normal nerve supply is interrupted and when the gland is transplanted to unnatural sites indicates that the most important function of the nerve supply is to regulate the flow of blood through the organ. The thyrotrophic hormone (TSH) of the anterior hypophysis is the principal factor that controls the rate of release of thyroid hormone.

Thyroid tissue regenerates rapidly after subtotal thyroidectomy if the dietary intake of iodine is low, but regeneration does not occur if exogenous thyroid hormone is administered.

Microscopic Anatomy

The thyroid has a greater capacity than any other endocrine gland for storing its secretions, and this is reflected in its histologic structure. The gland is composed of an aggregation of spherical or ovate cystlike *follicles* of variable size (Figs. 7–2 and 7–3). The interfollicular areas are occupied by a highly vascularized network of connective tissue, in which a few lymphocytes and histiocytes may be found. Also in interfollicular areas, as well as in the basal region of the follicles, are ovoid cells containing many granules and an irregularly shaped nucleus. These parafollicular cells, or C-cells, are responsible for the secretion of calcitonin and are of neural crest origin (see p. 229). Each follicle is a microscopic unit and is lined by a secretory epithelium composed of a single layer of cuboidal or low columnar cells. The closed cavities of the follicles normally contain a homogeneous, gelatinous, amber-colored globulin. This secretion is the so-called *colloid,* which gives to the gland its most distinguishing histologic peculiarity. The colloid is a storage product of the secretory epithelium. Its density varies in different glands and in different follicles of the same gland. The amount of colloid fluctuates in pathologic glands and may be reduced or increased by controlled experimental conditions. The thyroid of the normal rat contains in the neighborhood of 100,000 follicles, and these vary widely in size. The larger follicles are generally located near the periphery and the smaller ones in the center.

When the thyroid is inactive, there is a tendency for colloid to accumulate and for the epithelium to become low cuboidal or squamous; when it is overactive, the colloid stores are depleted, and the epithelium becomes columnar and plicated. There are, however, many exceptions, and histolog-

Figure 7–2. Histologic features of the normal thyroid gland of the rat. All normal thyroid glands are structurally similar, though slight variations occur with age, diet, habitation, and sexual status. The normal animals of this colony were maintained on a high protein ration, which probably accounts for the slight hypertrophic condition of the secretory epithelium.

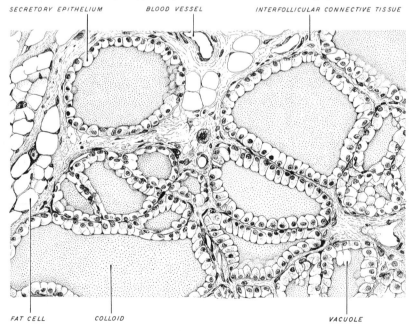

SECRETORY EPITHELIUM   BLOOD VESSEL   INTERFOLLICULAR CONNECTIVE TISSUE

FAT CELL   COLLOID   VACUOLE

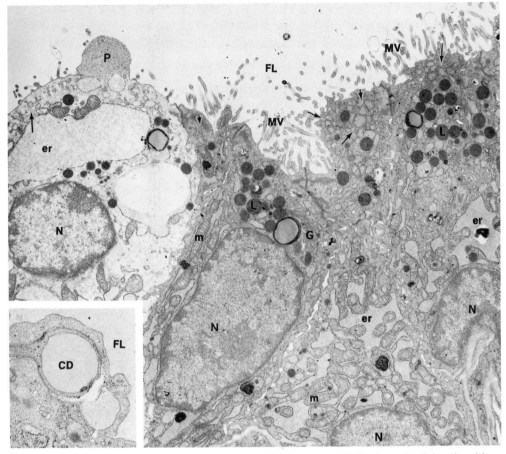

Figure 7–3. Low-powered electron micrograph of a group of follicular cells of dog thyroid, demonstrating their contents following stimulation with thyroid stimulating hormone (TSH). A number of microvilli (MV) projecting into the follicular lumen (FL) are demonstrated. In the cytoplasm, numerous single membrane-limited vacuoles, representing colloid droplets (arrows), are seen. Besides nuclei (N), Golgi apparatus (G), endoplasmic reticulum (er) and mitochondria (m), numerous lysosomes (L) are also seen. A pseudopod is shown (inset) with colloid droplet (CD) formation. Note that the material in the droplets is similar to that found in the follicular lumen (FL). (Electron micrograph and its interpretation kindly provided by Dr. Nicholas A. Panagiotis.)

ic examination alone does not suffice to establish the functional state of the gland.

Electron microscopy of thyroid cells reveals that they have many features in common with other secretory cells. There is an extensive endoplasmic reticulum (ER)) with dilated cisternae and laden with microsomes. This active ER is apparently very much involved with the synthesis of thyro-globulin. A prominent Golgi apparatus is seen near the apical portion of the cell, and mitochondria and lysosomes are scattered throughout the cytoplasm. Microvilli are prominent along the apical surfaces of the cells, and their number is increased following the administration of TSH (Fig. 7–3). In addition to uniodinated globulin, the thyroid cells probably secrete several enzymes into the follicular cavities. While merocrine secretion is probably employed most commonly, the release of entire secretion-laden cells (holo-crine secretion) may occur to some extent in all vertebrates, but evidence of this is most often observed in the thyroids of cyclostomes and teleosts.

Developmental Anatomy

The thyroid is an embryonic derivative of the alimentary tract. It first appears as a median, unpaired evagination from the floor of the embryonic pharynx at the level of the first pair of pharyngeal pouches (Fig. 8–3). The distal end of this outgrowth gradually expands and becomes bilobed, while the stalked attachment narrows to form the *thyroglossal duct.* The branched terminal end of the thyroid primordium assumes a position on the anterior surface of the trachea, and the thyroglossal duct is normally obliterated. The *foramen caecum,* a slight depression at the root of the tongue near the apex of the sulcus terminalis, persists in adult human beings and marks the point where the thyroglossal duct opened into the embryonic pharynx.

Studies on the embryos of several vertebrates indicate that a kind of biochemical maturation occurs in thyroid tissue. In the chick embryo, for example, the immature thyroid can accumulate iodide after incubation for 7 to 8 days, but it cannot form iodinated organic compounds. A brief monoio-dotyrosine stage occurs on the ninth day, and this is followed by the suc-cessive appearance of diiodotyrosine and thyroxine. Similar work on mice embryos has shown that colloid formation begins before the thyroid cells are organized into follicles, and that the synthesis of thyroxine begins later than the collection and organic binding of iodine.[89]

EVOLUTION OF THYROIDAL FUNCTION

Vertebrates

Thyroid glands are present in all vertebrate groups. In adult cyclostomes, the most primitive vertebrates, thyroid follicles are embedded in the fibrous tissue along the floor of the pharynx. The follicles of cyclostomes are his-tologically comparable to those of any other vertebrate, although they are scattered individually along the pharynx. The elasmobranch thyroid is an encapsulated organ usually located near the point where the afferent bran-chial arteries leave the ventral aorta. In most teleosts, the thyroid follicles are scattered along the ventral aorta, and the lack of an organ capsule prob-ably correlates with their tendency to disperse to remote sites. Thyroid folli-cles are often found in the head kidneys of the platyfish (*Platypoecilus*), the number increasing with age.[4, 5] In a few teleosts, such as the Bermuda parrotfish, the follicles are aggregated to form a compact, unpaired gland. The elasmobranch thyroid is typically an unpaired organ lying below the pharynx. The thyroids of amphibians (Fig. 7–4) and birds are paired and widely separated; in turtles and snakes, a single thyroid is found anterior to the heart (Figs. 8–4 and 8–5). Thyroid follicles are not present in the proto-chordates or in invertebrates.

Since the vertebrate thyroid originates as an outpocketing of the pha-ryngeal floor, it is not surprising to find that the endostyle of protochordates shares some functional properties with the thyroid. Autoradiographs pre-pared from *Amphioxus* after immersion in sea water containing ^{131}I demon-strate that the endostyle region does contain organically bound iodine. Some capacity for iodine binding has also been demonstrated in hemichor-dates and urochordates.[6, 8, 27, 88]

The life history of the cyclostomes seems to provide a connecting link between the endostyle organ of protochordates and the ductless glands of all higher chordates. The embryo of the lamprey develops into a larval stage

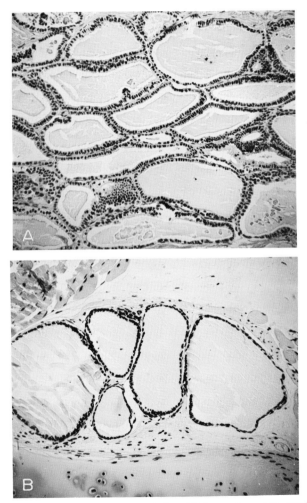

Figure 7–4. The histologic appearance of thyroid tissue from two urodele amphibians. *A, Amphiuma tridactylum; B, Necturus maculosus.* (From Kerkof, P. R., Tong, W., and Chaikoff, I. L.: Endocrinology 73:185, 1963.)

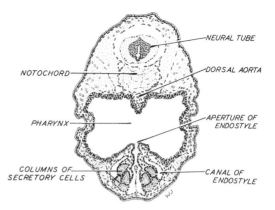

Figure 7–5. Transverse section through the pharynx and subpharyngeal gland (endostyle) of an *Ammocoetes.*

known as the *Ammocoetes,* which has a *subpharyngeal gland* (endostyle) and many other characteristics of *Amphioxus* (Fig. 7–5). Although the endostyle of *Amphioxus* communicates with the pharynx throughout its extent, the endostyle of *Ammocoetes* becomes roofed over both anteriorly and posteriorly, so that only a slitlike opening into the pharyngeal cavity remains at the level of the third gill pouch.

The endostyle of *Amphioxus* contains longitudinal glandular tracts, and it is generally held that its mucus-like secretions entrap particles of food material. It has been shown that the *Ammocoetes* endostyle functions in part, at least, as a holocrine gland; clumps of cells and amorphous materials may be traced through the endostylar duct and into the pharynx. These products from the endostyle are presumably passed into the intestine. After a period of three or more years, the *Ammocoetes* larva transforms into an adult lamprey. During this metamorphosis, some of the epithelial cells of the endostyle persist and transform into the follicles of the thyroid gland. While the endostyle of *Ammocoetes* contains nothing during its long larval life that resembles thyroid follicles, studies using radioiodine have shown that the endostylar epithelium functions similarly to thyroidal cells inasmuch as it accumulates and produces iodinated protein substances. Thyroid hormones have not been demonstrated to have any effect on the metamorphosis of *Ammocoetes.*[7, 19, 20]

Invertebrates

Diiodotyrosine, one of the precursors of thyroxine, was first identified in the organic skeleton or gorgonid corals. It is now known that the skeletons of sponges and corals contain monoiodotyrosine in addition to diiodotyrosine, monobromotyrosine, and dibromotyrosine. Although iodotyrosines have been detected in a great variety of invertebrate forms, thyroxine has been found in only a few invertebrates, notably gorgonians and tunicates.[10, 42, 43] It is especially striking that scyphozoan jellyfish can form thyroxine, which apparently functions in their metamorphosis.[11]

While it is surprising to find thyroxine so prevalent in the tissues of thyroidless invertebrates, it is known that mammalian tissues may produce thyroxine in the absence of the thyroid gland. Furthermore, the iodination of various proteins (*e.g.,* casein, blood proteins), followed by hydrolysis, yields crystals of thyroxine without enzymatic intervention. When iodine and proteins are incubated together under the proper conditions, the tyrosine in the protein molecule takes up this element and forms mono- and diiodotyrosine. The iodinated tyrosines are then coupled to yield thyroxine. Thus, the thyroid gland may not be the only tissue capable of synthesizing thyroxine. Since tissue proteins are certain to contain tyrosine, it is reasonable to assume that this amino acid can be converted to thyroxine if iodine is available and if suitable oxidizing systems are present. This view would regard the synthesis of thyroxine as a general biologic reaction, the thyroid gland being merely an organ highly specialized in this direction and capable of storing the hormone. There are indications that tyrosine iodination may occur in rainbow trout following the complete destruction of thyroid follicles by radiothyroidectomy.[34, 61, 78, 80]

Studies on the invertebrates indicate that thyroid hormones and their precursors became available to organisms long before a discrete thyroid gland developed. However, the mere presence of iodinated thyronines in the invertebrates does not mean that these substances are being used for any particular purpose. There is no clear evidence that the administration of thyroxine and similar substances to invertebrates produces any kind of response. It is probable that the phylogenetic appearance of a thyroid gland coincides with the development of a metabolic use for thyroxine and similar compounds.

Summary of Evolution

The diagrams in Figure 7–6 summarize the important events that appear to have occurred during evolution of the thyroid gland. Iodoproteins have been identified in most invertebrate phyla, but these have a tendency to be localized in hard exoskeletal structures, such as setae, byssus threads, periostracum, and pharyngeal teeth. It is supposed that the source of iodoproteins shifted into the pharyngeal region after such materials became of metabolic utility to the organism. It is possible that structures such as pharyngeal teeth provided a large and dependable source of iodoprotein, and that this material was digested in the intestine to form thyroxine and similar compounds. In *Amphioxus* and *Ammocoetes,* the iodoprotein is no longer a scleroprotein associated with pharyngeal teeth but emanates from a pharyngeal gland of exocrine type, the endostyle. While the endostyle of the lamprey contains a protease, it is more likely that hydrolysis of the iodoprotein occurs in the digestive tract. In contrast to *Amphioxus,* the iodoprotein-forming gland of *Ammocoetes* drains its products into the pharynx by means of a duct. When the endostylar duct closes at metamorphosis, the substance of the organ differentiates into a thyroid that already contains a thyroprotein-splitting enzyme (protease) like that of mammals. At this point in the life cycle of the lamprey, the vertebrate type of thyroid gland is differentiated; the presence of a local protease makes possible the closure of the

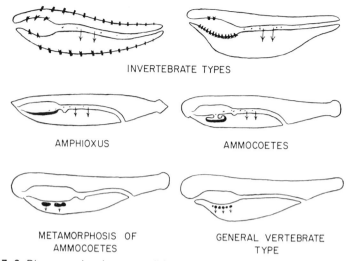

INVERTEBRATE TYPES

AMPHIOXUS   AMMOCOETES

METAMORPHOSIS OF   GENERAL VERTEBRATE
AMMOCOETES   TYPE

Figure 7–6. Diagrams showing a possible pattern of evolution of the thyroid gland. Iodoproteins are indicated as solid black. See text for explanation. (From Gorbman, A.: *In* Columbia
University Symposium on Comparative Endocrinology. New York, John Wiley & Sons, 1959.)

duct to the pharynx, the storage of iodoproteins, and the release of hormones directly into the circulation. It is reasonable to assume that these
changes occurring in the lamprey's endostyle at metamorphosis represent,
at least in part, the general pattern of changes that ensued during the evolution of the vertebrate thyroid.[40, 42]

BIOCHEMISTRY OF THYROID HORMONE

Thyroglobulin is the most important protein present in the colloid of the
thyroid follicle.[74] It is an iodinated glycoprotein having a molecular weight of
about 660,000 and is considered to be the storage form of the thyroid hormone. Thyroglobulin does not normally appear in the circulation. Under
physiologic conditions, this large protein is hydrolyzed by a mixture of cath-
eptases and yields a number of iodinated amino acids, *viz.*, mono- and
diiodotyrosine, 3,3'-diiodothyronine, 3,5,3'-triiodothyronine, 3,3',5'-triiodo-
thyronine, and 3,5,3',5'-tetraiodothyronine (thyroxine) (Fig. 7–7). Monoiodotyrosine (MIT) and diiodotyrosine (DIT) do not leave the follicle; they are rapidly deiodinated within the thyroid cells, the iodine being reutilized for a
recycling synthesis of thyroglobulin. This change is effected by the enzyme
deiodinase, which has only mono- and diiodotyrosine for its substrate. About
60 per cent of the iodine present in thyroglobulin is due to the iodotyrosines,
and 30 per cent to the iodothyronines. Of the thyronines that are secreted
into the circulation, only 3,5,3'-triiodothyronine and thyroxine are known to
have any biologic activity. In certain tests, 3,5,3'-triiodothyronine (T_3) is
found to be over seven times as active as thyroxine (T_4), and the latent period
required for it to produce its effect is less than with thyroxine.

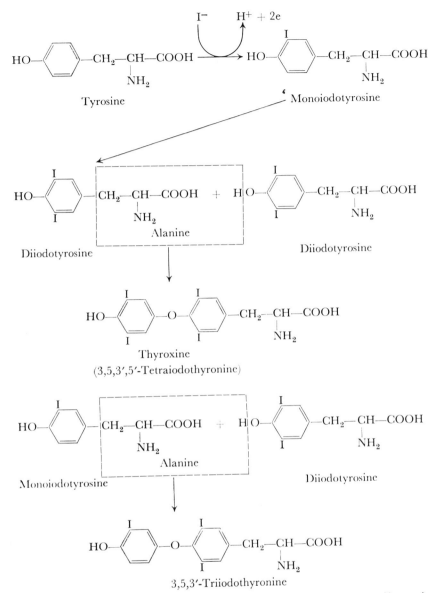

Figure 7-7. Proposed pathways in the biosynthesis of thyroid hormones. No mechanism has yet been discovered that explains the coupling of two molecules of diiodotyrosine.

The deaminated analogues, such as tetraiodothyroacetic acid (TETRAC) and triiodothyroacetic acid (TRIAC), have so far been demonstrated only in peripheral tissues. They have not been found in the blood and appear in the tissues only after the administration of radioactive thyroxine. They have not been found to appear in the tissues after the administration of radioiodide. The biologic effects of TETRAC and TRIAC are qualitatively different from those of the thyronines found in the blood. For example,

TRIAC is potent in inducing the metamorphosis of amphibian larvae, but it is relatively weak in preventing goiter and in elevating the consumption of oxygen in the rat. TETRAC, on the other hand, stimulates tissue metabolism, but is weak in promoting amphibian metamorphosis. TRIAC also exerts a selective lowering effect on serum cholesterol.

It is not known in what form the thyroid hormone acts upon the peripheral tissues, and this lack of information has hampered studies aimed at determining the mechanism of action of the hormone. It is known that both thyroxine and triiodothyronine are natural products of the gland, and that the latter has even greater potency than the former. Though thyroxine is present in the blood in far greater concentration than any other product of the thyroid, many investigators have felt that it may not be the active form of the hormone and have suggested that it may be converted to triiodothyronine or some other form before affecting peripheral tissues. There are indications that the kidney may play an important role in coverting thyroxine to a more active form of the hormone. Surviving kidney slices can deiodinate thyroxine to triiodothyronine, whereas homogenates of this organ do not. The mitochondrial fraction of rat kidney homogenates converts thyroxine and triiodothyronine to their respective acetic acid analogues, TETRAC and TRIAC. Both analogues uncouple oxidative phosphorylation in mitochondrial preparations, but they are less active by mammalian tests than are their respective precursors. It may be that a complex of thyroid compounds operates at the tissue level, or that the cellularly active form of the hormone has not yet been discovered.[62, 63]

The thyroid hormones are transported in the blood in close association with the albumin and α-globulin fractions of serum protein. The latter is referred to as thyroxine-binding protein (TBG). Thyroxine is bound very tightly to this protein, and only a small fraction is bound to albumin. Triiodothyronine is also bound to TBG, but the protein seems to have a higher affinity for T_4 than for T_3. TBG has been the subject of intensive investigation, and much has been learned about the nature of the molecule. Its relative affinities for various analogues of T_3 and T_4 have also been studied. The plasma contains more TBG than is necessary to bind normal concentrations of thyroxine, only about one-third of the protein-binding capacity of the serum proteins being used normally. During pregnancy and after the administration of estrogens, there is a profound increase in the thyroxine-binding capacity of the blood proteins. As the hormones circulate through the tissues, they are freed from their protein carriers, pass through the capillary walls, and impinge upon the tissue cells.[35, 46, 85]

Very little is known about the binding of thyroid hormones by tissue proteins. However, it has been reported that rat skeletal muscle contains a protein fraction that can bind physiologic concentrations of levorotatory thyroxine and 3,5,3'-triiodothyronine. This appears to be a specific protein and is not the same as TBG of the serum. It is important to note that both T_3 and T_4 have been shown to bind specifically to nuclei of cells of the rat liver and kidney. This has important implications in the mechanism of action of these hormones.

The naturally occurring thyroid hormones are levorotatory. Synthetic thyroxine is a mixture of the D- and L-isomers (racemic) and is much less active biologically than is L-thyroxine. It has been reported that enzyme systems from rat kidney do not deiodinate D-thyroxine to triiodothyronine. It might be that the failure of D-thyroxine to undergo these transformations correlates with its biologic inactivity.[31]

Biosynthesis of Thyroid Hormone

Knowledge of thyroid metabolism has been advanced by applying the techniques of chromatography and autoradiography of compounds labeled with [131]I. The first procedure makes it possible to separate minute amounts of material, and the second to locate iodinated products in tissues and to measure their rate of accumulation. The various antithyroid agents have also proved useful in investigating thyroid chemistry and physiology. The process of thyroid hormone formation may be divided into three stages: (1) the accumulation or trapping of iodide from the circulation, (2) the iodination of tyrosine, and (3) the proteolysis of thyroglobulin.[77, 88]

Iodide Accumulation

The diet may contain iodine in several forms. Most of it is reduced to iodide before it is absorbed from the gastrointestinal tract and appears in the blood as inorganic iodide. The concentration of inorganic iodide in the blood plasma is very low, but the cells of the thyroid epithelium have a greater avidity for it than does any other tissue. The concentration gradient

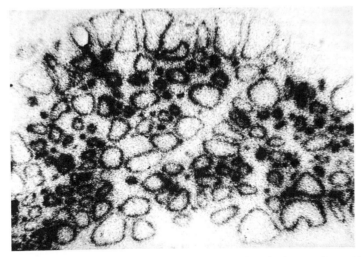

Figure 7–8. An autoradiogram of rat's thyroid 1 hour after the intraperitoneal injection of radioiodide. Note that at this early stage the radioiodide collects in the periphery of the follicles, rather than being distributed throughout the colloid. (From Nadler and Lebland: Brookhaven Symposia in Biology, No. 7, 1955.)

for iodide achieved by the normal thyroid is 20:1 or more, over the blood plasma. Inorganic iodide composes only about 1 per cent of the total iodine content of the thyroid under physiologic conditions. Within 15 minutes after the administration of radioiodide to the rat, 90 per cent of the radioactivity in the thyroid is present in organic compounds (Fig. 7–8). However, after the administration of certain antithyroid drugs that inhibit the iodination of tyrosine, high concentrations of inorganic iodide may accumulate in the gland.

Iodination of Tyrosine

The inorganic iodide that accumulates in the follicular epithelium is oxidized to I_2 (elemental iodine) or IO^-. This process is controlled by one or more enzyme systems, including a thyroid peroxidase. In the proposed pathway of thyroid hormone synthesis, tyrosine is first iodinated to monoiodotyrosine and then to diiodotyrosine (Fig. 7–7). The most popular belief is that this iodination takes place at the level of thyroglobulin rather than at the level of the free amino acids themselves (Fig. 7–9). It is easier to form T_4 in vitro by the iodination of protein than by the iodination of free tyrosine. Though the mechanism remains obscure, it has been postulated that thyroxine is formed by the coupling of two molecules of DIT, with the loss of one alanine side chain. Triiodothyronine may be produced by the coupling of one molecule of MIT with one of DIT, or by the loss of one iodine

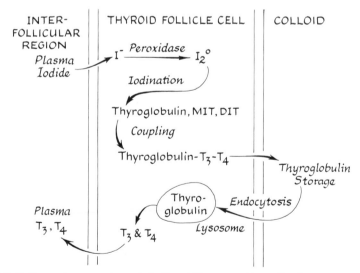

Figure 7–9. General survey of events in thyroid hormone biosynthesis, storage, and release. Reduced iodide enters the follicle cell, where it is oxidized to I_2 and where it iodinates tyrosyl residues of the thyroglobulin (Thyroglobulin MIT, DIT). The iodotyrosines are somehow coupled to form Thyroglobulin T_3, T_4 which passes to the colloid for storage. During T_3 and T_4 secretion, thyroglobulin is taken back from the colloid and is trapped in lysosomes. Subsequent enzymatic action leads to the release of T_3 and T_4.

atom from the T_4 molecule. How the coupling of iodinated tyrosines can occur while the amino acids are involved in peptide bonds in the thyroglobulin molecule is not understood. Apparently the thyroid cell produces thyroglobulin continuously and passes it into the lumen of the follicle, where it is stored. The synthesis of thyroid hormones is accelerated by pituitary thyrotrophin and is blocked by certain antithyroid agents. Certain forms of cretinism have been traced to an inability of the thyroid to couple iodotyrosines.[83]

Proteolysis of Thyroglobulin

The enzymatic elaboration and breakdown of thyroglobulin in the follicle occurs continuously, and this insures a regular turnover of thyroglobulin. During active thyroid hormone secretion, thyroglobulin stored in the colloid is apparently retrieved into the follicle cells by a kind of pinocytosis (Fig. 7–9). The retrieved globulin is presumably contained in many lysosomes in the follicular cytoplasm; because of enzymatic activity in these organelles, the thyroglobulin is split into smaller molecules, with the ultimate liberation of T_3 and T_4 into the circulation. Monoiodotyrosine and diiodotyrosine are deiodinated by the enzyme deiodinase, the resultant iodide being returned to the thyroid iodide pool. The synthesis of thyroid hormones in amphibians is similar to that of mammals.

It is clear that thyroglobulin is the storage form of the thyroid hormone, and thyroxine is the principal circulating hormone. Triiodothyronine is also present in the blood, but only in relatively small amounts. It is not known what form of the hormone is active at the level of the peripheral tissues. It may well be that a complex of hormones, including thyroxine, triiodothyronine, and their metabolites, is active in the peripheral tissues. The fact that thyroid functions are conditioned by the pituitary, adrenals, pancreas, and other endocrine glands suggests that secretions from multiple glands may be required at the tissue level in order for thyroid hormones to produce their characteristic effects.

Catabolism of Thyroid Hormones

The liver and kidneys are the chief organs concerned in the *catabolism* of thyroid hormones. Since the liver is an important organ in the destruction of excessive hormone and in the regulation of biliary excretion mechanisms, it appears to play an important role in regulating the thyroid hormone content of the body. Thyroxine and triiodothyronine are conjugated as glucuronides in the liver and are then passed through the bile into the intestine. An alternative pathway in the liver is the oxidative deamination of these hormones to form the corresponding pyruvic acid derivatives. Small amounts of thyroxine and triiodothyronine and their deaminated metabolites are excreted through the bile in an unconjugated form. Both free and conjugated forms of thyroxine are excreted in small amounts through the kidneys. Thyroidal compounds may be extensively deiodinated in the liver and in certain other organs, such as the salivary glands. There is also some evidence that certain metabolites of the thyroid hormones may be resorbed from the intestine and circulate repeatedly through the liver. The iodide produced from hormone degradation is reutilized by the thyroid gland or excreted by the kidney. Only minute amounts of organically bound iodine are lost through the kidneys. The body shows great economy in handling its iodine stores, and it normally retains most of the iodine freed through the metabolism of thyroid hormones.

Antithyroid Agents (Goitrogens)

A number of chemical agents can interfere, in one way or another, with the thyroid mechanisms involved in the synthesis of hormones. These antithyroid substances have the common property of causing a fall in the blood level of thyroxine, and this leads to an augmented output of thyrotrophin (TSH) by the anterior pituitary. The latter hormone causes hypertrophy of thyroid tissue, and, if there is conspicuous enlargement of the thyroid, it may be termed *goiter*. Hence, these agents are sometimes called *goitrogens*.

Iodine

Since iodine is an essential atom of the thyroid hormone molecule, the gland cannot synthesize its hormones without adequate quantities of iodide in the blood. Inadequate dietary intake of this element leads to thyroid hormone deficiency and to compensatory hypertrophy and hyperplasia of the thyroid epithelium, a condition known as simple hyperplastic goiter. Conversely, large doses of iodide, administered to those whose thyroids are hyperactive and secreting excessive hormone, reduce the hypertrophy and hyperplasia of the gland and promote the storage of colloid. High levels of blood iodide inhibit the thyroid of the normal subject in a comparable manner, although the effect is transitory and less pronounced. The mechanism whereby iodide produces this effect remains largely unknown. It is certain that its action is different from that of the goitrogens and that it does not interfere with the peripheral action of thyroid hormone.[44, 81, 95]

There are some suggestions that high levels of iodide may diminish thyroid function by antagonizing the action of TSH. It is known that the ability of the thyroid of the hypophysectomized rat to concentrate iodide in response to exogenous TSH is influenced by the iodine content of the diet. The thyroid concentrates radioiodide more effectively when iodine intake is low than when it is high. This effect is not due to the level of circulating iodide *per se* but rather to products arising through the organification of iodide within the thyroid itself. Probably organic iodine—containing compounds within the thyroid, possibly thyroid hormone itself, in some manner antagonize the stimulating action of TSH on the iodine-accumulating mechanism.

Prolonged iodine deficiency produces goiter in many species of laboratory animals. When rats are fed a diet low in iodine, the animals first develop hyperplastic thyroids owing to excessive stimulation by TSH; if the iodine deficiency persists, the thyroids become progressively larger and go on to develop nodules and different types of tumors. The histologic aspects of diffuse colloid goiter have been produced in hamsters by maintaining them on iodine-deficient diets and then administering iodine. The glands become very hyperplastic and lose colloid while the diet lacks iodine; when iodine is administered, large amounts of colloid distend the follicles.[3, 32]

Antithyroid Compounds

Goiters have been produced experimentally by feeding different kinds of natural foods and by administering chemical compounds that block the synthesis of thyroid hormone.[65] Two principal categories of compounds have been found to possess antithyroid activity. The first and most active group includes the thiocarbamide derivatives, such as thiourea, thiouracil, and propylthiouracil. The second category contains compounds that have an amino-benzene ring in their structure, including the sulfa drugs, paraaminobenzoic acid, paraaminosalicylic acid, etc. Other compounds, such as 5-vinyl-2-thiooxazolidine, from the seeds of rape, cabbage, kale, and turnips, are also active goitrogens. The sulfonylureas, a group of compounds used clinically in the treatment of diabetes mellitus, also have antithyroid properties.[73, 76]

Sulfonamides and Thioureas. It was first shown in 1941 that goiter could be produced in rats by the administration of sulfaguanidine. Shortly thereafter, it was found that other sulfonamides and thiourea also acted in a similar manner and produced large hyperplastic goiters in rats, mice, and dogs. Furthermore, the important observation was made that goiters of this type could not be prevented even by giving massive doses of iodide, leading to the conclusion that the drugs acted by suppressing the synthesis of thyroid hormone. Hyperplasia of the thyroid in response to these agents did not occur after hypophysectomy, indicating that the goiter was mediated by some pituitary factor, most probably TSH. These studies also provided convincing evidence that hormone synthesis by the thyroid could be divorced completely from the histologic picture of overactivity. Such enlarged, hyperplastic goiters produced little, if any, thyroid hormone, and the basal metabolic rates of the animals were at or near the thyroidectomy level. The administration of thyroxine to intact animals receiving antithyroid drugs restored the metabolic rate and completely prevented the thyroid hyperplasia.[70, 71]

The thioureas, sulfonamides, and related compounds apparently produce goiter in the following manner. The thyroids of treated animals can accumulate iodide normally, but the iodination of tyrosine in the gland is blocked. Thyroxine cannot be synthesized, and oxygen consumption falls. The low levels of circulating thyroxine elicit an augmented output of TSH by the anterior pituitary, and the latter hormone causes hypertrophy, hyperpla-

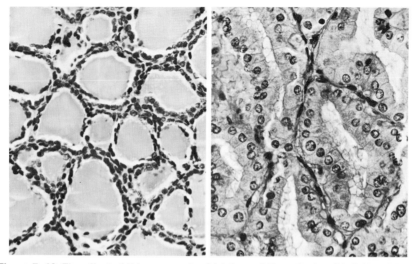

Figure 7–10. The effect of thiourea on the histology of the rat's thyroid. *A*, Normal thyroid; *B*, thyroid of rat fed 0.6 per cent thiourea for 21 days. Notice the loss of colloid and the hyperplastic epithelium in the gland of the treated animal. (From Mackenzie, C. G.: Fed. Proc. *17*, 1958.)

sia, and loss of colloid from the thyroid. Although the thyrotrophin causes enormous enlargement of the thyroid and an increased secretory surface, it still cannot synthesize thyroxine (Fig. 7–10). The goiter can be relieved only by administering thyroxine or by withdrawing the antithyroid drug. The enlarged thyroid (goiter) could be made to shrink below normal size by removing the pituitary, the source of TSH, but such glands would not produce any thyroxine so long as the goitrogen was administered.

While the thioureas and sulfonamides both prevent the iodination of tyrosine, the goiters produced by these two classes of compounds respond differently to dietary iodine. The goiters resulting from relatively low levels of thiourea and thiouracil can be reduced in weight by feeding small amounts of iodide, but no such effect is observed in the goiters resulting from administration of the sulfonamides. The dietary iodide reduces the hyperplasia and loss of colloid in the thiourea- and thiouracil-induced goiters, but in the sulfonamide-induced goiters, these changes are intensified by the same amounts of dietary iodide.

The mechanisms involved in the production of goiter by the antithyroid agents seem to be essentially the same in warm-blooded and in cold-blooded vertebrates. Thyroid tumors appear frequently on the gills and in the leg cartilages of *Ambystoma maculatum* reared in solutions of propylthiouracil.[22] Cells from the hyperplastic thyroids apparently are carried through the heart to the gill capillaries, from where they are filtered out and differentiate into thyroid follicles. Similar thyroid growths have been found in the lungs of mice after thiouracil feeding.[13, 17, 24, 26]

Thiocyanate.   Goiters may be produced by the administration of thiocyanate, if the blood iodide concentration is low. Its goitrogenic activity can be abolished by adding iodide to the diet. Thiocyanate, perchlorate, periodate, and other oxyacids of the two latter substances produce goiter by interfering with the "trapping" of iodide ions by the thyroid gland and by causing a discharge of concentrated iodide already in the gland at the time of their administration. These substances do not block any of the synthetic mechanisms in the thyroid (*i.e.,* oxidation, iodination of tyrosine, and coupling), but act in some way to inhibit the accumulation of iodide within the gland. If the dietary intake of iodide is high, enough may enter the gland to permit the synthesis of adequate amounts of thyroxine, and goiter does not occur. The mechanism involved in the reduced iodide accumulation is unknown.

CALCITONIN AND THE THYROID

Much experimental evidence has accumulated since 1961 indicating that the thyroid-parathyroid complex in mammals is the source of a fast-acting hormone which lowers the level of serum calcium. The hormone is released in response to hypercalcemia, and it opposes the action of the parathyroid hormone. The main points of controversy at present are whether the calcium-lowering principle originates in any of the parathyroids as well as in the thyroid gland, and whether the cells which supposedly secrete the hormone are of ultimobranchial origin.

Copp and his co-workers first identified a calcium-lowering factor which existed as an impurity in commercial parathyroid extracts, and called it "calcitonin." Munson reported that removal of the parathyroids of the rat by cautery produced a greater fall in serum calcium than did removal of the same glands by surgical excision. Hirsch and his colleagues found that cautery of the thyroid produces hypocalcemia in the rat, and this was offered as an explanation of the earlier findings of Munson. They adduced evidence that the calcium-lowering principle originated in the thyroid, rather than in the parathyroid, and called the substance "thyrocalcitonin." By using rats carrying functional parathyroid grafts, Talmage and his colleagues substantiated the presence of a hypocalcemic factor from the thyroid and demonstrated that it is normally conveyed by the blood. This hypocalcemic factor is calcitonin; it is produced and secreted from the parafollicular cells (C-cells).

PHYSIOLOGY OF THE THYROID GLAND

Control of Thyroid Secretion

Pituitary Thyrotrophin (TSH)

Pituitary thyrotrophin is the main factor controlling thyroid function under normal conditions (Figs. 7–11 and 7–12). After hypophysectomy, the

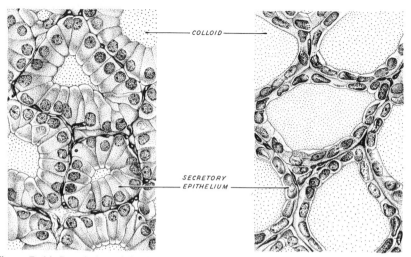

COLLOID

SECRETORY EPITHELIUM

Figure 7–11. Regulation of the functional state of the rat's thyroid gland by means of thyrotrophic hormone from the anterior lobe of the hypophysis. *A,* Thyroid from a normal rat which had received 10 daily injections of thyrotrophic hormone. Notice the high columnar cells of the secretory epithelium and the loss of colloid. *B,* Thyroid from a rat 6 months after complete removal of the pituitary gland. When an animal is deprived of thyrotrophic hormone, the thyroid gland becomes inactive; the cells of the secretory epithelium become low cuboidal or nearly squamous in type, and colloid distends the follicles. The two glands are drawn to scale.

capacity of the thyroid to trap ^{131}I is greatly decreased, and only traces of thyroxine appear in the circulation. The synthesis and discharge of thyroid hormone are automatically adjusted to the demand in accordance with the levels of hormone present in the blood. High circulating levels of thyroid hormone depress the output of pituitary TSH, whereas low levels increase it. As mentioned previously, goiter develops when the thyroid cannot meet the demands of the organism for thyroxine and TSH stimulates it at an excessive rate for prolonged periods. Furthermore, derangement of the physiologic feedback mechanism can produce neoplastic growths in the anterior hypophysis. A marked and sustained deficiency of thyroid hormone in the circulation may induce tumors involving the pituitary thyrotrophs, the cells that appear to be responsible for the secretion of TSH. Pituitary tumors of this type have been produced in laboratory rodents by surgical thyroidectomy, by radiothyroidectomy, and by giving propylthiouracil for long periods.[37, 41]

It has not been finally decided whether the pituitary gland produces one or several types of thyrotrophin. Clinical studies have suggested that abnormal kinds of thyrotrophins may appear in the serum of some thyrotoxic patients.[1] A substance closely related to TSH has been found in pituitary extracts; it is especially potent in producing exophthalmos, an abnormal protrusion of the eyeball. Most workers feel that the "exophthalmos-producing substance" is not a distinct anterior pituitary hormone, but that it may be an abnormal kind of TSH involved in the etiology of this eye defect.[48]

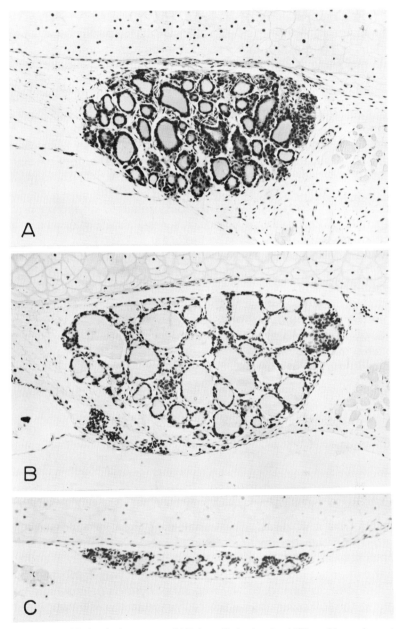

Figure 7–12. Thyroid glands from normal *(A)*, hypothalectomized *(B)*, and hypophysectomized *(C)* tadpoles of *Rana pipiens*. The hypothalectomized animals possess a pars distalis which is not connected with the brain. Since the thyroid glands from such animals have follicles with very flat epithelia and contain abundant colloid, it may be concluded that the output of TSH by the disconnected pars distalis is subnormal. In the hypophysectomized animal, TSH is lacking and the thyroids are very small and atrophic *(C)*. (Courtesy of Dr. Y. Hanaoka, Gunma University, Maebashi, Japan.)

Compensatory Adjustments

Unless adequate amounts of iodide are provided, the thyroid cannot meet the requirements of the body for thyroid hormone. During periods of iodine deficiency, the pituitary secretes augmented amounts of TSH and, under its influence, a compensatory adjustment occurs that results in the production of a more extensive secretory epithelium. The thyroid cells enlarge (hypertrophy) and increase mitotically (hyperplasia); thus the gland enlarges in an attempt to make up for the deficient activity of the individual cells. While the hyperplastic gland loses colloid, the epithelial cells increase in height, the follicular walls become plicated, vascularity is increased, and the gland generally increases in weight. *Goiter* is the term generally applied to the various types of thyroid enlargement. These morphologic changes indicate excitation and, so far as is known, TSH is the sole instrument that induces them. Since transplanted thyroids react to changing physiologic states exactly as do the intact glands, it seems that hormones are more essential than are regulatory nerves to the organ.

If, over a period of time, the pituitary stimulation does not succeed in restoring the thyroid secretion to normal, the gland enters into a phase of exhaustion from which it may never recover. The secretory cells of the exhausted gland decrease in size, and some of the cells degenerate and are lost from the epithelium (atrophy). On the other hand, if a more adequate iodine supply becomes available, pituitary stimulation is reduced and the hyperplastic gland subsides. The thyroid gland may repeat this cycle many times during the life of the individual:

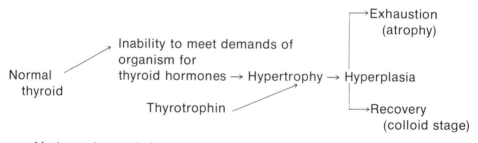

Marine advanced the concept that large colloid goiters might result from subjecting the thyroid repeatedly to hyperplasia and regression. This theory has been tested by administering sulfaguanidine to rats and withholding the treatment at intervals. When the goitrogen was withdrawn at the end of the third feeding period, the hyperplastic thyroids promptly accumulated colloid and the follicular epithelium regressed to the low cuboidal type. After a month with no sulfaguanidine being given, the thyroids continued to be two and a half times the normal size. Similar results have been obtained in the hamster, the animals being placed repeatedly on iodine-deficient diets.

Environment and Thyroid Function

It is known that many kinds of environmental stimuli can affect the release of hormones from the thyroid gland. The exposure of warm-blooded animals to cold environments increases thyroid activity. On the other hand, emotional and systemic stressors exert inhibitory effects on thyroid function. While noxious stimuli promote an augmented release of ACTH and a consequent activation of the adrenal cortex, the same stimuli apparently reduce the pituitary release of TSH and diminish thyroid functions.

Temperature. When rats are exposed to cold, an increase in metabolic rate occurs rapidly and thyroid hyperplasia becomes apparent after prolonged exposure. Thyroidectomized animals survive only for relatively short periods at low environmental temperatures. Survival apparently depends on the presence of thyroid hormone and on an increase in metabolic rate. Histologic changes in the thyroid gland of the guinea pig, indicating TSH stimulation, occur within 30 minutes after exposure to cold. When TSH is administered to rabbits pretreated with ^{131}I, labeled thyroxine appears in the thyroid vein blood after a very short latent period. These results indicate that the response of the pituitary-thyroid axis to cold is too rapid to be explained on the basis of increased utilization of thyroxine by the peripheral tissues and on the operation of a feedback mechanism. It is more probable that the cold stimulus activates a nervous reflex, which operates through the hypothalamus to augment and maintain the release of pituitary thyrotrophin.[14, 30, 50, 84]

Emotional and Systemic Stressors. Physical stressors, such as hemorrhage, trauma, and the injection of irritating substances, induce a prompt and prolonged inhibition of thyroid secretion, presumably as a consequence of diminished release of TSH. Changing illumination, pain, restraint, and other emotional situations likewise cause a prompt reduction of thyroid hormone secretion. This inhibitory influence on the thyroid also occurs rapidly and most probably involves the nervous system. During the period of thyroid inhibition, the concentration of thyroxine in the circulation is diminished; if the response were due to the operation of a feedback mechanism, the blood levels of thyroxine would be expected to rise, in order to reduce the output of TSH. It is difficult to account for the observation that surgical trauma in the rabbit continues to cause thyroid inhibition after the pituitary stalk has been sectioned.[15]

Hypothalamus and TSH Secretion

It is well known that reducing the secretory surface of the thyroid gland by subtotal thyroidectomy diminishes the blood thyroxine levels, and the pituitary gland accordingly augments its release of TSH. When about three-fourths of the rat's thyroid is removed, the remaining fragment undergoes hypertrophy and the thyroid-serum iodide ratio (T:S ratio) increases. After destroying proper areas of the hypothalamus by electrolytic lesions, the compensatory hypertrophy of the thyroid fragment does not occur. This indicates that the hypothalamic lesions may prevent the elevated output of TSH by the pituitary gland. Much evidence from different mammalian species indicates that the pituitary gonadotrophins, corticotrophin, and thyrotrophin may be independently affected, depending upon the specific area of the hypothalamus that is destroyed. The implication of these studies is that

nervous impulses discharged in hypothalamic centers result in the formation of release factors (TRF) that are carried to the anterior hypophysis via
the hypophysial portal veins.

Using the remote control method, it is possible to apply localized electrical stimuli to the hypothalamus for prolonged periods of time. A coil of
wire is implanted subcutaneously in the lumbar region, and leads are
passed under the skin to connect this coil with electrodes implanted in
the brain with the aid of a stereotactic instrument. The hypothalamic area of
the unanesthetized animal may be stimulated by remote control by placing
it in an electromagnetic field and inducing a certain voltage in the coil implanted under the skin. Particular areas of the hypothalamus may be stimulated continuously for several days in this manner. Since hypothalamic stimulation may cause ACTH release and since the adrenal cortical hormones
are known to depress thyroid activity in the rabbit, adrenalectomized animals give the most reliable results in studies with TSH. Stimulation of the
anterior median eminence results in an accelerated release of thyrotrophin
from the anterior pituitary, as determined by the release of radioactive materials from the thyroid. There is general agreement that a neural mechanism concerned with TSH secretion is located in the median eminence region of the hypothalamus.[47]

The problem of how the circulating thyroid hormones regulate the pituitary release of TSH is a very complicated one and has not been settled.
The fact that radioactive thyroxine and triiodothyronine tend to collect in
the paraventricular region of the hypothalamus, as well as in the neuro- and
adenohypophysis, is an interesting observation, but of unknown significance. It is quite possible that the blood level of thyroid hormone affects the
release of TSH by way of a hypothalamic mechanism ("long-loop feedback"), as well as by action directly on the pituitary gland. The hypothalamic mechanism appears to influence TSH secretion in both an excitatory and
an inhibitory manner, and there are strong indications that the integrity of
the hypophysial portal system is essential for this control. On the other
hand, injected thyroxine effectively decreases the output of TSH by pituitary
transplants persisting in the anterior eye chambers of hypophysectomized
rabbits. Thyroxine exerts the same effect in rabbits after sectioning of the
pituitary stalk. Thus, it seems reasonably well established that high levels of
blood thyroxine can act directly on the pituitary to inhibit the release of
TSH, and, in this regard, the data seem stronger for TSH than for any other
adenohypophysial hormone. In the light of these observations, it seems
rather paradoxical that the first hypothalamic releasing factor to be purified
and identified, TRF, is involved with an adenohypophysial hormone whose
control system may, under some circumstances, bypass the hypothalamus.
At present we can only assume that TSH secretion can be controlled both at
the level of the pituitary and at the level of the hypothalamus.

Physiologic Effects of Thyroid Hormone

The effects of thyroid hormones are multiple and, while this is a claim
that can be made for many other hormones, none truly has the breadth of

action of thyroid hormone. In part this broad spectrum of action is based upon the well-documented metabolic effects of thyroid hormones; however, in recent years, much has been added to our knowledge of the role of the thyroid in developmental processes. At present, it seems reasonable to categorize the actions of thyroid hormone into two general groups: (1) metabolic effects, and (2) growth-promoting developmental actions. Metabolic effects include calorigenesis, regulation of water and ion transport, and the regulation of intermediary metabolism. Developmental actions include influences on the growth rate of tissues of homoiotherms, regulation of amphibian metamorphosis, and the control of protein synthesis. Most developmental effects of thyroid hormone are probably mediated through the genetic control of RNA and protein biosynthesis.

Calorigenesis

Homoiotherms. In warm-blooded animals, the most characteristic effect of thyroid hormone is to increase the energy production and oxygen consumption of most normal tissues. The basal metabolic rate (BMR) falls rapidly after thyroidectomy or hypophysectomy and may be elevated above the normal level by administration of thyroid hormone. The increased metabolism of hyperthyroid animals is reflected in the accelerated respiration of its excised tissues; tissues taken from thyroidectomized animals respire at a comparatively low rate. After administration of thyroid hormone to the animal, the respiration of surviving liver, kidney, skeletal muscle, cardiac muscle, gastric mucosa, and diaphragm is strikingly increased. Several workers have found that the respiration of surviving brain, spleen, and testis is not enhanced by hormone administered to the animal and that the respiration of thyroid tissue is decreased by the same procedure. A number of enzyme systems, notably cytochrome oxidase, cytochrome c, and succinoxidase, increase in the tissues after thyroxine administration to the animal and are diminished by thyroidectomy or thiouracil feeding.

Calorigenesis in the normal organism is regulated by a balance of hormonal factors, thyroid hormone not being the only hormone involved. Heat production in the rat declines more abruptly after hypophysectomy than after thyroidectomy. Thyroxine and triiodothyronine elevate the BMR more effectively in thyroidectomized animals than in hypophysectomized animals. Doses of TSH sufficient to cause thyroid hypertrophy in hypophysectomized rats increase the BMR but do not restore it to normal. It is apparent that the anterior pituitary affects calorigenesis in some other manner in addition to its production of TSH. Corticotrophin (ACTH), acting to promote the secretion of adrenal steroids, appears to be an important factor. Certain adrenal cortical hormones (and ACTH) are calorigenic in the absence of the pituitary, of the thyroid, or of both glands. There is a gradual decline in ACTH production after thyroidectomy, and the adrenal cortices undergo considerable involution. When thyroxine is administered to the thyroidectomized animal, it not only restores the functional capacity of the adrenal cortex but also promotes the release of somatotrophin (STH) by the anterior pituitary and intensifies the action of this hormone on peripheral tissues. The decline in growth rate that follows thyroidectomy of the young rat parallels the decline in BMR. Hypophysectomized rats stop growing almost immediately, whereas thyroidectomized animals are capable of growing at a reduced rate. It is probable that the immediate loss of STH after hypophysectomy accounts, in part at least, for the more rapid decline in BMR and growth than occurs after thyroidectomy.

Experiments on the rat provide evidence that STH augments the action of exogenous TSH on the thyroid gland of the hypophysectomized rat, both hormones increasing calorigenesis more effectively than when TSH is given alone. Somatotrophic hormone also potentiates the calorigenic action of thyroxine in hypophysectomized rats, indicating that the calorigenic effect of STH is exerted in part at the level of the peripheral tissues.

Epinephrine, a hormone of the adrenal medulla, also has a calorigenic effect. It has been proposed that an important role of thyroxine in cold acclimatization of the rat is to potentiate the calorigenic action of endogenous epinephrine. Observations of this type provide an excellent example of the interaction of multiple hormones in conditioning metabolic processes.

Poikilotherms. While thyroid hormones are identifiable in the thyroids of all vertebrate classes, it has been difficult to demonstrate calorigenic effects in the poikilotherms, or cold-blooded vertebrates. Both positive and negative results have been reported with fishes and amphibians. Unfortunately, these results were often obtained from experiments performed at temperatures markedly different from the optimal operating temperatures for the species being tested. Numerous observations on fishes seem to imply that the piscine thyroid is more involved in the metabolism of salts and water than in oxidative metabolism. The thyroid gland of the goldfish (*Carassius auratus*) appears to be very inactive throught the year, and at no season does it undergo hypertrophy after the administration of thiourea and other goitrogens. It does, however, respond strongly to the administration of TSH. It has been suggested that the inactive thyroid in this species may enable it to tolerate an exceptionally wide range of temperatures (0 to 41°C.). The thyroid of *Notophthalmus viridescens,* an aquatic urodele, is more inactive than that of *Desmognathus fuscus,* a terrestrial urodele, and the thyroids of the two species respond differently to goitrogenic agents.[24] The thyroidal differences may correlate with the temperature ranges of the two amphibians. Thyroidectomy of the teleost parrotfish does not diminish oxygen consumption, nor does the administration of L-thyroxine elevate it.[9, 33, 72]

While birds and mammals can maintain their body temperatures in the cold, the reptile can only demonstrate a temperature sensitivity. There is evidence that the turtle, a poikilotherm, is sensitive to temperature changes, although it cannot regulate its body temperature. Exposing turtles to cold stress produces eosinopenia, whereas injecting them with epinephrine causes eosinophilia. Cold stress appears to activate nervous and hormonal mechanisms, but the animal fails to maintain a fixed body temperature; this may indicate that the stress hormones cannot stimulate heat production, or that the animal cannot reduce heat loss at low temperatures.

There are strong indications that environmental temperature may be a very important factor in conditioning thyroidal responses in the poikilotherms. If the lizard, *Anolis carolinensis,* is maintained at room temperature (20 to 24°C.), neither thyroidectomy nor the administration of thyroxine or TSH has an effect on oxygen consumption. When these lizards are maintained at a constant temperature of 30°C., thyroidectomy reduces oxygen consumption, and thyroxine or TSH elevates it. Cold has a profound effect on the sensitivity of tadpole tissues to thyroid hormone by elevating the threshold required to achieve a response. Concentrations of thyroxine which normally evoke a rapid metamorphic response may fail to do so at low temperatures.[60]

Hibernation. In warm-blooded animals that are active throughout the year, the thyroids are generally more active during the cold winter months than during the summer. However, in hibernating mammals, the thyroid tends to be inactive during the winter and reaches a high peak of activity in the spring as the animals emerge from hibernation. Most observations indicate that the reverse is true among hibernating poikilotherms. In hibernating frogs and toads, for example, the thyroid is moderately active during the winter and is most inactive during the summer.

Electrolytes and Water

In hypothyroidism, there is an extracellular retention of sodium and chloride and water, the blood volume being considerably reduced. When thyroid hormone is administered under these conditions, it causes diuresis and urinary loss of sodium. The plasma volume is elevated. Administration of the hormone to normal subjects also produces excessive water loss through the kidney, but under these conditions the urine is especially rich in potassium. This suggests that there has been a mobilization of intracellular fluid. When small amounts of thyroxine are given to young growing animals, they enhance calcium retention. This is probably a secondary effect resulting from the protein anabolic action of the hormone, which facilitates the deposition of new bone matrix. In hyperthyroid states there is increased mobilization of calcium from the skeleton and increased loss through the urine and feces. The calcium concentration of the blood is not appreciably changed.

Protein Metabolism

One of the most characteristic effects of cretinism and myxedema in human subjects is the deposition of a mucoprotein substance in the skin and other tissues. This protein is thought to be the same as that which constitutes the intercellular cement normally found between tissue cells. It is similar in composition to the mucin in which the fetal tissues are embedded. Thyroid hormones relieve the excessive accumulation of mucoprotein in the tissues of hypothyroid subjects.

Thyroid hormone may produce either a protein anabolic or a protein catabolic effect. Human cretinism may be simulated experimentally by removing the thyroid gland of the young animal or by feeding antithyroid drugs. Cretinic rats may be produced by feeding thiouracil to the pregnant mother and continuing administration during the course of lactation. At the time of weaning (22 days), the cretinic rats weigh about 19 gm, as compared with 42 gm for normal controls. The subnormal growth of these animals is due partly to the voluntary reduction of food intake consequent upon a low BMR, but it also suggests a deficiency in protein synthesis. The carcasses of young thyroidectomized rats contain less protein and more fat than normal controls. When such animals are force-fed to cause a weight gain, there is a further reduction in carcass protein and a further increase in carcass fat. Although thyroid deficiency favors increased nitrogen excretion, thyroidectomized rats are able to maintain a positive nitrogen balance. Profound shifts in protein stores occur in the thyroidectomized animal. The total plasma protein of the rat increases as much as 30 per cent after thyroidectomy, whereas the liver and kidneys are small and deficient in protein. The deficiencies of hypothyroidism can be corrected by adequate doses of thyroid hormone. Nitrogen retention is obtained and growth occurs at a normal rate; liver enlargement and the elevated plasma globulin are corrected.[64]

A protein anabolic effect of thyroxine has been demonstrated in the young hypophysectomized rat. The growth of nearly all tissues may be stimulated by thyroxine in the absence of pituitary hormones. The protein content of the pelt, including hair, is greatly increased. Physiologic doses of thyroxine must be employed in order to demonstrate protein anabolic effects; toxic amounts of the hormone do not stimulate growth.[79]

Fat Metabolism

Hypothyroidism is generally associated with a rise in serum cholesterol and phospholipid, which may be restored to normal levels by administering thyroxine. Since thyroid hormone increases the oxidative processes of the body, the carbohydrate stores may be depleted. If this occurs, fat is mobilized from the tissue deposits to the liver, and the rate of ketone body formation is augmented. Depot fat is usually not increased appreciably during thyroid deficiency because of reduced caloric intake.

Carbohydrate Metabolism

Thyroid hormone accelerates the rate of absorption of monosaccharides from the alimentary tract. Liver glycogen stores are diminished as a consequence of hepatic glycogenolysis, and the blood sugar levels tend to rise. The hyperglycemic effect of thyroid hormone is partially offset by the simultaneous increase in the oxidation of sugar by the tissues. Hypothyroidism increases hepatic glycogen without altering the fat content. The administration of thyroid hormone can produce diabetes mellitus in animals after the removal of a portion of the pancreas, but it does not produce diabetes in animals having an intact and healthy pancreas. Insulin requirements generally increase in hyperthyroidism and decrease in hypothyroidism. The administration of thyroxine or triiodothyronine to the rat increases the rate of degradation of insulin-^{131}I, and removal of the thyroid decreases it. Pancreatic diabetes in the cat and dog is not ameliorated by thyroidectomy, as it is by hypophysectomy or adrenalectomy.

Effects of Thyroid on Reproduction

There is ample evidence that normal reproductive functions depend upon thyroid activity, although there appear to be many species and age differences. Testicular functions are more easily impaired in young animals than in adults. Histologic defects, produced by feeding thiouracil to the mother during pregnancy and lactation, have been observed in the testes of cretinic rats. At 40 days of age, the testes from the cretinic animals weigh about 112 mg, as compared with 893 mg for the controls. The cretinic testes contain spermatozoa, but the infantile nature of the sex accessory organs indicates that androgens are not being secreted at this age. Hypothyroidism appears to delay sexual development in the young male and toxic levels of thyroxine appear to impair reproductive functions. However, moderate amounts of thyroid hormone have been reported to stimulate spermatogenesis in the rabbit, mouse, ram, and human subject, even when there is no demonstrable thyroid deficiency.

Thyroid deficiencies or excesses in the female may impair the ovaries and cause the cycles to cease or to become irregular. Reproduction in most species may occur after removal of the thyroid, but fecundity is usually subnormal. The litter size of hypothyroid rats is reduced and many of the young die because of insufficient lactation by the mother. There is evidence that thyroid deficiency may render the ovary particularly susceptible to cyst formation, a disorder frequently associated with infertility in man and domestic animals. At 40 days of age, the ovaries of cretinic rats do not contain vesicular follicles and lack lipid and cholesterol. When equine gonadotrophin is administered to the cretinic animals, the ovaries respond by forming large follicles without luteinization; normal ovaries respond to this gonadotrophin by forming both follicles and corpora lutea. Thus, hypothyroidism in the rat brings about some change in the ovary that favors the development of cystic follicles.[49, 66, 75]

The relationship between the reproductive system and thyroid function in birds is still unclear. Hypo- and hyperthyroidism have been reported to have no effect on testis weight of cockerels; however, uptake of ^{32}P was greater in hypothyroid birds than in controls.[67] Gonadotrophic assays of pituitaries of hypothyroid cockerels did not differ from those of normal birds, but those of thyroxine-treated birds demonstrate a significant decline in pituitary gonadotrophic activity.

Little is known about the exact manner in which thyroid hormones influence reproductive processes. Some of the impairments may be consequent upon disturbances in protein metabolism; others may be attributable to pituitary malfunctions. The anterior pituitary secretes large amounts of TSH after thyroidectomy, and under these conditions the gland enlarges and vacuoles appear in the basophils (thyrotrophs). The vacuolated basophils are generally regarded as active rather than degenerating elements. Thyroxine not only reinstates growth in the thyroidless rat, but also repairs the pituitary defects. In the hypophysectomized animal, thyroxine increases the rate of oxygen consumption, accelerates the heart rate, etc., but it does not restore normal body growth, adrenocortical growth, or reproductive development. These facts suggest that thyroid hormones exert some control over the release from the hypophysis of somatotrophin, corticotrophin, and gonadotrophins. There is no direct evidence indicating whether these defects of the thyroidectomized animal result from reduced ability of the pituitary to secrete gonadotrophins, ACTH, and STH, or to an inability of the target organs to respond normally in the absence of thyroid hormone.

Effects on Cardiovascular and Nervous Systems

In hypothyroidism, the heart enlarges and its rate and amplitude are diminished. Under these conditions, the mass movement of blood is less than normal. The isolated perfused heart increases in rate and stroke volume when thyroxine is added to the perfusion medium. In hyperthyroidism, there are typically a tachycardia, increased stroke volume, peripheral vasodilatation, and an increase in pulse pressure.

Numerous controlled experiments have demonstrated that thyroid hormone sensitizes the nervous system. There is good correlation between the basal metabolic rate and the rate of emanation of alpha waves from the brain. That a functional impairment of the nervous system results from hypothyroidism is indicated by the lowered resistance to narcotics, the increased thresholds to light and sound stimulations, the diminished alpha rhythms, and the decreased speed of reaction to electric shocks.

In hyperthyroid patients, as well as in rats receiving thyroxine injections, the BMR is elevated but the oxygen consumption of the brain remains normal. Dinitrophenol elevates the BMR but has no effect on brain excitability. These facts indicate that the increased excitability of the central nervous system after thyroid hormone administration is separable from the metabolic effects of the hormone. Changes in electrolyte distribution brought about by the hormone appear to be associated with brain excitability. Triiodothyronine is about five times more effective than thyroxine in increasing brain excitability in the rat. However, the effects of triiodothyronine are more transient than those of thyroxine.

Developmental Effects of Thyroid Hormone

Most vertebrates cannot attain normal adult form and dimensions in the absence of thyroid secretions. There is evidence that thyroid hormone and

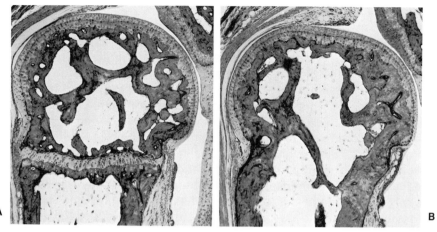

Figure 7–13. The effect of thyroid hormone on the epiphyseal plates of the hypophysectomized rat. *A*, Distal end of third metacarpal of a rat 1 year after removal of the pituitary gland. Hypophysectomy retards skeletal maturation; the epiphyseal cartilage plates persist in the hypophysectomized subject, but in the normal animal, they close at about 100 days of age. *B*, Comparable bone from a hypophysectomized animal that received thyroxine injections for 1 year. Note that the epiphyseal cartilages have been resorbed. (From Asling C. W., Simpson, M. E., Li, C. H., and Evans, H. M.: Anat. Rec. *119*:101, 1954.)

somatotrophin act synergistically in promoting normal skeletal growth. The arrest of endochondral ossification that occurs in the young hypophysectomized rat may be prevented by the administration of thyroxine. In the absence of pituitary hormones, thyroxine permits the erosion of cartilage and its replacement by bone to continue, but chondrogenesis itself is not maintained (Fig. 7–13).[2]

Thyroxine has been shown to have a direct effect on skeletal tissue of the chick grown *in vitro*. In these experiments, it was found that the same concentration of hormone may be stimulatory or toxic, depending upon the stage of differentiation of the tissue and upon the particular bone rudiment treated.

Thyroid hormone is essential for the metamorphosis of amphibian larvae, and this response has provided a useful method for bioassaying the hormone. The capacity of thyroid hormone to promote tissue differentiation is not directly related to its calorigenic action. Dinitrophenol increases the metabolic rate, but it does not produce this morphogenetic effect. Furthermore, certain stages of amphibian metamorphosis are promoted by thyroid hormone without being accompanied by an elevated metabolic rate.

Evidence is accumulating rapidly that morphogenetic effects of thyroid hormone are based upon cellular responses involving the selective regulation of protein synthesis. This has been best studied on the growth of the rat liver, the liver of the metamorphosing tadpole, and the regression of the isolated tadpole tail.[21, 86, 94]

Hormones and Molting

In mammals without seasonal molts (*e.g.,* mouse and man), the replacement of hair is an autonomous property of the hair follicle, but endocrine factors influence the process to some extent. Thyroidectomy of the mouse retards hair replacement, whereas adrenalectomy or gonadectomy accelerates it. Seasonal molting is characteristic of many mammals (*e.g.,* ferret), and in these species, neuroendocrine mechanisms play a very important role in the mediation of environmental stimuli.[51]

Molting has been extensively studied in birds; it is a very complex process involving the interaction of genetic and neuroendocrine factors. There are many species differences, and not all areas of the body respond in the same way. Thyroxine acts to promote molting, though in some species it is not absolutely essential; thyroidectomy has the reverse effect. Estrogens and androgens counteract the molt-inducing effects of thyroxine; progesterone encourages molting, especially in those species that breed throughout the year.[58] Prolactin also causes molting in some birds.[53] Seasonal molting is apparently controlled by external factors, acting via the hypothalamus, to induce variations in the endocrine system.

Molting in amphibians is a dual process involving (1) an inherent tendency of the skin to stratify and to keratinize, and (2) the periodic removal of the slough, which is regulated by neuroendocrine mechanisms. The specific hormonal controls differ in the anurans and urodeles.

Toads (Bufonidae) molt at intervals varying from one to two weeks, each animal maintaining its own individual rhythm rather precisely under uniform environmental conditions. Normal molting is abolished by hypophysectomy and is not restored by the administration of thyroxine. Adrenocortical steroids, on the other hand, induce molting in hypophysectomized toads. Molting can be produced in toads carrying ectopic autotransplants of the anterior pituitary by administering vasopressin. The neurohypophysial principle apparently stimulates the graft to release ACTH, which causes the adrenocortical tissue to discharge its steroids. Autonomous cyclic processes seem to be inherent in the skin, but these are sensitive to varying levels of hormones in the circulation. The hormones of the steroidogenic component of the adrenal, rather than those of the thyroid, seem to be the major ones affecting the anuran integument.[52]

Among urodeles, the thyroid hormones seem to perform a more important role in the molting process. Thyroidectomy or hypophysectomy prevents molting in urodeles; after these operations, the keratinized layers accumulate but are not sloughed. Thyroid-stimulating hormone induces shedding when administered to hypophysectomized urodeles; exogenous thyroxine is effective in both hypophysectomized and thyroidectomized animals. Prolactin has been reported to produce shedding in hypophysectomized urodeles. The implantation of thyroxine pellets into the skin of thyroidectomized newts produces localized molting (Fig. 7–14). This indicates that thyroxine acts directly upon the skin in these amphibians.[18, 55, 57]

Just as with amphibians, it is known that the shedding of the outer surface layer of lizards is dependent upon thyroid hormone. In marked con-

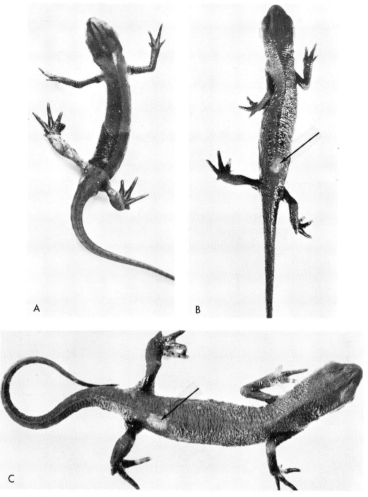

Figure 7–14. Thyroidectomized newts *(Notophthalmus viridescens)* undergoing molts following the subcutaneous implantation of thyroxine-cholesterol pellets. *A,* General molt produced by 0.96 μgm thyroxine; *B,* local molt (arrow) over an implant containing 0.03 μgm thyroxine; *C,* local molt (arrow) over an implant containing 0.07 μgm thyroxine. (From Clark, N. B., and Kaltenbach, J. C.: Gen. Comp. Endocr. *1*:513, 1961.)

trast, however, it has been discovered that increased skin sloughing occurs in thyroidectomized snakes.[16] Sloughing of the skin can be prevented in both intact and thyroidectomized snakes by the injection of thyroxine.

Amphibian Metamorphosis

The best-known function of the thyroid gland in poikilotherms is the control of amphibian metamorphosis (Fig. 7–15 and frontispiece). This effect was discovered by Gudernatsch (1912), who fed many kinds of mammalian tissues to amphibian larvae and found that thyroid tissue, unlike all others, caused suppression of growth and precocious metamorphosis (frontispiece).[45] Thyroid feeding produced this effect in both anurans and urodeles. Other workers devised methods for removing the anlage of the thyroid in early larval stages and showed that thyroidless larvae continued to grow normally but failed to metamorphose. Such larvae may become gigantic in size, since they continue to grow long after the unoperated controls have metamorphosed into adults. Adler (1914) found that hypophysectomy of the larvae prevented accumulation of colloid in the thyroid and that such animals fail to metamorphose. These findings have been confirmed and extended by many investigators, and it is now definitely established that thyroid activity is controlled by TSH from the anterior pituitary. Iodine and various iodine compounds can replace the thyroid secretions in promoting amphibian metamorphosis, but this probably results from the formation of thyroid hormone through the combination of iodine with tyrosine present in body tissues other than the thyroid itself.

Before the onset of metamorphosis, the frog tadpole is an aquatic animal having well-developed gills, a long flattened tail, and lidless eyes, and, being herbivorous, it has horny rasping teeth and a relatively long intestine.

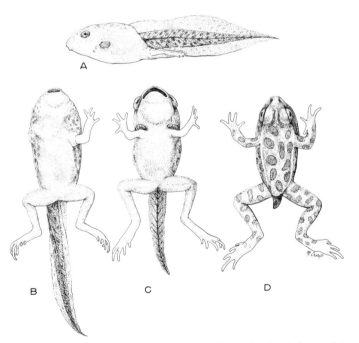

Figure 7–15. The effect of thyroxine upon the metamorphosis of *Rana pipiens* tadpoles. *A*, Untreated control removed at the end of the experiment (about life size). *D*, A metamorphosed tadpole killed 2 weeks after the first thyroxine was added to the aquarium water. Animals *B* and *C* were removed at intervals during this period. *B, C,* and *D* are a little larger than life size. Note the changes in the mouth, paired appendages, and tail.

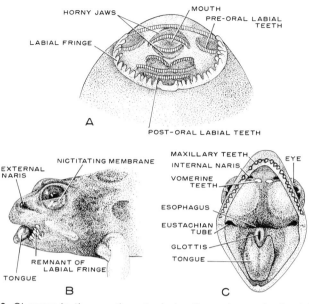

Figure 7–16. Changes in the mouth parts during the metamorphosis of *Rana pipiens*. *A*, The mouth of a young tadpole at an early stage of metamorphosis. The mouth is bounded above and below by horny beaks; two rows of pre-oral labial teeth and three rows of post-oral labial teeth are present, and the labial fringe is prominent. *B*, A tadpole at about stage 21, showing a remnant of the labial fringe at each corner of the mouth. *C*, The mouth parts of a completely metamorphosed frog.

The adult frog is adapted to terrestrial life, breathes by means of lungs, has well-developed limbs and no tail, and is carnivorous. During metamorphosis, therefore, larval structures such as gills, tail, and horny teeth are lost, whereas eyelids, lungs, and limbs develop (Fig. 7–16 and Table 7–1). Many of the larval structures that are carried over to the adult undergo extensive changes. The skin thickens and becomes more glandular, the brain becomes more highly differentiated, the gill arches become modified into the hyoid apparatus, and the intestine becomes proportionately shorter. It is obvious that certain tissues do not respond to thyroid hormone at metamorphosis; some exhibit marked growth, whereas others degenerate.[69] Certain tissues show a sharp rise in mitotic activity during the period of metamorphic climax. The metamorphic changes in specific tissues are direct effects of thyroxine and are not achieved indirectly through an elevation of the BMR. This has been demonstrated by the topical application of thyroid hormone. For example, localized regression of the dorsal fin of the tadpole may be produced by inserting pellets of thyroxine or its analogues into this region of the tail (Fig. 7–17).[55, 56] Adrenal cortical steroids, mixed with the thyroid hormone in the pellet, have been found to render the thyroid hormone more effective in producing localized regression of the fin.

The pellet implantation technique has been used for a variety of purposes, including studies on the effectiveness of thyroxine analogues (Fig.

Table 7-1 SUMMARY OF SOME METAMORPHIC CHANGES
IN ANURANS

SYSTEM	LARVA	ADULT
Locomotory	Aquatic; tail fins	Terrestrial; tailless tetrapod
Respiratory	Gills, skin, lungs; larval hemoglobins	Skin, lungs; adult hemoglobins
Circulatory	Aortic arches; aorta; anterior, posterior, and common cardinal veins	Carotid arch; systemic arch; pulmocutaneous arch; jugular veins, caval veins
Nutritional	*Vegetarian:* Long spiral gut—intestinal symbionts, carbohydrases; small mouth—horny jaws, labial teeth	*Carnivore:* Short gut—proteases; large mouth—long tongue
Nervous	No corneal reflex, lack of nictitating membrane, porphyropsin, lateral line system—Mauthner's neurons; bronchial columella	Corneal reflex—development of ocular muscles, nictitating membrane, rhodopsin, loss of lateral line system—degeneration of Mauthner's neurons, enlargment of mesencephalic V nucleus, enlargement of lateral motor columns, tympanic columella—tympanic membrane
Excretory	Mesonephros: Largely ammonia, some urea (ammonotelic)	Mesonephros: Largely urea, high activity of enzymes of ornithine-urea cycle (ureotelic)

7-17). Such studies have been done in conjunction with others in which tadpoles are immersed in solutions containing the hormones. A large number of thyroxine analogues have been prepared, and many of these exhibit biologic potencies quite different from those of the hormones secreted by the thyroid. Moreover, the observed potencies of these preparations are highly variable, depending upon the mode of administration.[91] For example, when tadpoles are tested by immersion in the test solution, triiodothyropropionic acid is some 300 times more potent than thyroxine in stimulating metamorphosis of *Rana pipiens*. However, when the hormone is administered by injection, this disparity is much reduced, indicating that differing results are due to the fact that the analogue is much more rapidly absorbed than is thyroxine. Difficulties such as this are inherent in *in vivo* studies, but can be circumvented, in part, by localized observations (as with pellet implantation). Small variations in the thyroxine molecule may greatly alter its potency. Thyroxine declines in potency if more than one atom of iodine is replaced by another halogen. The iodine atoms must be attached to positions 3 and 5; the analogues with iodine at positions 2 and 6 actually inhibit certain thyroxine effects (Fig. 7-18). Biologic activity is not lost if no iodine atoms are present in the β-ring. The hydroxyl group (OH) must occupy the 4′ position; physiologic activity is lost if it is moved to another position on the aromatic nucleus. The side chain at position 1 may be modified in various ways without impairing biologic potency. In fact, triiodothyropropionic acid is more effective than thyroxine in inducing localized resorption of the fin.[56]

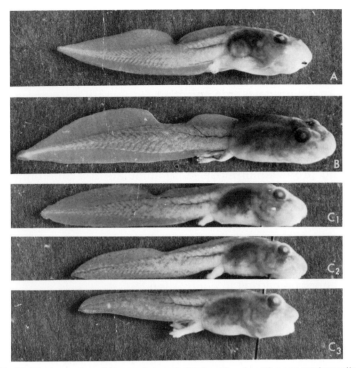

Figure 7–17. Photographs of *Rana pipiens* tadpoles (fixed in 10 per cent formalin), showing localized tail fin resorption induced by thyroxine analogue—cholesterol implants. *A,* Six days after implantation of a pellet containing 40 per cent diiodothyroacetic acid. *B,* Twenty days after implantation of a pellet containing 0.5 per cent tetraiodothyropropionic acid. The resorbed area is larger than that in *A. C,* Seven days after implantation of pellets containing 0.5 per cent isopropyldiiodothyronine. Due to the high metamorphosing activity of this compound, the localized reaction in the dorsal fin (C_1) was sometimes obscured by generalized fin resorption, part of an overall metamorphic response (C_2, C_3). (From Kaltenbach, J. C.: J. Exp. Zool. *174,* 1970.)

Some analogues with modifications at position 1 may exert negligible tail fin resorption, but do bring about metamorphic changes in the skin when implanted near the eye. Since this region is known to have a lower threshold of response to thyroxine, the implication is that such analogues exert normal, nonpathologic effects.

The local action of thyroxine has been tested on many specific metamorphic events, many of which take place in deeper tissues. For example, the hindbrain of amphibian larvae contains a pair of giant neurons, called Mauthner's cells, and they regress at metamorphosis instead of undergoing further differentiation, as the neighboring neurons do. The implantation of thyroid tissue or thyroid pellets into the hindbrain causes Mauthner's cells to regress promptly, whereas the adjacent nervous tissue responds by enlarging and increased mitotic activity.

The functional activity of the amphibian thyroid, as in mammals, is regulated by hypophysial thyrotrophin. The concentration of thyroid hormone in the blood of the anuran tadpole is extremely low during the early phases of metamorphosis, but it rises slowly, reaches a peak at the height of the metamorphic changes, and then drops rapidly after the transformations are completed. The metamorphosing tadpole must be regarded as a mosaic of parts, some of which develop a sensitivity to thyroid hormone and respond in characteristic ways to it. Exogenous hormones produce no changes until the tissues have developed a *readiness to respond.* There is apparently a progressive increase in sensitivity to the hormone, and not all of the tissues become reactive at the same time. A very important action of thyroid hormones during prometamorphosis is to stimulate the differentiation of the median eminence and its neurosecretory mechanism.[28, 90] The *increasing* concentrations of thyroid hormone in the blood, after metamorphosis starts, are probably an important factor since different thresholds are required by different tissues. This may be demonstrated by keeping the larvae at constant temperature and administering a constant dosage of hormone. If these thresholds are not exceeded, metamorphosis progresses to a particular stage and cannot be carried to completion.[59]

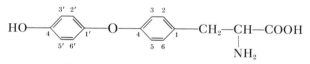

β-Ring   α-Ring

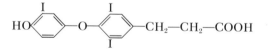

Triiodothyropropionic acid

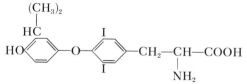

3. Isopropyldiiodo-L-thyronine

Figure 7–18. System of numbering of the thyroxine nucleus and two thyroxine analogues.

Temperature is a factor of great importance in amphibian metamorphosis. Metamorphic changes do not occur in either anurans or urodeles at temperatures below 5°C. Tadpoles of *Rana pipiens* attain larger body sizes when maintained in cold water than when kept in warm water. When thyroxine is administered to hypophysectomized tadpoles and some are maintained at high temperatures and others at low temperatures, the latter animals take longer to transform and never progress as far as the ones kept at high temperatures. This suggests that the temperature effect on metamorphosis is largely independent of thyroid function. It is thoroughly established that the effectiveness of thyroxine analogues in promoting amphibian metamorphosis is not necessarily correlated with their capacity to elevate the metabolic rate in mammals.

Anuran and urodele larvae differ with respect to the quantity of thyroxine required for development of the corneal reflex. This is a reflexive retraction of the eye into the orbit and elevation of the nictitating membrane in response to touching the cornea. The neural center regulating this action is located in the medullary portion of the brain. A relatively high concentration of thyroid hormone is required for the full development of the corneal reflex in frog larvae, but, in urodele larvae, it appears even after the quantity of thyroid hormone is radically reduced by hypophysectomy. The local application of thyroxine to the medulla, through the implantation of pellets, accelerates the development of this reflex in relation to other metamorphic changes occurring in the remainder of the body.

While most amphibians have an aquatic larval stage and a terrestrial adult stage, there are several groups in which the aquatic stage is abbreviated or omitted entirely. Members of the genus *Eleutherodactylus* lay their eggs on land, and the young are hatched as tiny, fully formed frogs.[68] External gills and other features of an aquatic tadpole are greatly suppressed or are lacking entirely. In such forms exhibiting direct development, the changes can occur after thyroid hormone synthesis has been blocked by antithyroid agents, and they are not stimulated by the administration of thyroxine. Although thyroxine has some effect in hastening tail resorption, pronephros degeneration, and loss of the egg tooth, these are all retrogressive processes that are characteristic of late embryonic stages.

Nectophrynoides occidentalis is a small viviparous toad inhabiting the summits of Mount Nimba in Africa. The ovaries develop corpora lutea, and the young are retained in the maternal uterus during the nine months of pregnancy. An aquatic stage is omitted entirely, and some larval structures fail to appear or are vestigial. External and internal gills, spiracle, branchial cavity, tail fin, and horny teeth do not develop in this species. The thyroid glands of the young *in utero* grow and progressively accumulate colloid during the early months of gestation. At about the eighth month of gestation, limbs are developed quickly and the tail regresses; these events correlate with the disappearance of colloid from the thyroid follicles. The thyroid begins to store colloid again after birth.[38]

Biochemical Aspects.   While amphibian metamorphosis entails a considerable degree of morphologic change, it must be remembered that profound physiologic adjustments must be made to accommodate the transition from an aquatic to a terrestrial existence. Biochemical alterations underlie this transition. The best known of these biochemical changes are related to respiration, excretion, vision, and tissue resorption; all may be induced experimentally by the administration of thyroid hormones.[21, 36, 87, 93]

Separate hemoglobins exist in larval and adult forms. Using various methods of extraction, several distinctive larval hemoglobins can be distinguished, not only by differences in chromatographic and electrophoretic mobilities, but by immunological properties as well, from an array of adult components. Probably these separate larval and adult hemoglobins provide the basis for the well-known differences in the oxygen dissociation curves between larvae and adults. While it is assumed that these differences have evolved in order to provide more efficient respiration for larvae and adults, the possibility that they also entail phylogenetic recapitulation cannot be totally excluded. It is interesting to note that during metamorphosis the transition from larval to adult hemoglobins is gradual and that red blood cells containing both larval and adult forms of the molecule can be found.[54]

Most species of amphibians excrete ammonia (ammonotelism) during larval stages, but begin to utilize urea (ureotelism) as an excretory product after the onset of metamorphosis. The biosynthesis of urea from bicarbonate and ammonia involves a number of enzymes, and their activity rises abruptly during metamorphic climax. Synthesis of important enzymes of the ornithine-urea cycle, such as carbamyl phosphate synthetase, can be induced in tadpoles exposed to thyroxine.[21] The visual pigments of tadpoles, just as with other fresh water poikilotherms, is porphyropsin (retinene$_2$). During metamorphosis, there is a shift to the use of rhodopsin (retinene$_1$) as a visual pigment. A prominent event in amphibian metamorphosis is the resorption of the tail fin, which can be induced even in the isolated tail that is exposed to thyroid hormone (Fig. 7–19). Involution of tail tissue occurs through the action of lysosomal enzymes.[94] In the presence of thyroxine, the activity of key enzymes such as cathepsin, phosphatase, and β-glucuronidase increases, leading to tail resorption.

Neoteny and Other Effects. It is well known that certain urodeles fail to metamorphose and retain the larval body form throughout life. The animals become sexually mature and are able to reproduce without "adults" ever appearing. Neoteny was first described in the American axolotl, *Ambystoma tigrinum,* in which it was noted that members of this species inhabiting high mountain lakes failed to metamorphose, whereas specimens of the same species living at lower altitudes metamorphosed, as do most other amphibians. Axolotls can be induced to metamorphose by treating them with thyroxine or various iodine compounds. Inorganic iodine is also effective if it is implanted under the skin or into the peritoneal cavity so that it is rapidly absorbed (Fig. 7–20). These observations suggest that the failure of metamorphosis in the axolotl is due to the inability of the thyroid to secrete hormone or to a decreased sensitivity of the tissues to the hormone.

It is reasonably certain that the Mexican axolotl, *Ambystoma mexicanum,* never undergoes metamorphosis in its natural habitat. When pituitary glands of *A. tigrinum,* a readily metamorphosing form, are transplanted into *A. mexicanum* larvae, metamorphosis is induced. On the other hand, pitui-

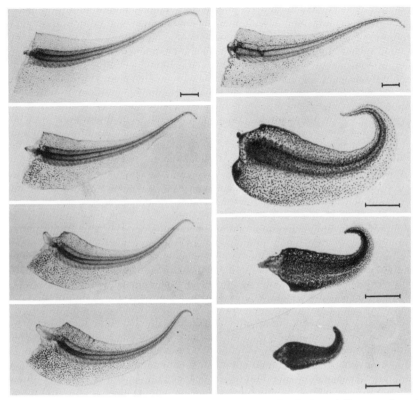

Figure 7–19. Hormonally induced involution of isolated tail tips of *Xenopus* in culture. *Left, from top to bottom:* Control tips maintained in Holtfreter solution for 6, 8, 10, and 12 days after amputation. *Right, from top to bottom:* Tail tips of the same age as the controls but treated for 3, 5, 7, and 9 days with DL-thyroxine. (From Weber, R.: Helv. Physiol. Pharmakol. Acta *21*, 1963.)

taries of *A. mexicanum* do not promote metamorphosis when transplanted to the larvae of *A. tigrinum.* This indicates that the pituitary gland of the Mexican axolotl is defective and apparently does not release the proper thyrotrophin.[12]

The perennibranchiate salamanders (*e.g., Necturus, Amphiuma*) are not known to undergo metamorphosis. They retain gills, tail fins, and other larval traits throughout their lives. Even large doses of thyroid hormone or other iodine compounds fail to produce any appreciable morphologic change in these species. The indications are that the perennibranchiate amphibians retain larval characters chiefly because their tissues have not developed a responsiveness to thyroid hormone. Studies have shown that the thyroids of *Necturus* and *Amphiuma* are very slow in accumulating radioiodine and in synthesizing thyroid hormone. In salamanders, as well as in certain fishes and reptiles, great variations are observed in the capacity of the thyroid to bind iodine and synthesize hormone; undoubtedly, complex factors such as seasonal changes and the accompanying fluctuations in endocrine balance are involved.

The influence of other hormones, especially prolactin, on metamorphic

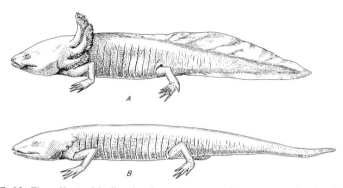

Figure 7–20. The effect of iodine implantation upon the metamorphosis of the American axolotl *(Ambystoma tigrinum). A,* Untreated gilled or axolotl stage; *B,* a similar specimen 30 days after the implantation of iodine crystals below the skin. Observe the atrophy of the gills and the loss of the tail fin.

events has attracted wide interest. The possible role of a hypophysial hormone in development was inferred from experiments in which excessive tadpole growth was obtained following transplantation of the hypophysial anlage.[29] Duplication of this effect following the injection of mammalian prolactin into tadpoles led to the conclusion that prolactin is indeed a growth-promoting hormone in tadpoles. Because prolactin administration also delayed metamorphosis, it was contended that this hormone acts as a goitrogen in amphibians. Following this, an array of experiments demonstrated that prolactin preparations have the capacity to inhibit the metamorphic action of thyroid hormone at the peripheral tissue level. Such experiments utilized the isolated tadpole tail or discs of tail tissue incubated in tissue culture with appropriate combinations of thyroid hormone and prolactin preparations.[25] A striking example of an exception to a prolactin-thyroxine antagonism at the peripheral level has been demonstrated to occur in the eye of bullfrog tadpoles, wherein prolactin failed to antagonize thyroxine-induced rhodopsin production.[23] While most studies on thyroxine-prolactin interaction in metamorphosis have involved anurans, it appears that prolactin preparations also inhibit urodele metamorphosis. It has been demonstrated that while larvae of the tiger salamander *(Ambystoma tigrinum)* injected with TSH metamorphose rapidly, others receiving TSH and prolactin undergo a metamorphic stasis.[39]

While the results of all of these experiments seem relatively clear, the fundamental question remains of whether the hypophysial agent that affects growth and metamorphosis is really prolactin and not somatotrophin. This question is difficult to solve because of the known close relationship between these two hypophysial principles. Nevertheless, there is an increasing body of evidence favoring the view that prolactin is a growth hormone in amphibian larvae.

Metamorphosis in Fishes

It is well known that cyclostomes and certain teleost fish undergo metamorphic changes during their life histories, but the hormonal mechanisms involved are not so clear as in amphibians. Metamorphosis of the lamprey is striking, but it has not been possible to influence this process through the administration of exogenous thyroxine to the larvae. There are some reasons for believing that adrenocortical hormones, rather than thyroid hormones, may be involved in the metamorphic process of cyclostomes.

While metamorphosis in teleost fishes is not so impressive as in amphibians, it does occur in certain species. In the salmon, for example, the freshwater parr transforms into the migratory, marine smolt. This involves a silvering of the integument, due to the deposition of guanine, and certain physiologic adjustments which equip the smolt for life in the sea. These transformations are accompanied by increased metabolic rate and hyperactivity of the thyroid. These facts imply that thyroid hormones are important in bringing about these changes in salmonids, though it is probable that other hormones play some part.

Mode of Action of Thyroid Hormone

Though much biochemical information has accumulated on the mechanism of action of thyroxine, the literature is tenuous, often contradictory, and subject to objections. Since we are dealing with hormones which produce many and varied effects in different species, some of the actions apparently being indirect, it is difficult to decide what cellular response could be most profitably investigated. Most of the early biochemical studies centered on the capacity of thyroxine to elevate the consumption of oxygen, even though this response is largely limited to warm-blooded vertebrates; it is not readily demonstrable in tissues cultured *in vitro,* and even the "tissue" form of the hormone remains unknown.

A number of studies have suggested that thyroid hormone may affect the rate of metabolism by acting at one or more points in the citric acid cycle. Since the enzymes involved in this cycle are localized in the mitochondria, there have been suggestions that thyroid hormone may act by altering the permeability of the cell membrane or the membrane system of the mitochondrion. One concept that has received much attention is that the hormones act to "uncouple oxidative phosphorylation." The mitochondria are known to be the sites at which the energy released by oxidative processes is incorporated into adenosine triphosphate (ATP). The increased oxygen consumption occurring in hyperthyroid states is accounted for, according to this view, as resulting from an impairment of the phosphorylation of ATP. How these effects are to be interpreted in the general action of thyroid hormone is as yet unknown.

The fact that a latent period intervenes between the administration of thyroxine and the onset of its actions has led many workers to believe that the hormone may stimulate the synthesis or activation of enzymes, processes that require time. This view is supported by the fact that some effects of thyroid hormone, for example, that on brain tissue, occur without affecting the metabolic rate. Moreover, as was pointed out, metamorphic events induced by the administration of small amounts of thyroid hormone lead to profound catabolic responses in some tissues, such as the tail, and to profound growth effects in other tissues. These facts set the stage for a variety of studies directed at unveiling the effects of thyroxine on the chain of events involved in protein synthesis. Tissues such as the rat liver, the liver of the metamorphosing tadpole, and the tadpole tail in organ culture have been especially fruitful targets of investigation.[87]

Administration of thyroid hormones to the thyroidectomized rat or to tadpoles leads to a number of effects on the liver, which can be readily assessed. In both systems, a prominent latent period exists between hormone injection and the observed effects. One of the prominent effects is the stimulation of nuclear RNA synthesis as determined by the synthesis of rapidly labeled RNA in both rat and tadpole and by the increased activity of RNA polymerase in the rat. These events were followed by the increased incorporation of amino acids into protein by mitochondria and microsomes in the

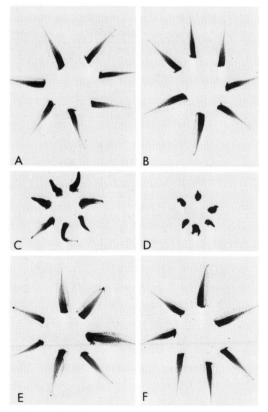

Figure 7–21. Triiodothyronine (T_3)-induced regression of amputated tails of *Rana temporaria* in organ culture. *A*, Control samples on the first day of culture; *B*, control, after 8 days of culture; *C*, on day 4 of culture in medium containing 1 microgm of T_3 per milliliter; *D*, on day 8 of culture with T_3; *E*, the same as *C* but with 2.5 gm of actinomycin per milliliter; *F*, same as *D* and with actinomycin. (From Tata, J. R.: Gen. Comp. Endocr., Suppl. 2:385, 1969.)

rat and by the synthesis of microsomal phospholipids and mitochondrial respiratory enzymes in both rat and tadpole. In the tadpole liver, there was a profound synthesis of serum albumin, adult hemoglobin, and urea cycle enzymes. Presumably, in both rat and tadpole livers the latter events result from the effects on RNA synthesis. It seems likely that the thyroid-hormone induced RNA effects are largely directed at the synthesis of ribosomal RNA. This is supported by the fact that the protein stimulating effects of thyroid hormone are inhibited by doses of actinomycin D, to which ribosomal RNA synthesis is more sensitive than is m-RNA synthesis. In tadpoles, the effects of thyroid hormone on RNA synthesis are apparently not restricted to the liver. This has been shown by the prevention of hormone induced tadpole tail involution by actinomycin D, an inhibitor of RNA synthesis[86] (Fig. 7–21). The degree of involution is paralleled by the activity of lysosomal enzymes.[94] Presumably, the synthesis or the activity of these enzymes is based upon the action of thyroid hormones on RNA synthesis.

REFERENCES

1. Adams, D. D.: The presence of an abnormal thyroid-stimulating hormone in the serum of some thyrotoxic patients. J. Clin. Endocr. *18*:699, 1958.
2. Asling, C. W., Simpson, M. E., Li, C. H., and Evans, H. M.: The effects of chronic administration of thyroxin to hypophysectomized rats on their skeletal growth, maturation and response to growth hormone. Anat. Rec. *119*:101, 1954.
3. Axelrad, A. A., and Leblond, C. P.: Induction of thyroid tumors in rats by a low iodine diet. Cancer *8*:339, 1955.
4. Baker, K. F.: Heterotopic thyroid tissue in fishes. J. Exp. Zool. *138*:329, 1958.
5. Baker-Cohen, K. F.: Renal and other heterotopic thyroid tissue in fishes. *In* A. Gorbman (ed.): Comparative Endocrinology. New York, John Wiley & Sons, 1959, p. 283.
6. Barrington, E. J. W.: Hormones and vertebrate evolution. Experientia *18*:201, 1962.
7. Barrington, E. J. W.: On the responses of the glandular tracts and associated regions of the endostyle of the larval lamprey to goitrogens and thyroxine. Gen. Comp. Endocr. *3*:153, 1963.
8. Barrington, E. J. W.: The Biology of Hemichordata and Protochordata. London, Oliver and Boyd, 1965, p. 133.
9. Berg, O. A., and Gorbman, A.: Normal and altered thyroidal function in domesticated goldfish *Carassius auratus.* Proc. Soc. Exp. Biol. Med. *86*:156, 1954.
10. Berg, O., Gorbman, A., and Kobayashi H.: The thyroid hormones in invertebrates and lower vertebrates. *In* A. Gorbman (ed.): Comparative Endocrinology, New York, John Wiley & Sons, 1959, p. 302.
11. Black, R. E., and Webb, K. L.: Metabolism of ^{131}I in relation to strobilation of *Chrysaora quinquecirrha* (Scyphozoa). Comp. Biochem. Physiol. *45A*:1023, 1973.
12. Blount, R. F.: The effects of heteroplastic hypophyseal grafts upon the axolotl, *Ambystoma mexicanum.* J. Exp. Zool. *113*:717, 1950.
13. Bradley, W. O.: The effects of certain antithyroid drugs on the uptake of radioactive iodine by the frog thyroid. Biol. Bull. *101*:62, 1951.
14. Brown-Grant, K.: Changes in the thyroid activity of rats exposed to cold. J. Physiol. *131*:52, 1956.
15. Brown-Grant, K., Harris, G. W., and Reichlin, S.: The effect of emotional and physical stress on thyroid activity in the rabbit. J. Physiol. *126*:29, 1954.
16. Chiu, K. W., and Lynn, W. G.: The role of the thyroid in skin-shedding in the shovel-nosed snake, *Chionactis occipitalis.* Gen. Comp. Endocr. *14*:467, 1970.
17. Claire, Sister M. The uptake of ^{131}I by the thyroid gland of turtles after treatment with thiourea. Biol. Bull. *111*:190, 1956.
18. Clark, N. B., and Kaltenbach, J. C.: Direct action of thyroxine on skin of the adult newt. Gen. Comp. Endocr. *1*:513, 1961.

19. Clements, M., and Gorbman, A.: Protease in ammocoetes endostyle. Biol. Bull. *108*:258, 1955.
20. Clements-Merlini, M.: The secretory cycle of iodoproteins in ammocoetes. II. A. radioautographic study of the transforming larval thyroid gland. J. Morph. *106*:357, 1960.
21. Cohen, P. P.: Biochemical differentiation during amphibian metamorphosis. Science *168*: 533, 1970.
22. Copenhaver, W. M.: Growth of thyroid tissue in the gills of *Amblystoma punctatum* reared in propylthiouracil. J. Exp. Zool. *129*:291, 1955.
23. Crim, J. W.: Prolactin-thyroxine antagonism and the metamorphosis of visual pigments in *Rana catesbeiana* tadpoles. J. Exp. Zool. *192*:355, 1975.
24. Dent, J. N., and Lynn, W. G.: A comparison of the effects of goitrogens on thyroid activity in *Triturus viridescens* and *Desmognathus fuscus*. Biol. Bull. *115*:411, 1958.
25. Derby, A., and Etkin, W.: Thyroxine induced tail resorption *in vitro* as affected by anterior pituitary hormones. J. Exp. Zool. *169*:1, 1968.
26. Dimond, Sister M. T.: The reactions of developing snapping turtles, *Chelydra serpentina serpentina* (Linné), to thiourea. J. Exp. Zool. *127*:93, 1954.
27. Dunn, A. D.: Iodine metabolism in the ascidian, *Molgula manhattensis*. Gen. Comp. Endocr. *25*:83, 1975.
28. Etkin, W.: Metamorphosis-activating system of the frog. Science *139*:810, 1963.
29. Etkin, W., and Lehrer, R.: Excess growth in tadpoles after transplantation of the adenohypophysis. Endocrinology *67*:457, 1960.
30. Evans, E. S., Contopoulos, A. N., and Simpson, M. E.: Hormonal factors influencing calorigenesis. Endocrinology *60*:403, 1957.
31. Flock, E. V., David, C., Hallenbeck, G. A., and Owen, C. A., Jr.: Metabolism of D-thyroxine. Endocrinology *73*:764, 1963.
32. Follis, R. H., Jr.: Experimental colloid goiter in the hamster. Proc. Soc. Exp. Biol. Med. *100*: 203, 1959.
33. Fortune, P. Y.: Comparative studies of the thyroid function in teleosts of tropical and temperate habitats. J. Exp. Biol. *32*:504, 1955.
34. Fraser, R. C.: Acceleration of frog metamorphosis with iodinated proteins. J. Exp. Zool. *133*:519, 1956.
35. Freinkel, N., Dowling, J. T., and Ingbar, S. H.: The interaction of thyroxine with plasma proteins: Localization of thyroxine-binding protein in Cohn fractions of plasma. J. Clin. Invest. *34*:1698, 1955.
36. Frieden, E.: Thyroid hormones and the biochemistry of amphibian metamorphosis. Rec. Progr. Hormone Res. *27*:139, 1967.
37. Furth, J.: Experimental pituitary tumors. Rec. Progr. Hormone Res. *11*:221, 1955.
38. Gallien, L.: Endocrine basis for reproductive adaptations in Amphibia. *In* A. Gorbman (ed.): Comparative Endocrinology. New York, John Wiley & Sons, 1959, p. 479.
39. Gona, A. G., and Etkin, W.: Inhibition of metamorphosis in *Ambystoma tigrinum* by prolactin. Gen. Comp. Endocr. *14*:589, 1970.
40. Gorbman, A.: Some aspects of the comparative biochemistry of iodine utilization and evolution of thyroidal function. Physiol. Rev. *35*:336, 1955.
41. Gorbman, A.: Pituitary tumors in rodents following changes in thyroidal function: A review. Cancer Res. *16*:99, 1956.
42. Gorbman, A.: Problems in the comparative morphology and physiology of the vertebrate thyroid gland. *In* A. Gorbman (ed.): Comparative Endocrinology. New York, John Wiley & Sons, 1959, p. 266.
43. Gorbman, A., Clements, M., and O'Brien, R.: Utilization of radioiodine by invertebrates with special study of several Annelida and Mollusca. J. Exp. Zool. *127*:75, 1954.
44. Greer, M. A., and De Groot, L. J.: The effect of stable iodide on thyroid secretion in man. Metabolism *5*:682, 1956.
45. Gudernatsch, J. F.: Feeding experiments on tadpoles. Arch. Entwicklungsmech. Organ. *35*: 457, 1912.
46. Hamolsky, M. W., Stein, M., Fischer, D. B., and Freedberg, A. S.: Further studies of factors affecting the plasma protein-thyroid hormone complex. Endocrinology *68*:662, 1961.
47. Harris, G. W.: Neuroendocrine control of TSH regulation. *In* A. Gorbman (ed.): Comparative Endocrinology. New York, John Wiley & Sons, 1959, p. 202.
48. Haynie, T. P., Winzler, R. J., Matovinovich, J., Carr, E. A., Jr., and Beierwaltes, W. H.: Thyroid-stimulating and exophthalmos-producing activity of biochemically altered thyrotropin. Endocrinology *71*:782, 1962.
49. Hopper, A. F.: Uptake of ^{32}P by cystic ovary of the rat. Endocrinology *71*:740, 1962.

50. Hsieh, A. C. L., and Carlson, L. D.: Role of the thyroid in metabolic response to low temperature. Amer. J. Physiol. *188*:40, 1957.
51. Jørgensen, C. B., and Larsen, L. O.: Molting and its hormonal control in toads. Gen. Comp. Endocr. *1*:145, 1961.
52. Jørgensen, C. B., Larsen, L. O., and Rosenkilde, P.: Hormonal dependency of molting in amphibians: Effect of radiothyroidectomy in the toad *Bufo bufo* (L). Gen. Comp. Endocr. *5*:248, 1965.
53. Juhn, M., and Harris, P. C.: Molt of capon feathering with prolactin. Proc. Soc. Exp. Biol. Med. *98*:669, 1958.
54. Jurd, R. D., and Maclean, N.: An immunofluorescent study of the haemoglobins in metamorphosing *Xenopus laevis*. J. Embryol. Exp. Morph. *23*:299, 1970.
55. Kaltenbach, J. C.: Direct action of thyroxine analogues on peripheral tissues of anuran larvae. Anat. Rec. *128*:572, 1957.
56. Kaltenbach, J. C.: Local metamorphic action of thyroxine analogues in *Rana pipiens* larvae. J. Exp. Zool. *174*:55, 1970.
57. Kaltenbach, J. C., and Clark, N. B.: Direct action of thyroxine analogues on molting in the adult newt. Gen. Comp. Endocr. *5*:74, 1965.
58. Kobayashi, H.: On the induction of molt in birds by 17α-oxyprogesterone-17-capronate. Endocrinology *63*:420, 1958.
59. Kollros, J. J.: Thyroid gland function in developing cold-blooded vertebrates. *In* A. Gorbman (ed.): Comparative Endocrinology. New York, John Wiley & Sons, 1959, p. 340.
60. Kollros, J. J.: Mechanisms of amphibian metamorphosis: Hormones. Amer. Zool. *1*:107, 1961.
61. La Roche, G., Johnson, C. L., and Woodall, A. N.: Thyroid function in rainbow trout (*Salmo gairdneri*, Rich.). I. Biochemical and histological evidence of radiothyroidectomy. Gen. Comp. Endocr. *5*:145, 1965.
62. Lardy, H., Tomita, K., Larson, F. C., and Albright, E. C.: The metabolism of thyroid hormones by kidney and the biological activity of the products. Ciba Found. Colloq. Endocr. *10*:156, 1957.
63. Larson, F. C., and Albright, E. C.: Distribution of 3:5:3'-triiodothyroacetic acid in the rat. Endocrinology *63*:183, 1958.
64. Leathem. J. H.: Relationships between the thyroid and protein metabolism. *In* W. H. Cole (ed.): Protein Metabolism, Hormones and Growth. New Brunswick, N.J., Rurgers University Press, 1953, p. 17.
65. Leathem, J. H.: Goitrogen-induced thyroid tumors. Ciba Found. Colloq. Endocr. *12*:50, 1958.
66. Leathem, J. H.: Nutritional effects on endocrine secretions. *In* W. C. Young (ed.): Sex and Internal Secretions, Vol. 1. Baltimore, the Williams & Wilkins Co., 1961, p. 666.
67. Lehman, G. C.: The effects of hypo- and hyperthyroidism on the testes and anterior pituitary glands of cockerels. Gen. Comp. Endocr. *14*:567, 1970.
68. Lynn, W. G., and Peadon, A. M.: The role of the thyroid gland in the anuran *Eleutherodactylus martinicensis*. Growth *19*:263, 1955.
69. Lynn, W. G., and Wachowski, H. E.: The thyroid gland and its functions in cold-blooded vertebrates. Quart. Rev. Biol. *26*:123, 1951.
70. Mackenzie, C. G.: Experimental goiter. Fed. Proc. *17*:72, 1958.
71. Mackenzie, J. B., Mackenzie, C. G., and McCollum, E. V.: The effect of sulfanilylguanidine on the thyroid of the rat. Science *94*:518, 1941.
72. Matty, A. J.: Thyroidectomy and its effect upon oxygen consumption of a teleost fish, *Pseudoscarus guacamaia*. J. Endocr. *15*:1, 1957.
73. Mulvey, P. F., Jr., and Slingerland, D. W.: The *in vitro* stimulation of thyroidal activity by propylthiouracil. Endocrinology *70*:7, 1962.
74. Nadler, N. J., Young, B. A., Leblond, C. P., and Mitmaker, B.: Elaboration of thyroglobin in the thyroid follicle. Endocrinology *74*:333, 1964.
75. Parrott, M. W., Johnston, M. E., and Durbin, P. W.: The effects of thyroid and parathyroid deficiency on reproduction in the rat. Endocrinology *67*:467, 1960.
76. Pitt-Rivers, R.: Mode of action of antithyroid compounds. Physiol. Rev. *30*:194, 1950.
77. Pitt-Rivers, R.: Iodine metabolism in the thyroid gland. Mem. Soc. Endocr., No. 11, 71, 1961.
78. Reineke, E. P.: The formation of thyroxine in iodinated proteins. Ann. N. Y. Acad. Sci. *50*:450, 1949.
79. Scow, R. O.: Effect of thyroxine on the weight and composition of muscle, pelt and other tissues in young hypophysectomized rats. Endocrinology *53*:344, 1955.

80. Selenkow, H. A., and Asper, S. P., Jr.: Biological activity of compounds structurally related to thyroxine. Physiol. Rev. *35*:426, 1955.
81. Serif, G. S., and Kirkwood, S.: The metabolism of the antithyroid action of iodide ion. Endocrinology *58*:23, 1956.
82. Shellabarger, C. J., and Brown, J. R.: The biosynthesis of thyroxine and 3:5:3′-triiodothyronine in larval and adult toads. J. Endocr. *18*:98, 1959.
83. Stanbury, J. B., Ohela, K., and Pitt-Rivers, R.: The metabolism of iodine in 2 goitrous cretins compared with that in 2 patients receiving methiomazole. J. Clin. Endocr. *15*:54, 1955.
84. Swanson, H. E.: The effect of temperature on the potentiation of adrenalin by thyroxine in the albino rat. Endocrinology *60*:205, 1957.
85. Tata, J. R.: A cellular thyroxine-binding protein fraction. Biochim. Biophys. Acta *28*:91, 1958.
86. Tata, J. R.: Requirement for RNA and protein synthesis for induced regression of the tadpole tail in organ culture. Develop. Biol. *13*:77, 1966.
87. Tata, J. R.: The action of thyroid hormones. Gen. Comp. Endocr., Suppl. *2*:385, 1969.
88. Tong, W., Kerkof, P., and Chaikoff, I. L.: Identification of labeled thyroxine and triiodothyronine in *Amphioxus* treated with [131]I. Biochim. Biophys. Acta *56*:326, 1962.
89. van Heynigen, H. E.: The initiation of thyroid function in the mouse. Endocrinology *69*:720, 1961.
90. Voitkevich, A. A.: Neurosecretory control of the amphibian metamorphosis. Gen. Comp. Endocr., Suppl. *1*:133, 1962.
91. Wahlborg, A., Bright, C., and Frieden, E.: Activity of some new triiodothyronine analogs in the tadpole. Endocrinology *75*:561, 1964.
92. Weber, R.: Zur Aktivierung der Kathepsine im Schwanzgewebe von Xenopuslarven bei spontaner und "in vitro" induzierter Rückbildung. Helv. Physiol. Pharmakol. Acta *21*:277, 1963.
93. Weber, R.: Biochemistry of amphibian metamorphosis. *In* R. Weber (ed.): The Biochemistry of Animal Development, Vol. 2. New York, Academic Press, 1967, p. 227.
94. Weber, R., Hagenbüchle, O., and Ryffel, G.: Thyroid hormones and RNA metabolism in anuran metamorphosis. Fortsch. Zool. *20*(3):419, 1974.
95. Yamada, T., Iino, S., and Schichijo, K.: Inhibitory effect of excess iodide on thyroidal radioiodine release in the rat. Endocrinology *72*:83, 1963.

CHAPTER 8

Parathyroid and Ultimobranchial Glands: PTH, Calcitonin, and the Cholecalciferols

The first anatomic description of the parathyroids was provided by Sandström (1880). Prior to and during this period, surgeons performed thyroidectomies without being aware that they were also removing some or all of the parathyroid glands. Gley (1891) discovered that the rabbit possesses an external pair of parathyroids, in addition to the pair that is closely applied to the thyroid lobes, and demonstrated that total thyroidectomy (external parathyroids remaining intact) did not result in tetany, as was commonly supposed. Erdheim (1903) associated these glands with bone diseases such as rickets, and, in 1908, MacCallum and Voegtlin were able to relieve parathyroprivic tetany by administering calcium salts. The latter workers proposed that the parathyroids were involved in the regulation of calcium exchange. Physiologically active parathyroid extracts were prepared by Hanson (1924) and Collip (1925). Since that time there has been intense interest in the relationship between the parathyroid glands and vitamin D.

An event of great importance in endocrinology was the introduction of the radioimmunoassay technique, which makes it possible to measure minute amounts of peptides in tissues and body fluids. This type of assay was first applied to insulin in the 1960's, and good use has been made of it in elucidating the chemistry and physiology of the peptide hormones of the parathyroid, thyroid, and ultimobranchial glands. Current interest is being focused on a steroid hormone, 1,25-dihydroxycholecalciferol, which is metabolized from vitamin D in the kidney. Its actions are integrated with those of parathyroid hormone (PTH) and calcitonin (CT) in the regulation of skeletal and mineral metabolism.

ANATOMY OF THE GLANDS

Structure and Location

The human parathyroids are flattened, ovate, or pyriform bodies situated on the posterior surfaces of the lateral lobes of the thyroid, near their

225

mesial edges. There are usually four glands in man, a superior pair and an inferior pair (Fig. 7–1). Ultimobranchial glands are absent in the human, as they are in other mammals. The number and location of the parathyroids are quite variable in all vertebrates that have them. Occasionally, some of them may be buried deeply in the substance of the thyroid or thymus; this association stems from the close origin of these structures in the embryo. Though one or both of the inferior parathyroids may be located some distance caudad to the thyroid, they usually follow the branches of the inferior thyroid arteries. Parathyroid rests may be scattered widely in the adipose and connective tissues of the neck or in the mediastinum.

Blood supply is chiefly from the inferior thyroid arteries, but a certain amount of blood may be received through anastomosing branches of the superior thyroid arteries. Veins from the parathyroids enter those that drain the thyroid glands. Transplanted glands appear to function quite normally in the absence of the usual nervous connections. The parathyroids undergo no conspicuous change after hypophysectomy and are not controlled by any of the pituitary trophic hormones.

Each parathyroid is surrounded by a connective tissue capsule, from which septa extend into the substance of the gland and divide it imperfectly into lobules. The gland consists of densely packed masses and cords of epithelial cells, between which are interspersed numerous small blood vessels (Fig. 8–1). Mammalian glands contain mostly chief cells, and these are the

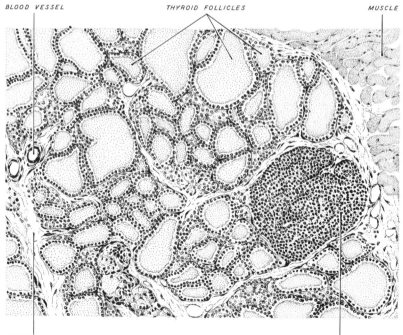

BLOOD VESSEL   THYROID FOLLICLES   MUSCLE

INTERFOLLICULAR CONNECTIVE TISSUE   PARATHYROID

Figure 8–1. A section of the thyroid and parathyroid glands of the rat as seen under low power of the microscope. Notice that the parathyroid gland lies near the surface and is surrounded on three sides by the thyroid follicles.

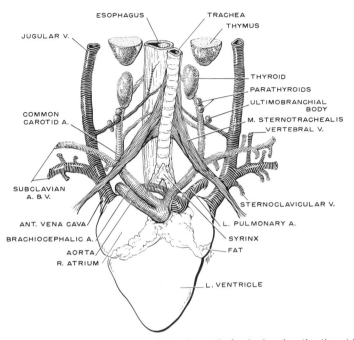

ESOPHAGUS TRACHEA
THYMUS
JUGULAR V.
THYROID
PARATHYROIDS
ULTIMOBRANCHIAL
BODY
COMMON
CAROTID A.
M. STERNOTRACHEALIS
VERTEBRAL V.
SUBCLAVIAN
A. & V.
STERNOCLAVICULAR V.
ANT. VENA CAVA
L. PULMONARY A.
BRACHIOCEPHALIC A.
SYRINX
AORTA
FAT
R. ATRIUM
L. VENTRICLE

Figure 8–2. Dissection of the thorax of the domestic fowl, showing the thyroids, parathyroids, and ultimobranchial bodies in relation to the heart and major blood vessels.

source of PTH. Follicle-like groups of cells enclosing colloid are found frequently in the parathyroids of many vertebrates, but the colloid does not contain iodine. Seasonal changes in histology and secretory activity occur in the parathyroids of many amphibians and reptiles; their heterothermic nature is an important factor in conditioning the way they respond to endocrine manipulations.[14, 28]

Phylogenetically, the parathyroids first appear in amphibians. In frogs, they are small, rounded bodies lying posterior to the thyroids in close association with branches of the external jugular vein. Since they are spatially separated from the thyroids, they may be removed without interfering with other glands. Most reptiles have two pairs of parathyroids, though three pairs or one pair may be found in certain species. Birds usually have two separate parathyroids located caudad of each thyroid lobe, but in some species the glands on each side tend to fuse (Fig. 8–2).

Well-defined ultimobranchials are present in fishes, and they are known to contain plentiful amounts of calcitonin. The utility of this hormone in fishes, presumably functioning in the absence of PTH, is poorly understood.

Developmental Anatomy

The parathyroids of mammals originate from the dorsal halves of the third and fourth pairs of pharyngeal pouches (Fig. 8–3); thymic tissue dif-

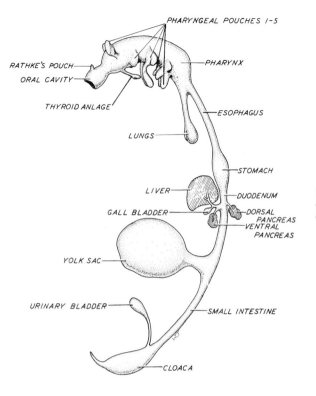

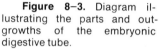

Figure 8–3. Diagram illustrating the parts and outgrowths of the embryonic digestive tube.

ferentiates from the ventral halves of the same pouches. In amphibians, reptiles and birds, unlike mammals, the parathyroids arise from the *ventral* portions of pouches 2, 3, and 4, and thymic tissue from the *dorsal* portions of the same pouches. Some of the parathyroid anlagen may disappear or fuse during the course of development. In amphibians, for example, the anlagen from pouch 2 generally disappear, so that the adults typically have only two pairs of parathyroids, arising from pouches 3 and 4. This also happens in turtles, but in other reptiles, all three pairs of anlagen may persist and give rise to adult parathyroids. In crocodiles, only the anlagen from pouch 3 survive. In the chicken embryo, the parathyroid anlagen from pouches 3 and 4 remain together and often fuse; the adult glands are easily identifiable on the common carotid arteries a short distance caudad of the thyroids (Fig. 8–2).

The parathyroids of amphibians arise from the pharyngeal pouches during metamorphosis. They have not been found in permanently neotenous amphibians, such as the Mexican axolotl and *Necturus,* and presumably are absent. Parathyroids are not present in fishes.

It should be noted that the embryonic pharynx gives rise to the thyroids, parathyroids, thymus, and ultimobranchial glands. Since all of these structures are intimately associated during development, there are many opportunities for their tissues to adhere or intermingle during embryonic migrations.[13, 19, 23] In turtles, for example, the anterior parathyroids are deeply embedded in the thymus, whereas the posterior pair is closely associated with the ultimobranchial glands (Fig. 8–4). In fish, amphibians, reptiles, and birds, the fifth pair of pharyngeal pouches contributes to the formation of the ultimobranchial glands, which are populated by C cells and secrete calcitonin. In mammals, where ultimobranchials are absent, the C cells lodge in the thyroid, thus making this gland the main source of calcitonin.[12, 29]

A new dimension has been added to our understanding of the embryonic origin of the secretory cells found in glands of pharyngeal origin. It has been suggested that most polypeptide hormone secreting cells belong to the APUD series (see p. 53, Chap. 2), and it is proposed that these cells are of neural crest origin.[35] Thus, the pre-endocrine cells could migrate into the pharynx and gut to populate various glands. The best evidence for this hypothesis is derived from studies on the avian thymus, and an extension of these results could explain the presence of calcitonin secreting cells not only in the thyroid gland of mammals, which lack ultimobranchial bodies, but in various atypical locations such as parathyroid, thymus, thyroglossal duct, and along the main vessels of the neck. Definitive proof of the neural crest origin of C cells of the ultimobranchial glands was obtained by the embryonic transplantation of neural tissue from the quail to the chick.[27] The donor quail nuclei are clearly distinguishable from those of the host chick because their nucleoli contain a condensation of heterochromatin, which is prominent and which serves as an excellent marker. Examination of the host ultimobranchial bodies reveals the presence of both quail and chick

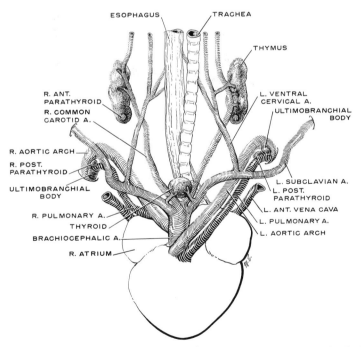

Figure 8–4. Heart and major blood vessels of the turtle *(Pseudemys scripta),* showing the thyroid gland and the usual locations of parathyroid and ultimobranchial glands.

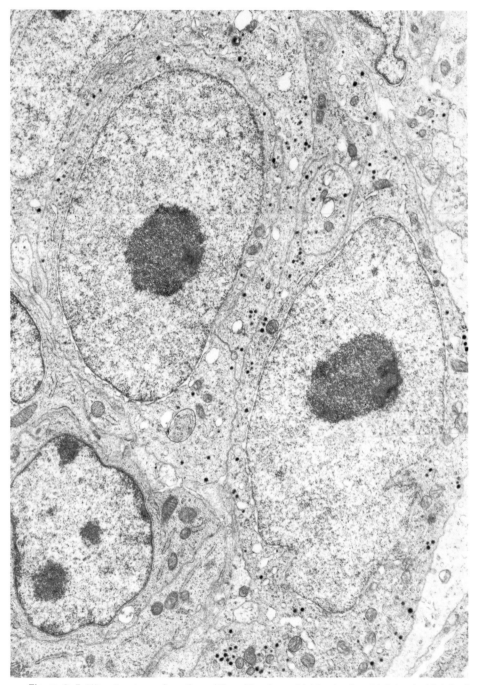

Figure 8–5. Ultrastructure of portion of the ultimobranchial body of a chick host which had received a graft of quail rhombencephalon. Cells of quail origin, characterized by their large DNA-rich nucleoli, contain secretory granules involved with the secretion of calcitonin. Cells of the glandular cords that contain no secretory granules contain the chick type nucleus (lower left). (Courtesy of N. Le Douarin.)

cells, and it is important to note that those of the quail contain secretory granules whereas those of the chick are limited to a supporting role (Fig. 8–5).

BONE AND MINERAL METABOLISM

Parathyroid hormone, calcitonin, and dihydroxycholecalciferol are the principal hormones concerned with the metabolism of ions such as calcium, phosphate, pyrophosphate, citrate, and magnesium, and with regulation of the metabolism of bone and its organic constituents. Without attempting to give a detailed and exhaustive treatment of the subject, some aspects of mineral metabolism in relation to the skeletal system are presented as an aid to understanding parathyroid and ultimobranchial physiology.

Calcium Metabolism

The human body contains more calcium than any other cation, and about 99 per cent of this is present in the mineral crystals (hydroxyapatite) of bone. A human adult of average size contains 1200 to 1400 gm of calcium. Most of this resides in the skeleton; about 12 gm is present in the soft tissues and is chiefly intracellular, and less than 1 gm is found in blood and extracellular fluid. The amount of ionized calcium in the plasma is accurately maintained despite the enormous reservoir of calcium present in the skeleton, and despite the wide fluctuations in intake and excretion of calcium. Although the concentration of calcium ions in the body fluids is low, it performs a vital role in neuromuscular excitability, membrane permeability, enzyme activity, the clotting of blood, and the responses of the organism to fluctuations in acid-base balance. Minor variations in the plasma concentration of ionized calcium produce profound effects on neuromuscular irritability. Tetany (tonic spasms of the skeletal muscles) occurs when the Ca^{++} in the body fluids falls too low. The magnitude of contraction of the isolated frog's heart is directly proportional to the amount of Ca^{++} present, up to a certain concentration. In the absence of Ca^{++}, the heart remains in diastole, but if the concentration is too great, the heart goes into a state of sustained contraction or rigor. Potassium and magnesium ions antagonize the effects of Ca^{++} on the contraction of the heart.

Calcium performs at least three general functions at the cellular level. (1) It is a key component of the cell membrane and conditions its permeability and electrical properties. Hypercalcemia in amphibians decreases the permeability of the skin and urinary bladder, thus reducing the transport of sodium ion, urea, and water across these surfaces. Hypocalcemia, on the other hand, is associated with increased membrane permeability, and this leads to increased neuromuscular irritability. (2) Calcium is known to serve as a coupling factor during excitation and contraction in all forms of muscle. (3) There are indications that calcium ions participate at an early stage to couple hormone and target-cell response. A clear instance is the action of oxytocin on uterine muscle: The hormone promotes increased entry of calcium through the cell membrane of the uterine cell, just as nervous excitation (via acetylcholine) brings about the contraction of skeletal muscle. There is abundant evidence that calcium ions perform significant roles in mediating the actions of a variety of hormones, but the sequence of events following the initial hormone-receptor interaction is largely unknown. Isolated mitochondria from a variety of organs accumulate calcium when incubated under proper conditions. The electron-dense granules that accumulate within the mitochondria of osteoblasts as they engage in bone resorption consist of calcium phosphate.

By using radiocalcium (^{45}Ca) and radiophosphorus (^{32}P), it is possible to follow the movement of these elements from the blood into the tissues. Intravenous ^{45}Ca leaves the blood very rapidly and is deposited in the skeleton. Long-term studies on the retention of ^{45}Ca indicate that the turnover of total bone calcium occurs very slowly.

Calcium is absorbed largely from the upper part of the small intestine, and factors that hasten the passage of intestinal contents through this part of the tract reduce the amount of calcium that can be absorbed. Since hydrochloric acid has a solubilizing effect on dietary calcium, the efficiency of calcium absorption may be influenced by the reservoir function of the stomach and its frequency of emptying (Fig. 8–6).[2] 1,25-Dihydroxycholecalciferol (1,25-$(OH)_2D_3$), a vitamin D_3 metabolite synthesized in the

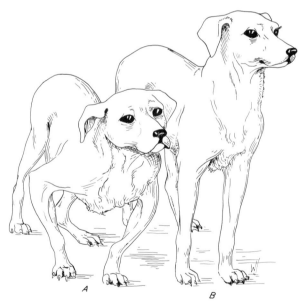

A   *B*

Figure 8–6. Homogeneous osteoporosis produced in the dog by the surgical removal of the stomach. The animal on the left (*A*) was gastrectomized at 103 days of age and appeared as in this sketch 510 days after the operation. The animal on the right (*B*) is an unoperated control. Both puppies were given the same opportunities for feeding. The bowing of the front legs and the swaying of the back become pronounced after gastrectomy in this species and are indicative of a weakened skeleton. (Drawn from taxidermic mounts provided by Dr. A. C. Ivy.)

kidney, is essential for the transport of calcium from the intestine. The presence of alkali, an excess of fat, or a high calcium-to-phosphate ratio in the diet may make calcium absorption difficult and raise the requirement for $1,25\text{-}(OH)_2D_3$. On the other hand, an excess of dietary phosphate has no striking effect on the absorption of calcium; factors that reduce calcium absorption generally impede phosphate absorption. There is practically no movement of calcium through the intestinal mucosa of parathyroidectomized animals. This is due to the fact that PTH controls the production and secretion of $1,25\text{-}(OH)_2D_3$ by the kidney.[39]

The human erythrocyte does not contain calcium. The normal level of serum calcium is about 10 mg per 100 ml, with a range of 9 to 11 mg per 100 ml; in infants and during early childhood, the range is slightly higher. Approximately 55 to 60 per cent of the calcium in the serum is ultrafiltrable and diffusible; the remaining 40 to 45 per cent is bound to serum proteins, largely to the albumin fraction. The diffusible fraction of serum calcium is generally considered to be ionized, although some of the diffusible calcium may be in the nonionized form. Citrate forms a nonionized compound with diffusible calcium. If the citrate levels of the serum are high, all of the serum calcium may become diffusible, although not ionized. The cerebrospinal fluid contains about 5 mg per 100 ml of calcium, and this is the diffusible fraction since the protein-bound portion is not free to leave the circulation.

The blood plasma of laying hens contains both "ionic" (diffusible) and organically bound (nondiffusible) calcium. The latter is bound to phosphoprotein and forms a readily dissociable complex. While the egg is in the shell gland (the region of the oviduct that secretes the shell), the protein-bound fraction is appreciably reduced, whereas the diffusible calcium varies only slightly. It is probable that the "ionic" calcium leaves the bloodstream by diffusion as the shell is formed and its concentration in the plasma is maintained by a dissociation of the organically bound fraction. During the egg-laying cycle, the diffusible fraction increases cyclically relative to the total calcium, but the increase is relatively small.

The amount of calcium in the blood depends on a balance between (1) the amount received by intestinal absorption and by the resorption of bone, and (2) the amount lost by excretion in the urine and feces and by deposition in bone salt. Bone resorption in the young animal occurs principally in the areas in which growth and remodeling are occurring, but some deposition of new bone takes place in the normal adult. Despite the large and variable movements of calcium into and out of the blood, the level of serum calcium is held remarkably constant. Within a few hours after parathyroidectomy, the total calcium falls to 5 to 7 mg per 100 ml, whereas hyperparathyroidism elevates it above 10 mg per 100 ml.

An interesting syndrome may be produced experimentally by gastrectomy of puppies. After surgical removal of the stomach of the dog, skeletal deformities similar to those of rickets become apparent as the animal ages (Fig. 8–6). The achlorhydria consequent upon gastrectomy interferes with the absorption of calcium from the upper intestine. Furthermore, in the absence of the stomach, incompletely digested food passes so rapidly along the intestine that insufficient amounts of calcium and phosphorus are absorbed. An acidosis ensues in such gastrectomized animals after the ingestion of food, and increased amounts of calcium and phosphate are excreted in the urine. While the levels of serum calcium and phosphate are within normal limits, the animals are not absorbing and retaining sufficient minerals to permit proper hardening of the skeletal system. The skeleton therefore is exceptionally spongy, a condition called "homogeneous osteoporosis."

Disuse osteoporosis, called "cage fatigue," often occurs in domestic chickens when they are reared in small cages which do not allow ample room for exercise. The bones become spongy and the femurs often fracture from supporting the weight of the body. When such osteoporotic birds are allowed to exercise in more spacious quarters, the weakened skeleton generally undergoes repair.[54]

Phosphate Metabolism

Elemental phosphorus is highly toxic and is present in the body only as organic or inorganic phosphates. The adult human body contains 500 to 600 gm of phosphate, and around 85 per cent of this is in the skeleton. In infants and young children, the inorganic phosphate of the blood serum ranges from 5 to 7 mg per 100 ml. This diminishes with age and 3 to 4.5 mg per 100 ml is the range generally stated for normal adults. Nearly all the inorganic phosphate of the serum is diffusible. The level of serum phosphate is a poor reflection of the rapid phosphate exchanges that go on continuously within the living organism. The phosphate radical is present in every cell and is of vital importance in a multitude of cellular activities. The adenine and guanine nucleotides are phosphorylated compounds that provide most of the chemical energy for intracellular work. Inorganic phosphate performs a key role in the regulation of glycolysis and energy metabolism. The ribonucleic acids of the cell are polyphosphate polymers, and the phospholipids are important constituents of the plasma membrane and the various intracellular membranes. Phosphate is an important ingredient of bone salts, and also acts as a buffer in the preservation of normal acid-base balance.

Phosphorus in the form of inorganic phosphate is absorbed from the small intestine, and this is facilitated by acid. In alkaline media there is a tendency for it to be precipitated as insoluble phosphates, such as calcium phosphate. Phosphate absorption is improved by diets low in calcium; insoluble phosphates are formed if there is an excess of calcium in the diet. Since $1,25\text{-}(OH)_2D_3$ promotes calcium absorption, it indirectly facilitates phosphate absorption. The phosphate that reaches the circulation may be stored in bone or in the form of such compounds as nucleic acid, phospholipids, nucleoprotein, and phosphoproteins. Phosphate excretion occurs chiefly through the kidney, about 66 per cent of the ingested phosphorus appearing in the urine; fecal excretion accounts for the remainder. The kidneys are important organs in controlling phosphate balance. Hyperphosphatemia is characteristic of kidney failure since phosphate continues to be absorbed from the intestine and is retained.

Severe skeletal defects develop in rats when they are maintained on a phosphate-deficient diet. There may be little or no change in the serum calcium level, but the serum phosphate may reach a value of less than 1 mg per 100 ml. Despite a deficiency in the blood, the phosphate in the liver, muscle, and other soft tissues remains normal. The requirements of the soft tissues are met at the expense of the skeleton, and this leads to a progressive osteoporosis. The ribs and vertebrae become very thin and low in minerals, but the teeth are relatively unaffected.

The Chemistry and Histology of Bone

Chemistry

Bone consists of an organic matrix (35 per cent) and inorganic material (65 per cent). If the mineral component of bone is removed by letting it stand in dilute acid, there remains a strong flexible matrix of organic material, which retains the shape of the original bone. The matrix consists chiefly of collagen, a protein which is rich in glycine, proline, and hydroxyproline; mucopolysaccharides and mucoproteins are also contained in this phase of bone. Bone collagen seems to be structurally similar to that found in cartilage, tendons, and other connective tissues. Collagen from sources other than bone can serve as a template for hydroxyapatite formation, and this suggests that the collagen of bone is not structurally unique. It is not clear what factors determine whether or not collagen becomes mineralized *in vivo;* one possibility is that pyrophosphate inhibits crystal initiation and its enzymatic destruction in bone could therefore permit hydroxyapatite nucleation to occur.

The skeleton may be regarded as a mass of protein that has become heavily impregnated with mineral crystals. In addition to calcium and phosphate, the inorganic phase contains small quantities of magnesium, potassium, sodium, fluorine, and strontium. The same minerals are found in teeth, but the water content in teeth is lower than in bone. Dentine and enamel contain more calcium phosphate and less calcium carbonate than does bone. The mineral matter of the skeleton is in the form of crystals, and this suggests that it is deposited as a consequence of precipitation. The mineral exists as an apatite, a double salt of calcium phosphate and calcium carbonate. These crystals are oriented with reference to the fibrous latticework of the matrix and to the mechanical stresses and strains applied to the bone in performing its function. Disuse of the skeleton may cause a loss of minerals and matrix from the bones that normally bear the weight of the body. A lengthy period of complete bed rest in a previously active individual may cause enough demineralization of the skeleton to elevate the calcium levels of the blood. This effect may result in part from an increased flow of blood through the bones in relation to function.

In adults, as well as in young organisms, the skeletal system undergoes constant structural and metabolic changes. Bone is being formed in some areas and is simultaneously resorbed in other areas, the two processes taking place side by side. The whole skeleton is in a state of dynamic equilibrium, matrix formation and calcium salt deposition adding to it, and matrix destruction and calcium salt removal subtracting from it. Thus, the bones are plastic structures and are able to undergo a certain degree of remodeling in accordance with the everyday stresses to which they are subjected.

Since the introduction of radioactive isotope methods, it has been amply demonstrated that the mineral salts of bone are metabolically active. There is a continuous and rapid exhange of calcium and phosphate between the tissue fluids that bathe the bone trabeculae and the crystals of calcium phosphate that compose the bone. The greatest exchange occurs in the areas of the bone in which the circulation is greatest. Furthermore, the rate of exchange between body fluids and bone varies in different sites in the bone and in different bones of the body. For example, the rate of renewal of calcium in the ribs and sternum of the dog is much more rapid than that in the calvarium or in the diaphysis of the femur or tibia. Radioactive phosphorus has been found to remain in the body of an adult rat for about two months; 30 per cent of the ^{32}P taken up by the skeleton is lost within 20 days. Even the molar teeth, which do not grow in the adult rat, take up small amounts of ^{32}P and lose it very slowly. These and many other observations show that mineral matter of bone is constantly changing.

Histology

In order to understand how hormones and other regulatory agents influence the transport of minerals between bone and body fluids, it is essential to keep in mind certain general features of bone structure, particularly the various types of cells and the fluid compartments present in bone.[47] Within the fibrillar matrix of the haversian system there are numerous lacunae which are interconnected by means of canaliculi. *Osteocytes* occupy the lacunae and communicate with one another by means of small cytoplasmic processes that extend into the canaliculi. This system of canaliculi provides the only means of transfer between the body fluids and mineralized bone. All of the surfaces in bone are covered by an endosteal or osteoblastic membrane which changes dramatically during different physiologic states. In the areas of active bone formation, the *osteoblasts* constituting this membrane undergo hypertrophy and actively synthesize collagen. When bone destruction occurs, the osteoblastic membrane atrophies and is difficult to visualize. This surface layer of osteoblasts communicates with the deeper osteocytes via canaliculi which penetrate the inorganic phase of the bone (Fig. 8–7). The *osteoclasts* are multinucleated macrophages that resorb all components of bone; they are most conspicuous in the region undergoing resorption. Though osteoclasts can transport calcium into the extracellular fluid, their action is slow and they probably do not have much influence on the fine control of this ion.

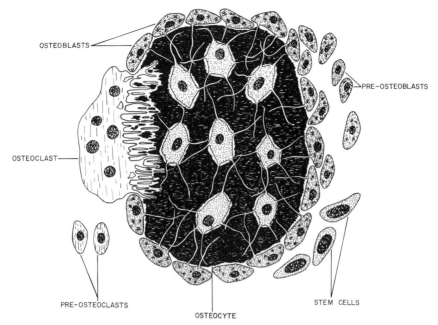

OSTEOBLASTS

PRE–OSTEOBLASTS

OSTEOCLAST

PRE–OSTEOCLASTS

STEM CELLS

OSTEOCYTE

Figure 8–7. Diagram showing the various types of cells present in bone and illustrating the two fluid compartments in this tissue. One fluid space is in direct contact with the solid inorganic phase of bone and consists of the spaces present around the osteocytes, within the canaliculi, within vascular channels of the haversian system, and immediately internal to the osteoblast layer. The other compartment is exterior to the osteoblast layer and is continuous with the extracellular fluid spaces of the body. The mineralized matrix is shown in black. (Redrawn from Talmage, R. V.: Clin. Orthopaed., No. 67, 1969.)

It is certain now that the exchange of ions between bone and the major extracellular fluid compartment is regulated by the activities of the bone cells, and hence is not purely a physicochemical phenomenon. All the surfaces of bone are lined by a cellular layer, considered by some specialists to consist of a "family" of osteoblasts, but some question remains as to whether or not this envelope functions as a typical epithelial membrane. Another problem is whether or not the envelope of cells is complete; there may be areas at which the apatite crystal is devoid of a cellular covering. If the compartmentalization concept is correct, there are actually two fluid compartments in bone: One compartment, consisting of the fluid-filled spaces around the osteocytes, in the canaliculi, and below the layer of osteoblasts, is in direct contact with the mineralized tissue; the other compartment is exterior to the enveloping layer of osteoblasts and is continuous with the main extracellular fluid spaces of the body (Fig 8–7). The fact that the pH on the mineralized side of the membrane is lower (about 6.8) than that on the opposite side (about 7.4) suggests that the two compartments must be fairly tight.

Bone Formation and Resorption

Bones are very active structures, contrary to popular opinion, and are constantly being reshaped through the combined effects of the formation of new bone and the resorption of old bone. These processes occur simultaneously and continuously in the same bone. There is a very high degree of skeletal remodeling in young subjects but, in normal adults, it occurs mostly in response to disuse and to ordinary mechanical stresses and strains. The initial step in the building of new bone is elaboration of an extracellular collagen matrix by the osteoblastic layer of cells. This new matrix, or osteoid, begins to mineralize quite rapidly, but the process slows down and is generally not completed for weeks or months. The macromolecular elements of the matrix, *i.e.,* collagen and possibly associated proteins, serve as templates for the *nucleation* of the mineral crystals. As mineral accretion in the matrix progresses there is a displacement of water, and this decreases the rate of movement of minerals into and out of the bone.

The resorption of mineralized bone is not fully understood, but the major factor associated with its extent seems to be the requirements of the organism in maintaining normal levels of blood calcium and phosphate. It was formerly supposed that the osteoclasts were solely responsible for bone dissolution or resorption, but there is also convincing evidence that the osteoblasts and osteocytes are likewise involved. Though the osteoclasts secrete enzymes capable of hydrolyzing collagen, it is probable that their main function is to remove all breakdown products of bone resorption during the terminal phases.

The two basic events occurring during resorption are the dissolution of the organic matrix and the breakdown of bone crystal; it is difficult to determine which is the initial event, or even whether the two processes occur simultaneously. It is quite obvious that, when bone crystal *per se* is broken down, both calcium and phosphate must be released and in the same proportions as they are combined in the crystal. Different kinds of ions may displace calcium and phosphate ions from the crystal surface.

There are indications that a solubility relationship exists between the concentrations of calcium and phosphate ions in blood plasma and those in bone mineral crystals. This can be demonstrated in mammals and certain other vertebrates by incubating chips of dead or live bone with plasma from a member of the same species.[49] If the concentrations of calcium and phosphate in the plasma are within normal ranges, the bone fragments withdraw both kinds of ions from the plasma. If the contents of these ions in the plasma are subnormal, they are withdrawn from bone and added to the plasma. There has been a long-standing belief that the *solubility product,* or the product of the concentrations of calcium and phosphate ions in the extracellular fluid, was the major factor regulating mineral accretion in bone. There are abundant reasons for believing that bone cells are quite instrumental in regulating mineral homeostasis and that more is involved than a simple solubility product.

Enzymatic analyses of bone are difficult to make because there are great local differences in metabolic activities, a heterogeneous population of bone cells, and a large mass of mineralized matrix to contend with. *Alkaline phosphatase* is abundant in bone and has been studied by many workers, but there is still uncertainty regarding its role in this tissue. Some have found the activity of this enzyme to be greatest in the areas of new bone formation, where collagen is being synthesized and mineral accretion is beginning. However, histochemical methods reveal that it is present in the osteocytes that are involved in bone destruction. Though not all of the plasma alkaline phosphatase is derived from the skeleton, there are marked variations in the circulating titers of this enzyme in certain bone diseases. Histochemical techniques show that *acid phosphatase* is most abundant in the areas undergoing osteoclastic resorption. Enzymes of the citric acid cycle are present in bone. *Protease* activity likewise is highest in the areas of bone undergoing resorption. When the collagen of the bone matrix is destroyed, a portion of it is degraded into hydroxyproline-containing peptides, which reach the blood and are eliminated in the urine. Since collagen breakdown may occur in tissues other than bone, some of the urinary hydroxyproline may be of extraosseous origin. However, the amounts being excreted provide a reasonably valid method of estimating the degree of altered bone resorption. The administration of parathyroid hormone increases hydroxyproline excretion, whereas calcitonin diminishes it.

HORMONES IN MINERAL HOMEOSTASIS

Parathyroid Hormone (PTH)

Chemistry, Biosynthesis, and Assay

Bovine, porcine, and human PTH each contain 84 amino acid residues in a single peptide chain, and these sequences have been elucidated. This form of the hormone has a molecular weight of about 9600. Hormone molecules of comparable size have been found in the rat and chicken; the amino acid sequence varies with the species. There is no information on the chemistry of PTH in amphibians and reptiles and, since parathyroids are absent in fishes, PTH would not be expected in that class. The porcine PTH differs from the bovine by the substitution of seven amino acids in the 84-residue chain. This is the molecular species that is stored in the gland and released into the circulation as the need arises. A fragment of this molecule, consisting of 33 or 34 amino acids at the N-terminus, contains the structural requirements for full biologic activity (Fig. 8–8). A peptide consisting of the first 20 residues of PTH is inactive; activity is completely lost following deletion of residues 1 and 2. Several immunoreactive subfragments are present in the peripheral circulation, but the chemical composition and biologic potency of these are unknown. Little is known regarding the manner in which the hormone is transported in the blood or the sites of its inactivation.[4, 6, 7, 8, 53]

Proparathyroid hormone (proPTH), a biosynthetic precursor of PTH,

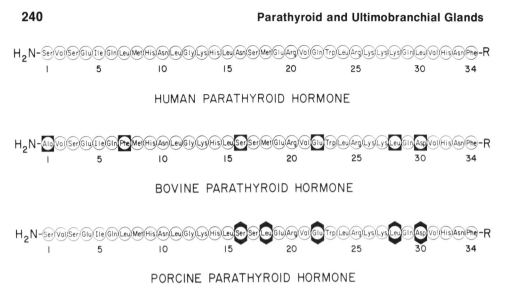

HUMAN PARATHYROID HORMONE

BOVINE PARATHYROID HORMONE

PORCINE PARATHYROID HORMONE

Figure 8–8. Structure of the first 34 N-terminal residues of human, bovine, and porcine parathyroid hormone. The boxed amino acids indicate the loci at which bovine and porcine hormones differ from that of the human. (From H. Rasmussen, in Textbook of Endocrinology, R. H. Williams, ed. Fifth edition, 1974. W. B. Saunders Co., Philadelphia.)

has been found in parathyroid tissue from cattle, swine, rats, chickens, and human beings. It has a molecular weight of about 12,000, and differs in part from PTH by having an additional hexapeptide linked to the N-terminus of the hormone; this bond is susceptible to cleavage by trypsin or trypsin-like enzymes. The amino acid sequences for the hexapeptides that precede the PTH molecules of several species are:

human: Lys-Ser-Val-Lys-Lys-Arg — R

bovine: Lys-Ser-Val-Lys-Lys-Arg — R

porcine: Lys-Pro-Ile-Lys-Lys-Arg — R

Since proPTH has a molecular weight of 12,000, compared with 9600 for PTH, it appears that the amino-terminal hexapeptide accounts for only part of this difference in molecular weight. It is being found that the proPTH molecule contains another peptide segment affixed to the carboxy-termi-nus.[11, 21, 24]

The biologic activity of proPTH is 3 to 50 per cent less than that of PTH, as determined by different bioassay procedures. The prohormone also shows reduced immunologic reactivity with most antisera to the hormone, particularly with antisera which are directed toward the biologically active end (1 – 34 N-terminal sequence) of PTH. When parathyroid tissue is incu-bated with certain amines, the conversion of proPTH to PTH is inhibited. Ul-tramicroscopic studies indicate that the inhibitory amines may exert their effects by impairing intracellular organelles such as microtubles or the Gol-gi complex.[26, 41]

In vitro and ultrastructural observations of parathyroid cells indicate that the microtubules perform an important role in the intracellular trans-port and processing of the hormone before it is released. Agents such as colchicine, vinblastine, and D_2O are known to damage microtubules and inhibit the secretion *in vitro* of several polypeptide hormones. Colchicine treatment of the rat causes a loss of microtubules from the parathyroid cells, which is followed by a fall in serum calcium and an accumulation of secretory granules within the cells. Assembled microtubules increase in parathyroid cells during experimental hypocalcemia, and secretory granules do not accumulate. Microtubular blockade does not interfere with secretion *in vitro* in those cases (*e.g.,* adrenal steroids) in which the product is not packaged into secretion granules. *In vitro* studies on bovine parathyroid tissue indicate that microtubular inhibitors produce a delay in the secretion of PTH and increase the ratio of biosynthetic precursor (proPTH) to the finished hormone (PTH). The results are consistent with the view that the microtubules participate in the transport of proPTH from the rough endoplasmic reticulum, where it is synthesized, to the Golgi complex; the prohormone is converted to PTH at some intracellular site before it is packaged into secretion granules.[26]

The rate of secretion of PTH is inversely proportional to the ambient calcium concentration of the blood plasma. Using radioimmunoassay techniques, it has been shown in many species that PTH in the blood increases when calcium levels are low, and decreases when calcium levels are high. This has been amply confirmed by many types of experiments performed with parathyroid tissue cultured *in vitro*. The plasma levels of magnesium and phosphate ions may directly or indirectly affect parathyroid secretion in certain circumstances. For example, the production of PTH can be stimulated by elevating the plasma phosphate, either through nephrectomy or through the feeding of high phosphate-to-calcium ratios, the levels of serum calcium remaining within normal limits. In some mammals, a severe deficiency of Mg^{++} may lead to a hypocalcemic state in which the expected elevation of PTH fails to occur.

Since the skeleton and kidneys are the main targets for PTH, various parameters may be employed in assaying the hormone. The four most common methods are: (1) *in vivo* procedures utilizing either the calcium-mobilizing or the phosphaturic effects of the hormone, (2) an *in vitro* bioassay based on the capacity of PTH to stimulate the uptake of phosphate by isolated liver mitochondria, (3) an *in vitro* procedure which determines the capacity of the test material to release radiation from Ca^{45}-labeled bones of rat fetuses in tissue culture, and (4) a very sensitive radioimmunoassay similar to that employed for detecting other peptide hormones.

Parathyroidectomy: Hypoparathyroidism

Total removal of parathyroid glands from mammals such as the dog, cat, and rat, produces a characteristic train of disturbances that increases in severity after the operation. The serum calcium drops from a normal of about 10 mg per 100 ml to between 4 and 7 mg per 100 ml. This hypocalcemia results from impaired ability to mobilize calcium from the bones, kidneys, and intestine. The fall in blood calcium is accompanied by a reduced excretion of phosphate and a consequent elevation of inorganic phosphate in the blood (hyperphosphatemia). The reduced concentration of calcium ions in the extracellular fluid produces hyperexcitability of the neuromuscular system, and this leads to *tetany,* an involuntary twitching of the muscles. Unless measures are taken to elevate calcium levels in the blood, death often results from asphyxiation due to spasm of the laryngeal muscles. Studies on bones of hypoparathyroid animals indicate that both bone formation and resorption are diminished; the osteoblast and osteoclast pools on the interior bone surfaces are slowly reduced. The diminished transport of calcium from the intestine is due in part, at least, to the inability of the kidney to form 1,25-dihydroxycholecalciferol, an essential hormone derived from vitamin D_3.

It is necessary for oviparous vertebrates to mobilize enormous quantities of calcium and phosphate from the skeleton and intestine for the formation of yolk and secretion of the eggshell. During incubation calcium is moved from the inner wall of the eggshell to the skeleton of the developing embryo. The serum calcium of the parathyroidectomized rooster falls promptly to 6 to 8 mg per 100 ml. White Leghorn hens in heavy lay have a serum calcium level of 12 to 47 mg per 100 ml; this fluctuates markedly after parathyroidectomy. The operated hens lay soft-shelled eggs for a while, and finally egg production ceases. The majority of such birds die within a few days, but they can survive if given vitamin D, high calcium diets, or exogenous PTH.

Total parathyroidectomy of lizards and snakes reduces serum calcium and leads to tetanic convulsions.[9, 10] Tetany does not ensue in parathyroidectomized turtles, possibly because of the large calcium stores in the bones of the carapace and plastron. Parathyroidectomy of the frog *(Rana pipiens)* elicits a fall in serum calcium and a transient hypercalciuria. PTH is necessary for the mobilization of calcium carbonate from the paravertebral lime sacs of the frog, whereas CT prevents excessive mobilization.[43] Hypoparathyroidism diminishes serum calcium in all species of amphibians studied, but in several species this is not sufficient to induce tetany.

Hyperparathyroidism

All of the dysfunctions resulting from removal of the parathyroids can be repaired by the administration of PTH. However, excessive amounts of the hormone lead to dysfunctions in the opposite direction. One of the first changes to occur is an increase in the renal excretion of phosphate and a diminished loss of calcium through the urine. The serum citrate level rises. The hypercalcemia results from an excessive rate of bone resorption, the decreased renal elimination of calcium and, possibly, an improved intestinal transport of calcium. One of the early effects of PTH is to increase the activity of osteocytes and osteoclasts, producing a prompt dissolution of bone mineral. Osteoblastic activity is diminished reducing the synthesis of new collagen matrix. If bone resorption exceeds bone formation for long periods, profound effects upon the osseous system result (Fig. 8–9). The bones

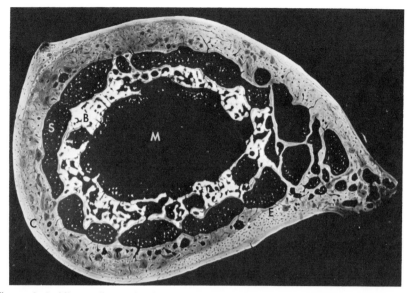

Figure 8–9. Microradiograph of cross section of the tibia of a laying hen following the administration of parathyroid extract. The hormone produces bone resorption mainly in the area between the endosteum (E) and the intramedullary bone deposits (B), leaving spaces (S) which become filled with osteoclasts, mesenchymal cells, and blood vessels. Note also the absorption cavities in the cortical bone (C). The higher radiodensity of the intramedullary bone (B) results from the fact that it contains more mineral and less collagen. This kind of bone lesion is called *osteitis fibrosa cystica*. M, marrow cavity. (Courtesy of M. R. Urist, University of California School of Medicine, Los Angeles.)

may be softened so greatly by the loss of minerals that fractures and disabling deformities are unavoidable. Longstanding hyperparathyroidism often leads to metastatic calcium deposits in kidney tubules, the gastric and intestinal walls, the heart, lesser arteries, liver, bronchi, and lungs.

In summarizing the foregoing observations on hypo- and hyperparathyroidism, it may be concluded that PTH increases the levels of plasma calcium and decreases the levels of plasma phosphate by (1) acting on the kidneys to reduce the excretion of calcium and to increase the excretion of phosphate, and to promote the conversion of $25\text{-}OH\text{-}D_3$ to $1,25\text{-}(OH)_2D_3$ by the kidney;[33] (2) by acting on bone, in conjunction with $1,25\text{-}(OH)_2D_3$, to promote bone resorption, thus moving calcium from the skeleton to the extracellular fluid; and (3) by acting indirectly, at least, to facilitate the intestinal absorption of calcium (Fig. 8–11). Following the administration of PTH, the level of cAMP rises rapidly and markedly in bone and kidney before the physiologic effects of the hormone become apparent, and this is followed by a transitory elevation of the nucleotide in the plasma and urine. These and other observations provide strong evidence that cAMP serves as a second messenger in these targets.[1, 31]

Calcitonin (CT)

Chemistry, Assay, and Secretion

Calcitonin is a polypeptide chain consisting of 32 amino acid residues and has a molecular weight of 3000.[3, 15, 37, 38] In all species, the first 7 resi-

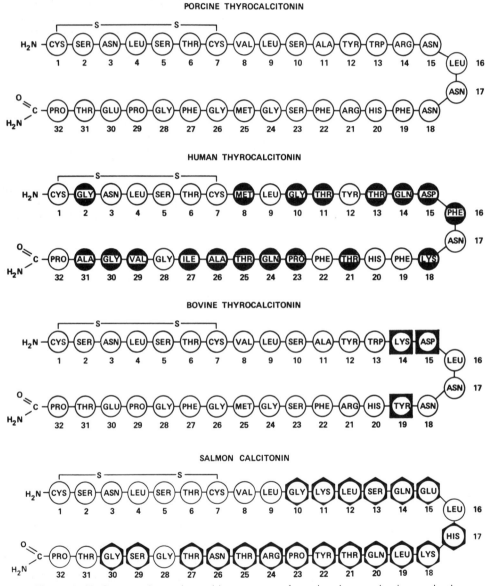

Figure 8–10. Comparative amino acid sequences of porcine, human, bovine, and salmon calcitonins. The darkened or boxed symbols represent loci that are different from those of the porcine hormone. (From H. Rasmussen, in Textbook of Endocrinology, R. H. Williams, ed. Fifth edition, 1974. W. B. Saunders Co., Philadelphia.)

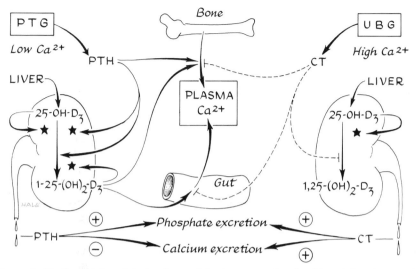

Figure 8–11. Some interrelated actions of the hormones involved in calcium homeostasis. The parathyroid glands release PTH in response to low serum calcium; the ultimobranchial glands (or thyroid) secrete CT when calcium is high. The liver metabolizes vitamin D_3 to produce 25-OH-D_3 which supplements the action of PTH in promoting reabsorption of calcium by the renal tubules (see stars). A PTH-dependent kidney enzyme converts 25-OH-D_3 to 1,25-$(OH)_2D_3$, a steroid hormone which is especially potent in promoting the transport of calcium from the intestine to the body fluids. Calcitonin blocks the renal synthesis of 1,25-$(OH)_2$ D_3, thus acting indirectly to inhibit the intestinal absorption of calcium. Under certain physiologic conditions, calcitonin may act directly on the intestine to produce the same effect. The steroid hormone from the kidney also supplements the action of PTH in enhancing bone resorption; CT prevents bone resorption. Broken lines indicate inhibitory actions; stars signify promotion of calcium resorption by nephrons.

dues at the N-terminus are included in an intrachain disulfide bridge (Fig. 8–10). Human, porcine, ovine, bovine, and salmon calcitonins are well known chemically, and progress is being made in purifying rat and chicken calcitonins. Chemical synthesis of human, porcine, and salmon hormones has been accomplished, and adequate amounts of these have been available for experimental purposes and for clinical trials. Unlike PTH, there is no biologically active subfragment in the CT molecule; in other words, the entire molecule is essential for activity. The amino acid sequences are quite variable among the molecules that have been studied most carefully. Comparison of the residues of human, ovine, bovine, porcine, and salmon calcitonins reveals that in these five species only 9 of the 32 residues are homologous, and these tend to occur at the two ends of the molecule. There are 16 homologous positions in human and salmon calcitonins.

Structural studies of rat CT indicate that it is more similar to human CT than it is to those of the pig or salmon. In both hormones the C-terminal amide is necessary for immunoreactivity; the main antigenic determinants are located in the C-terminal regions of the molecules.[3]

The known calcitonins vary greatly in biologic potency. The salmon CT is a much more potent hypoglycemic agent when tested on higher vertebrates than any that has been isolated; this is due in part to the fact that it is comparatively resistant to metabolic degradation. In man, the salmon hormone is far more potent in lowering the level of blood calcium than is the human hormone or that obtained from any other mammalian species. The level of CT in normal human blood is extremely low, but it rises following an infusion of calcium. Abnormally high concentrations are found in patients with medullary thyroid carcinoma, a tumor consisting largely of C cells.[29] Glucagon and several of the gastrointestinal hormones stimulate CT secretion, indicating that factors other than blood calcium levels have to be considered.

Calcitonin may be assayed by an *in vivo* procedure which is based on its capacity to lower the plasma calcium in rats or other mammals. Radioimmunoassay is commonly used for quantitating the hormone in blood, urine, cell extracts, or tissue culture media.

In vitro studies on CT secretion have been facilitated by the use of homogeneous monolayer cultures of C cells isolated from the ultimobranchial (UB) glands of trout.[44] Cultures of avian UB glands have been used, but these are sometimes contaminated by parathyroid cells, and a specific immunoassay for avian CT has not been available. Calcitonin-secreting cells constitute a very small percentage of those present in cultures of mammalian thyroid. Using trout C cells, several gastrointestinal hormones (*e.g.*, gastrin, cholecystokinin), prostaglandin E_2, and dibutyryl cyclic AMP were found to exert marked secretagogic effects. Calcium is the best documented secretagogue for mammalian systems, whereas it is a relatively mild stimulant when applied to the trout C cells. This suggests that there may be some differences as well as similarities in the regulation of CT secretion among different vertebrate classes. Human C cells derived from medullary thyroid carcinoma have been similarly cultured.[45]

Main Actions of CT

The physiologic utility of CT remains ambiguous. The prevailing tenet continues to be that the hormone is released mainly in response to elevated serum calcium and that it acts upon bones and kidneys to produce effects that are opposite to those of PTH.[22] In certain species and under certain physiologic conditions, CT may act to inhibit intestinal absorption of calcium (Fig. 8–11).[34, 42] CT is a very effective hypocalcemic agent, especially when administered to young birds and mammals. It prevents softening of the skeleton in animals maintained on low calcium rations (Fig. 8–12).[25] Experiments on the rat show that the ingestion of food or the anticipation of food initiate a chain of interrelated events, probably involving both the nervous system and some of the gastrointestinal hormones, which prepare the organism in advance for increasing levels of calcium and phosphate in the blood. The plasma calcitonin and gastrin rise rapidly in the rats after the initiation of feeding. The implication of these studies is that calcitonin secretion is augmented by an intestinal stimulus rather than by a rise in plasma calcium.[30, 50, 51]

Since fishes have no parathyroids, PTH is presumably absent; the function of CT in these vertebrates is by no means clear. Though salmon CT has marked hypoglycemic effects in higher vertebrates, the same hormone has

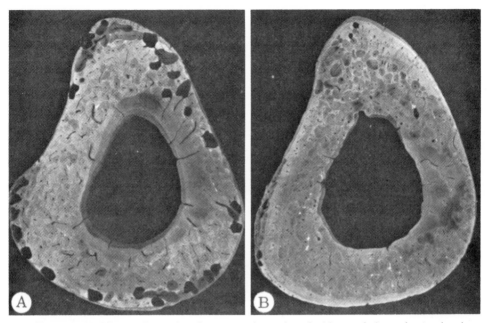

Figure 8–12. Microradiographs of cross sections of cortical bone of ulnas of cats, showing the capacity of porcine calcitonin to prevent dietary osteoporosis. *A,* From a control cat fed a low calcium diet for 5 months. Many resorption spaces are visible. *B,* From a cat fed the same low calcium diet and injected with calcitonin (5.0 U/kg. per day) for 5 months. Note that resorption spaces are practically absent. (From Jowsey, J.: Endocrinology *85*:1196, 1969.)

little or no effect on the levels of blood calcium in salmon and other teleosts. Hyperglycemic conditions in both trout and salmon produce no consistent increase in the rate of secretion of CT. Some studies suggest that CT in fishes may perform a role in enabling them to adjust to changing hydromineral environments.[20]

The Cholecalciferols

Chemistry

Vitamin D has long been recognized as an important factor in skeletal and mineral homeostasis. There has been much recent research which elucidates its complex metabolic pathways, and this had aided in understanding its mechanism of action. A metabolite of cholecalciferol, 1,25-dihydroxycholecalciferol ($1,25-(OH)_2D_3$), is generally recognized as having the greatest biologic activity and, on the basis of its structure and mode of action, is considered to be a steroid hormone.[16, 17, 40]

Cholecalciferol may be synthesized in the skin from 7-dehydrocholesterol, under the influence of ultraviolet light, or ingested dietarily (Fig. 3–3).

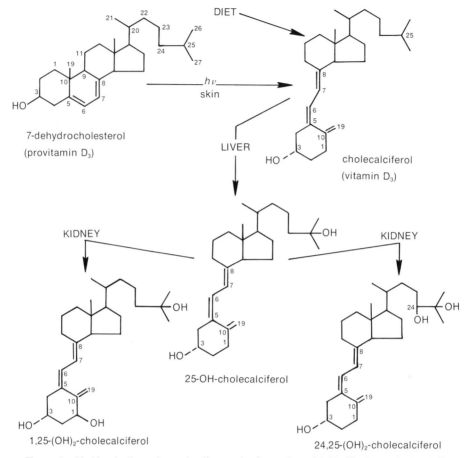

7-dehydrocholesterol
(provitamin D₃)

cholecalciferol
(vitamin D₃)

25-OH-cholecalciferol

1,25-(OH)₂-cholecalciferol

24,25-(OH)₂-cholecalciferol

Figure 8–13. Metabolic pathway leading to the formation of 1,25-dihydroxycholecalciferol, the hormonally active form of vitamin D. Cholecalciferol (vitamin D₃) may be ingested with food or synthesized in the skin; it is acted upon by a hydroxylase in the liver to form 25-OH-chole- calciferol. The latter is carried by the blood to the kidney, where the steroid hormone is produced. In some species and under certain conditions, the kidney may also produce 24,25-dihydroxy- cholecalciferol, but its physiologic significance is not clear. (After A. W. Norman and H. Henry.)

This is conveyed to the liver, where it is hydroxylated at position 25 to pro- duce 25-OH-cholecalciferol. This is then passed to the kidney, where it is further metabolized to produce the active hormone, 1,25-(OH)₂D₃. The 1- hydroxylase effecting this transformation is exclusively present in the kidney cortex and is contained in the mitochondrial fraction. This enzyme is present in the kidneys of many vertebrates, from teleosts to mammals. The consensus is that PTH is involved in the signal to the kidney to release 1,25-(OH)₂D₃, but there is disagreement as to whether this is a direct or indirect effect. After the steroid is released from the kidney, it associates with binding proteins present in the plasma and is carried to the target organs, principally bone and intestinal mucosa (Fig. 8–13). Secretion of this steroid by the kidney in response to skeletal needs for calcium, and its selective uptake by the target organs, support the view that it is a hormonal regulator of calcium metabolism.[33]

Main Functions of 1,25-Dihydroxycholecalciferol

This hormone (1) acts in concert with PTH to control the mineralization of bone, (2) increases the reabsorption of calcium and phosphate by the kidney tubules, and (3) increases the transport of calcium and the calcium-dependent transport of phosphate across the cells of the intestinal mucosa. This possibly involves facilitated entry of calcium across the brush border of the mucosal cell, increased uptake of calcium by mitochondria, and the synthesis of a calcium-binding protein.[33]

Mineral homeostasis is accomplished largely through the integrated actions of PTH, CT, and the metabolites of cholecalciferol. These relationships may be reviewed by referring to Figures 8–11 and 8–14. The diagrams are based on current information which is very incomplete, and hence must be regarded as tentative.

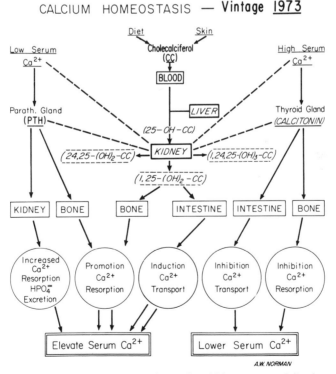

Figure 8–14. The interrelated actions of parathyroid hormone, calcitonin, and 1,25-dihydroxycholecalciferol in the maintenance of calcium homeostasis. (From A. W. Norman and H. Henry, Rec. Prog. Horm. Res. 30:431, 1974.)

Other Hormones Affecting the Skeleton

Pituitary growth hormone increases the rate of bone formation and remodeling and is especially important in young, growing organisms. The hormone promotes the synthesis of collagen and encourages adjustments which provide adequate calcium and phosphate for its mineralization.

The gonadal steroids affect bone growth and maturation, and many of their actions are interrelated with adenohypophysial hormones. The estrogens are known to have profound effects on mineral and skeletal homeostasis in birds. The glucocorticoids of the adrenal gland promote gluconeogenesis by increasing the rate of protein breakdown and the conversion of the resulting amino acids to glucose. The antianabolic action of these steroids shows up in bone as a profound decrease in collagen synthesis and accelerated bone resorption; this may lead to *osteoporosis*.

The thyroid hormones are clearly necessary for the normal growth and maturation of the skeleton. They accelerate both the formation and resorption of bone; these effects may take place partly through a direct action on the skeleton, but it is probable that they increase the responsiveness of osteolytic bone cells to PTH. It is also possible that the thyroid hormones may exert effects on the intestinal and renal transport of calcium and phosphate, but the published research reports are conflicting.

Estrogen Hypercalcemia in Birds

Dramatic changes in calcium metabolism occur in oviparous and ovoviviparous vertebrates during the reproductive periods, and these are associated with increased estrogen production by the ovaries. As birds approach the laying period, large amounts of calcium are stored in the intramedullary deposits that appear in the cavities of the long bones. New bone is added from the endosteum and reduces or obliterates the marrow cavity. This is the avian method of storing large amounts of calcium for egg production. The hen's egg contains about 2.0 gm of calcium in the shell and approximately 30 mg in the yolk. Isotopic techniques have shown that 40 to 50 per cent of the calcium in the shell is turned over from the skeleton and that the remainder is passed from the intestine through the blood plasma to the shell gland. The hypercalcemia due to estrogen action results in large measure from the large amounts of phosphoprotein-calcium complex in transit from the liver to the ovary, where it is used in the formation of yolk.[54]

The long bones of young chicks and cocks contain little if any intramedullary bone, and it becomes very sparse in resting hens or in hens at the end of a long period of egg production. The deposition of intramedullary bone in cocks and young birds may be induced by the administration of estrogens. No other hormone has this effect. The intramedullary bone is promptly resorbed upon withdrawal of the hormone. This bone serves as a special substrate for the rapid turnover of calcium required by the ovary and oviduct for the formation of eggs.

Adult chickens can maintain a total serum calcium level of 10 mg per

100 ml for at least a month when deprived of calcium in the diet. This is accomplished by resorption of bone mineral, especially from the flat bones of the body. About 25 per cent of the total bone mass may be lost in this manner, though the long bones of the appendages are not severely affected except in prolonged calcium deficiency. Rapidly growing chicks cannot survive long in the absence of calcium. In hens deprived of both calcium and vitamin D, egg production is discontinued within 5 days.

In order to store very large amounts of calcium, birds move calcium in the form of protein-calcium complexes through the blood to and from the skeleton, and this transport is accomplished rapidly. Very large amounts of calcium are required for the deposition of the shell and some for the formation of yolk. Even in fishes, amphibians, and viviparous snakes, in whom eggshells are not produced, a hypercalcemia occurs during the reproductive periods that is associated with the transport of yolk proteins. This indicates that the estrogen-induced hypercalcemia in birds is a reflection of the transport of protein-calcium complexes for the formation of yolk, and is not entirely the result of the movement of calcium from bone for the calcification of eggshells, as was formerly believed. Neither hypercalcemia nor the formation of a phosphoprotein-calcium complex is known to occur during the reproductive cycles of mammals.[54]

Estrogens produce conspicuous skeletal modifications in mice.[55] The effect is proportional to the amount of estrogen administered, and new spongy bone may entirely fill the marrow cavities. Estrogen does not have this effect in adult rats but, in young animals, there may be some increase in the spongy bone below the growing epiphysis.

MECHANISMS OF HORMONE ACTION

Parathyroid Hormone

The main targets of PTH are bone and kidney: both of these are complex organs containing multiple tissues and types of cells. Tissue cultures prepared from these organs typically contain a heterologous cell population and cells at various stages of differentiation; under these conditions it is difficult to assign hormonal responses to specific cell types. The hormone activates basically similar intracellular mechanisms in the two target organs.[5, 18, 32, 36]

Much evidence is consistent with the hypothesis that cyclic 3′,5′-adenosine monophosphate (cAMP) is a second messenger involved in the action of PTH. One of the early effects observed after the injection of PTH is a transient movement of calcium into bone cells. Application of the hormone to isolated kidney cells also increases the intracellular content of calcium. After activation of adenylate cyclase and the generation of cAMP, the cytosol calcium is increased by efflux of this ion from the mitochondria.

Many kinds of experiments have shown that PTH increases the content of cAMP in target cells of bone and kidney. *In vitro* and *in vivo* experiments on rat calvaria have demonstrated a rapid and marked accumulation of cAMP in these bones following the application of PTH. The addition of dibutyryl-cyclic AMP (dbcAMP) to bone explants mimics many of the actions of PTH on the same preparations; it promotes bone resorption and causes the release of calcium and certain enzymes. The injection of dbcAMP into the rat produces bone resorption and hypercalcemia, and increases the urinary excretion of phosphate. Many of the actions of PTH on the kidney are reproduced by the intravenous injection of cAMP or the dibutyryl analogue. The fact that cAMP levels within the target cells of bone and kidney rise promptly, before the physiologic effects of the hormone become apparent, suggests the importance of this nucleotide as a second messenger.

The effects of PTH on uridine metabolism are at least partly mediated by cAMP. It appears that the hormone promotes bone resorption partly through a process involving the synthesis of new RNA. *In vivo* and *in vitro* studies show that PTH enhances the incorporation of radioactive precursors into skeletal RNA. A brief exposure of organ-cultured rat bones to PTH causes a prolonged increase in bone resorption; this effect is blocked by actinomycin D and other inhibitors of RNA synthesis. These inhibitors also block the hypercalcemic effect of PTH *in vivo*.

The precise nature and sequence of events occurring within the target cells in response to PTH are not completely understood, but they involve the following: (1) binding of the hormone to receptors at the cell surface, (2) activation of adenylate cyclase, (3) increased concentrations of cAMP within the cell, (4) stimulation of a kinase or phosphorylating enzyme, and (5) enhanced transport of calcium into the target cells.

Calcitonin

CT and PTH are both peptide hormones employing targets in bone and kidney, and these facts would lead one to suspect that their mechanisms of action would be similar in certain respects; but, since their physiologic effects are radically different, the intracellular mechanisms employed by the two hormones would have to be different. In both bone and kidney, CT apparently activates adenylate cyclase, and this leads to increased levels of cAMP in the cells. To get around this enigma, some investigators have proposed that the receptors for PTH and CT might be located on different cell types, or that particular target cells might contain a unique kind of adenylate cyclase that would respond to only one of the hormones. Neither point of view has been conclusively established for both bone and kidney.

Using cultured preparations of periosteum, osteocytes, osteoblasts, and marrow cells separated from the skeletons of adult rats, adenylate cyclase responsiveness to PTH and CT has been tested.[46] Cultures of periosteum and marrow cells do not respond to either hormone. The adenylate cyclase of osteoblasts and osteocytes responds to both PTH and CT. PTH-stimulated activity in osteocytes was increased by adding CT, and this suggests that the culture may have contained different types of osteocytes. No additive effect is observed with osteoblasts. In the case of osteoblasts, at least, one is faced with the problem of explaining how two hormones can produce opposite effects by stimulating adenylate cyclase and elevating the levels of cAMP in the same cell. It is apparent that the mechanism of CT action involves a unique metabolism of calcium and phosphate or, perhaps, unidentified intracellular mediators.

1,25-Dihydroxycholecalciferol

An important target of this steroid hormone is the intestinal mucosa, where it facilitates the synthesis of a calcium-binding protein that is essential for the transcellular movement of calcium and calcium-dependent phosphate. A current hypothesis is that $1,25\text{-}(OH)_2D_3$ acts in the same general manner as other steroid hormones, such as those from the gonads or adrenal cortices. Specifically, this would include binding of the hormone to a cytoplasmic receptor, movement of the steroid-receptor complex to the nucleus where it binds to the chromatin, activation of a specific gene locus, increased synthesis of the mRNA required for the production of calcium-binding protein, and finally increased transport of calcium across the mucosal cell as a consequence of increased production of protein. Mechanisms within the mucosal cell are complex and undoubtedly involve many factors in addition to calcium-binding protein.

Cytosol and nuclear receptors have been identified in the mucosal cells.[33] After the hormone becomes associated with the chromatin, new RNA is synthesized. This produces calcium-binding protein and other proteins necessary for the physiologic response. Actinomycin D inhibits RNA synthesis and blocks the intestinal response to 1,25-dihydroxycholecalciferol. This indicates that at least some of the actions of this steroid hormone depend upon gene activation. The precise manner by which it stimulates osteoclastic proliferation and bone resorption is not known.

A Unifying Hypothesis[47, 48]

Talmage and associates have formulated a working hypothesis intended to account for the manner in which PTH and related hormones control calcium and phosphate homeostasis in the skeleton and blood plasma. The main emphasis has been upon the capacity of PTH to increase the flow of calcium into its target cells, whether in bone, kidney, or other soft tissue, and upon the presence of a layer of cells that separates two fluid compartments (Fig. 8–7). This cellular interface in bone contains active osteoblasts and lines most of the bone surfaces. Since all of the bone lining cells are connected by cytoplasmic extensions to osteocytes within the lacunae, the osteoblast-osteocyte complex forms a functional unit. The electrolyte content of the bone fluid compartment (BFC) is distinct and different from that of the extracellular fluid compartment (ECF).

The osteoblast-osteocyte areas of compact bone respond promptly both to PTH and to CT; PTH hastens the rate of transfer of calcium back to the ECF, whereas CT interferes with the rate of transfer of calcium out of the bone compartment. If there is prompt need for calcium, the osteocytes can provide it (osteocytic osteolysis); if the need for calcium is prolonged, PTH can eventually stimulate bone resorption by osteoclasts. It is clear that PTH increases RNA synthesis in the mesenchyme family of bone cells and accelerates the differentiation of these into osteoclasts and osteoblasts. As mentioned earlier, PTH may indirectly increase the intestinal absorption of calcium by controlling the synthesis of 1,25-dihydroxycholecalciferol by the kidney. It is not known how these various target cell activities relate to the activation of adenylate cyclase and the elevated intracellular cAMP.

According to this postulate, the cells of the osteoblastic membrane are polarized and possess a calcium pump that is restricted to the side of the cell coming in contact with the ECF (Fig. 8–15). This position of the pump confines the escape of calcium to one edge of the osteoblast, enabling this ion to move out of bone against the concentration gradient. This is similar to the manner in which calcium is transported from the intes-

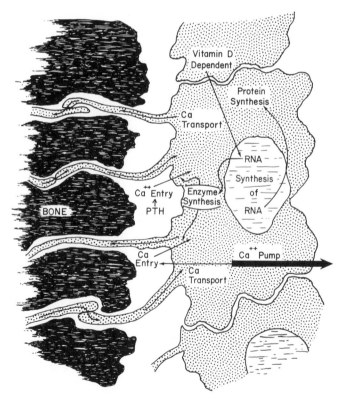

Figure 8–15. Diagram illustrating some factors involved in the mechanism of action of PTH on bone cells. The hormone is throught to promote the entry of calcium ions (CA++) into cells of the osteoblast membrane, and a calcium pump on the opposite side of the cell passes the ions into the extracellular fluid compartment. Note the open channels existing between contiguous osteoblast cells; these should permit fluid and ions to leak back into the mineralized compartment. (Redrawn from Talmage, R. V.: Clin. Orthopaed., No. 67, 1969.)

tinal lumen across the mucosa into the blood, and from the lumen of the renal tubule across the lining cells into blood. The quantities of intracellular calcium are extremely low in all cells, and higher concentrations are present in the surrounding tissue fluids. Excessive accumulation of this ion within cells is prevented by the relative impermeability of the cell membrane and by the action of a pumping system that eliminates it. It is probable that dangerous increases in intracellular calcium and phosphate are prevented in all cells by the temporary storage of these ions in mitochondria, or by the storage of nonionized complexes of the membranes of the endoplasmic reticulum. The side of the osteoblast next to the mineralized compartment is more permeable to calcium ions than is the side possessing the pump. Thus, the membrane on the mineralized side of the osteoblast permits calcium ions to enter according to the gradient between the cell and its environment, and these ions are pumped out through the membrane on the opposite side of the cell, against the normal gradient prevailing between blood and bone. Since the concentration of calcium is much higher in the ECF than in the BFC, it is believed that the intercellular channels between the contiguous osteoblasts are open and permit the movement of ions from the ECF into the BFC (Fig. 8–15).

Talmage and others believe that calcitonin is related to ions other than calcium, and that it is probably secreted in response to hormonal and possibly neural signals originating in the alimentary tract. Calcitonin may be important in the homeostatic control of phosphate, since it can influence these ions in the plasma independently of its effect on calcium. In mammals, CT acts upon the osteocyte-osteoblast complex of compact bone to decrease the release of calcium from these areas, and this effect is augmented by phosphate.[30, 50, 51, 52]

REFERENCES

1. Aurbach, G. D., Keutmann, H. T., Niall, H. D., Tregear, G. W., O'Riordan, J. L. H., Marcus, R., Marx, S. J., and Potts, J. T., Jr.: Structure, synthesis, and mechanism of action of parathyroid hormone. Rec. Prog. Horm. Res. *28*: 353, 1972.
2. Bassabarger, R. A., Freeman, S., and Ivy, A. C.: The experimental production of severe homogeneous osteoporosis by gastrectomy in puppies. Amer. J. Physiol. *121*: 137, 1938.
3. Burford, H. J., Ontjes, D. A., Cooper, C. W., Parlow, A. F., and Hirsch, P. F.: Purification, characterization and radioimmunoassay of thyrocalcitonin from rat thyroid glands. Endocr. *96*: 340, 1975.
4. Care, A. D., and Bates, R. F. L.: Control of secretion of parathyroid hormone and calcitonin in mammals and birds. Gen. Comp. Endocr. Suppl: *3*: 448, 1972.
5. Care, A. D., Bates, R. F. L., and Gitelman, H. J.: A possible role for the adenyl cyclase system in calcitonin release. J. Endocr. *48*: 1, 1970.
6. Chu, L. L. H., Forte, L. D., Anast, C. S., and Cohn, D. V.: Interaction of parathyroid hormone with membranes of kidney cortex: degradation of the hormone and activation of adenyl cyclase. Endocr. (In press – 1975 or 1976)
7. Chu, L. L. H., MacGregor, R. R., Anast, C. S., Hamilton, J. W., and Cohn, D. V.: Studies on the biosynthesis of rat parathyroid hormone and proparathyroid hormone: adaptation of the parathyroid gland to dietary restriction of calcium. Endocr. *93*: 915, 1973.
8. Chu, L. L. H., Macgregor, R. R., Hamilton, J. W., and Cohn, D. V.: Conversion of proparathyroid hormone to parathyroid hormone: the use of amines as specific inhibitors. Endocr. *95*: 1431, 1974.
9. Clark, N. B.: Calcium regulation in reptiles. Gen. Comp. Endocr. Suppl. *3*: 430, 1972.

10. Clark, N. B., and Dantzler, W. H.: Renal tubular transport of calcium and phosphate in snakes: role of calcitonin. Gen. Comp. Endocr. *26*: 321, 1975.
11. Cohn, D. V., MacGregor, R. R., Sinha, D., Huang, D. W. Y., Edelhoch, H., and Hamilton, J. W.: The migratory behavior of proparathyroid hormone, parathyroid hormone and their peptide fragments during gel filtration. Arch. Biochem. Biophys. *164*: 669, 1974.
12. Copp, D. H.: Calcium regulation in birds. Gen. Comp. Endocr. Suppl. *3*: 441, 1972.
13. Copp, D. H.: Endocrine regulation of calcium metabolism. Ann. Rev. Physiol. *32*: 61, 1970.
14. Cortelyou, J. R., and McWhinnie, D. J.: Parathyroid glands in amphibians. Parathyroid structure and function in the amphibians, with emphasis on regulation of mineral ions in body fluids. Amer. Zool. *7*:843, 1967.
15. Cutler, G. B., Jr., Habener, J. F., and Potts, J. T., Jr.: Comparative immunochemical studies on chicken ultimobranchial calcitonin. Gen. Comp. Endocr. *24*: 183, 1974.
16. DeLuca, H. F.: The kidney as an endocrine organ for the production of 1,25-dihydroxyvitamin D_3, a calcium-mobilizing hormone. New Engl. J. Med. *289*: 359, 1973.
17. DeLuca, H. F.: The metabolism and function of vitamin D. Trans. & Studies College Physicians of Philadelphia *39*:1, 1971.
18. Feinblatt, J. D., and Raisz, L. G.: Secretion of thyrocalcitonin in organ culture. Endocr. *88*: 797, 1971.
19. Feinblatt, J. D., Tai, L-R., and Kenny, D. D.: Avian parathyroid glands in organ culture: secretion of parathyroid hormone and calcitonin. Endocr. *96*: 282, 1975.
20. Fenwick, J. C.: Effect of partial ultimobranchialectomy on plasma calcium concentration and on some related parameters in goldfish (*Carassius auratus* L.) during acute transfer from fresh water to 30% sea water. Gen. Comp. Endocr. *25*: 60, 1975.
21. Hamilton, J. W., Niall, H. D., Jacobs, J. W., Keutmann, H. T., Potts, J. T., Jr., and Cohn, D. V.: The N-terminal amino-acid sequence of bovine proparathyroid hormone. Proc. Nat. Acad. Sci. *71*: 653, 1974.
22. Hirsch, P. F., Sliwowski, A., Orimo, H., Darago, L. S., and Mewborn, Q. A.: On the mode of the hypocalcemic action of thyrocalcitonin and its enhancement of phosphate in rats. Endocr. 93:12, 1973.
23. Hoyt, R. F., Jr., Tashjian, A. H., Jr., and Hamilton, D. W.: Distribution of thyroid, parathyroid and ultimobranchial hypocalcemic factors in birds. Thyroid and ultimobranchial calcitonins in pigeons and pullets. Endocr. *91*: 770, 1972.
24. Huang, W-Y., Chu, L. L. H., Hamilton, J. W., McGregor, D. H., and Cohn, D. V.: The NH_2-terminal amino acid sequence of human proparathyroid hormone by radioisotope microanalysis. Arch. Biochem. Biophys. *166*: 67, 1975.
25. Jowsey, J.: Effect of long-term administration of porcine calcitonin in the development of dietary osteoporosis in cats. Endocr. *85*: 1196, 1969.
26. Kemper, B., Habener, J. F., Rich, A., and Potts, J. T., Jr.: Microtubules and the intracellular conversion of proparathyroid hormone to parathyroid hormone. Endocr. *96*: 903, 1975.
27. Le Douarin, N. M.: Cell recognition based on natural morphological nuclear markers. Medical Biology *52*: 281, 1974.
28. McWhinnie, D. J., and Cortelyou, J. R.: Influence of parathyroid extract on blood and urine mineral levels in iguanid lizards. Gen. Comp. Endocr. *11*: 78, 1968.
29. Melvin, K. E. W., Tashjian, A. H., Jr., and Miller, H. H.: Studies in familial (medullary) thyroid carcinoma. Rec. Prog. Horm. Res. *28*: 399, 1972.
30. Milhaud, G., Perault-Staub, A. M., and Staub, J-F.: Diurnal variation of plasma calcium and calcitonin function in the rat. J. Physiol. (Lond.) *222*: 559, 1972.
31. Nagata, N., Sasaki, M., Kimura, N., and Nakane, K.: The hypercalcemic effect of parathyroid hormone and skeletal cyclic AMP. Endocr. *96*: 725, 1975.
32. Nieto, A., Fando, J. J. L., and Candela, J. L. R.: Biosynthesis and secretion of calcitonin *in vitro* in chicken ultimobranchial gland. Gen. Comp. Endocr. *25*: 259, 1975.
33. Norman, A. W., and Henry, H.: 1,25-Dihydroxycholecalciferol — a hormonally active form of vitamin D. Rec. Prog. Horm. Res. *30*: 431, 1974.
34. Olson, E. B., Jr., DeLuca, H. F., and Potts, J. T., Jr.: Calcitonin inhibition of vitamin D-induced intestinal absorption. Endocr. *90*: 151, 1972.
35. Pearse, A. G. E.: Common cytochemical and ultrastructural characteristics of cells producing polypeptide hormones (the APUD series) and their relevance to thyroid and ultimobranchial C cells and calcitonin. Proc. Roy. Soc. Ser. B. *170*: 71, 1968.
36. Peck, W. A., Messinger, K., Kimmich, G., and Carpenter, J.: Stimulation of uridine incorporation in isolated bone cells by parathyroid hormone and cyclic AMP. Endocr. *95*: 289, 1974.
37. Potts, J. T., Jr., Keutmann, H. T., Niall, H. D., Habener, J. F., and Tregear, G. W.: Comparative biochemistry of parathyroid hormone and calcitonin. Gen. Comp. Endocr. Suppl. *3*: 405, 1972.

38. Potts, J. T., Jr., Niall, H. D., and Deftos, L. J.: Calcitonin. *In* L. Martini and V. H. T. James, eds.: Experimental Endocrinology, Vol. 1, Academic Press, New York, 1971.

39. Rasmussen, H., Bordier, P., Kurokawa, K., Nagata, N., and Ogata, E.: Hormonal control of skeletal and mineral homeostasis. Amer. J. Med. *56*: 751, 1974.

40. Rasmussen, H., Wong, M., Bikle, D., and Goodman, D. B. P.: Hormonal control of the renal conversion of 25-hydroxycholecalciferol to 1,25-dihydroxycholecalciferol. J. Clin. Inv. *51*: 2502, 1972.

41. Reaven, E. P., and Reaven, G. M.: A quantitative ultrastructural study of microtubule assembly and granule accumulation in parathyroid glands of control, phosphate, and colchicine treated rats. Proc. 56th Ann. Meeting Endocr. Soc., 1974, p. A182.

42. Robertson, D. R.: Effects of the ultimobranchial and parathyroid glands and vitamins D_2, D_3 and dihydrotachysterol$_2$ on blood calcium and intestinal calcium transport in the frog. Endocr. *96*: 934, 1975.

43. Robertson, D. R.: Influence of parathyroids and ultimobranchial glands in the frog (*Rana pipiens*) during respiratory acidosis. Gen. Comp. Endocr. Suppl. *3*: 421, 1972.

44. Roos, B. A., Bundy, L. L., Bailey, R., and Deftos, L. J.: Calcitonin secretion *in vitro*. Preparation of monolayer C-cell cultures. Endocr. *95*: 1142, 1974.

45. Roos, B. A., Bundy, L. L., Miller, E. A., and Deftos, L. J.: Calcitonin secretion by monolayer cultures of human C-cells derived from medullary thyroid carcinoma. Endocr. *97*: 39, 1975.

46. Smith, D. M., and Johnston, C. C., Jr.: Hormonal responsiveness to adenyl cyclase activity of separated bone cells. Endocr. *95*: 130, 1974.

47. Talmage, R. V.: Morphological and physiological considerations in a new concept of calcium transport in bone. Amer. J. Anat. *129*: 467, 1970.

48. Talmage, R. V.: Calcium homeostasis — calcium transport — parathyroid action. The effects of parathyroid hormone on the movement of calcium between bone and fluid. Clin. Orthop., No. *67*: 210, 1969.

49. Talmage, R. V.: Aspects of parathyroid physiology in mammals. Amer. Zool. *7*: 825, 1967.

50. Talmage, R. V., Doppelt, S. H., and Cooper, C. W.: Relationship of blood concentrations of calcium, phosphate, gastrin and calcitonin to the onset of feeding in the rat. Proc. Soc. Exper. Biol. Med. *149*:855, 1975.

51. Talmage, R. V., Roycroft, J. H., and Anderson, J. J. B.: Daily fluctuations in plasma calcium, phosphate, and their radionuclide concentrations in the rat. Calcif. Tiss. Res. *17*: 91, 1975.

52. Talmage, R. V., Whitehurst, L. A., and Anderson, J. J. B.: Effect of calcitonin and calcium infusion on plasma phosphate. Endocr. *92*:792, 1973.

53. Tregear, G. W., Van Rietschoten, J., Greene, E., Keutmann, H. T., Niall, H. D., Reit, B., Parsons, J. A., and Potts, J. T., Jr.: Bovine parathyroid hormone: minimum chain length of synthetic peptide required for biological activity. Endocr. *93*: 1349, 1973.

54. Urist, M. R.: Avian parathyroid physiology: Including a special comment on calcitonin. Amer. Zool. *7*: 883, 1967.

55. Urist, M. R., Budy, A. M., and McLean, F. C.: Endosteal-bone formation in estrogen-treated mice. J. Bone Joint Surg. 32-A: 143, 1950.

CHAPTER 9

The Pancreatic Islets

Langerhans (1869) described small clusters of cells in the pancreas that were richly vascularized but, unlike the digestive acini, did not establish connections with the duct system of the organ. The experiments of von Mering and Minkowski (1886–1889) demonstrated that total pancreatectomy of the dog leads to severe metabolic disturbances that simulate those prevailing in human subjects suffering from diabetes mellitus. [68] It was not until 1921 that Banting and Best prepared islet extracts which had insulin effects. Crystallization of insulin was accomplished by Abel (1926), and this made possible many chemical and biologic studies.

The pancreas is a compound gland consisting of exocrine and endocrine tissues (Fig. 9–1). The exocrine constituent secretes pancreatic juice which is poured into the duodenum via the pancreatic ducts; the islets of Langerhans are aggregations of cells which liberate their hormones directly into the circulation. The human pancreas contains up to 2 million islets scattered widely throughout the acinar tissue; they measure from 20 to 300 microns in diameter, and the total islet tissue constitutes only 1 or 2 per cent of the pancreatic mass. The islet cells are arranged in irregular cords which are separated by a very rich system of capillary vessels or sinusoids (Fig. 9–1). The gland is supplied by sympathetic and parasympathetic fibers, and these terminate on or near both exocrine and endocrine cells. It is now recognized that these nerves perform important roles in controlling the synthesis and release of islet hormones.[24]

ANATOMY OF THE PANCREATIC ISLETS

Embryonic Origin

The pancreas forms in mammalian embryos through the fusion of two duodenal outgrowths arising close to the hepatic diverticulum (Fig. 8–3). Despite many experimental and ultrastructural studies, the precise source of the cells from which the islets originate remains uncertain. There have been reports that endocrine cells of the islets may arise from surrounding acinar cells, but this is doubted by many workers. It is generally agreed that some, if not all, of the islet cells are budded off from the epithelial lining of the pancreatic ductules. The origin of the endocrine cells comprising the

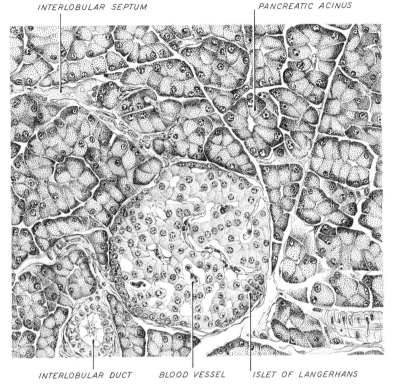

INTERLOBULAR SEPTUM   PANCREATIC ACINUS

INTERLOBULAR DUCT   BLOOD VESSEL   ISLET OF LANGERHANS

Figure 9–1. Section through the pancreas of the rat. The islet of Langerhans is a gland of internal secretion, whereas the surrounding acinar tissue forms an exocrine gland.

buds is not clear: they may arise *in situ* from endodermal cells of the gut mucosa, or they may be neuroectodermal cells that migrated into the foregut mucosa at an earlier stage of development. According to the APUD hypothesis, cells from the neural crest populate the foregut and are carried into its derivatives, including the developing pancreatic anlagen. Some of the APUD cells remain in the alimentary mucosa and are thought to secrete the various kinds of gastrointestinal hormones.[46, 47, 48] There are so many structural and functional relationships between the peptide hormone secreting cells of the alimentary tract and those of the pancreatic islets that some specialists refer to them collectively as the gastro-entero-pancreatic endocrine system.[19]

Biogenic amine-storing (APUD) cells have been demonstrated in the duodenal mucosa of chick embryos from day 13 or 14 of incubation. The cells become concentrated at the site where the dorsal pancreatic evagination will form a little later and are eventually found grouped and scattered in the pancreas. In this instance it is clear that the APUD cells in the duodenal mucosa are the precursors of islet cells of one or more types.[1]

Microscopic Anatomy

The islet tissue of all vertebrates above the cyclostomes contains at least three functionally different types of cells: A-cells producing glucagon (termed A_2-cells in Aves), B-cells producing insulin, and D-cells (A_1-cells in Aves) which may elaborate a third islet hormone. Enteroglucagon is a glucagon-like hormone secreted by endocrine cells in the gastrointestinal mucosa.[39] These cells have essentially the same light microscopical and ultrastructural features as the A-cells within the islets. In mammals, the B-cells are most abundant and contain granules which are soluble in alcohol and acetic acid; since these cells contain insulin, they may be specifically stained with pseudoisocyanin. The content of insulin in the B-cells and of glucagon in the A-cells can be visualized by immunofluorescence techniques.

The assignment of secretory functions to the islet cells has been facilitated by the electron microscope and by the employment of histochemical and fractional procedures. The islet hormones are polypeptidal in nature, and it has always been difficult to extract them from pancreatic tissue owing to their rapid destruction by the proteolytic enzymes contained in the acinar cells. The small size of the islets, coupled with their scattered location in another type of tissue, has discouraged many kinds of cellular observations that should have been made earlier. Techniques have been perfected for isolating the islets and maintaining them *in vitro*. Islets surviving in organ culture have been shown to release hormones in response to glucose and other agents known to regulate their production. Such tissue from a number of mammalian species has been successfully cultured in monolayer and found to be functional.[36]

Ultrastructural studies reveal that the secretory granules originate in the vicinity of the Golgi apparatus and are surrounded by smooth membranes (Fig. 9–2). Continuous pericapillary spaces are conspicuous in the islets, and it is probable that these spaces facilitate the spread of secretions from one type of islet cell to another. There is evidence that both glucagon and gastrin effect the release of insulin from B-cells. Secretin, another gastrointestinal hormone, stimulates the B-cells both *in vivo* and *in vitro,* and this is of interest since secretin possesses some of the same amino acid sequences as glucagon. It may well be that the pancreatic islet is a functional unit, the constituent cells not being wholly independent of each other.

Ultrastructural and fractional studies indicate that the secretory activities of the islet cells are similar in many ways to acinar cells and to others which specialize in the synthesis and release of exportable polypeptides or proteins. The synthetic activities of the B-cells have been examined most extensively. Current evidence indicates that a conventional RNA-directed mechanism is involved in the synthesis of a single polypeptide chain precursor (proinsulin) by ribosomes on the rough-surfaced endoplasmic reticulum (ER). The precursor is passed across the membrane of the ER into the cisternae, and the final storage form is contained within membrane-bound granules. The Golgi apparatus is involved in the genesis of the granules, but some workers think the granules arise from vesicular formations of the

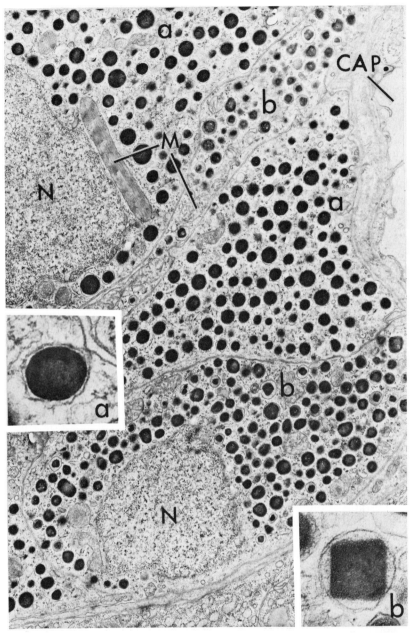

Figure 9–2. Electron micrograph of pancreatic islet cells of the lizard, *Eumeces fasciatus.* Alpha (a) and beta (b) cells are clustered about a capillary (CAP) and can be distinguished by structural differences in their secretion granules and mitochondria. An alpha granule (left inset) is homogeneously dense and has a round profile, whereas a beta granule (right inset) is crystalline when fully condensed. The density of the beta granules depends on their degree of condensation. Many alpha cell mitochondria (M) possess tubular cristae oriented longitudinally, as shown beside the nucleus (N) in the upper left corner of the figure, whereas beta cell mitochondria are typical in appearance. Golgi elements and endoplasmic reticulum are usually more abundant in the beta cells. Micrograph ×12,000; insets ×54,000. (Courtesy of Dr. Paul R. Burton.)

ER. During formation of the granules, the proinsulin is converted to at least one intermediate product and, finally, to insulin. The enzymes for these conversions are probably present in the Golgi apparatus or early secretion granules. When the B-cells are challenged, as by an elevation of blood glucose, the granules are moved to the surface of the cell and fuse with the cell membrane; the granule then ruptures to release insulin into the pericapillary space without leaving a break in the cell membrane.[7, 26, 32, 61]

Alloxan exerts a diabetogenic effect by promptly and selectively destroying the B-cells, thus reducing or preventing the production of insulin. The administration of exogenous insulin tends to reduce the secretion of the B-cells. Anti-insulin serum neutralizes the insulin in the blood and induces a diabetic state. The effect of the antibody is to stimulate insulin synthesis and release and, if this prevails, severe degranulation of the B-cells occurs. The prolonged administration of neutral red to the rat produces hypoglycemia after fasting; this is thought to be related to degenerative changes in the A-cells and a consequent deficiency of glucagon.

Phylogenesis[13]

The basic arrangement of exocrine and endocrine tissues in mammalian pancreata is preserved throughout the gnathostomes. The avian pancreas consists of four distinct lobes, the splenic lobe being especially rich in islet tissue. Unlike the mammalian pancreas, the avian islets are populated by either A_2- or B-cells, thus giving rise to A-islets or B-islets. The A_1-cell (D-cell) is present in both types of islets as well as scattered in the exocrine tissue surrounding the islets. Total pancreatectomy of the chicken, duck and goose leads to a profound hypoglycemia which results in death unless glucose or glucagon is administered.[60] The content of glucagon in the avian pancreas is 8 to 10 times higher, on a unit weight basis, than that of the mammalian pancreas. Such observations suggest that glucagon, not insulin, is the dominant islet hormone in birds.[21, 42, 58]

In reptiles, as in birds, glucagon-secreting A-cells are generally more abundant than the B-cells. Several groups show a tendency to concentrate islet tissue in the caudal pancreas. Large intrasplenic islets occur in some members of this class.

Both A- and B-cells are present in amphibian islets, but glucagon production does not appear to exceed the production of insulin.

Much diversity is encountered among bony fishes, but, in some of them *(e.g., Ameiurus, Lophius, Cottus)*, most of the islet tissue is concentrated in one or more principal islets or Brockmann corpuscles (Fig. 9–3). Exocrine pancreatic cells may form a thin layer around the periphery of the principal islet, but the remainder is composed purely of A- and B-cells. In the initial attempts to isolate insulin, proteolytic enzymes from the exocrine pancreas often destroyed the hormone during extraction; the principal islets of the anglerfish *(Lophius)* contain few acinar cells, and high yields of insulin could be extracted from them. As in other gnathostomes, the exocrine and endocrine tissues of the pancreata are intermingled in the great majority of bony fishes.[44, 59, 65]

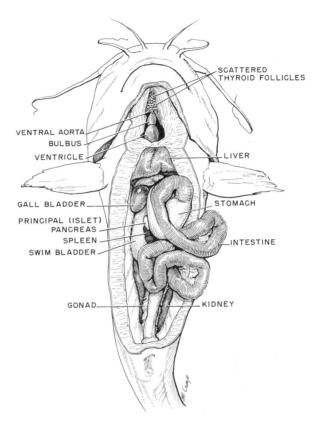

SCATTERED
THYROID FOLLICLES

VENTRAL AORTA
BULBUS
VENTRICLE

LIVER

GALL BLADDER

STOMACH

PRINCIPAL (ISLET)
PANCREAS
SPLEEN
SWIM BLADDER

INTESTINE

GONAD

KIDNEY

Figure 9–3. Ventral dissection of the catfish (*Ameiurus*), showing the location of the principal (islet) pancreas with reference to other organs. Scattered thyroid follicles are shown diagrammatically around the ventral aorta.

The islet cells of cartilaginous fish are localized mainly in the outer layer of the epithelium which lines the pancreatic ducts. In adult sharks and rays, the B-cells are slightly more abundant than the A-cells. Both insulin and glucagon have been extracted from the pancreas of the spiny dogfish, *Squalus acanthias.*[16]

The cyclostomes (Agnatha) are the most primitive living vertebrates, but they constitute a separate evolutionary line and cannot be regarded as immediate ancestors of the gnathostomes. Two important changes occur in the pancreata of the lampreys and hagfishes: (1) A- and D-cells are absent from the islet organs, and (2) there is no compact exocrine pancreas with small islets of Langerhans embedded in it. In the ammocete larva of the lamprey, clusters of cells are found in the submucosa at the junction of the esophagus and intestine.[29, 69] These follicles were described by Langerhans in 1873 and are known to consist of islet tissue. The cells comprising the follicles react to pseudoisocyanin and other differential staining procedures in the same way as the B-cells of mammalian islets, and there is no doubt that they contain insulin. Islet tissue is more extensive in adult lampreys than in the larvae, but, as in the larva, it contains only B-cells. The exocrine part of the pancreas is represented by zymogen cells, which are scattered in the intestinal mucosa. In the adult hagfish *(Myxine glutinosa),* the islet organ is a compact nodule lying in the submucosa of the intestine near the point of entrance of the bile duct, and is known to contain insulin. Insulin-producing B-cells are also found in the bile duct mucosa; though no A- or D-cells are present in the islet organ, a few scattered glucagon-immuno-reactive cells are present in the intestinal epithelium.[12, 16, 43]

No structure comparable to the pancreas is found among invertebrates, though insulin-secreting cells have been reported in the gastrointestinal epithelium of certain echinoderms, tunicates, molluscs, and crustaceans. Glucagon-producing cells have not been found in any of the inverte-brates.[16, 17]

PANCREATIC HORMONES AND RELATED FACTORS

Insulin: Chemistry and Assay

Sanger and co-workers, in the period between 1945 and 1955, deter-mined the complete amino acid sequences and overall structure of insulins from several different species.[55, 56] This was a brilliant achievement in pro-tein chemistry because it was the first time that a well-defined protein had been totally elucidated in terms of primary structure. Sheep insulin was syn-thesized in 1963 by Katsoyannis and his colleagues, and this represented the first synthesis of a naturally occurring protein.[25] It was also the first time that the proposed primary structure of a protein was confirmed by chemical synthesis. The two polypeptide chains were synthesized separately, and the protein produced by the combination of the two chains duplicated the bio-logic activity possessed by the natural hormone. The synthesis of human in-sulin was achieved in 1966, largely through the separate contributions of Dixon, Du, Katsoyannis, Zahn, and their respective colleagues.

The structure of a molecule of ox insulin is shown in Figure 9–4. It consists of an A chain containing 21 amino acid residues with glycine as the N-terminal residue, and a B chain containing 30 residues with phenylala-nine as the N-terminal amino acid. The two chains are linked by two disulfide bridges at positions 7 and 20 in the A chain and at positions 7 and 19 in the B chain. A disulfide bridge in the A chain links the cysteine residues at posi-tions 6 and 11.

Zinc-free insulin has a molecular weight of 6,000 in basic media and of 12,000 in acid media. The crystalline hormone usually contains from 0.15 to 0.6 per cent of zinc, and it is necessary to add zinc or other metal ions in order to crystallize it. When insulin in aqueous solution is heated at a pH below 3.5, the molecules aggregate to form fibers; these fibers return to solution in highly alkaline media without any loss of biologic potency. This tendency for two or more insulin molecules to become associated is influ-enced by such factors as temperature, pH, and the presence of metal ions. Insulin molecules adsorb quickly, but rather loosely, to glassware, filter paper, agar, and certain blood proteins; they bind very strongly to specific antibodies. The hormone is inactivated by proteolytic enzymes or acid hy-drolysis, and hence preparations are ineffective when given orally. The three disulfide bonds are essential for stable configuration of the molecule,

(a)

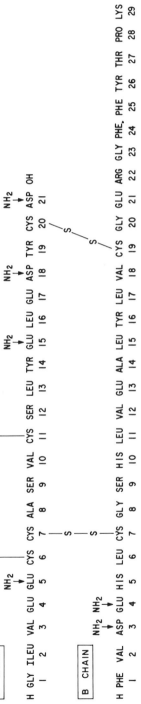

(b)

Figure 9-4. *A,* The sequence of amino acids in a molecule of ox insulin. *B,* The sequence of amino acids in the glucagon molecule.

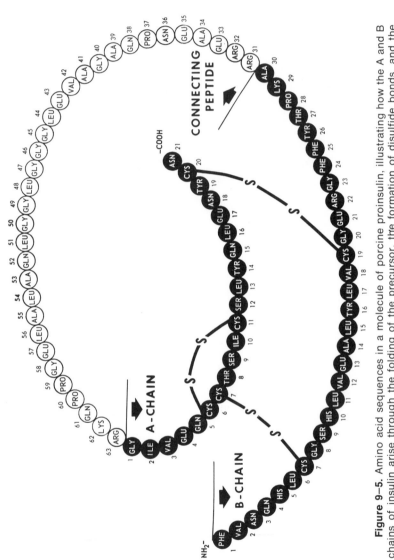

Figure 9–5. Amino acid sequences in a molecule of porcine proinsulin, illustrating how the A and B chains of insulin arise through the folding of the precursor, the formation of disulfide bonds, and the deletion of a connecting peptide. Dark circles represent the insulin moiety. ARG, arginine; ALA, alanine; ASN, asparagine; CYS, cysteine, cystine or one-half of residual; GLN, glutamine; GLU, glutamic acid; GLY, glycine; HIS, histidine; ILE, isoleucine; LYS, lysine; PRO, proline; PHE, phenylalanine; SER, serine; TYR, tyrosine; THR, threonine; VAL, valine. (From Chance, R. E.: Rec. Progr. Horm. Res. 25:274, 1969; position 35 corrected in accordance with a personal communication.)

and these are invariable in insulins obtained from vertebrates ranging from cyclostomes to man.

Studies on human B-cell adenomata and isolated islet tissue of the rat indicate that insulin is synthesized within the B-cells from a single-chain polypeptide precursor called *proinsulin*.[7, 62] The N-terminus of proinsulin begins with the 30 amino acid residues of insulin, continues through a segment of about 33 residues (connecting peptide), and terminates with the 21 amino acid sequence of the A chain (Fig. 9–5). After formation of the disulfide bridges, the connecting peptide is enzymatically deleted to form the insulin molecule. Thus, the insulin molecule is naturally derived from a single-chain polypeptide and not through the union of two independently synthesized chains. Small amounts of proinsulin are present in commercial insulin preparations, but such precursors have very little, if any, biologic potency. Human, porcine, rat, and fish proinsulins have been characterized, and species differences are known to occur in the amino acid sequences of the connecting peptide as well as in the A and B chains.

By extracting the islet organs of several thousand hagfish, enough insulin has been obtained to allow the determination of amino acid sequences and to compare the molecule with other known insulins from mammals, birds, and teleost fishes. With one exception, all of the 21 residues known to be invariant among other known insulins are invariant in the hagfish molecule (Table 9–1). The exception is position 18 in the B chain, where alanine is substituted for valine. Thus, there are 20 invariant residues common to porcine and hagfish insulins. Of the 16 conservative amino acid sites, 9 residues are identical in pig and hagfish insulins. Compared to pig insulin, 12 radical substitutions occur, but all of these are in positions where substitutions can be made without loss of biological activity. As in mammals, the hagfish insulin is synthesized on the rough endoplasmic reticulum of the B-cells as a large single chain precursor, proinsulin, which is cleaved in the newly formed secretion granules to yield the more active two-chain hormone.[45, 51] It is interesting that a hormone as ancient as hagfish insulin still has some ability to lower blood glucose and promote lipogenesis when applied to mammalian test systems, but its potency is low in these systems as compared with pig insulin.[16, 63, 66]

All insulin-treated patients develop antibodies to insulin, but there are variations in the antigenicity of insulins and in the ability of individuals to form antibodies. Although pig and sperm whale insulins are identical with respect to amino acid sequences, some insulin antisera can distinguish between the two molecules. Human and porcine insulins have the same amino acid compositions, except for position 30 in the B chain (threonine in man, alanine in pig), but they can be distinguished by antibodies. Removal of this alanine residue from the porcine molecule causes only a slight reduction in biologic potency in man; it reduces but does not eliminate the antigenicity. Antigenicity of the protein obviously may depend upon factors other than primary structure.

Circulating insulin is largely bound to protein carriers of the plasma. It is rapidly degraded in the body and only traces appear in the urine of normal subjects. The portal vein conveys pancreatic blood first to the liver, and

Table 9–1 Results of studies of the amino-acid sequence of hagfish insulin (Peterson et al., 1975) compared with that of pig insulin. Variations known from insulins in other mammals, as well as those in some birds and teleost fish, are also included (Dayhoff, 1972; Blundell & Wood, 1975).

A-Chains

Positions: 1 … 5 … 10 … 15 … 20 … 22

Hagfish: **GLY-ILE**-VAL-GLU-**GLN-CYS-CYS**-His-Lys-Arg-**CYS**-SER-Ile- **TYR**-Asn-**LEU**-Gln-**ASN-TYR-CYS-ASN**

Pig: **GLY-ILE**-VAL-GLU-**GLN-CYS-CYS**-Thr-Ser-Ile- **CYS**-SER-Leu-**TYR**-Gln- **LEU**-Glu-**ASN-TYR-CYS-ASN**

Other residues:
(His) [circled] … Ala Gly Val / Glu Asn Thr / (His)(Lys)(Pro) [circled] / (Arg) [circled] … Thr Arg His Asp / Asn (Lys)Asn [Lys circled] / (Asp) (Ile)(Phe) [circled] … Met (Ser) [circled] / (Gln) [circled] … Asp

B-Chains

Positions: 0 1 … 5 … 10 … 15 … 20

Hagfish: Arg-Thr-Thr-*Gly*-*HIS*-**LEU-CYS-GLY**-Lys-Asp-**LEU-VAL**-*Asn*-*ALA*-**LEU-TYR**-*Ile*-*Ala*-**CYS**-*GLY*-

Pig: Phe-Val-Asn-*Gln*-*HIS*-**LEU-CYS-GLY**-Ser-His-**LEU-VAL**-*Glu*-*ALA*-**LEU-TYR**-*Leu*-*Val*-**CYS**-*GLY*-

Other residues:
(Met) [circled] Tyr (Ala) [circled] Lys Arg Arg / (Val)(Ala)(Pro) [circled] Ser Lys / (Ala)(Pro) [circled] … Pro Asn / Gln … (Asp) [circled] Thr / Ser / Gln Arg

Positions: 21 … 25 … 30 31

Hagfish: *Val*-**ARG-GLY-PHE**-*PHE*-*TYR*-Asp-**PRO**-Thr-Lys-Met

Pig: *Glu*-**ARG-GLY-PHE**-*PHE*-*TYR*-Thr-**PRO**-Lys-Ala

Other residues:
His Asp / (Asp) [circled] … Tyr Arg Ser Asn Met Thr / Pro (Ser) [circled] Asp Ser / Ile / (Gln) [circled] / (Asn) [circled]

INVARIANT (boldface)
CONSERVATIVE (italics)
HIGHLY VARIABLE (circled)

Boldface indicates amino-acid residues known to be invariant in species above hagfish. Residues given in *italics* are generally considered to be conservative. The remaining residues are known to be highly variable (as shown in the table). Residues designated by capital letters seem to be common to hagfish and pig insulins. Encircled residues among "other residues" are found in teleost fish.

References: Blundell, T. L., and Wood, S. P.: Is the evolution of insulin Darwinian or due to selectivity neutral mutation? Nature 257:197–203, 1975.

Dayhoff, M.: Atlas of protein sequence and structure. Vol. 5, pp. D 186–187. National Biomed. Res. Found., Wash., D.C., 1972.

Peterson, J. D., Steiner, D. F., Emdin, S. O., and Falkmer, S.: The amino acid sequence of the insulin from a primitive vertebrate, the Atlantic hagfish (*Myxine glutinosa*). J. Biol. Chem. 250:5183–5191, 1975.

this organ traps about 50 per cent of the insulin delivered to it. The half-life of insulin in the peripheral circulation is estimated to be from 15 to 35 minutes. The inactivation and degradation of insulin by homogenates and slices of liver have been shown to be accomplished by an enzyme, insulinase, which is relatively specific in cleaving the disulfide bridges connecting A and B chains. An insulin-degrading enzyme has been isolated in a highly purified state from beef liver. Liver extracts also contain a factor that can competitively inhibit the action of insulinase both *in vitro* and *in vivo*. This has been referred to as "insulinase inhibitor." The effectiveness of insulin depends upon the balance between these two principles — the binding of insulin by antibodies and other proteins, and various factors that compete with or antagonize the action of the hormone at the cellular level.[41]

It has been shown that insulin becomes firmly bound to certain target tissues. The metabolic effects on the diaphragm, mammary gland, and adipose tissue may be demonstrated after a short immersion of each tissue in a solution of the hormone, and prolonged washings do not remove the hormone from the tissues. These results have been confirmed by using isotopic insulin, and the indications are that the hormone becomes chemically bound to the cells as a prerequisite to its action.

Radioimmunologic methods are the most sensitive and specific for measuring insulin in the body fluids. Bovine or porcine insulins are generally administered to guinea pigs in order to obtain an antiinsulin serum. The extent to which known amounts of crystalline insulin and insulin labeled with I^{131} or I^{125} are bound to the antibody is then determined. The unlabeled insulin in the specimen is allowed to compete with labeled insulin for binding sites on the antibody, care being taken not to allow all of the labeled insulin to combine with the antibody. It is essentially a matter of determining the extent to which the labeled insulin in the incubation medium is diluted by the unlabeled insulin in the sample being tested. Different procedures may be used to determine how much of the labeled insulin is bound to antibody and how much is not. A second antibody may be produced by immunizing rabbits with guinea pig gamma globulin, and this may be used to precipitate the insulin-insulin antibody complex. It thus becomes relatively easy to centrifuge the mixture and determine the amount of radioactivity in the precipitate.

Other assay procedures depend upon the ability of unknown samples to behave like insulin in *in vitro* systems. Since insulin promotes the uptake of glucose by muscle, rat or mouse diaphragms may be indubated in a medium containing glucose; the insulin-like activity (ILA) may be determined on the basis of glucose uptake or glycogen deposition. Insulin has many effects on adipose tissue, and these parameters may be determined on the basis of glucose uptake or glycogen deposition. Insulin has many effects on adipose tissue, and these parameters may be employed for assay purposes.[14, 53, 43] The production of carbon dioxide from glucose by epididymal fat pads of the rat correlates well with the concentrations of insulin in the incubation medium. One of the most sensitive *in vitro* procedures is based on the capacity of insulin to inhibit lipolysis in adipose tissue or isolated adipose cells. Since some ILA remains in plasma after total pancreatectomy and after the action of specific insulin antibodies, it is not entirely clear what the *in vitro* tests measure in addition to showing the presence of insulin molecules.

Glucagon: Chemistry and Assay

This hyperglycemic-glycogenolytic factor is found in extracts of the pancreas and, like insulin, brings about many important biochemical alterations in the liver. It causes a rise in blood sugar upon intravenous injection and is frequently present in insulin preparations as an impurity. Biochemically and physiologically, it is quite different from insulin. The glucagon molecule is a straight-chain polypeptide containing 29 amino acid residues and has a molecular weight of 3485 (Fig. 9–4). It may be noted that only a few dipeptide sequences are similar to those in insulin and that disulfide bridges are lacking in the glucagon molecule. It does not contain cystine and this probably accounts for its relative resistance to alkali treatment, a property that facilitates the preparation of glucagon solutions free from insulin activity.[4, 6]

Glucagon may be bioassayed by either *in vivo* or *in vitro* methods. A satisfactory method is to determine the height and duration of the hyperglycemic response after administering the test preparation intravenously to fasting, anesthetized cats. By using the cat assay, a unit of glucagon is defined as the amount capable of causing a blood sugar rise of 30 mg per 100 ml, and this is about equal to the activity of 0.1 microgram (μg) of crystalline glucagon per kilogram of body weight. The rate of glycogenolysis in liver slices and the reactivation of phosphorylase in liver slices or homogenates provide sensitive *in vitro* methods of assay. Radioimmunoassay, similar to that used for insulin, is commonly employed.

Glucagon loses its biologic activity when perfused through the liver or when incubated with extracts of liver, kidney, or muscle. It is also inactivated by incubation with blood. The indications are that glucagon is destroyed by the same enzyme system that destroys insulin and other proteins. Degredation products retain no hyperglycemic activity, indicating that the whole molecule is essential.

Pancreatic Polypeptides

Avian pancreatic polypeptide (APP) is a single chain consisting of 36 amino acid residues and has a molecular weight of about 4200. The amino acid sequence differs from insulin, glucagon, C-peptide, and mammalian gastrin. APP is present in pancreatic extracts of the chicken and in at least seven other avian species; it also occurs in extracts of turtle and alligator pancreas. Though positive proof is lacking, this hormone is generally regarded as a product of the A_1-cell (D-cell). Islet cell adenomas in man (Zollinger-Ellison syndrome) are known to secrete large quantities of gastrin I and II, and these tumors consist mostly of D-cells. Intravenous injection of

APP to chickens causes the depletion of liver glycogen, but has no effect on the levels of plasma glucose. The secretagogic effects of APP are quite profound in birds; after cannulation of the proventriculus, it can be shown that the hormone promotes pepsin secretion, total acid secretion, and the volume flow of digestive juices.

There has been much speculation as to whether or not APP is avian gastrin, but there is still no final answer to this question. Gastrin has not been isolated from the alimentary mucosa of birds. It is difficult to account for the structural disparity between APP, containing 36 amino acid residues, and mammalian gastrins which contain 17 residues. Polypeptides containing 36 amino acid residues are also found in bovine, ovine, porcine, and human pancreata, in addition to gastrin (17 residues) in the stomach mucosa. Bovine pancreatic polypeptide (BPP) inhibits previously induced gastric secretion in dogs, whereas APP has the oppposite effect. Both APP and BPP have tyrosine amide at the carboxyl-terminal position. The cellular origin and physiological significance of these hormones await clarification.[21, 22, 27]

Nonpancreatic Factors with Insulin-like Activity

The Somatomedins

The blood plasma contains a protein with insulin-like biologic activity (ILA) but, unlike insulin, its actions are not suppressed by insulin antibody. This compound with nonsuppressible insulin-like activity (NSILA) is not a product of the pancreas, and hence does not disappear following pancreatectomy. Its concentration in the blood is reduced by hypophysectomy. NSILA lowers blood sugar and affects adipose tissue and skeletal muscle in much the same way as insulin. Its molecular weight and physical-chemical characteristics depend upon methods of extraction and isolation. A low molecular weight fraction of NSILA is now considered to be somatomedin (SM). This includes a family of low molecular weight (4500–10,000) heat stable polypeptides under control of pituitary growth hormone. These were formerly referred to as the "sulfation factor." Physiologic concentrations of SM compete with I^{125}-insulin for receptor sites on the various cells that respond to insulin. With the exception of proinsulin, SM polypeptides are the only compounds known to compete in this manner. This competition for insulin-binding sites indicates that insulin and SM possess certain structural and functional features in common. In addition to mimicking the actions of insulin, SM is known to be a potent stimulator of cell growth in tissue culture. Nerve growth and epithelial growth factors, both extracted from mouse salivary glands, mimic insulin in certain ways, but their dependency on growth hormone has not been demonstrated.[8, 67]

The Regulation of Islet Secretions

Glucose is clearly the major factor promoting release of insulin by mammalian islets, but profound species variations are encountered among vertebrates. Fatty acids markedly stimulate insulin secretion in ruminants, whereas arginine and other amino acids are especially effective in teleosts and certain birds (*e.g.,* penguins).[2] Glucagon from the islet A-cells also promotes insulin secretion from the B-cells. Glucose regulates insulin and glucagon reciprocally, so that one falls as the other rises. Amino acids stimulate A- and B-cell secretions simultaneously, and it is probable that in these circumstances glucagon potentiates the insulin-stimulating effect of amino acids. Various substances such as beta-adrenergic stimulants, the hypoglycemic sulfonylureas, theophylline, and cAMP elicit insulin secretion both *in vivo* and *in vitro.*[11, 15, 37, 38] The importance of calcium in the secretory process of the B-cell is indicated by the fact that the stimulating action of glucose and other insulin secretagogues is reversibly blocked by the absence of calcium ions.[23]

Augmenting Effect of Gastrointestinal Hormones

The passage of food along the alimentary tract releases a number of gastrointestinal hormones — enteroglucagon, secretin, gastrin, cholecystokinin — and each of these has been reported to promote the release of insulin from the B-cells. It has been shown that the effectiveness of insulin secretagogues such as glucose and amino acids is augmented by the simultaneous administration of gastrointestinal hormones. Feeding glucose or introducing it into the alimentary tract produces a far greater increment in plasma insulin than when the same amount of glucose is given intravenously. Since the augmenting gastrointestinal hormones are secreted into the blood at the beginning of intestinal absorption, the pancreatic islets are alerted to the subsequent nutrient load and there is a far greater increment in plasma insulin than would occur without the gastrointestinal involvement. It is probable that the autonomic nervous system also participates in this gastrointestinal anticipation phenomenon by regulating the output of gastrointestinal hormones and by direct stimulation of the endocrine cells of the islets.

Neural Control of the Endocrine Pancreas

Hormone-producing cells of the islets are adequately supplied with autonomic nerve endings, and there are indications that these are involved in the mechanisms that control the release of both insulin and glucagon. A "cephalic" release of insulin can be demonstrated in the dog by merely introducing food into the esophagus. Stimulation of the dorsal vagus or the pancreatic nerve of the dog increases the output of insulin and glucagon, and this response is abolished by atropine. Acetylcholine, the parasympathetic transmitter, releases insulin from the B-cells *in vivo* and *in vitro.* Epinephrine and norepinephrine, from the adrenal medulla or released by adrenergic terminals, inhibit insulin release, and are the only endogenous substances known to do so. The B-cells of the islets possess both *alpha-* and *beta-* adrenergic receptors, and activation of the *alpha*-receptor by the catecholamines suppresses insulin secretion. Insulin output is enhanced by stimulation of the *beta* receptor; this can be prevented by *beta* blocking agents such as propranolol, sotalol, and butoxamine. Though the monoaminergic mechanisms exert potent inhibitory effects on the release of insulin, they do not affect the biosynthesis of insulin. It is probable that the autonomic nervous system acts continuously to modulate the basal secretion of islet hormones.[5, 40]

PHYSIOLOGY OF THE PANCREATIC HORMONES

General Actions of Insulin and Glucagon

Insulin has broad influences within the body and acts directly or indirectly to affect many kinds of biochemical processes. An overall effect of the hormone is to facilitate the utilization of glucose by the cells and to prevent the excessive breakdown of glycogen (glycogenolysis) stored in liver and muscle. Consequently, it is a powerful hypoglycemic agent. In addition to affecting carbohydrate metabolism, it has extremely important regulatory actions on the metabolism of fats and proteins. Glucose is the most important precursor of fat since its degradation yields glycerol, acetate units, and reduced ADPH, and these are the essentials for fat synthesis (lipogenesis). Insulin favors lipogenesis by promoting the uptake and metabolic utilization of glucose by adipose cells, and also discourages the breakdown and mobilization of stored fat (antilipolysis). An abundance of glucose in the plasma, as in the diabetic or pancreatectomized subject, is ineffective in stimulating lipogenesis in the absence of insulin. In normal subjects, high carbohydrate rations lead to elevated levels of blood glucose which in turn stimulate insulin secretion, and the hormone promotes lipogenesis and inhibits lipolysis. Conversely, carbohydrate-deficient rations limit the availability of glucose, reduce insulin secretion, and encourage the mobilization and oxidation of fat.

Insulin facilitates the movement of amino acids into cells, promotes a positive nitrogen balance, and favors the synthesis of proteins (proteogenesis). In the insulin-deficient subject, proteogenesis is reduced and amino acids are catabolized as a source of energy; the administration of insulin promotes protein anabolism and discourages excessive breakdown (proteolysis) of tissue protein. Pituitary growth hormone and testosterone are also important protein anabolic hormones and some of their actions are remarkably similar to those of insulin.

In most instances, the actions of glucagon are contrary to those of insulin.[18] While glucagon produces hyperglycemia, it decreases glucose oxidation. Acting in the liver, it stimulates glycogenolysis and gluconeogenesis, and these effects have been demonstrated both *in vivo* and *in vitro*. It produces lipolysis in the liver and also in adipose tissue, and, as a consequence of this action, there is increased ketogenesis and gluconeogenesis.

Under certain conditions, the hormone exerts a mild proteolytic effect. Glucagon elevates cyclic AMP in liver, whereas insulin has the reverse effect.

As was mentioned previously, glucagon acts on the B-cells of the islets to accelerate the secretion of insulin. Intensive treatment of young rabbits with glucagon results eventually (in about five months) in a true metaglucagon diabetes. The pancreatic islets decrease in size and the B-cells undergo hydropic degeneration. The hyperglycemia, glycogenolysis, and negative nitrogen balance persist after the glucagon is discontinued, and these disturbances result from insulin deficiency consequent upon destruction of the B-cells.[33]

When pure insulin-free glucagon is administered to an animal, the most outstanding effect is an elevation in the concentration of blood glucose. The levels of potassium in the blood plasma rise, probably as a consequence of glycogen breakdown in the liver. The severity and duration of the hyperglycemia depend upon the amount of hormone given, the manner of administration, and the nutritional status of the test animal. Glucagon is more effective when given intravenously or intraperitoneally than when given subcutaneously or intramuscularly. The most effective way to administer the hormone is to inject it into the portal vein, which carries it directly to the liver. Glucagon has no effect on blood sugar after circulation through the liver is blocked or after the liver is removed. The capacity of the hormone to produce hyperglycemia is reduced by prolonged fasting, diabetic acidosis, or other conditions that lower the glycogen reserves of the liver.

The main action of glucagon is to promote hepatic glycogenolysis. This has been demonstrated in perfused livers, liver slices, and liver homogenates. The hormone also promotes gluconeogenesis from protein. The liver cannot hold glycogen and the blood glucose rises sharply. Glucagon-treated animals fail to gain weight, and this correlated with the protein catabolic effect of the hormone and with a diminished consumption of food. Prolonged treatment results in increased nitrogen excretion, a negative nitrogen balance, and a reduced concentration of amino acids in the blood. Under glucagon treatment, the volume of gastric juice is reduced and its content of hydrochloric acid is quite low. Motility of the gastrointestinal tract is reduced, and practically no pancreatic juice is secreted.

Experimental Diabetes Mellitus

Diabetic states, simulating those that occur spontaneously in the human subject, may be produced by a number of experimental procedures. Since insulin is produced by the B-cells of the pancreatic islets, total pancreatectomy produces an immediate onset of diabetes. The Thiroloix-Sandmeyer type of diabetes may follow subtotal removal of the pancreas. The diabetic symptoms are mild immediately after the operation, but either increase in severity with the lapse of time, or gradually subside. The B-cells may be selectively damaged by the administration of toxic agents, such as alloxan, although it is doubtful whether such agents can completely prevent the production of insulin. The administration of excessive glucose for prolonged periods may result in exhaustion atrophy of the B-cells. There is also evidence that damage to the B-cells may result from the prolonged administration of excessive insulin. Temporary or permanent damage to the B-cells, resulting in diabetic states, may be produced by the repeated administration of large doses of anterior pituitary, adrenocortical, or thyroid hormones.

Total Pancreatectomy

Removal of the pancreas has been accomplished in many vertebrates and the intensity of the resulting diabetic state is quite variable. Pancreatectomy of the toad *(Bufo arenarum)* produces a prompt hyperglycemia, and the untreated animals survive for about 10 days.[49] Reptiles and birds are extremely sensitive to the hyperglycemic action of glucagon and vary in their sensitivity to insulin; some species exhibit hypoglycemia for several days or weeks following pancreatectomy. Tortoises develop an intense hyperglycemia immediately following removal of the pancreas. In pancreatectomized snakes *(e.g., Xenodon merremii)* and lizards *(e.g., Tupinambis teguixim, T. refescens),* the blood sugar falls for a few days after the operation, returns to normal, and eventually remains much above the normal level. The blood sugar of pancreatectomized alligators may rise within 24 hours from a normal level of 73 per 100 ml to 321 mg per 100 ml. The animals die with ketosis by 2 to 4 months after the operation and may attain blood sugar levels of 606 mg per 100 ml.[50] In the duck, only a transitory hyperglycemia follows pancreatectomy and a hypoglycemia may occur. A diabetic syndrome, however, develops in geese in the absence of the pancreas. Very severe diabetes follows ablation of the pancreas in dogs, cats, rats, and other mammals. The metabolic defects occurring in the depancreatized dog will be considered in some detail since they are essentially the same as those appearing in the human diabetic.

Hyperglycemia and Glycosuria. Shortly after the supply of insulin is cut off by pancreatectomy, the blood sugar begins to rise and sugar appears in the urine after the renal threshold (160 to 180 mg per 100 ml) is surpassed. The hyperglycemia and glycosuria in the pancreatectomized dog may be severe, blood sugar levels reaching 300 to 400 mg per 100 ml and the animals losing 3 to 4 gm of glucose per kilogram of body weight through the urine per day. Even in fasting animals, the blood sugar generally remains above the renal threshold and glycosuria occurs continuously. The diabetic animal passes abnormally large amounts of urine (polyuria) and consequently is thirsty and consumes much fluid (polydipsia). Since the tissues cannot utilize glucose normally, even though they need fuel, the diabetic animal is constantly hungry and tends to eat excessively (polyphagia). There is an increased urinary elimination of nitrogen, and the continued loss of water from the body results in a state of dehydration, together with profound disturbances in tissue electrolyte balance. Ketone bodies in the blood and urine are at a high level. Wounds are easily infected in the diabetic subject. The untreated animal gradually becomes weaker and loses weight, despite a voracious appetite, and, when diabetic coma ensues, the plasma volume decreases and shock and kidney failure develop. Pancreatectomized dogs usually do not live for more than one or two weeks without insulin. Even when given adequate insulin they do not live indefinitely; they eventually develop a fatty infiltration of the liver, which is fatal. This liver defect in the pancreatectomized dog can be prevented or cured by feeding lipotropic factors such as choline, methionine, or betaine.

The glycogen stores of the diabetic liver are low, and little if any increase occurs after administration of glucose. The hyperglycemia is largely a consequence of increased liver glycogenolysis and deficient glycogenesis by muscle. While the tissues of the diabetic subject receive a generous supply of glucose, they are unable to utilize it properly. The muscle glycogen falls during exercise, as in normal animals, but the resynthesis of glycogen occurs at a very slow rate in the pancreatectomized dog. In such animals, however, glycogen deposition may occur in such tissues as heart muscle, kidney tubules, and leukocytes. The so-called hydropic degeneration of the B-cells of the islets appears to be an actual deposition of glycogen in the cytoplasm. The subnormal utilization of glucose by the diabetic is indicated by reduced glucose tolerance, decreased respiratory quotient (R.Q.), and fasting hyperglycemia and glycosuria. When extra glucose is injected into a diabetic subject, the R.Q. does not rise as it does in normal animals, and there is a prolonged hyperglycemia and glycosuria. Excised organs from diabetic animals consume some glucose, though at a much slower rate than comparable tissues from normal animals. That the diabetic animal produces excessive glucose from protein (gluconeogenesis) is indicated by the negative nitrogen balance and the elevated urinary glucose-nitrogen (G:N) ratio.

The hyperglycemia so characteristic of pancreatic diabetes is due in large measure to metabolic defects in the liver. No type of pancreatic diabetes can be produced after removal of the liver (hepatectomy). In the pancreatectomized-hepatectomized dog, the blood levels fall rapidly and severe hypoglycemia develops.

Fat and Protein Utilization. Since the diabetic organism cannot use glucose properly, the fat and protein stores of the body are drawn upon as sources of energy. As the fat stores are mobilized, the fat content of the blood rises; the blood cholesterol is also elevated. When a sample of blood from an individual with a severe case of diabetes is allowed to stand, a thick creamy layer of fatty material may be detectable. Protein is also utilized excessively by the diabetic, and as a consequence there is severe tissue wasting. The antiketogenic amino acids derived from dietary and tissue proteins are converted to glucose, but this cannot be stored as glycogen or utilized properly by the tissues and hence is eliminated through the urine. In the diabetic individual, there is also a diminished capacity to convert sugar into fatty acids. In severe diabetes, fatty acid synthesis ceases and such compounds cannot be completely oxidized to carbon dioxide. Thus, an abnormal type of fatty acid oxidation ensues that results in an excessive production of ketone bodies; these appear in the blood (ketonemia) and in the urine (ketonuria). The ketone bodies are acetoacetic acid, β-hydroxybutyric acid, and acetone, and the process of their formation is called "ketogenesis." In human patients in diabetic coma, the breath and urine may have the odor of acetone. Since two of the ketone bodies are acids, the alkali reserve of the blood is reduced and the carbon dioxide combining power is diminished. The breathing becomes slow and deep (air hunger) and the alveolar CO_2 tension falls. The content of ammonium salts increases in the urine; the pH of the urine remains normal if the acidosis is compensated for, or falls if it is uncompensated for.

From the foregoing, it appears that the main defect consequent upon insulin deficiency is the reduced ability to utilize extracellular glucose for oxidation to CO_2 and for the synthesis of fatty acids, and probably also for the deposition of glycogen. Body fats and to some extent proteins are then utilized to an increased extent, but a portion of these materials is lost in the urine as ketone bodies and glucose. Lipogenesis is seriously impaired in the diabetic animal. It is possible that the inability to synthesize fatty acids and to oxidize them completely results secondarily from impaired glucose metabolism, but some evidence has accumulated indicating that insulin deficiency causes a defect in fat metabolism *per se.* The body economy of the untreated diabetic resembles that prevailing during chronic starvation, and even if acidotic crises are avoided, death eventually results from tissue wastage.

Subtotal Pancreatectomy

If one-eighth of the dog's pancreas is left intact, the animal maintains normal blood sugar and does not become diabetic. After surgical reduction of the pancreas, the intact fragment is less resistant than the whole pancreas and can be damaged easily by the administration of anterior pituitary extracts or adrenocortical or thyroid hormones, thus producing diabetes. After such an operation in the cat, permanent diabetes can be produced by the prolonged administration of excessive glucose. The elevated blood sugar overworks the remaining B-cells in the fragment, causing them to undergo functional exhaustion and destruction. Such lesions in the pancreatic islets of the intact fragment do not develop if hyperglycemia is prevented by giving insulin along with the glucose.

When more than seven-eighths of the dog's pancreas is removed, Thiroloix-Sandmeyer diabetes ensues. This is a mild type of diabetes that is not stationary. The B-cells of the fragment may degenerate progressively and cause the diabetic state to increase in severity until death results, or the islet cells may increase in number and volume and eventually secrete enough insulin to return the blood sugar level to normal.

Diabetes in the Rat

Methods have been perfected for total pancreatectomy of the rat, and such animals die within two days from diabetic coma unless replacement therapy is employed.[57] When about 5 per cent of the rat's pancreas is left intact, a very slow type of diabetes develops. For one or two months after the operation, there are no apparent indications of diabetes. An incipient state develops, during which blood sugar levels are normal during fasting, but hyperglycemia and glycosuria become apparent after feeding. A manifest diabetes eventually develops and becomes more severe until the animals succumb. This slow and gradually developing type of diabetes facilitates the study of certain problems, such as factors that tend to ameliorate the condition or factors that cause it to increase in severity. It has been found that the incidence of this type of diabetes in rats is less in females than in males. Ovariectomy increases the incidence of diabetes after subtotal pancreatectomy of the female, and the opposite effect is obtained by administering estrogens. Estrogens and adrenocortical steroids may at first increase the severity of the diabetic state, and later exert a preventive effect on the diabetes of subtotally pancreatectomized rats. Estrogens have a curative effect when administered to rats made diabetic with alloxan; the hormone causes an increase in the number of pancreatic islets and of B-cells. This stimulating action of estrogen on the pancreas is especially pronounced when it acts in the presence of insulin.

Alloxan Administration

Alloxan provides a quick and convenient method for producing experimental diabetes in a variety of vertebrates. Three phases are generally observed after the administration of alloxan: transitory periods of hyperglycemia and hypoglycemia, followed by permanent hyperglycemia and other diabetic symptoms. Alloxan is thought to act directly and specifically on the B-cells, causing them to undergo degeneration and resorption; the A-cells and the acinar tissue remain relatively unaffected. The alloxan diabetic animal, however, is not totally deprived of insulin. Dehydroascorbic and dehydroisoascorbic acids resemble alloxan in chemical structure and produce similar diabetogenic effects.

Progressive hyperglycemia and B-cell destruction have been observed in alloxanized catfish. Permanent diabetes occurs in a small percentage of turtles treated with alloxan, and typical B-cell lesions are observed. Alloxan apparently does not produce diabetes in birds, such as ducks, chickens, pigeons, and owls. The B-cells of the avian pancreas generally do not seem to show such conspicuous changes as in mammals, although there may be some slight indications of hydropic degeneration. The islets of the alloxanized duck may show necrotic lesions, but diabetic symptoms do not appear. Among mammals, alloxan diabetes has been studied most extensively in rats, mice, hamsters, and guinea pigs.

There are certain very conspicuous differences between the diabetes produced by alloxan and that produced by removal of the pancreas. In alloxan diabetes, the hyperglycemia and glycosuria are generally more severe than in totally pancreatectomized animals. Alloxanized animals survive longer without insulin than do the pancreatectomized animals, and ketonemia and ketonuria may be mild and transitory. When dogs are made diabetic with alloxan and then undergo pancreatectomy, the glycosuria is reduced and less insulin is required to maintain normal blood sugar levels.

In these animals, however, ketonuria and coma supervene promptly when insulin is discontinued. It may well be that some of these differences result from the fact that the alloxanized animal is not deprived of glucagon from the A-cells, whereas the totally pancreatectomized animal lacks both insulin and glucagon.

Adrenal Cortex and Diabetes

Metabolic processes are regulated by a complicated interplay of multiple hormones, and in the organism, one hormone never acts completely alone. The metabolism of carbohydrates is related to that of fats and proteins, and these processes are regulated by a balance of hormones from the pancreas, anterior pituitary, adrenal cortex and medulla, and thyroid, and, in some instances, the gonadal steroids. It has been known for a long time that the diabetic symptoms of pancreatectomized dogs and cats tend to clear up if the adrenal glands are also removed.[34] In certain human diseases, such as Cushing's syndrome, in which there is an increased secretion of 11-oxygenated steroids by the adrenal cortex, a diminished tolerance to glucose or even overt diabetes is frequently found. These diabetic symptoms are ameliorated or cured by surgical removal of the adrenal.

The 11-oxygenated steroids of the cortex probably influence blood glucose in two ways. They inhibit the incorporation of amino acids into protein and stimulate protein mobilization, thus augmenting the supply of gluconeogenic materials. There is also evidence that these steroids retard the utilization of glucose by peripheral tissues, although the mechanism of this effect remains unknown. The net effect of administering cortisol and similar cortical hormones is an elevation of the blood sugar. Conversely, in adrenalectomized animals, the blood sugar falls to low levels when food is withheld.

A transitory (corticoid) diabetes can be produced in normal rats, rabbits, and guinea pigs by the administration of adrenocortical oxysteroids; resistance to insulin is increased and the blood sugar rises. While some lesions may develop in the pancreatic islets of these species after such treatment, a permanent diabetic state does not ensue. Dogs and cats may be made sensitive to diabetogenic agents by removing 80 to 85 per cent of the pancreas, the intact fragment being capable of maintaining normal blood sugar levels under usual conditions. Temporary (corticoid) or permanent (metacorticoid) diabetes may be produced in these animals by administering such adrenal cortical hormones as cortisol or cortisone. At first, these hormones appear to cause islet hypertrophy or hyperplasia that probably results in an augmented output of insulin; after prolonged administration, the B-cells are permanently damaged and metacorticoid diabetes results.

Thyroid Administration

The general effect of thyroid hormones is to enhance many catabolic pathways and to augment oxidative processes in the body. Hyperthyroidism in man increases the intensity of the diabetic state. The administration of thyroxine to laboratory animals may lead to a complete absence of glycogen in the liver. Toxic goiters are often accompanied by symptoms of mild diabetes. Permanent (metathyroid) diabetes can be produced in subtotally pancreatectomized dogs by the repeated administration of thyroid hormone. As with other hormones that produce a hyperglycemic state, there is an increase in insulin production at first, but this decreases later as the islet cells are damaged.

Anterior Pituitary and Diabetes

Corticotrophin (ACTH), acting to promote the secretion of adrenal cortical hormones, may increase the supply of carbohydrate as a consequence of augmented gluconeogenesis. Another hormone of anterior hypophysial origin, probably somatotrophin, elevates the blood glucose by some mechanism that remains unexplained.

Transitory (hypophysial) or permanent (metahypophysial) diabetes may be produced in a variety of vertebrates by the administration of pituitary extracts or hormones to the intact animal.[3] The prolonged administration of excessive somatotrophin to normal dogs or cats causes irreversible damage to the B-cells, and a permanent diabetes follows withdrawal of the hormone. This pancreatic lesion leading to permanent diabetes is a direct consequence of the prolonged hyperglycemia rather than of the presence of the hypophysial hormone itself. After surgical reduction of the pancreas in cats and dogs, transitory or permanent diabetes may be produced by the injection of corticotrophin or prolactin. This is a pancreatic diabetes resulting from exhaustion and degeneration of the B-cells, the source of insulin. There are indications that the production of insulin is not completely suppressed in any type of metahormonal diabetes.

The role of the anterior hypophysis in carbohydrate metabolism and diabetes has been extensively studied by a number of workers. The main facts are: (1) Hypophysectomized animals tend to develop hypoglycemia when fasting. Sensitivity to insulin is greatly increased; that is, a given dose of insulin produces a larger fall of blood sugar than it does in normal animals. The ability of the hypophysectomized animal to release glucose from the liver in response to hypoglycemia is impaired. (2) Removal of the hypophysis from an animal rendered diabetic by total pancreatectomy diminishes the intensity of the diabetic state ("Houssay animals"). (3) Certain anterior pituitary hormones increase the resistance of normal, hypophysectomized, or pancreatectomized animals to the antagonism between the pancreas and the anterior hypophysis; this is indicated by the fact that hypophysectomized subjects are strikingly sensitive to insulin, whereas certain anterior lobe hormones produce insulin resistance. (4) Pituitary extracts or partially purified hormones increase the intensity of the diabetic state when administered to pancreatectomized or pancreatectomized-hypophysectomized animals. (5) Prolonged administration of certain anterior lobe hormones can produce pancreatic diabetes in intact or partially pancreatectomized animals.

The Houssay Effect in Animals. Work with the pancreatectomized-hypophysectomized dog emphasizes the physiologic importance of a balance between insulin on the one hand and the anterior hypophysial hormones on the other. Although the diabetic condition is attenuated, the Houssay animal is far from normal; it seems to be precariously balanced between hypoglycemia and hyperglycemia. There are wide fluctuations in the levels of blood sugar, whereas the administration of carbohydrate causes marked hyperglycemia. Compared with animals lacking pancreas only, the doubly operated animal survives longer without insulin and is more resistant to infections. In the Houssay animal the nitrogen balance is not so profoundly negative, and there is less tissue wastage than in the pancreatectomized subject. Blood sugar may remain within normal limits for prolonged periods, and the glycosuria and polyuria are diminished or occasionally are absent. Ketosis is less severe than in singly operated animals. Liver and muscle glycogen may be within normal limits and, after the injection of glucose, the respiratory quotient (R. Q.) may be increased almost as in normal animals. Like animals lacking pituitary glands only, the Houssay animal is extremely sensitive to insulin. The ameliorating effects of hypophysectomy on pancreatic diabetes are mainly due to reduced gluconeogenesis and ketogenesis and to the increased ability of the tissues to utilize glucose when the blood sugar is held to lower levels.

The Houssay Phenomenon *In Vitro.* Liver slices from normal cats, pancreatectomized cats, and pancreatectomized-hypophysectomized cats (Houssay animals) have been studied for their capacity to incorporate isotopic acetate into the higher fatty acids. Fat synthesis by liver slices from pancreatectomized animals is reduced to a very low level; removal of the pituitary in addition to the pancreas restores the synthesis of fatty acids to normal ranges. Liver slices from pancreatectomized cats also produce large quantities of ketone bodies *in vitro,* but similar slices from Houssay cats produce almost none. *In vitro* measurements have shown that the uptake of glucose by liver from diabetic animals is below normal. It may be increased until it approximates the normal level by removing the pituitary gland or by injecting insulin at suitable times before removing the liver for the *in vitro* measurements. Livers from diabetic animals lose glucose faster than do those from normal subjects. Apparently, in the intact organism certain metabolic processes proceed under the balanced influence of insulin and pituitary factors; imbalance results when the animal is deprived of one or the other, and in the Houssay animal, the balance is reinstated by reducing the hormones from both sources to zero.

Actions of Insulin in Diabetic Subjects

The pancreatectomized animal can be kept in good health for long periods by the administration of insulin, provided the animal is given a suitable diet. Insulin has been of great value in treating diabetes mellitus in man, especially in those cases in which the islets are damaged and cannot secrete insulin. It should be stressed, however, that not all cases of diabetes result from defects in the islets of Langerhans and an insufficiency of insulin production by the pancreas. Many factors other than pancreatic defects can enter in human diabetes, and these extrapancreatic features of the disease have not been fully clarified. Insulin is acidic and is fairly soluble in plasma and tissue fluids, and hence it rapidly diffuses away from the site of injection. Much progress has been made in preparing slowly absorbed insulins that exert prolonged effects. The rate of absorption can be reduced by combining insulin with a basic protein (*e.g.*, protamine from fish sperm), and the addition of zinc makes it still less soluble in tissue fluids. Zinc preparations of insulin have also been devised in which the duration of effectiveness in the body is correlated with the form and size of the particles in suspension.

When insulin is administered to a pancreatectomized animal, the principal effects are: (1) reduction of the blood sugar and a consequent disappearance of the glycosuria and polyuria; (2) increased utilization of glucose by the tissues; (3) increased conversion of glucose to fat; (4) increased rate of protein synthesis; (5) inhibition of excessive ketogenesis; (6) reduced gluconeogenesis by the liver; (7) increased storage of glycogen by the liver and muscles; and (8) decreased concentration of potassium and inorganic phosphate in the blood. This electrolyte effect is probably a consequence of an increased uptake of glucose and other hexoses into the tissue cells and of the deposition of potassium and phosphate with glycogen in the liver and muscles. The concentration of these electrolytes (K and PO_4) closely parallels the blood glucose, suggesting that their titers in the circulation are dependent upon metabolic mechanisms involving phosphorylation.

The increased oxidation of glucose in the tissues and its utilization for the synthesis of fat and glycogen encourage its removal from the circulation. Furthermore, in the presence of insulin, the liver is more competent to retain glycogen. Whether insulin exerts a direct effect on the synthesis of hepatic glycogen or whether it opposes the glycogenolytic action of other hormones has not been clearly determined. In any case, insulin facilitates the utilization of glucose and diminishes its production, and these two phenomena serve to reduce the blood sugar levels. That extrapancreatic hormonal factors are involved in the regulation of blood sugar has already been indicated.

After an overdose of insulin, the blood sugar may fall to levels low enough to produce convulsions and coma. A comparable condition occurs in hyperinsulinism, during which the pancreatic islets liberate an excess of insulin. When the blood sugar drops to about 40 mg per 100 ml, there are likely to be symptoms such as headache, a feeling of apprehension, inability to concentrate, tremor, sweating, and eventual coma. The condition can be relieved by giving sugar orally or by injecting glucose or epinephrine. The action of epinephrine depends upon the presence of ample stores of glycogen in the body from which glucose can be formed. Some of the symptoms of hypoglycemia result from the increased secretion of epinephrine from the adrenal medulla.

The Hypoglycemic Sulfonamides and Diabetes

There were suggestions that guanidine derivatives might be useful in the treatment of diabetes, but some were found to have many toxic side effects. Interest in the sulfonamides began in 1941 when it was fortuitously observed that certain of these agents produced hypoglycemic effects in man and in experimental animals, with a minimum of undesirable side reactions. Loubatières and others extended these observations, and some progress has been made in analyzing the mechanism of action of such compounds.[9, 10, 35] The sulfonylureas were originally produced and tested as more soluble sulfa drugs that would give prolonged chemotherapeutic effects; their hypoglycemic actions in diabetes were unexpected or accidental findings. The potentialities of this discovery as an approach to the oral treatment of diabetes were quickly appreciated by investigators all over the world, and the problem has been studied very intensively since 1954. One important aspect of the research on hypoglycemic compounds has been a reinvestigation of the etiology of diabetes mellitus and the recognition that there are different forms of the disease.

Middle-aged obese diabetics (maturity-onset type) often have normal levels of pancreatic insulin and adequate amounts in the blood, but for unknown reasons this insulin does not reach the tissues and act in the normal way. Young diabetics (growth-onset type), on the other hand, more frequently have little if any insulin in the blood or in pancreatic tissue, reflecting an actual deficiency of the hormone. Some diabetic patients require more insulin than is necessary to maintain a totally pancreatectomized person. Many middle-aged and elderly diabetics are relatively insensitive to insulin, compared to most juvenile diabetics, and this suggests that contrainsulin factors may play a role in the etiology and course of the maturity-onset type.

With the development of isotope techniques it has become possible to introduce small amounts of labeled insulin into living organisms and trace its distribution and eventual fate. Insulin labeled with I^{131} generally disappears less rapidly from the blood of diabetics who have taken insulin for long periods of time than from the blood of normal persons. This and other observations suggest the presence of a plasma-binding factor in many insulin-treated persons, which hinders the entry of the hormone into the tissues and depresses its enzymatic degradation. It has been proposed that the plasma factor that binds insulin may be an antibody that arises as a consequence of insulin therapy. Among the factors that may interfere with the normal action of insulin are: (1) hormones from the pituitary and adrenal glands that antagonize the action of insulin, (2) enzymatic destruction of insulin, (3) development of antibodies to exogenous or even endogenous insulin, and (4) extracellular factors that may interfere with the distribution of insulin to the peripheral tissues.

It is of great interest that the hypoglycemic sulfonamide derivatives act almost exclusively in the maturity-onset type of diabetes, in which there is available — although it is nonuseful — insulin emanating from the pancreatic islets. The mechanisms whereby the sulfonamides act have not been established with certainty. There is considerable evidence that such compounds act primarily on the B-cells to promote the production of endogenous insulin; thus, their effectiveness depends upon the number of B-cells remaining in the islets or the number that can be regenerated. Significant effects have not been demonstrated in pancreatectomized mammals. Since the effectiveness of exogenous insulin is potentiated by the sulfonamides, it is possible that they prevent insulin degradation by inhibiting the insulinase action of the liver. Under certain conditions, sulfonylurealike drugs may suppress the production of glucose by the liver. Destruction of the A-cells, with a decrease in glucagon production, has been suggested as a possible mechanism of action of these drugs. The response of the duck to sulfonamides appears not to be altered by either total pancreatectomy or enterectomy. This suggests that hypoglycemic compounds may act by different mechanisms in birds and in mammals. Studies on the domestic fowl indicate that tolbutamide reduces the level of blood sugar by acting mainly through extrapancreatic and extrahepatic mechanisms. Thus, it appears that no one action can explain the antidiabetic effects of these drugs in man and animals.

Hereditary Obesity and Hyperinsulinism in Mice

A mutant mouse strain having an autosomal recessive trait for obesity has been obtained; these mice have been studied extensively since the islets of Langerhans function excessively and contain about 10 times more insulin than do islets of normal mice of the same age. The obese syndrome appears only in homozygous recessive individuals, and, by 6 to 8 weeks of age, the excessive accumulation of abdominal fat serves to distinguish them from the nonobese heterozygous and homozygous dominant littermates. The islets of these mice increase greatly in size and number due to hyperplasia and degranulation of the B-cells. Multiplication of the B-cells in these islets seems to be a compensatory reaction to counteract the hyperglycemia of extrapancreatic origin. Since A-cells are extremely sparse, such islets are particularly suitable for *in vitro* studies on the synthesis and secretion of insulin.[20, 28]

The quantities of immunoreactive insulin are elevated and insulin-like activity is increased in individual pancreata as well as in the pooled sera of these mice. The insulin obtained from these animals does not differ from normal hormone in biologic and immunologic effectiveness. In spite of the sustained hyperinsulinism, there is a severe and persistent hyperglycemia and glycosuria; there is no evidence of ketosis. Refractoriness to exogenous insulin has been demonstrated both *in vivo* and *in vitro;* however, sensitivity to exogenous insulin can be restored by restricting food intake sufficiently to hold the animals to normal weight.

When hereditary obese mice are parabiotically united with nonobese littermates, they lose weight or fail to gain weight; after separation, the obese parabionts gain weight rapidly. This could be interpreted as indicating that a blood-borne factor characterizes the defect. The transplantation of islet tissue from normal donors relieves the hyperglycemia and stabilizes the weight gains of the obese hosts. This has been interpreted as indicating that a pancreatic abnormality is involved in the obese syndrome.[64]

Preliminary studies have shown that insulin levels in the obese mouse are not elevated by intravenous glucose, but they are consistently elevated by feeding glucose. It has also been reported that moderate fasting of the obese animals reduces plasma insulin markedly, but has little effect on glucose levels. There are indications that some of the gastrointestinal hormones, secreted into the blood in response to carbohydrate feeding, may stimulate the B-cells to release insulin. The interesting possibility has been suggested that an intestinal agent of this kind, produced in excess in response to eating, might be the main defect in the obese mouse leading to hyperinsulinism, resistance to insulin, and hyperglycemia.[20]

MECHANISMS OF ACTION OF ISLET HORMONES

Insulin

There are indications that homeostatic efficiency has increased during the evolution of organisms through the addition of chemical messengers which serve the organism by supplementing basic or fundamental means of cellular regulation. The implication is that hormones do not initiate new biochemical reactions, but function at the cellular level to condition the speed and extent of preexisting reactions. Four general types of concepts have been proposed to account for the action of insulin: (1) It may regulate the permeability of membrane systems of the target cells, (2) it may have direct effects upon intracellular enzyme systems, (3) it may act through an energy-conferring metabolic agency, or (4) it may act directly upon the chromosomes to activate or inhibit particular genes. It is important to note that these various concepts are not necessarily mutually exclusive; in fact, considerable experimental support can be found for all of them.

The insulin receptor is a protein having a molecular weight of about 300,000. These binding sites are located on the cell membrane, and are absent from nuclei, microsomes, mitochondria, and other internal components. The receptors on blood cells seem to be similar to those on the plasma membranes of fat and liver cells. If insulin is bound to glass beads or to agarose and then added to a suspension of fat or liver plasma membranes, particles containing the insulin receptor complex can be extracted. Each target cell possesses a limited number of receptor sites, estimated to be sufficient to bind 11,000 molecules of insulin. The degree of binding is proportional to the insulin-type potency of each constituent; for example, the concentration of proinsulin must be 20 times greater than that of insulin before it attains the maximal action exerted by insulin. This indicates that the receptors have a twenty-fold greater affinity for insulin than for proinsulin.

Insulin is essentially an anabolic hormone having profound effects on carbohydrate, protein, and fat metabolism. Though few cells in the organism escape its effects, its principal targets are liver, muscle, and adipose tissues. The cellular effects of insulin have probably been studied more intensively than have those for any other hormone, and a tremendous amount of scattered information has accumulated; nevertheless, insulin's mechanism of action remains far from clear. The sequences and interrelationships of the intracellular changes have not been determined, and different workers interpret many of the established facts differently. As with other hormones, it is difficult to determine which actions are primary (initial) and which ones are subsidiary or consequential. A single, unique action of insulin, leading to all of the varied intracellular adjustments resulting from the hormone, has not been discovered. Consideration of targets as diverse and complex in structure and function as liver cells, muscle cells, and fat cells does not seem to encourage the view that an all-encompassing, primary action will be found. For example, insulin does enhance the entrance of glucose and amino acids into certain receptor cells, but this is not an essential action for all effects of the hormone.

The concept that insulin stimulates the transport of glucose, amino acids, and electrolytes through cell membranes has received some support, but does not accommodate all of the information now available.[30, 31] Since nonmetabolizable sugars (e.g., xylose, arabinose) may enter cells but not become involved in metabolic pathways, any effect of insulin on such sugars would necessarily be on transport. Various experiments have shown unequivocally that sugars enter certain target cells slowly in the absence of insulin and rapidly in its presence. Insulin-sensitive transport systems have been demonstrated in skeletal muscle, cardiac muscle, and adipose tissue. Insulin does not stimulate glucose transport into nerve cells or erythrocytes, nor does it promote intestinal absorption of glucose or reabsorption from the renal tubule. Glucose transport into liver cells is not altered by insulin; liver cells are permeable to glucose in the absence of insulin, but the hormone rapidly stimulates hepatic utilization of glucose. Insulin also stimulates the uptake of amino acids by the liver and promotes their incorporation into protein. There is no doubt that insulin does augment glucose transport in certain target tissues; this could correlate with many effects of insulin as increased oxidation of glucose, increased glycogenesis, enhanced lipogenesis and proteogenesis, decreased lipolysis, and decreased formation of ketone bodies.

Insulin has two major effects on fat cells: (1) It stimulates the entry of glucose, and this correlates with an accelerated metabolism of glucose and the synthesis and esterification of fatty acids; and (2) it exerts a potent antilipolytic effect, opposing the lipolytic actions of certain pituitary hormones and the catecholamines. There is evidence, however, that insulin affects glycogen, lipid, and protein metabolism in adipose cells in ways that are not related to the transport of glucose and amino acids. Studies on fat cells indicate that ions have important effects on substrate transport and on the hormonal activation of adenylate cyclase at cell surfaces. Magnesium ions seem to be essential for all effects of insulin.

Though it has been amply demonstrated that insulin facilitates the transport of amino acids and glucose into skeletal and cardiac muscle, there is convincing evidence that insulin-induced proteogenesis does not depend upon this transport. Insulin increases the synthesis of RNA in muscle, but this apparently is not the manner in which it accelerates protein anabolism. Actinomycin, an antibotic that selectively inhibits the formation of all kinds of RNA, does not block insulin-induced proteogenesis in muscle. This shows that an increase in RNA is not essential for insulin to be effective. In other words, sufficient RNA is already present, and insulin effects do not depend upon the synthesis of any new RNA. Actinomycin does not interfere with insulin-induced acceleration of glucose uptake by muscle. The protein anabolic effect of insulin seems to be independent of its effects on substrate transport, high-energy phosphate formation, and glycogenesis. Studies with puromycin and cycloheximide, compounds that block the ribosomal synthesis of protein, strongly suggest that insulin acts in striated muscle at the ribosomal (translational) level to facilitate protein synthesis. These agents effectively prevent the stimulating action of insulin upon protein synthesis in muscle.[70]

Since some of the catabolic peptides and amines (*e.g.,* ACTH, glucagon, epinephrine) employ cyclic AMP as a second messenger in their target cells, there has been much interest in determining whether or not adenylate cyclase and the nucleotide mediate any of the effects of insulin. The levels of cyclic AMP in a tissue can be altered by both production and destruction, and the nucleotide is known to be an important factor in regulating enzyme systems as diverse as glycogen synthetase, phosphorylase, and lipases. It is known that insulin diminishes the concentration of cyclic AMP in liver and adipose tissue. It has also been reported that the nucleotide inhibits the incorporation of labeled amino acids into protein in diaphragm muscle.[70] Cyclic AMP is known to decrease such activities as glycogenesis, proteogenesis, and lipogenesis, and it might be noted that these are processes that are stimulated by insulin. It is probable that cyclic AMP is involved in the responses of the major insulin targets, but it does not seem to function as a special intracellular mediator or informational molecule, as it does in the case of certain catabolic hormones (*e.g.,* glucagon).

Though we still do not know the complete story of how insulin acts, or, for that matter, the complete details of how any hormone acts, rapid progress is being made. The problem of how hormones affect intracellular reactions is a difficult one, but the answers are of such fundamental importance as to justify the expenditure of time and effort.

Glucagon

Glucagon stimulates adenylate cyclase activity and it is thought that cyclic AMP, in turn, acts as a second messenger within the target cells to alter the enzymatic and metabolic processes affected by the hormone. There is evidence that adenylate cyclase is firmly bound to the plasma membrane of liver cells, and stimulation of this enzyme appears to be one of the earliest ef-
liver and other tissues as active (phosphorylase *a*) and inactive (phosphorylase *b*) forms. The phosphorylase *a* contains phosphate and its inactivation involves the removal of phosphate to form dephosphophosphorylase. Inactivation is accomplished by phosphorylase phosphatase, and activation by dephosphophosphorylase kinase, both enzymes being present in liver tissue. All of the phosphorylase kinases require a nucleotide, cyclic AMP, as

cofactor or activator. The enzyme adenylate cyclase, in the presence of Mg^{++}, generates cyclic AMP from ATP. Both *in vivo* and *in vitro* experiments have shown that glucagon increases cyclic AMP in liver, whereas insulin decreases it.

Glucagon stimulates adenylate cyclase activity and it is thought that cyclic AMP, in turn, acts as a second messenger within the target cells to alter the enzymatic and metabolic processes affected by the hormone. There is evidence that adenylate cyclase is firmly bound to the plasma membrane of liver cells, and stimulation of this enzyme appears to be one of the earliest effects of glucagon. Thus, the over-all effect of glucagon is to facilitate the activation of phosphorylase, the enzyme which catalyzes the first step in the breakdown of liver glycogen to form blood glucose.

The formation of liver phosphorylase *a* by dephosphophosphorylase in cell-free homogenates of dog and cat liver is increased markedly by the addition of small amounts of glucagon. This is one of the few instances in which hormones are found to affect enzyme systems in the absence of intact cell structure.

It is now known that enzymes from different tissues of the *same animal* may possess different chemical structures, but still exert the same catalytic activities. Both glucagon and epinephrine activate liver phosphorylase, but muscle phosphorylase is activated only by epinephrine. Tissue differences in the enzyme apparently explain why phosphorylase of liver responds to glucagon, whereas phosphorylase of muscle does not. It is a curious fact that two hormones as different in chemical structure as glucagon and epinephrine can share the common ability of activating liver phosphorylase.[52]

REFERENCES

1. Andrew, A.: APUD cells in the endocrine pancreas and the intestine of chick embryos. Gen. Comp. Endocr. *26*:485, 1975.
2. Basabe, J. C., Farina, J. M. S., and Chieri, R. A.: *In vitro* insulin secretion from the penguin *(Pygoscelis papua)* pancreas. Gen. Comp. Endocr. *27*:43, 1975.
3. Bates, R. W., Scow, R. O., and Lacy, P. E.: Induction of permanent diabetes in rats by pituitary hormones from transplantable mammotropic tumor. Endocrinology *78*:826, 1966.
4. Behrens, O. K., and Bromer, W. W.: Glucagon. Vitam. Horm. *16*:263, 1958.
5. Brinn, J. E., Jr. The pancreatic islets of bony fishes. Amer. Zool. *13*:653, 1973.
6. Bromer, W. W., Sinn, L. G., and Behrens, O. K.: The amino acid sequence of glucagon. J. Amer. Chem. Soc. *79*:2807, 1957.
7. Chance, R. E., Ellis, R. M., and Bromer, W. W.: Procine proinsulin: Characterization and amino acid sequence. Science *161*:165, 1968.
8. Cohen, K. L., and Nissley, S. P.: Comparison of somatomedin activity in rat serum and lymph. Endocrinology *97*:654, 1975.
9. Colwell, A. R., Jr., and Colwell, J. A.: Pancreatic action of the sulfonylureas. J. Lab. Clin. Med. *53*:376, 1959.
10. Duncan, L. J. P., and Clarke, B. F.: Pharmacology and mode of action of the hypoglycaemic sulphonylureas and diguanides. Ann. Rev. Pharmacol. *5*:151, 1965.
11. Edgar, P., Rabinowitz, D., and Merimee, T. J.: Effects of amino acids on insulin release from excised rabbit pancreas. Endocrinology *84*:835, 1969.
12. Epple, A.: The endocrine pancreas. *In* W. S. Hoar and D. J. Randall (eds.): Fish Physiology, Vol. 2, New York, Academic Press, 1969, p. 275.
13. Epple, A., and Lewis, T. L.: Comparative histophysiology of the pancreatic islets. Amer. Zool. *13*:567, 1973.
14. Fain, J. N., Kovacev, V. P., and Scow, R. O.: Antilipolytic effect of insulin in isolated fat cells of the rat. Endocrinology *78*:773, 1966.

15. Fajans, S. S., and Floyd, J. C., Jr., Knopf, R. F., and Conn, J. W.: Effect of amino acids and proteins on insulin secretion in man. Rec. Progr. Horm. Res. 23:617, 1967.
16. Falkmer, S., Cutfield, J. F., Cutfield, S. M., Dodson, G. G.,' Gliemann, J., Gammeltoft, S., Marques, M., Peterson J. D., Steiner, D. F., Sundby, F., Emdin, S. O., Havu, N., Östberg, Y., and Winbladh, L.: Comparative endocrinology of insulin and glucagon production. Amer. Zool. 15(Supply. 1):255, 1975.
17. Falkmer, S., Emdin, S., Havu, N., Lundgren, G., Marques, M., Östberg, Y., Steiner, D. F., and Thomas, N. W.: Insulin in invertebrates and cyclostomes. Amer. Zool. 13:625, 1973.
18. Foà, P. P.: Glucagon: an incomplete and biased review with selected references. Amer. Zool. 13:613, 1973.
19. Fujita, T. (ed.): Gastro-entero-pancreatic endocrine system. A cell-biological approach. Igaku Shoin Lt., Tokyo, 1973.
20. Genuth, S. M.: Hyperinsulinism in mice with genetically determined obesity. Endocrinology 84:386, 1969.
21. Hazelwood, R. L.: The avian endocrine pancreas. Amer. Zool. 13:699, 1973.
22. Hazelwood, R. L., Turner, S. D., Kimmel, J. R., and Pollock, H. G.: Spectrum effects of a new polypeptide (third hormone?) isolated from chicken pancreas. Gen. Comp. Endocr. 21:485, 1973.
23. Hellman, B.: The significance of calcium for glucose stimulation of insulin release. Endocrinology 97:392, 1975.
24. Kaneto, A., Miki, E., and Kosaka, K.: Effects of vagal stimulation on glucagon and insulin secretion. Endocrinology 95:1005, 1974.
25. Katsoyannis, P. G.: Synthetic insulins. Rec. Progr. Horm. Res. 23:505, 1967.
26. Lacy, P. E., Klein, N. J., and Fink, C. J.: Effect of cytochalasin B on the biphasic release of insulin in perifused rat islets. Endocrinology 92:1458, 1973.
27. Langslow, D. R., Kimmel, J. R., and Pollock, H. G.: Studies of the distribution of a new avian pancreatic polypeptide and insulin among birds, reptiles, amphibians and mammals. Endocrinology 93:558, 1973.
28. Lavine, R. L., Voyles, N., Perrino, P. V., and Recant, L.: The effect of fasting on tissue cyclic AMP and plasma glucagon in the obese hyperglycemic mouse. Endocrinology 97:615, 1975.
29. Leibson, L., and Plisetskaya, E. M.: Effect of insulin on blood sugar level and glycogen content in organs of some cyclostomes and fish. Gen. Comp. Endocr. 11:381, 1968.
30. Levine, R., and Goldstein, M. S.: On the mechanism of action of insulin. Rec. Progr. Horm. Res. 11:343, 1955.
31. Levine, R.: The action of insulin at the cell membrane. Amer. J. Med. 40:691, 1966.
32. Lin, B. J., and Haist, R. E.: Insulin biosynthesis: the monoaminergic mechanisms and the specificity of "Glucoreceptor." Endocrinology 96:1247, 1975.
33. Logothetopoulos, J., Sharma, B. B., Salter, J. M., and Best, C. H.: Glucagon and metaglucagon diabetes in rabbits. Diabetes 9:278, 1960.
34. Long, C. N. H., and Lukens, F. D. W.: Effects of adrenalectomy and hypophysectomy on experimental diabetes in the cat. J. Exp. Med. 63:465, 1936.
35. Loubatières, A.: The hypoglycemic sulfonamides: History and development of the problem from 1942 to 1955. Ann. N. Y. Acad. Sci. 71:4, 1957.
36. Macchi, I. A., and Blaustein, E. H.: Cytostructure and endocrine function of monolayer cultures of neonatal hamster pancreas. Endocrinology 84:208, 1969.
37. Malaisse, W., Malaisse-Lagae, F., Wright, P. H., and Ashmore, J.: Effects of adrenergic and cholinergic agents upon insulin secretion in vitro. Endocrinology 80:975, 1967.
38. Marques, M.: Effects of prolonged glucagon administration to turtles (Chrysemys d'Orbignyi). Gen. Comp. Endocr. 9:102, 1967.
39. Mashiter, K., Harding, P. E., Chou, M., Mashiter, G. D., Stout, J., Diamond, D., and Field, J. B.: Persistent pancreatic glucagon but not insulin response to arginine in pancreatectomized dogs. Endocrinology 96:678, 1975.
40. Miller, R. E.: Effects of vagotomy or splanchnicotomy on blood insulin and sugar concentrations in the conscious monkey. Endocrinology 86:642, 1970.
41. Mirsky, I. A.: Insulinase, insulinase-inhibitors, and diabetes mellitus. Rec. Progr. Horm. Res. 13:429, 1957.
42. Mirsky, I. A., and Gitelson, S.: The diabetic response of geese to pancreatectomy. Endocrinology 63:345, 1958.
43. Morris, R., and Islam, D. S.: Histochemical studies on the follicles of Langerhans of the ammocoete larva of Lampetra planeri (Bloch). Gen. Comp. Endocr. 12:72, 1969.
44. Nakamura, M., Yamada, K., and Yokote, M.: Ultrastructural aspect of the pancreatic islets in carps of spontaneous diabetes mellitus. Experientia 27:75, 1971.
45. Östberg, Y., Van Noorden, S., and Pearse, A. G. E.: Cytochemical, immunofluorescence,

and ultrastructural investigations on polypeptide hormone localization in the islet parenchyma and bile duct mucosa of a cyclostome, *Myxine glutinosa.* Gen. Comp. Endocr. *25:* 274, 1975.

46. Pearse, A. G. E., and Polak, J. M.: Neural crest origin of the endocrine polypeptide (APUD) cells of the gastrointestinal tract and pancreas. Gut*12:*783, 1971.
47. Pearse, A. G. E., Polak, J. M., and Bussolati, G.: The neural crest origin of gastrointestinal and pancreatic endocrine polypeptide cells and their distinction by sequential immunofluorescence. Folia Histochem. Cytochem. *10:*115, 1972.
48. Pearse, A. G. E., Polak, J. M., and Heath, C. M.: Development, differentiation and derivation of the endocrine polypeptide cells of the mouse pancreas. Diabetologia *9:*120, 1973.
49. Penhos, J. C., and Lavintman, N: Total pancreatectomy in toads: Effect of hypophysectomy and glucagon. Gen. Comp. Endocr. *4:*264, 1964.
50. Penhos, J. C., Wu, C. H., Reitman, M., Sodero, E., White, R., and Levine, R.: Effects of several hormones after total pancreatectomy in alligators. Gen. Comp. Endocr. *8:*32, 1967.
51. Peterson, J. D., Coulter, C. I., Steiner, D. F., Emdin, S. O., and Falkmer, S.: Hagfish insulin: Structural and crystallographic observations on a primitive protein hormone. Nature *251:* 239, 1974.
52. Rall, T. W., Sutherland, E. W., and Berthet, J.: The relationship of epinephrine and glucagon to liver phosphorylase. J. Biol. Chem. *224:*463, 1957.
53. Rodbell, M., Jones, A. B., Chiappe de Cingolani, G. E., and Birnbaumer, L.: The action of insulin and catabolic hormones on the plasma membrane of the fat cells. Rec. Progr. Horm. Res. *24:*215, 1968.
54. Rudman, D., and Shank, P. W.: Comparison of the responsiveness of perirenal adipose tissue of the rat, hamster, guinea pig and rabbit to the antilipolytic action of insulin. Endocrinology *79:*565, 1966.
55. Sanger, F.: Chemistry of insulin. Science. *129:*1340, 1959.
56. Sanger, F., Thompson, E. O. P., and Kitai, R.: The amide groups of insulin. Biochem. J. *59:* 509, 1955.
57. Scow, R. O.: "Total" pancreatectomy in the rat: Operation, effects, and postoperative care. Endocrinology *60:*359, 1957.
58. Simon, J., Freychet, P., and Rosselin, G.: Chicken insulin: radioimmunological characterization and enhanced activity in rat fat cells and liver plasma membranes. Endocrinology *95:*1439, 1974.
59. Sivadas, P.: The occurrence of *β*-cells in the islets of Langerhans of *Tilapia mosambica* (Peters) (Teleostei). Gen. Comp. Endocr. *4:*295, 1964.
60. Smith, P. H.: The effects of selective partial pancreatectomy on pancreatic islet cell morphology in the Japanese quail. Gen. Comp. Endocr. *26:*310, 1975.
61. Sorenson, R. L., Steffes, M. W., and Lindall, A. W.: Subcellular localization of proinsulin to insulin conversion in isolated rat islets. Endocrinology *86:*88, 1970.
62. Steiner, D. F., Clark, J. L., Nolan, C., Rubenstein, A. H., Margoliash, E., Aten, B., and Oyer, P. E.: Proinsulin and the biosynthesis of insulin. Rec. Progr. Horm. Res. *25:*207, 1969.
63. Steiner, D. F., Peterson, J. D., Tager, H., Emdin, S., Östberg, Y., and Falkmer, S.: Comparative aspects of proinsulin and insulin structure and biosynthesis. Amer. Zool. *13:*591, 1973.
64. Strautz, R. L.: Islet implants: Reduction of glucose levels in the hereditary obese mouse. Endocrinology *83:*975, 1968.
65. Thomas, N. W.: Observations on the cell types present in the principal islet of the dab *Limanda limanda.* Gen. Comp. Endocr. *26:*496, 1975.
66. Van Noorden, S., and Pearse, A. G. E.: Immunoreactive polypeptide hormones in the pancreas and gut of the lamprey. Gen. Comp. Endocr. *23:*311, 1974.
67. Van Wyk, J. J., Underwood, L. E., Hintz, R. L., Clemmons, D. R., Voina, S. J., and Weaver, R. P.: The somatomedins: a family of insulinlike hormones under growth hormone control. Rec. Progr. Horm. Res. *30:*259, 1974.
68. Von Mering, J., and Minkowski, O.: Diabetes Mellitus nach Pankreasextirpation. Arch. Exp. Path. Pharmakol. *26:*371, 1889.
69. Winbladh, L.: Light microscopical and ultrastructural studies of the pancreatic islet tissue of the lamprey (*Lampetra fluviatilis*). Gen. Comp. Endocr. *6:*534, 1966.
70. Wool, I. G., Stirewalt, W. S., Kurihara, K., Low, R. B., Bailey, P., and Oyer, D.: Mode of action of insulin in the regulation of protein biosynthesis in muscle. Rec. Progr. Horm. Res. *24:*139, 1968.

CHAPTER 10

The Adrenal Medulla: Chromaffin Tissue

The adrenal glands were first described in man by Eustachius in 1563. Other anatomists, dissecting poorly preserved cadavers, identified these organs along the anterior borders of the kidneys and were impressed by the fact that they were generally filled with fluid. Not fully appreciating the effects of postmortem decay, they used the term suprarenal "capsules" to describe them. Cuvier (1805) recognized that each gland consists of an inner and outer region, now referred to as the medulla and cortex, respectively. The first hint that these glands might be of functional significance came from Thomas Addison's description (1849) of a clinical condition resulting from their deterioration, a syndrome now bearing his name.

ANATOMY OF THE ADRENALS

The Mammalian Adrenal

This gland is a compound structure consisting of an outer *cortex* and an inner *medulla*. The hormones of the cortex are steroids, whereas those of the medulla are amines. The two components of the organ originate from different embryonic primordia. The cortex is derived from lateral mesoderm in close association with the developing gonads. The medulla differentiates from neural crest cells along with the sympathetic ganglia. The medullary cells are modified ganglion cells and remain in intimate contact with the preganglionic fibers of the sympathetic system. Secretion from the medulla is regulated very largely by means of these nerves. The cortex, on the other hand, resembles the anterior hypophysis in being practically devoid of secretory nerve terminals.

Like other endocrine glands, the adrenals receive a rich blood supply (Fig. 10–1). The human organs are flattened bodies situated in the retroperitoneal tissue along the cranial ends of the kidneys. They vary considerably in shape, but are usually described as being triangular or crescentic. Accessory deposits of cortical tissue are frequently found in many mammalian species, most commonly in the perirenal fat and along the path of descent of the gonads.

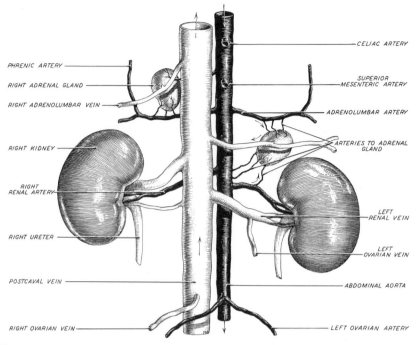

Figure 10–1. A dissection of the kidneys and adnexa of the cat, showing the position of the adrenal glands and their blood supply. The adrenals receive blood through numerous small arteries arising from the adrenolumbar arteries, the aorta, and the renal arteries. The venous drainage of the cat's adrenal is into the adrenolumbar vein, which passes over or through the gland. The arterial system is indicated in black.

During the third month of intrauterine life, the human adrenal reaches its maximum relative size and exceeds that of the kidney. This large size of the fetal adrenal is due to the presence of a thick *boundary* zone (fetal cortex or X zone) between the *definitive* cortex and the medulla. During late prenatal and early postnatal life, the fetal zone involutes and is not present to any appreciable extent in the glands of normal adults. In the adult human, the adrenal is only one-thirtieth as large as the kidney. Studies have shown that the fetal cortex is capable of secreting adrenal steriods, and there are suggestions that chorionic gonadotrophin may perform a role in the development and maintenance of this zone, possibly by influencing the release of ACTH from the fetal pituitary.[39] A comparable zone has been described in the adrenals of mice, hamsters, and certain other mammalian species.[33]

The mammalian gland is surrounded by a relatively heavy connective tissue capsule, from which trabeculae extend into the substance of the cortex. The epithelioid cells of the cortex are supported by a loose framework of reticular tissue. Histologically, the cells of the cortex are arranged into three vaguely defined layers: the *zona glomerulosa, zona fasciculata,* and *zona reticularis* (Fig. 10–2). The glomerulosa is a thin layer lying immediately below the capsule, and it is composed of irregular groups of cells. The

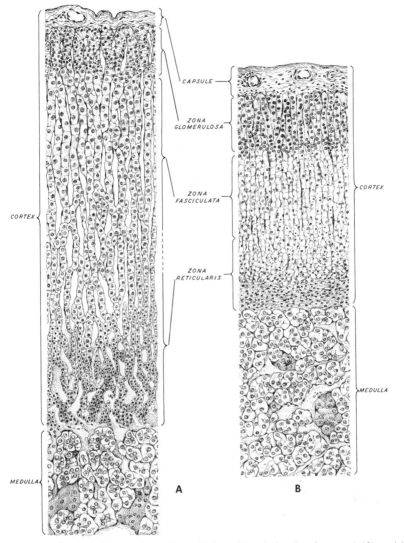

Figure 10–2. Comparable sections through the adrenal glands of normal (*A*) and hypophysectomized (*B*) rats. Since the functional capacity of the adrenal cortex is conditioned by the release of ACTH, hypophysectomy results in tremendous shrinkage of the cortex. The medulla is not influenced by hypophysectomy. Both sections are drawn to scale.

fasciculata, the widest layer of the cortex, is composed of radially disposed cords of polyhedral cells. The reticularis is the innermost layer of the cortex, and the radial arrangement of its cells is usually not so obvious as in the fasciculata. The zona glomerulosa is the source of steroid hormones that function in the regulation of electrolyte metabolism and, depending upon the species, it may or may not be affected by hypophysectomy. The fasciculata and reticularis are highly dependent on the presence of the pituitary gland and are thought to be responsible for the formation of carbohydrate-regulating steroids. Studies on the bovine adrenal suggest that the zones of the cortex possess different enzyme systems and hence can effect the biosynthesis of different steroid hormones.

Although the cortical cells are particularly susceptible to injury, they have a marked capacity for regeneration. One method of producing demedullated animals is to sever the capsule and express as much of the contents as possible; a complete cortex is regenerated from the capsule and the few glomerulosa cells that adhere to it. Like nervous tissue, however, the medullary cells are highly differentiated and there is no provision for their replacement. Mitotic divisions may be observed in all zones of the cortex, but there is a tendency for them to occur most frequently in the outermost regions of the zona fasciculata. Whether or not there is normally a centripetal movement of cells from the outer fasciculata into the inner reticularis remains a contended point.[13, 56]

Unlike the cortex, the medulla is not essential for life since demedullated animals survive quite well (although they are under the sheltered conditions of laboratory environments). The medulla is composed of irregular strands and masses of cells separated by sinusoidal vessels. Most of the medullary cells contain fine cytoplasmic granules that stain with chromates and hence are called "chromaffin cells." They also give a green color reaction when treated with ferric chloride. Sympathetic ganglion cells, occurring singly or in groups, may be found interspersed among the medullary cells. In aging birds, the medullary cells may undergo structural modifications in the direction of ganglion cells.[46]

There are widely scattered accumulations of cells in both vertebrate and invertebrate organisms that resemble the medullary cells in origin, structure, and staining reactions. These include the paraganglia found within or adjacent to the capsules of the sympathetic ganglia; the carotid glands located near the bifurcation of the common carotid arteries; the organs of Zuckerkandl near the origin of the inferior mesenteric artery; and scattered chromaffin cells within the liver, heart, kidney, gonads, and elsewhere. Chromaffin cells and catecholamines have been identified in the mantles of certain molluscs, the nervous system of leeches, and the cutaneous glands of certain amphibians. Serotonin is an indole amine that, like epinephrine, originates in chromaffin cells.

The adrenal medullary cells are generally regarded as modified postganglionic neurons, and their functional activity seems to be controlled largely by nervous mechanisms. Secretion by the medullary cells may be prevented by sectioning the splanchnic nerve or by applying nicotine directly to the gland itself. Stimulation of the splanchnic nerve elicits a marked outpouring of medullary hormones. Centers in the posterior hypothalamus are known to relay impulses to the adrenal medulla by way of the splanchnic nerves.

Comparative Morphology

Adrenal tissues are present in all vertebrates from cyclostomes to mammals, but profound differences are encountered in the arrangement of

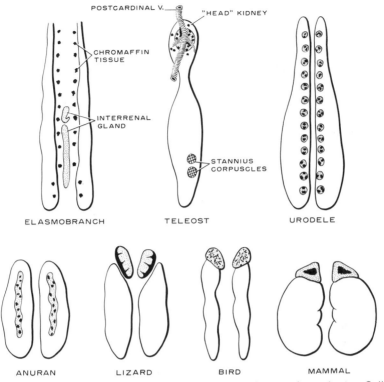

Figure 10–3. Comparative morphology of the adrenal tissues of vertebrates. Solid black indicates chromaffin tissue; stippling indicates steroidogenic tissue. Note that chromaffin tissue and steroidogenic tissue (interrenal gland) are spatially separate in the elasmobranch. The adrenal tissues of bony fishes are typically found in the "head" kidneys, around branches of the postcardinal veins; there may be some spatial separation of the two kinds of tissues, but they are usually intermingled. Note that a cortex (steroidogenic tissue) and medulla (chromaffin tissue) are present only in mammalian adrenals. (Based on Gorbman, A., and Bern, H. A.: Textbook of Comparative Endocrinology. New York, John Wiley & Sons, 1962.)

the functional components, *i.e.,* the steroid-producing cells and the catecholamine-producing cells. Histologic studies indicate that the two kinds of adrenal tissue coexist in cyclostomes: cells, presumed to be steroidogenic, are scattered along the walls of the postcardinal veins and in the mesonephric kidneys; small clusters of chromaffin cells are found in the same areas, and these occasionally come into contact with the steroidogenic cells. In elasmobranchs, the steroidogenic tissue is condensed into several well-formed bodies lying between the caudal ends of the kidneys; these are the *interrenal glands.* Paired aggregations of chromaffin cells are present between the kidneys, the more posterior ones being embedded in the kidneys (Fig. 10–3). The two components of the chondrichthyean adrenal are typically separated, though small islets of chromaffin cells have been described in the interrenal glands of the ray *Raja clavata.* It should be noted that the chondrichthyes are the only vertebrates having an adrenal component which is accurately described as an "interrenal" gland, meaning located between the kidneys, and these fishes are not in the main evolutionary line leading to tetrapods.[6, 12]

Great variation is found among actinopterygian fishes with respect to the condensation and dispersal of the adrenal tissues. These are generally located within or just anterior to the "cephalic kidneys," and occur around the postcardinal veins and their branches (Fig. 10–4). In many species, the so-called "cephalic kidneys" consist largely of lymphoid or myeloid tissue, or both, and hence are blood-forming organs. The two types of adrenal cells are entirely separated in certain species *(Salmo),* but in others they are intermingled *(Cottus).* Branches of the postcardinal veins may be lined with chromaffin cells, which are surrounded by steroidogenic cells.[40, 43]

The corpuscles of Stannius are bodies within the mesonephric kidneys of some teleosts and are thought to arise as proliferations from the urinary ducts (Fig. 10–3). These corpuscles have been considered to play a physiologic role comparable to that of the adrenal cortices of mammals. However, the fact that they differ in embryonic origin and in mode of secretion from established patterns of steriodogenic tissue in teleosts has led many investigators to abandon the view that they are comparable to adrenal cortices.[25] This is supported by the failure of some workers to identify steroids in this tissue. Moreover, the profile of effects that occurs after removal of the corpuscles of Stannius is not consistent with adrenocortical function in fishes.[10] Current information favors the view that the corpuscles of Stannius function primarily in the maintenance of serum calcium levels in environ-

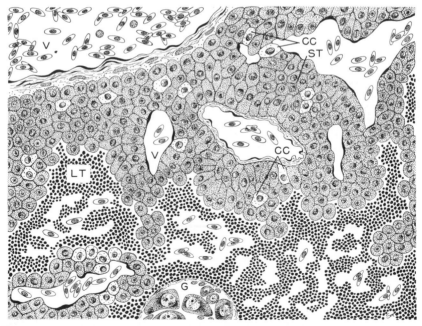

Figure 10–4. Histology of the carp adrenal gland. CC, chromaffin cells; G, ganglion; LT, lymphoid tissue of "head" kidney; ST, steroidogenic tissue; V, vein containing red corpuscles. Camera lucida, ×540.

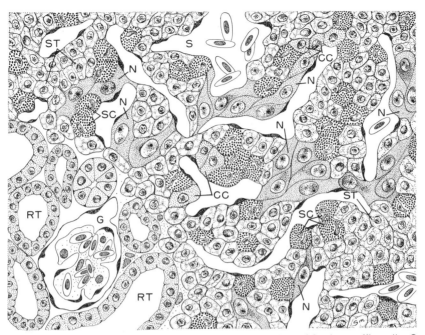

Figure 10–5. Histology of the adrenal gland of *Rana pipiens*. CC, chromaffin cells; G, glomerulus of kidney; N, neuron; RT, renal tubule; S, sinusoid containing red corpuscles; SC, Stilling cells; ST, steroidogenic tissue. Camera lucida, ×540.

ments of high calcium content.[44] Possibly this is accomplished by the release of a protein hormone from these corpuscles. Stanniectomy in several teleosts results in hypercalcemia. This effect can be corrected by injections of extracts of the corpuscle of Stannius or by homotransplants of the gland.

The amphibian adrenal consists of more or less discrete bodies along the ventral surfaces of the kidneys, with the chromaffin and steroidogenic cells being interspersed (Fig. 10–3). At certain points, the adrenal tissue may be completely buried within the kidney, making adrenalectomy practically impossible. The steroidogenic cells are organized into cords which are separated by conspicuous blood sinuses; the chromaffin cells occur singly or in small clusters; and many neurons are present throughout the gland. A characteristic feature of the adrenals of aquatic anurans is the presence of many "Stilling cells" scattered throughout the organs. These cells resemble mast cells and are PAS-positive and eosinophilic (Fig. 10–5). The functional role of the Stilling cells is unknown, but they are said to be absent in three genera of terrestrial toads.[38]

The adrenal glands of reptiles and birds are more compact than in lower forms, and the two types of tissue are intermingled. The adrenals of turtles are discrete bodies on the anterior ventral surfaces of the kidneys; in snakes, the adrenals are some distance anterior to the kidneys (Figs. 10–6 and 10–7). In certain lizards and snakes, the chromaffin cells aggregate to form a distinct band of tissue at the periphery of the organ, partly surrounding the central mass of steroidogenic tissue (Fig. 10–3). The avian adrenals

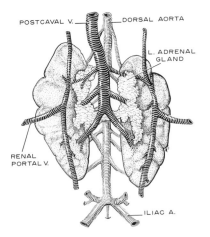
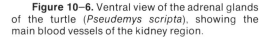

Figure 10–6. Ventral view of the adrenal glands of the turtle (*Pseudemys scripta*), showing the main blood vessels of the kidney region.

are located near the anterior poles of the kidneys and consist of cords of steroidogenic tissue and clusters of chromaffin cells (Figs. 10–8 and 10–9). It is only in mammals that distinct cortices and medullae are present, and even here, there may be considerable interdigitation and intermingling of the two kinds of tissue.[11, 26, 57, 61, 62]

Studies on the adrenal gland of the rat suggest that the production of epinephrine by the medullary cells is regulated by the pituitary-adrenocortical system. The conversion of norepinephrine to epinephrine requires the transfer of a methyl group, and this process is catalyzed by the enzyme phenylethanolamine-N-methyl transferase (PNMT). The activity of this medullary enzyme is markedly reduced after hypophysectomy, but it may be restored by administering either ACTH or glucocorticoids. The ACTH produces its effect by increasing the availability of glucocorticoids from the steroidogenic tissue. Since the glucocorticoids are known to promote protein synthesis in a variety of tissues, it is probable that they elevate PNMT activity by regulating the conditions which are necessary for its synthesis. The evolutionary trend has been toward a closer association of catecholamine-

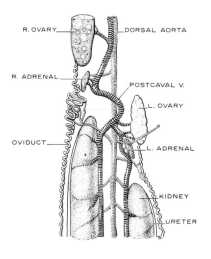

Figure 10–7. Adrenal glands and adnexa of the snake (*Natrix*), from ventral view.

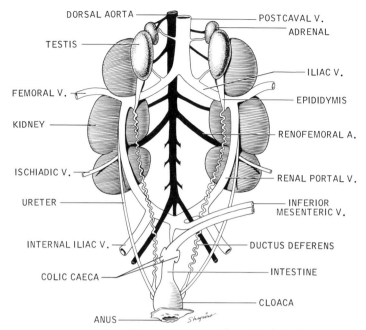

Figure 10–8. Urogenital organs of the male pigeon (*Columba livia*). Both testes are retracted laterally to expose the adrenal glands.

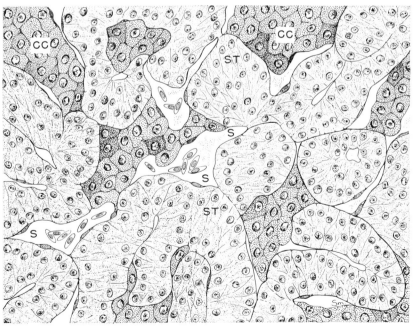

Figure 10-9. Histology of the chicken adrenal gland. CC, chromaffin cells; S, sinusoids containing red corpuscles; ST, steroidogenic tissue. Camera lucida, ×540.

producing tissue and steroid-producing tissue, and, in light of the above observations, this relationship may have some functional significance.[63] The ability of chromaffin cells, and possibly adrenergic neurons, to form epinephrine through the methylation of norepinephrine might conceivably be enhanced by their nearness to the cells that secrete adrenal steroids.

Adrenal Terminology

These glands have been named with reference to their positions with respect to the kidneys, using such prefixes as *ad* (to or near), *inter* (between), *intra* (within), and *supra* (above or over). Confusion often arises through the establishment of a morphologic nomenclature suitable for mammals, before anything is known about the lower vertebrate classes. Since the steroid-producing constituent of the adrenal forms a cortex only in mammals, it is misleading to refer to it as "adrenocortical tissue" in sub-mammalian forms, which have no cortex. Furthermore, *interrenal glands* are present only in chondrichthyean fishes, and, even though they secrete some of the same steroids as the mammalian cortex, it is equally misleading to apply the term "interrenal tissue" to this component in teleosts, amphibians, reptiles, birds, and mammals, in whom the adrenals are not situated between the kidneys, and in whom the glands are a composite of both chromaffin and steroidogenic tissues. There can be no doubt that the interrenal glands of elasmobranchs are homologous and analogous to the adrenal cortices of mammals; and that the scattered aggregations of chromaffin cells in elasmobranchs and other fishes are homologous and analogous to the mammalian medullae. As the situation stands at present, there is no adequate morphologic designation for the steroid-producing tissue in the adrenals of teleosts, amphibians, reptiles, and birds. Perhaps the time has come when it would be desirable to describe the two adrenal components in physiologic rather than morphologic terms.

It is probable that there are extra-adrenal deposits of chromaffin cells in all vertebrates. Catecholamine-containing cells stain brownish with bichromate solutions, and this is generally called the "chromaffin reaction." Other reactions have been utilized, such as the production of a green color with ferric chloride, production of a blue color with ferric-ferricyanide, blackening with osmium tetroxide, and reduction of silver salts and gold chloride. Though there have been recent improvements in staining techniques, there remains some doubt as to how specifically these procedures are capable of identifying epinephrine and norepinephrine in cells.[22, 31] Since the identification of chromaffin cells presents difficulties and yields doubtful results, it seems that more extensive use should be made of the sensitive biologic and chemical assay methods which are now available for the identification of catecholamines in tissue extracts. The cytochemical procedures for identifying "chromaffin cells" are not ideal, and they may stain other elements (mastlike cells), which are capable of storing dopamine and other catecholamines, but probably do not synthesize them. As information accumulates, it may be advantageous to replace the term "chromaffin cells" by a more precise term, such as "catecholamine-containing" cells.

There is no justification for calling the adrenal glands of teleosts, amphibians, reptiles, and birds "interrenal glands," nor does it make sense to refer to the steroid-producing tissue in these groups as "interrenal" or "adrenocortical" tissue. "Steroidogenic" would seem to be a more precise designation for this tissue, though the terms "interrenal tissue" and "adrenocortical tissue" could be retained for chondrichthyeans and mammals, respectively. The term "catecholamine tissue" could safely be applied to the chromaffin cells which comprise integral parts of the adrenal glands.

BIOCHEMISTRY OF THE CATECHOLAMINES

The cells of the adrenal medulla elaborate epinephrine and norepinephrine, often referred to collectively as *catecholamines.* Both hormone molecules contain an asymmetric carbon atom and therefore can exist in two optically active forms. The hormones secreted by the gland are levorotatory (L-forms), whereas those produced by laboratory synthesis are racemic (DL-forms). The mixture is resolved after preparation and the L-form is supplied for clinical use. The L-isomer of epinephrine is about 15 times more active than the D-isomer in elevating the blood pressure of the spinal cat. Commercial preparations made from ox adrenals may contain as much as 20 per cent of norepinephrine. The two hormones are very similar in chemical properties, but the presence of an additional methyl group in epinephrine changes the side chain from a primary amine (norepinephrine) to a secondary amine (epinephrine) (Fig. 10–10). Considerable quantities of ascorbic acid, which is thought to play an important role in maintaining the medullary hormones in the reduced state, are present in the medulla. It has been shown that the vitamin acts *in vitro* to protect these pressor amines from oxidation.

Adrenal extracts contain both epinephrine and norepinephrine, the proportions of which are fairly constant and characteristic for the species. Dopamine, a precursor of norepinephrine, is also found in medullary extracts. The adult human adrenals secrete about 10 times more epinephrine than norepinephrine; the adrenergic nerves of the sympathetic division release only traces of epinephrine. During prenatal life, the human adrenals and the organs of Zuckerkandl contain only norepinephrine. Epinephrine appears after birth, and at 1 year of age the two hormones are present in about equal proportions. The amount of epinephrine gradually increases until it becomes the major amine of the adult adrenal. The reverse appears to be true in chickens; during early life, the adrenal contains mostly epinephrine, whereas norepinephrine predominates in the adult. Chromaffin tumors sometimes appear in the adrenal medulla or wherever chromaffin tissue is found in the body, and in these cases, the quantities of pressor amines in the blood may be increased tremendously.

Since norepinephrine is a transmitter substance released by certain nerve terminals, its distribution in the body is not limited to the adrenal medulla and chromaffin deposits.[50] It has been demonstrated in almost all

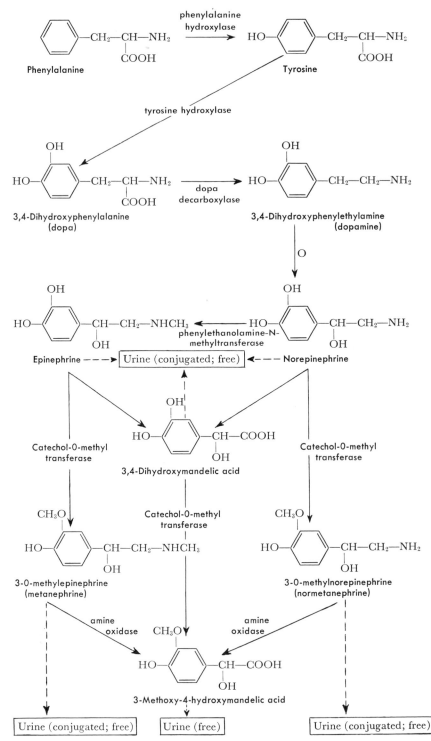

Figure 10–10. Biosynthesis and metabolism of adrenal medullary hormones. (Modified from Cantarow, A., and Schepartz, B.: Biochemistry, 3rd ed. Philadelphia, W. B. Saunders Co., 1962.)

mammalian tissues except the placenta, which lacks nerve fibers. Norepi-nephrine is present in the central nervous system and attains a relatively high concentration in the hypothalamus. The norepinephrine content is highest in nerves that are rich in adrenergic fibers, such as the sympathetic trunk and the splenic and splanchnic nerves. The amount of norepinephrine present in the splenic nerves increases from the proximal toward the distal portion. The amine is synthesized by the nerve cell and stored in the axonic terminals, whence it is passed to the exterior.[14, 17, 21, 23]

In recent years, a considerable amount of information about the distri-bution of catecholamines has been derived through the perfection of a technique by Hillarp and Falck for the histochemical demonstration of the presence of catecholamines and 5-hydroxytryptamine (5-HT, serotonin).[24] Under appropriate conditions, dopa, dopamine, epinephrine, and norepi-nephrine give rise to yellow or green fluorescent products by condensing with formaldehyde. While it is still somewhat risky to attempt to distinguish among the various amines on the basis of color production alone, the tech-niques can be used in conjunction with others.[48] With the use of the fluo-rescence technique, the distribution of these monoamines in the brain of several species of amphibians, reptiles, and mammals has been delineated.

Spindle-shaped cells giving the chromaffin reaction have been de-scribed in various tissues and are especially abundant in the skin and lungs. There is little direct information regarding the capacity of chromaffin cells outside the adrenal medulla to produce catechol hormones. After degenera-tion of the adrenergic nerves to an organ, almost all of the norepinephrine in the organ disappears, whereas the epinephrine content may be slightly increased. If the adrenergic fibers regenerate and re-establish connections with the organ, the level of norepinephrine in the organ is restored. This may indicate that chromaffin cells within the organ do not degenerate after denervation and continue to secrete epinephrine. Sectioning of the pregan-glionic sympathetic fibers does not diminish the norepinephrine content of an organ, showing that the synthesis of norepinephrine by the postgan-glionic neuron is not dependent on impulses delivered to it over the pregan-glionic fibers. The norepinephrine content of sympathetic effectors is closely correlated with the number of adrenergic fibers that supply them. Since adrenergic nerves can release norepinephrine continuously on re-peated stimulation over long periods, it must be synthesized rapidly and there would appear to be some provision for the intra-axonal storage of the neurohumor.

Cellular Origin of the Hormones

Electron microscopic studies of chromaffin cells have demonstrated that they contain large numbers of dense osmiophilic granules, ranging in diameter from 100 to 400 mμ. These granules are surrounded by mem-branes, and appear to originate in the Golgi region of the cell. They contain a very high content of catecholamines and adenosine triphosphate (ATP). The hormones are liberated rapidly when the granules are placed in hypotonic solutions. Exposure of the granules to high temperatures also causes a prompt release of pressor amines. It is probable that the granules do not leave the cell but only discharge their contents on stimulation. The normal stimulus for the discharge of medullary hormones is acetylcholine, which is liberated by the splanchnic nerve terminals that come in contact with the medullary cells. The mechanism of release remains unknown; however, it is possible that ATP is implicated. It is interesting to note that acetylcholine does not induce the liberation of pressor amines when added to a suspension of granules in isotonic sucrose solution.[48] However, the sympathomimetic amine *tyramine* does have this capacity. By comparing denervated adrenals with normal ones, it has been found that nerve impulses arriving at the gland do not appreciably change the distribution of pressor amines between the granules and the nongranular cytoplasm.[7, 19, 32]

As with other endocrine glands secreting multiple hormones, the question arises of whether both hormones are secreted by the same cell or whether there are separate cells for the production of each hormone. Evidence favoring the view that there are two cell types is based on: (1) histochemical studies indicating that different cells in the medulla stain selectively for either norepinephrine or epinephrine; (2) the isolation from medullary extracts of granules differing in their relative content of the two amines; and (3) the capacity of different stimuli to release epinephrine or norepinephrine selectively. Studies on human subjects indicate that active aggressive emotional displays are associated with the urinary excretion of norepinephrine, while tense, but passive, emotional displays increase the excretion of epinephrine without affecting the excretion of norepinephrine.[9, 20, 36]

The adrenal venous blood of the cat contains more norepinephrine than epinephrine. Stimulation of the sciatic nerve or the application of other painful stimuli encourages the secretion of epinephrine; clamping the carotid arteries produces a reflexive vasoconstriction and the adrenal medullae secrete mostly norepinephrine. After denervation of the cat's adrenal, the output of norepinephrine is reduced to very low levels. Reducing the blood sugar by administering insulin causes an augmented release of epinephrine, but the intravenous injection of excessive glucose diminishes the secretion of epinephrine without affecting the secretion of norepinephrine. This is consistent with the fact that epinephrine possesses more hyperglycemic activity than does norepinephrine. Stimulation of a particular area of the hypothalamus causes mainly epinephrine to appear in the adrenal venous blood; stimulation of another area promotes the appearance of norepinephrine in the venous effluent. These observations indicate that epinephrine and norepinephrine may be released separately by the medulla and support the concept that the hormones arise from different medullary components.

Whether the two hormones originate from one or two cell types cannot be stated at present. The various histochemical techniques lack absolute specificity. Furthermore, studies on depleted glands show that norepinephrine reappears in advance of epinephrine, and this suggests that previous functional activity would have an effect on the proportions of the two hormones extractable from them. Granular fractions containing mostly norepinephrine may represent immature stages that would eventually form epi-nephrine.[30, 37]

Biosynthesis and Metabolism of the Catecholamines

The amino acids are extremely important compounds since the body uses them for numerous purposes. The protein complex of the organism is constantly changing; some proteins are continuously being broken down and new tissue proteins are being synthesized. The products of tissue protein breakdown and the amino acids derived from dietary proteins produce a common metabolic pool of nitrogen from which the tissues may withdraw the necessary amino acids for their repair, maintenance and growth. Unless the amino acids are promptly incorporated into tissue or other proteins, they undergo deamination and are lost so far as protein synthesis is concerned. Amino acids, therefore, are essential for the repair and growth of tissues, as well as for the synthesis of normal supplies of hormones, vitamins, and other substances. Tyrosine or phenylalanine, for example, are essential for producing such hormones as thyroxine and epinephrine. The synthesis of insulin, glucagon, and the various hormones of the pituitary gland makes heavy demands on the amino acid pool of the body.[41]

The amino acids phenylalanine and tyrosine are generally regarded as precursors of epinephrine. The main biosynthetic pathway is phenylalanine → tyrosine → dopa → dopamine → norepinephrine → epinephrine, as shown in Figure 10–10. Tyrosine is oxidized to dopa, and this is decarboxylated to dopamine, which is oxidized to norepinephrine. The lattar is methylated to form epinephrine.[2] In nervous tissue, in which norepinephrine functions as a chemical transmitter, very little, if any, epinephrine is formed. It is believed by some workers that the end-product of catecholamine biosynthesis may be dopamine in certain tissues (*e.g.,* lungs, intestine, liver) where it acts as a local hormone. Epinephrine and norepinephrine may exist in the blood plasma in the free form or undergo conjugation with sulfate or glucuronide; most of the circulating epinephrine is bound to blood proteins, mainly albumin. Norepinephrine does not bind to blood proteins to such a great extent.

The catecholamines disappear very rapidly from the circulation. Both may be present in the urine as free or conjugated forms. Their metabolic degradation involves methylation, effected by the enzyme catechol-O-methyl transferase, and deamination and oxidation, effected by amine oxidase. The metabolites appearing in the blood and urine are inactive, and the most abundant ones are 3-methoxy-4-hydroxymandelic acid, metanephrine, and normetanephrine (Fig. 10–10).[3, 4, 18, 39, 47]

The Neurohumors

Evidence has accumulated to demonstrate convincingly that nerve cells release a variety of physiologically active agents. We have divided these into two classes: (1) *Neurohormones* are considered to be the products of neurosecretory cells which are discharged into the circulation to act as hormones upon distant target tissues and organs, and (2) *neurohumors* are the transmitter agents released at the synapse and are largely destroyed before reaching the blood.

Although epinephrine and norepinephrine are hormones of chromaffin tissue, norepinephrine is also released as a neurohumor by most postganglionic sympathetic nerve endings. It is possible that adrenergic nerves may release small amounts of epinephrine, but the great mass of evidence indicates that norepinephrine is the neurotransmitter. The postganglionic neurons in the splenic nerves contain large quantities of norepinephrine, but almost no epinephrine. Extracts of organs that receive sympathetic innervation usually contain both epinephrine and norepinephrine, but the latter amine disappears from these organs after the nerves are sectioned and allowed to degenerate. Epinephrine continues to be produced by such denervated organs and probably emanates from chromaffin cells within the organ rather than being contained in the neurons. These observations indicate that the transmitter agent of adrenergic nerves is norepinephrine only and not actually a mixture of norepinephrine and epinephrine. Some dopamine may be present with norepinephrine at the nerve terminals.[35]

Bilaterally adrenalectomized human beings excrete practically no epinephrine in the urine, but the urinary levels of norepinephrine remain within normal limits. The norepinephrine must come from some extra-adrenal source, most probably from the adrenergic nerves. Furthermore, in adrenalectomized subjects there continues to be a diurnal variation in the excretion of norepinephrine. More of the amine appears in the urine during wakefulness than during sleep, as in normal subjects. Even changes from the recumbent to the standing position increase the urinary output of norepinephrine. These observations strengthen the concept that norepinephrine, rather than epinephrine, is the neurohumoral transmitter of the sympathetic nervous system.

PHYSIOLOGY OF THE CHROMAFFIN CELL HORMONES

Comparative Effects of Epinephrine and Norepinephrine

Although these two medullary hormones are similar in some of their biologic actions, there are important differences in the nature and degree of their effects (Table 10–1). Both hormones increase the heart rate, although epinephrine is the more potent in this respect. Both increase systolic blood pressure, whereas epinephrine has no effect on diastolic pressure. The hypertensive effect of norepinephrine is a consequence of increased peripheral resistance; that of epinephrine results from an increased cardiac output in spite of decreased total peripheral resistance. Epinephrine increases the blood flow through skeletal muscle, liver, and brain, whereas norepinephrine either has no effect or decreases it. Both hormones pro-

Table 10–1 CONTRASTED ACTIONS OF EPINEPHRINE AND NOREPINEPHRINE

| SYSTEM | FUNCTION | EFFECT | | RELATIVE ACTIVITY |
		EPINEPHRINE	NOREPINEPHRINE	E/N*
Cardio-vascular	Peripheral resistance	Decreased	Increased	—
	Systolic B. P.	Increased	Increased	0.5
	Diastolic B. P.	No effect	Increased	—
	Heart rate	Increased	Slightly increased	20
	Cardiac output	Increased	No change	—
	Blood vessels in denervated limb	Vasodilatation	Vasoconstriction	—
	Coronary vessels	Vasodilatation	Vasodilatation	—
	Pulse rate	Increased	Decreased	—
	Eosinophil count	Increased	No effect	—
	Net peripheral vascular effect	Vasodilatation	Limited vasodilator actions; over-all vasoconstriction	—
Blood flow through individual organs	Skeletal muscle	100% increase	Unaltered or decreased	—
	Liver	100% increase	No material effect	—
	Brain	20% increase	Slight decrease	—
	Kidney	40% decrease	20% decrease	2
Respiratory system	Bronchial muscle	Inhibition	Inhibition	20
Carbohydrate metabolism	Blood sugar	Increased	Increased	4
Eye	Pupillary dilators	Excitation	Excitation	15
Intestine	Small	Inhibition	Inhibition	2
	Large	Inhibition	Inhibition	1
Genital system	Nonpregnant uterus (rat, cat)	Inhibition	Inhibition	100
Central nervous system (man)	Mental state	Anxiety	No effect	—

*E = epinephrine; N = norepinephrine.

duce constriction of the skin capillaries and cause pallor. Renal blood flow is diminished by both hormones. The net peripheral vascular effect of epinephrine is to cause vasodilation; norepinephrine exerts limited vasodilator actions, but its over-all effect is to produce vasoconstriction. Epinephrine is very potent in increasing oxygen consumption and glucose output from the liver, but norepinephrine is relatively weak in these respects.

The adrenal medulla functions in conjunction with the sympathetic nervous system and is intimately concerned with emotional adjustments. The medullary hormones are released in response to sympathetic stimulation, and this division of the autonomic system is integrated by components involving the cerebral cortices, midbrain, and hypothalamus. Although the two amines are related chemically and biologically, they appear to be released independently and to perform separate and distinct roles in the economy of the organism. Anticipatory states tend to elevate the release of norepinephrine more than epinephrine, but in intense emotional reactions, the release of both amines is elevated. The actions of epinephrine seem suitable to equip the organism to meet certain kinds of emergency situations: It acts to prevent hypoglycemia by stimulating metabolism and mobilizing glycogen as glucose; it redistributes the blood, draining it out of the skin and forcing it into important organs, such as skeletal muscle, liver, and brain. Norepinephrine is predominantly present at sympathetic endings and seems to function largely as a pressor hormone normally required for the maintenance of blood pressure. With the exception of the coronary arteries, norepinephrine produces general vasoconstriction and stimulates the heart, but it is relatively impotent in its metabolic actions.

Actions of Epinephrine

Carbohydrate Metabolism

Epinephrine increases the blood sugar level and is one of the most important factors in the normal organism for counteracting the hypoglycemic action of insulin[28] (Fig. 10–11). Emotional excitement, injury, and exercise, as well as the administration of certain anesthetics (ether, morphine), cause an augmented release of epinephrine and a consequent elevation of blood sugar. A low level of blood sugar, resulting from any cause, has a stimulatory effect on the adrenal medulla, and epinephrine operates to bring the glucose level back to normal. Epinephrine exerts its hyperglycemic action by increasing the rate of glycogenolysis in the liver and mus-

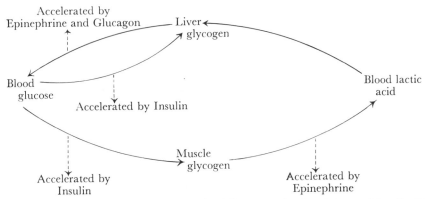

Figure 10–11. Diagram showing the major influences of epinephrine and insulin on the distribution of carbohydrate in the body. (After West and Todd: Textbook of Biochemistry.)

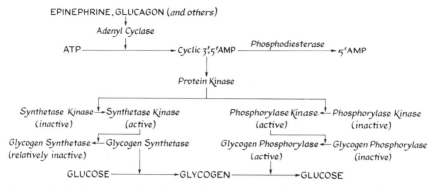

Figure 10–12. Diagrammatic interpretation of epinephrine and glucagon effects on glycogen mobilization.

cles. Under the influence of the hormone, both liver and muscle glycogen are converted to hexose phosphate and, in the liver, glucose is formed by the action of a phosphatase. Muscle lacks this phosphatase and completes the glycolytic process with the formation of lactic acid. The muscle may resynthesize some of the lactic acid to glycogen, but much of it escapes into the blood and is carried to the liver, where it is converted to glycogen or glucose. After the injection of epinephrine, the hepatic glycogen stores are generally higher than normal, owing to the synthesis of glycogen from lactate that had been released from the muscles.

According to current thought epinephrine and glucagon mediate their effects on glycogen metabolism by a scheme of enzyme activation operating through the "second messenger," cyclic AMP (Fig. 10–12).[51, 52, 53] Through an interaction with its receptor, the hormone activates the enzyme adenylate cyclase, leading to the synthesis of cylic AMP which, in turn, activates another group of enzymes generically designated as protein kinase (Fig. 10–12). Through the action of protein kinase, both the phosphorylase and synthetase systems are activated. Accordingly, glucose is ultimately released through the action of glycogen phosphorylase, and at the same time glycogen formation is reduced because glycogen synthetase is inactivated. The existence of this dual control system is necessary to regulate enhanced glycogen synthesis in the face of higher glucose levels following glycogen breakdown.

The chain of enzymatic events following activation of protein kinase by cylic AMP is part of biochemical amplification.[27] During the "cascade" of enzymatic steps, the initiating hormone stimulus is amplified some 100 times at each of the enzymatic events involved in the process (Fig. 10–13). This results from the fact that in each of the steps in this system the enzyme can transform about 100 molecules of substrate into product in a few seconds. Theoretically, following this 100-fold amplification by each of the four enzymes, one molecule of initiating hormone is responsible for the release of 100 million molecules of glucose.

Epinephrine also influences carbohydrate metabolism indirectly by

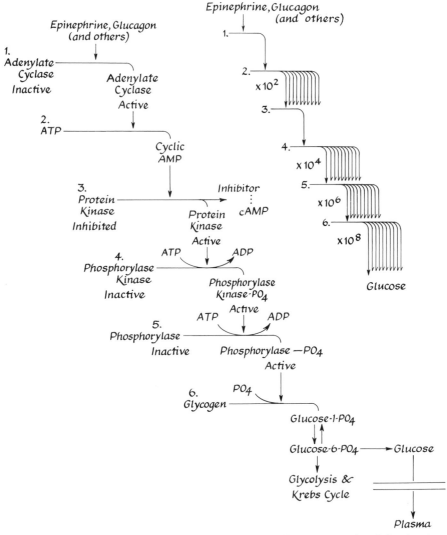

Figure 10–13. Formation of glucose in response to glucagon or epinephrine involves a "cascade" of enzymatic steps, beginning with the activation of adenylate cyclase. Biochemical "amplification" (sequence at right) occurs at four of the steps, through the capacity of a single estimated to be at least 10^2. Through this process, a single molecule of hormone can release at least 10^8 molecules of glucose. (From Goldberg, N. D., Hospital Practice, May 1974.)

stimulating the adenohypophysis to release ACTH. It is not known whether epinephrine activates the pituitary gland directly, or indirectly through connections in the hypothalamic portion of the brain. In any case, the ACTH augments the release of steroids from the adrenal cortex, and the 11-oxygenated hormones are extremely potent in promoting the synthesis of carbohydrate from protein.

Some workers have found that epinephrine depresses the rate at which the tissues use glucose. Epinephrine reduces glucose tolerance, and the arteriovenous glucose difference is slight even when the arterial blood contains much glucose. If there is an actual inhibition of glucose utilization, it may be due in part to the action of adrenocortical steroids. There is also some evidence that epinephrine may act at the level of the cell membrane and reduce the rate of entry of glucose into the cells.

Epinephrine exerts more marked effects on carbohydrate metabolism in some mammalian species than in others, the rabbit being much more sensitive than the human being, dog, cat, or rat. Hyperglycemia may result from doses that do not produce any elevation of blood pressure. Norepinephrine, in contrast to epinephrine, produces very slight changes in carbohydrate metabolism. Animals deprived of the adrenal medulla recover very slowly from hypoglycemia, which is probably accounted for on the basis of the relative inability of norepinephrine to mobilize glycogen stores. Muscle glycogenolysis fails to occur in demedullated animals, even when they are subjected to operative trauma or severe hypoglycemia. This suggests that the medulla is the principal source of circulating epinephrine and that the norepinephrine released by adrenergic nerves does not attain circulatory titers sufficient to have this effect.

The effects of epinephrine and norepinephrine on carbohydrate metabolism in some fishes have been studied and represent some of our best knowledge of the functions of the adrenal medulla in poikilotherms. Responses to epinephrine are somewhat variable; however, in general it can be said that epinephrine administration induces hyperglycemia in some chondrichthyean fishes,[45] lampreys,[5] and teleosts.[64] Norepinephrine seems to be less effective in this regard in some species, but it appears to have clear hypoglycemic activities in the holocephalian, *Hydrolagus.*

Epinephrine increases oxygen consumption and basal metabolic rate when given in moderate amounts; large doses may produce the opposite effect. Cold-adapted rats have an increased ability to produce heat by means other than muscular contraction. Although norepinephrine has little calorigenic effect in warm-adapted rats, it markedly elevates the oxygen consumption of cold-adapted rats without producing a hyperglycemia.[34] Hyperkalemia, or a rise in serum potassium, typically follows epinephrine treatment.

In summary, epinephrine elevates the blood sugar in three ways: (1) by mobilizing the carbohydrate stores of the liver; (2) by encouraging the transformation of muscle glycogen into lactic acid, from which the liver manufactures new carbohydrate; and (3) by stimulating the adenohypophysis to secrete ACTH, which causes the release of adrenal cortical hormones having an effect on glyconeogenesis. There is evidence that epinephrine acts in some manner to depress the utilization of carbohydrate by tissues. Since hypoglycemia elicits the secretion of epinephrine and hyperglycemia stimulates the secretion of insulin, it is apparent that these two hormones are important in the homestatic regulation of blood sugar levels (Fig. 10–11).

Cardiovascular System

The catecholamines affect the heart and blood vessels in many different ways, but it should be understood that these effects can be influenced by many factors, such as compensatory reflex adjustments, dosage, manner and rate of administration, and the species. Epinephrine is a powerful heart stimulant, increasing the frequency (positive chronotropic effect), force (positive inotropic effect), and amplitude of contraction. Systolic blood pressure, pulse rate, and cardiac output are increased. Small doses of epinephrine can increase the cardiac output without elevating the blood pressure. Norepinephrine, in contrast, is a powerful vasoconstrictor and raises both the systolic and diastolic pressures, but it does not produce much change in the cardiac output (Table 10–1). Tachycardia typically follows epinephrine treatment, but bradycardia often follows norepinephrine injections. The elevated blood pressure resulting from norepinephrine usually causes a reflexive increase in vagal tone and a slowing of the heart. These differences in the cardiovascular effects of the two amines are due largely to the fact that epinephrine reduces peripheral resistance by producing dilatation of the vascular bed of the skeletal muscles; norepinephrine causes a rise in total peripheral resistance by constricting the vessels in the muscles, skin, and viscera. When applied locally to the skin and mucous membranes, both hormones produce pallor by diverting blood away from the smaller capillaries and into a few main vascular channels.

The pharmacologic actions of epinephrine may be demonstrated by applying them to isolated organs, or strips of organs, suspended in physiologic solutions. When they are applied to isolated mammalian hearts, the contractions increase in rate and amplitude. The denervated mammalian heart is accelerated by as little as 1 part of epinephrine in 1.4 billion parts of fluid. Muscular contractions in intestinal strips from the rabbit are inhibited by the addition of small quantities of epinephrine or norepinephrine. It must be recognized that the reactions elicited in excised organs or in anesthetized animals are not necessarily indicative of the responses that would be obtained in the normal intact subject, in whom compensatory adjustments may be accomplished by nervous reflexes.

Nervous System

The injection of epinephrine to normal human subjects produces a feeling of restlessness and anxiety and a sense of fatigue, whereas norepinephrine does not produce such symptoms. Hence, the two hormones have different effects on the central nervous system.

It has been known for a long time that tissues and organs supplied by the sympathetic nerves are made more sensitive to the catechol hormones by denervation, but there is no satisfactory explanation of this phenomenon. Possibly the concentrations of enzymes that destroy the adrenergic transmitter (norepinephrine) may diminish in the organs after the nerves have degenerated. Ephedrine has been reported to inhibit the action of amine oxidase and thereby to potentiate the effects of the catechol hormones and also to increase the effects produced by stimulation of the adrenergic nerves.

Thyroid

There is general agreement that hyperthyroidism causes an increased sensitivity to epinephrine and that hypothyroidism causes tolerance to epinephrine. The ability of epinephrine to elevate the blood sugar in guinea pigs is strikingly reduced by thyroidectomy. There are reports that the level of amine oxidase in the liver and in blood is decreased by thyroxine injections and increased by thyroidectomy or the administration of antithyroid agents. This may account in part for the exaggerated effects of the catecholamines when they are administered to hyperthyroid animals.

Pigmentary Effectors

The pigment cells of many teleost fishes and reptiles are richly supplied with autonomic nerve fibers, and color changes may be effected by stimulating or sectioning these fibers. The release of neurohumoral agents by the nerve terminals appears to be the most important factor in regulating the chromatophores in those forms in which the chromatophores are directly innervated. Epinephrine-like compounds also affect chromatophores that are not innervated and generally evoke a concentration of pigment-containing organelles; however, in some cases, catecholamines cause a dispersal of these organelles.

Some Miscellaneous Actions

Epinephrine generally reduces the level of circulating eosinophils by its action on ACTH release and a consequent increase in the production of adrenocortical hormones. Mitotic activity in tissues *in vitro* is suppressed by epinephrine.[8] The clotting time of blood is reduced by exogenous epinephrine, but the mechanism of this action is poorly understood. The medullary hormones have important effects on water and electrolyte metabolism, but these reactions are complex and varied.

Nonesterified fatty acids are produced from rat adipose tissue when it is incubated *in vitro* with either epinephrine or norepinephrine. The hormones presumably promote the hydrolysis of neutral fats within the tissue. The L-isomers are much more active than the D-isomers, which suggests that this is the type of response that might occur within the organism.[60] Lipolysis induced by catecholamines seems to be mediated through cyclic AMP. Epinephrine differs from ACTH in not requiring ionized calcium for this lipolytic effect.

ADRENERGIC RECEPTOR CONCEPT[42]

The response of tissues to catecholamine stimulation depends upon the presence of adrenergic receptor sites. The existence of such receptors was suggested early by Sir Henry Dale following experiments which demonstrated that the alkaloid *ergot* blocked only some effects of epinephrine.[16] Subsequently, it was revealed that two separate sets of responses to an array of epinephrine-like compounds (sympathomimetic amines) occurs, and it was demonstrated that the response to one or more of these compounds could be blocked by certain drugs. On this basis, Ahlquist concluded that two different adrenergic receptor sites exist, which he designated *alpha* and *beta*.[1] The alpha receptors mediate responses of four common sympathomimetic amines having the following order of potency: Epinephrine (E)> norepinephrine (NE)> phenylephrine (PE)> isoproterenol (ISO), while beta receptors mediate responses for which the order of potency is ISO > E > NE > PE. Responses mediated by alpha receptors can be antagonized by a variety of agents, such as ergot alkaloids, phentolamine, dibenamine, and others, which exhibit little antagonism toward responses mediated by beta receptors. Similarly, another group of such blocking agents, including dichloroisoproterenol (DCI), propranolol, and pronethalol specifically block responses mediated through beta receptors.

In general, the alpha adrenergic receptor is associated with vasoconstriction, myometrial contraction, retraction of the third eyelid, contraction of the pupil, and relaxation of intestinal muscle. The beta receptor is associated with vasodilation, relaxation of smooth muscle of bronchi, intestine, and uterus, and the adrenergic-positive cardiac inotropic and chronotropic effects. Norepinephrine primarily mediates its responses through the alpha receptors, while epinephrine effects operate through both alpha and beta receptors. Synthetic compounds such as isoproterenol mediate their effects largely through the beta receptors. A responsive tissue may possess either or both alpha and beta receptors. The presence of both receptors on blood vessels can explain why epinephrine serves as a vasoconstrictor except in the presence of blocking agents, when it becomes vasodilatory. Heart muscles possess mainly beta receptors. Accordingly, exogenous norepinephrine has little effect on the heart because it does not operate through the beta receptor. On the other hand, exogenous epinephrine exerts both inotropic and chronotropic effects through the mediation of the beta receptor.

The presence of adrenergic receptors is not restricted only to tissues that are normally innervated. For example, the pigment cells of the amphibian *Rana* and the lizard *Anolis,* which are known to be noninnervated, possess either or both alpha and beta receptors. The unusual darkening of toads in response to catecholamine stimulation apparently is due to the presence of only beta receptors on their melanophores. Similarly, fat cells and toad bladder cells are known to contain adrenergic receptors. Recently, evidence has accumulated indicating that some cyclic AMP-mediated epinephrine effects are regulated through differential adrenergic receptor stimulation.[55] From an examination of epinephrine effects on isolated rat pancreas, isolated fat cells, and toad bladder in the presence and absence of alpha and beta blocking agents, it has been concluded that stimulation of the alpha adrenergic receptor decreases cyclic AMP synthesis while stimulation of the beta receptor leads to an elevation of the cyclic AMP level. The mechanism by which adrenergic receptor stimulation affects intracellular levels of cyclic AMP is not known; however, studies of the characteristics of the binding of epinephrine to the receptor show promise of helping to solve this problem as well as that of the nature of the adrenergic receptors, themselves. An investigation of the binding of epinephrine and glucagon to isolated rat liver membranes reveals that both hormones bind to specific receptor proteins that are distinct from adenylate cyclase.[54] Thus, at least one intervening step occurs between binding of the hormone and adenylate cyclase stimulation. At least two protein-epinephrine complexes are present in the membrane, and it seems that the two ring hydroxyls of epinephrine are important in the binding. The beta blocking agent, propranolol, inhibits the binding of epinephrine to the plasma membrane. The fact that both glucagon and epinephrine have a higher affinity for isolated plasma membranes than for other membranes, e.g., nuclear, mitochondrial, and endoplasmic reticulum, is consistent with the receptor concept.

THE AUTONOMIC NERVOUS SYSTEM

Some general features of the autonomic nervous system are mentioned here as an aid to understanding the roles performed by the catecholamines in the economy of the organism.

Anatomic Organization

The peripheral nervous system is composed of the craniospinal nerves and the components of the autonomic system. The latter is an aggregation of ganglia, nerves, and plexuses through which efferent innervation is supplied for the heart, glands, and smooth muscle in diverse locations. The autonomic fibers are connected so intimately with the central nervous system that the two cannot be delimited anatomically. The autonomic system is controlled mainly by the hypothalamic portion of the brain. Hence the autonomic nerves constitute a functional rather than an anatomic division of the nervous system. The general anatomic features are indicated in Figure 10–14. The sympathetic division, or the thoracolumbar outflow, is shown on the right side of the figure, while the parasympathetic division, or craniosacral outflow, is shown on the left.

Sympathetic Division. The sympathetic ganglia are of two types, vertebral and collateral. The vertebral group consists of approximately 22 pairs of ganglia united by intervening fiber tracts in such a manner as to form a chain along the right and left sides of the vertebral column. These sympathetic chains extend from the level of the first cervical vertebra to the anterior surface of the coccyx. The largest of the collateral (prevertebral) ganglia

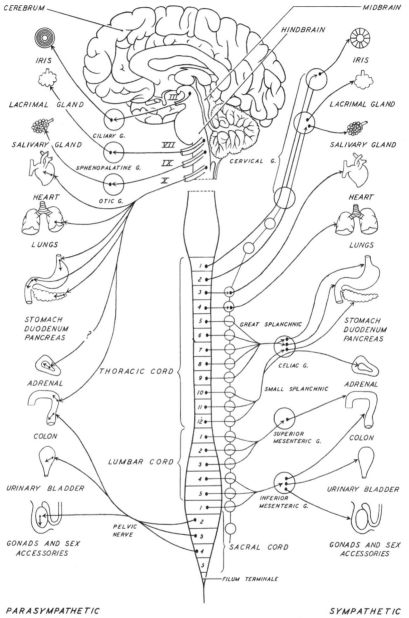

Figure 10–14. Diagram of the autonomic nervous system. The parasympathetic division is shown on the left, the sympathetic division on the right. Roman numerals refer to cranial nerves.

are the celiac, superior mesenteric, and inferior mesenteric. The *preganglionic neurons* extend from the gray matter of the central nervous system to one of the ganglia where they make synaptic connections with *postganglionic neurons* that extend from the ganglia to the effector organs. The cell bodies of the preganglionic neurons of the thoracolumbar outflow are contained within the gray matter of the thoracic and lumbar regions of the spinal cord. These fibers, together with ordinary somatic efferent fibers, emerge from the cord through the anterior roots of the spinal nerves. The preganglionic fibers soon separate from the somatic efferent fibers of the anterior roots and terminate in a ganglion.

Most of the spinal nerves emerging from these regions of the cord are connected with the vertebral ganglia by means of the *white rami communicantes.* The preganglionic neurons may form synapses with postganglionic neurons within the vertebral ganglia that they first enter, they may pass through one or more ganglia and form synapses within other vertebral ganglia at higher or lower levels, or they may pass uninterruptedly through the vertebral ganglia and establish synapses within one of the collateral ganglia. The cell bodies of the postganglionic neurons, together with their dendritic ramifications, lie within the sympathetic ganglia. The axons of the postganglionic neurons, unlike the preganglionic neurons, are usually unmyelinated. The postganglionic axons either course through the sympathetic nerves to the viscera or enter spinal nerves to reach the body wall and skin. All the spinal nerves are connected to corresponding ganglia of the sympathetic chains by means of the *gray rami communicantes,* through which they receive fibers from the sympathetic trunks.

There are usually many more postganglionic fibers leaving the sympathetic ganglia than there are preganglionics coming to them. The numerous synaptic connections in the sympathetic system make possible an extensive dissemination of impulses. The preganglionic sympathetic fibers to the adrenal are unusual inasmuch as they make no ganglionic connections before terminating in the medullary portion of the gland.

Parasympathetic Division. The cell bodies of the preganglionic neurons of the parasympathetic system or craniosacral outflow are situated within the midbrain, hindbrain, and sacral region of the spinal cord. The preganglionic fibers of the cranial component of the parasympathetic system are contained within the oculomotor, facial, glossopharyngeal, and vagus nerves. The preganglionic fibers of the sacral constituent emerge in the anterior roots of the corresponding sacral nerves and proceed to the pelvic organs as the pelvic nerves. It will be noted that the preganglionic fibers of the parasympathetic system are long and end within terminal ganglia located in or close to the effector organs. Thus, the postganglionic axons of the parasympathetic nerves are relatively short. Like the fibers of the sympathetic system, the preganglionics are myelinated, whereas the postganglionics are unmyelinated.

Visceral Sensory Nerve Supply. While it has been traditional to consider the autonomic system as purely efferent, it should not be inferred that the visceral organs lack a sensory or afferent nerve supply. The afferent fibers from the viscera transmit impulses from the various internal organs to the brain and spinal cord. Their cell bodies are located in the dorsal root ganglia or in similar cranial ganglia, and they have no synapses in either the spinal or sympathetic ganglia.

General Actions of the Autonomic System

Most of the visceral organs are doubly innervated, and in general, the sympathetic and parasympathetic components exert antagonistic actions. Thus, stimulation of the parasympathetic fibers within the vagi slows the rhythmic contractions of the heart, whereas sympathetic stimulation accelerates heart action. The contractility of the heart is due basically to a mechanism within its own walls, but the autonomic system modifies this activity. The parasympathetic fibers to the stomach and small intestine augment gastrointestinal processes, whereas the sympathetic fibers to the same organs are inhibitory. The term "autonomic" is not entirely appropriate when applied to this portion of the peripheral nervous system since it is dependent on the brain and cord and is unable to function as an independent unit. The term signifies, however, that this system of neurons is concerned with the regulation of physiologic processes that are beneath consciousness and hence proceed in the absence of voluntary control.

In spite of the diversified functions of the sympathetic division, this system is not essential for life. Large parts of it have been surgically removed from human subjects without serious impairment of function. Sympathectomized animals, particularly cats, have been maintained in good health for long periods under laboratory conditions, but the effects of the operation become evident when such animals are subjected to emergencies and to unfavorable environments. Obviously, these animals would succumb if forced to struggle for existence in a hazardous environment. They are incapable of arduous physical work, do not adjust properly to changing temperatures, and are unable to become physically aroused when attacked by enemies.

It is common practice to designate autonomic neurons as *adrenergic* or *cholinergic*. Neurons that release norepinephrine are adrenergic; those that release acetylcholine and similar agents are cholinergic. Most of the postganglionic neurons of the sympathetic system are adrenergic; all of the preganglionic neurons of both sympathetic and parasympathetic divisions are cholinergic. Most of the postganglionic neurons of the parasympathetics, as well as the ordinary somatic motor neurons terminating in skeletal muscles, are cholinergic.

In addition to the catecholamines and acetylcholine, 5-hydroxytryptamine and a number of other substances have been identified as neurohumoral substances. If neurons are to be identifed on the basis of the kind of neurohumor they produce, more categories than adrenergic and cholinergic are needed.[58]

Since the isolation of epinephrine in 1901, many similarities between the systemic effects of exogenous epinephrine and those produced by stimulation of the sympathetic nerves have been recognized. However, certain discrepancies between the two become apparent and could not be accounted for until norepinephrine became available for experimental purposes. For example, stimulation of the splenic nerve of the cat stimulates the denervated heart, but it does not cause relaxation of the uterus; small amounts of exogenous epinephrine produce both effects. It appears that this nerve produces norepinephrine in quantities sufficient to affect the denervated heart, but this amine is known to have very weak effects on the uterus of the cat. Norepinephrine is the only neurohumor convincingly demonstrated to be produced by the adrenergic terminals of mammals. Although traces of epinephrine are also present at these endings, it remains to be determined whether this amine arises from the nerve cells themselves or from extra-axonal chromaffin cells which may be closely associated with them.[21]

FUNCTIONAL UTILITY OF THE CATECHOLAMINES

Progress in understanding the functional role of the adrenal medulla has been slow for a number of reasons. Among these are: (1) the presence of extramedullary chromaffin deposits that presumably secrete catecholamines, (2) the production of no profound disturbances by removal of the adrenal medulla, (3) the former belief that the adrenal medulla secreted only epinephrine, (4) the uncertainty regarding the nature of the adrenergic neurohumor, and (5) the fact that the actions of exogenous epinephrine may be modified or reversed by several means. Although norepinephrine was synthesized in 1904, its importance as a medullary hormone and as a sympathetic neurhumor was not recognized until 1948. Since then, the functional roles of the adrenal medulla and sympathetic division have become clearer, though there are still many gaps.

The adrenal medulla is the source of two or more hormones and its functional state is regulated by a direct nerve supply. Centers in the hypothalamus control medullary secretion via the splanchnic nerves. While it is not known that the hormones are elaborated by separate medullary cells, they can be released independently. Since the medulla is under constant stimulation by nerve impulses originating throughout the body, it is generally agreed that there is a basal level of production of hormones. This basal rate of secretion fluctuates with normal body activities and is tremendously increased during emergencies. Medullary activity is accelerated chiefly by hypoglycemia and by exposure to stressor stimuli, such as severe temperature changes, trauma, hemorrhage, combat, attack, and so on.[4, 15]

There is much evidence to support the emergency theory of epinephrine function, as proposed by Cannon, and the concept appears to be generally accepted. The adrenal medulla usually secretes more epinephrine than norepinephrine, and the actions of the former hormone seem well suited to equip an organism for emergencies. Coping with a sudden emergency requires a massive response of the autonomic nervous system. The sympathetic division can produce a massive, widespread reaction, but the responses to parasympathetic stimulation are highly localized. Activation of the sympathicoadrenal system results in the release of large quantities of catecholamines. Since the preganglionic sympathetic fibers to the adrenal medulla are cholinergic, a comparable outpouring of medullary hormones may be induced by the administration of acetylcholine. Under these conditions, the animal shows typical signs of heightened emotion: cardiac acceleration, deep respiration, gastrointestinal inhibition, sweating, pallor of the skin, increased pilomotor activity, elevated blood sugar, and increased flow of blood through the muscles. All of these changes may occur to varying degrees under different circumstances.

There can be no doubt that noxious stimuli promote the secretion of medullary hormones and that many of the responses to epinephrine (*e.g.,* accelerated heart action, increased flow of blood through muscles) are of utility to the hard-pressed organism. It is not certain, however, that all of the physiologic actions of epinephrine are necessary to enable an organism to adjust to environmental changes. Much of the earlier work attempting to prove the emergency theory of epinephrine action failed to take into consideration the importance of the adrenal cortical hormones in emergency adjustments. It is known that epinephrine may operate under certain conditions to promote the release of ACTH from the anterior hypophysis, with a consequent release of certain adrenal cortical steroids, although pituitary activation may be only a minor function of epinephrine under stressful conditions. The mechanisms involved in the neuroendocrine adjustments to stressor stimuli are extremely complicated and await full clarification. Both norepinephrine and epinephrine are involved in stress adjustments, but the latter medullary hormone is regarded as being of more importance in this respect.

Norepinephrine is the chief neurohumor that mediates adrenergic impulses, and it acts mainly at these terminals. Though small amounts of it may diffuse from the nerve endings into the general circulation, and some is released from the adrenal medulla, this hormone is less well suited than epinephrine for promoting emergency adjustments. Norepinephrine is currently regarded as functioning in the normal organism in the maintenance of vascular tone and hence of blood pressure. It is probably secreted continuously by the sympathetic endings and acts locally to effect rapid adjustments essential for the maintenance of blood pressure. Various lines of evidence indicate that the release of norepinephrine is increased or decreased in response to conditions that threaten to alter normal blood pressure levels.

In summary, the chief functions of the catecholamines are to maintain blood pressure, to bring about alterations in carbohydrate metabolism, and to assist in systemic adjustments to certain kinds of stress. Norepinephrine is the transmitter substance of adrenergic nerves, and the neurohumor arising from this source can maintain normal vasomotor tone in the absence of adrenal medullary tissue. The differential release of the catechol hormones from the medulla probably depends on the functional requirements of the organism. Thus, norepinephrine is released in response to needs for circulatory adjustments, while epinephrine is of primary importance in metabolic adjustments and in the regional supply of blood to certain organs. Although both norepinephrine and epinephrine are involved in emotional expressions, epinephrine conforms more nearly to Cannon's concept of an emergency hormone.[59] Many actions of the catecholamines do not occur in the absence of adrenocortical hormones, the latter being necessary to maintain the integrity and responsiveness of the tissues.[49] Unlike the adrenal cortex, in which emphasis is on adjustments to nonspecific stress, the adrenal medulla maybe considered as a component of the sympathetic system, and its hormones participate in specific emotional reactions.

REFERENCES

1. Ahlquist, R. P.: A study of the adrenotropic receptors. Am. J. Physiol. *153*:586, 1948.
2. Axelrod, J.: Enzymatic formation of adrenaline and other catechols from monophenols. Science *140*:499, 1963.
3. Axelrod, J., and Tomchick, R.: Enzymatic O-methylation of epinephrine and other catechols, J. Biol. Chem. *233*:702, 1958.
4. Axelrod, J., and Whitby, L. G.: Effect of psychotic drugs on the uptake of H³-norepinephrine by tissues. Science *133*:383, 1961.
5. Bentley, P. J., and Follett, B. K.: The effects of hormones on the carbohydrate metabolism of the lamprey *Lampetra fluviatilis*. J. Endocr. *31*:127, 1965.
6. Bern, H. A., deRoos, C. C., and Biglieri, E. G.: Aldosterone and other corticosteroids from chondrichthyean interrenal glands. Gen. Comp. Endocr. *2*:490, 1962.
7. Blaschko, H., Hagen, P., and Welch, A. D.: Observations on the intracellular granules of the adrenal medulla. J. Physiol. *129*:27, 1955.
8. Bullough, W. S.: A study of the hormonal relations of epidermal mitotic activity *in vitro*. III. Adrenalin. Exp. Cell Res. *9*:108, 1955.
9. Burgos, M. H.: Histochemistry and electron microscopy of the three cell types in the adrenal gland of the frog. Anat. Rec. *133*:163, 1959.
10. Chan, D. K. O., Rankin, J. C., and Chester Jones, I.: Influences of the adrenal cortex and the corpuscles of Stannius on osmoregulation in the European eel (*Anguilla anguilla* L.) adapted to freshwater. Gen. Comp. Endocr., Suppl. *2*:342, 1969.
11. Chester Jones, I.: The Adrenal Cortex. London, Cambridge University Press, 1957.
12. Chester Jones, I., Phillips, J. G., and Bellamy, D.: Studies on water and electrolytes in cyclostomes and teleosts with special reference to *Myxine glutinosa* L. (the hagfish) and *Anguilla anguilla* L. (the Atlantic eel). Gen. Comp. Endocr., Suppl. *1*:36, 1962.
13. Chester Jones, I., and Spalding, M. H.: Some aspects of zonation and function of the adrenal cortex. J. Endocr. *10*:251, 1954.
14. Chidsey, C. A., Kaiser, G. A., and Braunwald, E.: Biosynthesis of norepinephrine in isolated canine heart. Science *139*:828, 1963.
15. Coleman, B., and Glaviano, V. V.: Tissue levels of norepinephrine and epinephrine in hemorrhagic schock. Science *139*:54, 1963.
16. Dale J. J.: On some physiological actions of ergot. J. Physiol. (London) *34*:163, 1906.
17. De Robertis, E., and vaz Ferreira, A.: Submicroscopic changes in the nerve endings in the adrenal medulla after stimulation of the splanchnic nerve. J. Biophys. Biochem. Cytol. *3*: 611, 1957.
18. De Schaepdryver, A. F., and Kirshner, N.: Metabolism of adrenaline after blockade of monoamine oxidase and catechol-O-methyltransferase. Science *133*:586, 1961.
19. Eade, N. R.: The distribution of the catechol amines in homogenates of the bovine adrenal medulla. J. Physiol. *141*:183, 1958.
20. Elmadjian, F., Hope, J. M., and Lamson, E. T.: Excretion of epinephrine and norepinephrine in various emotional states. J. Clin. Endocr. *17*:608, 1957.
21. von Euler, U. A.: Distribution and metabolism of catechol hormones in tissues and axones. Rec. Prog. Hormone Res. *14*:483, 1958.
22. von Euler, U. S.: Chromaffin cell hormones. *In* U. S. von Euler (ed.): Comparative Endocrinology, Vol. 1. New York, Academic Press, 1963, p. 258.
23. von Euler, U. S., and Fänge, R.: Catecholamines in nerves and organs of *Myxine glutinosa*, *Squalus acanthias* and *Gadus callarias*. Gen. Comp. Endocr. *1*:191, 1961.
24. Falck, B.: Observations on the possibilities of the cellular localization of monoamines by a fluorescene method. Acta Physiol. Scand. *56*:Suppl. 197:1, 1962.
25. Fontaine, M.: Evolution of form and function of endocrine organs with special reference to the adrenal gland. Proc. 16th Internat. Cong. Zool., Washington, D.C. *3*:25, 1963.

26. Gabe, M., and Martoja, M.: Contribution à l'histologie dela glande surrénale des Squamata (reptiles). Arch. Anat. Microscop. Morphol. Exp. *50*:1, 1961.
27. Goldberg, N. D.: Cyclic nucleotides and cell function. Hosp. Pract. *May*:127, 1974.
28. Goldfien, A., Zileli, M. S., Despointes, R. H., and Bethume, J. E.: The effect of hypoglycemia on the adrenal secretion of epinephrine and norepinephrine. Endocr. *62*:749, 1958.
29. Guyton, A. C., and Gillespie, W. M., Jr.: Constant infusion of epinephrine: Rate of epinephrine secretion and destruction in the body. Amer. J. Physiol. *165*:319, 1951.
30. Hagen, P.: The storage and release of catecholamines. Pharmacol. Rev. *11*:361, 1959.
31. Hale, A. J.: Observations on the nature of the chromaffin reaction. J. Physiol. *141*:193, 1958.
32. Hillarp, N. A., Lagerstedt, S., and Nilson, B.: The isolation of a granular fraction from the suprarenal medulla, containing the sympathomimetic catechol amines. Acta Physiol. Scand. *29*:251, 1953.
33. Holmes, W. N.: Histological variations in the adrenal cortex of the golden hamster with special reference to the X-zone. Anat. Rec. *122*:271, 1955.
34. Hsieh, A. C. L., and Carlson, L. D.: Role of adrenaline and noradrenaline in chemical regulation of heat production. Amer. J. Physiol. *190*:243, 1957.
35. Iverson, L. L.: The uptake and storage of noradrenaline in sympathetic nerves. Cambridge, England, Cambridge University Press, 1967.
36. Kirshner, N.: Uptake of catecholamines by a particular fraction of the adrenal medulla. Science *135*:107, 1962.
37. Kopin, I. J.: Storage and metabolism of catecholamines: The role of monoamine oxidase. Pharmacol. Rev. *16*:179, 1964.
38. Lakshman, A. B.: A descriptive study of the cytology of the adrenal glands of South Indian anurans. Endocrinologica Japonica *11*:169, 1964.
39. Lanman, J. T.: The adrenal fetal zone: Its occurrence in primates and a possible relationship to chorionic gonadotropin. Endocrinology *61*:684, 1957.
40. Mahon, E. F., Hoar, W. S., and Tabata, S.: Histophysiological studies of the adrenal tissues of the goldfish. Canadian J. Zool. *40*:449, 1962.
41. Meister, A.: Biochemistry of the Amino Acids. New York, Academic Press, 1957.
42. Moran, N. C. (ed): New adrenergic blocking drugs: Their pharmacological, biochemical, and clinical actions. Ann. N.Y. Acad. Sci. *139*:545, 1967.
43. Nandi, J.: New arrangement of interrenal and chromaffin tissues in teleost fishes. Science *134*:389, 1961.
44. Pang, P. K. T.: Endocrine control of calcium metabolism in teleosts. Amer. Zool. *13*:775, 1973.
45. Patent, G. J.: Comparison of some hormonal effects on carbohydrate metabolism in an elasmobranch *(Squalus acanthias)* and a holocephalan *(Hydrolagus colliei)*. Gen. Comp. Endocr. *14*:215, 1970.
46. Payne, F.: Adrenal ganglia and medullary cells in hypophysectomized and ageing fowl. J. Exp. Zool. *128*:259, 1955.
47. Poole, T. R., and Watts, D. T.: Peripheral blood epinephrine levels in dogs during intravenous infusion. Amer. J. Physiol. *196*:145, 1959.
48. Quay, W. B.: Catecholamines and tryptamines. J. Neuro-Visceral Rel., Suppl. IX:212, 1969.
49. Ramey, E. R., and Goldstein, M. S.: The adrenal cortex and the sympathetic nervous system. Physiol. Rev. *37*:155, 1957.
50. Richardson, J. A., and Woods, E. F.: Release of norepinephrine from the isolated heart. Proc. Soc. Exp. Biol. Med. *100*:149, 1959.
51. Sutherland, E. W., Øye, I., and Butcher, R. W.: The action of epinephrine and the role of the adenyl cyclase system in hormone action. Rec. Progr. Hormone Res. *21*:623, 1965.
52. Sutherland, E. W., and Rall, T. W.: The relation of adenosine-3', 5'-phosphate and phosphorylase to the actions of catecholamines and other hormones. Pharmacol. Rev. *12*:265, 1960.
53. Sutherland, E. W., Robison, G. A., and Butcher, R. W.: Some aspects of the biological role of adenosine 3', 5'-monophosphate (cyclic AMP). Circulation *37*:279, 1968.
54. Tomasi, V., Koretz, S., Ray, T. K., Dunnick, J., and Marinetti, G. V.: Hormone action at the membrane level. II. The binding of epinephrine and glucagon to the rat liver plasma membrane. Biochim. Biophys. Acta *211*:31, 1970.
55. Turtle, J. R., and Kipnis, D. M.: An adrenergic receptor mechanism for the control of cyclic 3', 5' adenosine monophosphate synthesis in tissues. Biochem. Biophys. Res. Commun. *28*:797, 1967.
56. Walker, B. E., and Rennels, E. G.: Adrenal cortical cell replacement in the mouse. Endocrinology *68*:365, 1961.
57. Wassermann, G., and Tramezzani, J. H.: Separate distribution of adrenaline- and noradrenaline-secreting cells in the adrenal of snakes. Gen. Comp. Endocr. *3*:480, 1963.

58. Welsh, J. H.: Neuroendocrine substances. *In* A. Gorbman (ed.): Comparative Endocrinology. New York, John Wiley & Sons, 1959, p. 121.
59. West, G. B.: The comparative pharmacology of the suprarenal medulla. Quart. Rev. Biol. *30*:116, 1955.
60. White, J. E., and Engel, F. L.: A lipolytic action of epinephrine and norepinephrine on rat adipose tissue *in vitro*. Proc. Soc. Exp. Biol. Med. *99*:375, 1958.
61. Wright, A., and Chester Jones, I.: The adrenal gland in lizards and snakes. J. Endocr. *15*:83, 1957.
62. Wright, A., Chester Jones I., and Phillips, J. G.: The histology of the adrenal gland of Prototheria. J. Endocr. *15*:100, 1957.
63. Wurtman, R. J., and Axelrod, J.: Adrenaline synthesis: Control by the pituitary gland and adrenal glucocorticoids. Science *150*:1464, 1965.
64. Young, J. E., and Chavin, W.: Effects of glucose, epinephrine or glucagon upon serum glucose levels in the goldfish (*Carassius auratus* L.). Amer. Zool. *5*:689, 1965.

CHAPTER 11

The Adrenal Cortex: Steroidogenic Tissue

STRUCTURE AND NOMENCLATURE OF STEROID HORMONES

Steroid hormones are secreted by the adrenal cortex, testis, ovary, and placenta, and some knowledge of their structure and nomenclature is essential. The steroids comprise a group of biologically active organic compounds which includes such substances as cholesterol, androgens, estrogens, and progestogens. The steroids have in common a cyclopentano-perhydro-phenanthrene nucleus consisting of a fully hydrogenated phenanthrene (rings A, B, and C), to which is fused a five-carbon cyclopentane ring (D) (see Fig. 11–1, B). The constituents in the nucleus and on the commonly occurring side chains are numbered as shown in Figure 11–1, B. Steroid chemists do not ordinarily write in all the carbon and hydrogen atoms as in Figure 11–1, A, but use a kind of shorthand for the steroid nucleus, and indicate only the most important characteristics of the compound. It is understood that the full complement of valence bonds for each carbon atom is satisfied by carbon or hydrogen atoms, or both. The angular methyl groups are indicated by straight lines at the junctures of the respective rings, and the unsaturated carbons are shown by double bonds.

By referring to Fig. 11–1, A, it may be seen that there are six asymmetric carbon atoms which are common to two different rings. The nucleus contains three types of carbon atoms: Those which are linked with two adjacent carbons and carry two hydrogen atoms (carbons 1, 2, 3, etc.); carbons 5, 8, 9, and 14, which are asymmetric carbon atoms that are linked to three carbon atoms and carry only one hydrogen atom; and finally carbons 10 and 13, to which the angular methyl groups are attached and which are linked to four carbon atoms and carry no hydrogen atoms.

The naturally occurring steroid molecules may be visualized as essentially flat structures, with some substituents projecting below them (away from the observer) and others projecting above them (toward the observer). The angular methyl groups are important for reference and may be regarded as arising from the nucleus and projecting above it. The positions of the two methyl groups above the plane of the molecule are indicated by using solid lines to attach them to carbons 10 and 13. When substituent groups are con-

324

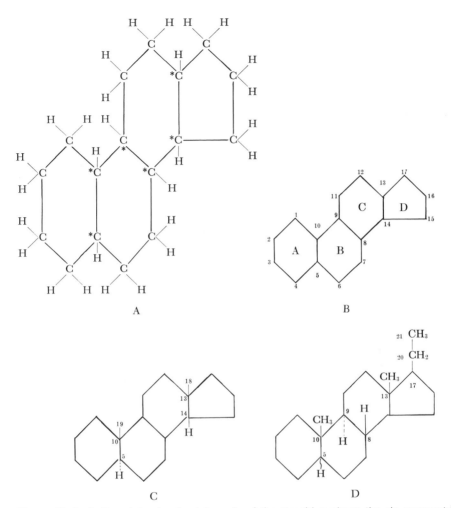

Figure 11-1. *A,* Complete structural formula of the steroid nucleus; the six asymmetric carbon atoms are indicated by asterisks. *B,* Numbering of the 17 carbon positions and designation of the four rings in gonane, a hypothetical parent compound. *C,* Angular methyl groups (numbered 18 and 19) are attached to carbons 10 and 13; these groups are indicated by a solid line since they project toward the observer (*cis* or β position). The hydrogen at carbon 5 is attached by a broken line since it projects away from the observer (*trans* or α); the hydrogen at carbon 14 is *cis* or β. *D,* In addition to the angular methyl groups (carbons 18 and 19), an ethyl group is attached at carbon 17, and its carbons are numbered 20 and 21. The hydrogen at position 5 is attached by a wavy line, indicating that it may be *cis* or *trans.*

nected to the nucleus by solid lines, this means that they lie on the same side of the molecule as the angular methyl groups. If a substituent is attached by a broken valence bond, it means that it projects downward below the plane of the nucleus and hence is on the opposite side with respect to the angular methyl groups. Groups that project in the same direction from the plane of the nucleus are said to be *cis* to each other; if they project in different directions they are *trans* to each other. Groups that are *cis* to the methyl reference points are designated as "β" and are indicated by solid valence lines; those that are *trans* to the same points are designated as "α" and are shown by broken valence lines. Wavy lines may be used when substituents may be either *cis* or *trans*.

Unfortunately, steroid nomenclature is quite confusing because a great variety of schemes have been followed by different workers. The common or trivial name for a compound has the advantage of being easy to remember, but it does not reveal anything about the nature of the substituents on the nucleus, their positions, or their spatial arrangements. Four hypothetical hydrocarbons on which nomenclature is based are shown in Figure 11–2. In addition to the stereoisomerism, often encountered at carbon atoms 3, 5, 11, and 17, nuclear modifications also occur and these have to be designated. The basic hydrocarbons are all saturated (no double bonds) and are given names that end with the suffix "*ane.*" They may become unsaturated by losing hydrogens, and this is indicated in the nucleus by double bonds, and in the nomenclature by changing the suffix "*an(e)*" to "*en(e).*" Two double bonds make the suffix "*dien(e),*" and three make it "*trien(e).*" In naming unsaturated compounds, the position of the double bond must be indicated; this is done by giving the number of the carbon atom where the double bond starts. Thus, "—3" indicates that the double bond extends between carbons 3 and 4. When double bonds exist between carbon atoms which are not numbered consecutively, as between carbons 9 and 11, both carbons are indicated. This double bond would be indicated as "—9(11)," the numbers being placed before part of the hydrocarbon name and followed by the suffix "*ene.*"

The basic hydrocarbon may be further modified by substituting oxygen

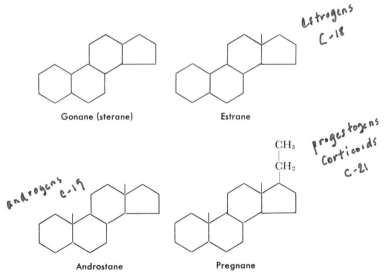

Gonane (sterane)   Estrane

estrogens
C-18

androgens
C-19

progestogens
Corticoids
C-21

CH₃
CH₂

Androstane   Pregnane

Figure 11–2. Four hypothetical hydrocarbons upon which nomenclature is based. Gonane lacks side chains and is a C-17 steroid. Estrane has an angular methyl group at carbon 13, giving a total of 18 carbons; androstane has an additional methyl group at carbon 10, giving a total of 19 carbon atoms; and pregnane has both methyl groups plus an ethyl side chain at carbon 17, making it a C-21 steroid.

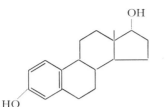

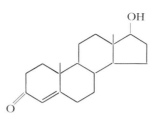

Estra-1,3,5(10)-triene-3,17β-diol
(Estradiol-17β, from ovary)

17β-Hydroxyandrost-4-en-3-one
(Testosterone, from testis)

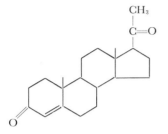

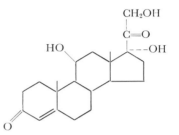

Pregn-4-ene-3,20-dione
(Progesterone, from ovary)

11β,17α,21-Trihydroxypregn-4-ene-3,20-dione
(Cortisol, from adrenal cortex)

Figure 11–3. Four naturally occuring steroid hormones.

for hydrogen. The suffix *"ol"* is used to indicate an alcohol or hydroxyl group, and this is preceded by the number of the carbon atom to which it is attached. This may also be shown by placing the term *"hydroxy"* before the name of the hydrocarbon. Ketone groups are indicated by the suffix *"one"* or by the prefix *"oxo"* preceding the hydrocarbon name. The prefix *"nor"* indicates shortening of a side chain or the contraction of a ring.

Four naturally occurring steroid hormones are shown in Figure 11–3, and both trivial and systematic names are given for each. The systematic name for estradiol-17β is estra-1,3,5(10)-triene-3,17β-diol; testosterone is 17β-hydroxyandrost-4-en-3-one; progesterone is pregn-4-ene-3,20-dione; and cortisol is 11β, 17α,21-trihydroxypregn-4-ene-3,20-dione.

The steroid hormones are conveniently classified according to the number of carbon atoms present in the nucleus and side chains. The androgens, estrogens, progestogens, and corticoids are derived from the basic hydrocarbons shown in Figure 11–2. The estrogens are derivatives of estrane and are C-18 steroids and generally have a high degree of unsaturation in the A ring; androgens derive from androstane and are C-19 compounds; progestogens and corticoids have the pregnane nucleus and are C-21 compounds.

Stereoisomerism

Steroid hormones may have the same molecular and structural formulas but different spatial or configurational formulas. Differences in molecu-

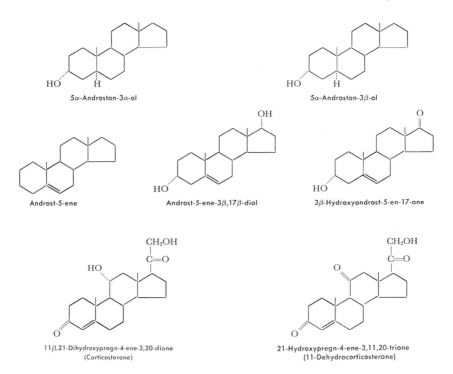

HO   H
5α-Androstan-3α-ol

HO   H
5α-Androstan-3β-ol

Androst-5-ene

Androst-5-ene-3β,17β-diol

3β-Hydroxyandrost-5-en-17-one

11β,21-Dihydroxypregn-4-ene-3,20-dione
(Corticosterone)

21-Hydroxypregn-4-ene-3,11,20-trione
(11-Dehydrocorticosterone)

Figure 11–4. Some steroids to illustrate isomerism, substitutions, and nomenclature.

lar shape, produced by the attachment of substituents in *cis* or *trans* positions, may have very important effects upon biologic activity. Isomerism at carbon atoms 3, 5, 11, and 17 is quite common among the steroid hormones. Isomerism at carbon 3 is illustrated by the first two compounds in Figure 11–4; 5α-androstan-3α-ol has a hydroxyl group at carbon 3 in the *trans* position, but in 5α-androstan-3β-ol, the hydroxyl group is in the *cis* position. In both compounds, the hydrogens at positions 5 are *trans* (α) with respect to the angular methyl groups. Among the adrenocortical steroids, a hydroxyl group is frequently found at carbon 11; it is generally *cis* to the angular methyl groups and is therefore the β configuration. When a hydroxyl group is present at position 17, it may take the α or β form, depending on whether or not an ethyl side chain is present at the same position. If there is an ethyl side chain at position 17, the hydroxyl group will be of the α type; if it is absent, the hydroxyl group has the β configuration.

Study the compounds shown in Figures 11–3 and 11–4. Notice how the chemical names used for the compounds allude to the parent hydrocarbon and designate the kind of change, the place of change, and the stereoisomerism involved in the change.

HORMONES FROM THE STEROIDOGENIC TISSUE OF THE ADRENAL GLAND

Nearly 50 steroids have been obtained from the cortical component of the mammalian adrenal gland. This mixture includes corticoids, possessing glycogenic and electrolytic activities, androgens, progestogens, estrogens, and, in addition, a large number of apparently inactive steroids that are precursors or metabolites of the active hormones. The adrenal cortex is a very versatile organ, and it is possible that more hormones of physiologic importance will be discovered in adrenal extracts and venous blood as better procedures are developed to test them.[25, 59, 64]

The most important adrenal corticoids, excluding androgens, estrogens, and progestogens, are shown in Figure 11–5. All of these are derivatives of pregnane and contain a total of 21 carbon atoms. Structures essential for activity are: (1) a double valence bond at C-4, (2) a ketonic group (C═O) at carbon 3, and (3) a ketonic group at carbon 20. The corticoids have profound effects on carbohydrate and mineral metabolism. Such compounds are sometimes called "glucocorticoids" and "mineralocorticoids," respectively. A hydroxyl group (OH) at carbon 21 enhances the capacity of the compound to encourage sodium retention and must be present for an effect on carbohydrate metabolism. Action on carbohydrate metabolism is heightened by the presence of a hydroxyl group at carbon 17. Corticoids having oxygen at carbon 11, either as hydroxyl or ketonic groups, exert major activity in carbohydrate metabolism. An oxygen function at position 11 generally decreases the capacity of the steroid to cause sodium retention, but aldosterone is an exception.

On the basis of chemical structure and biologic activity the hormones of the adrenal cortex may be grouped into four categories:

1. The 11-oxygenated corticosteroids that possess oxygen at carbon 11 are especially potent in affecting carbohydrate and protein metabolism, but have relatively little effect on water and electrolyte metabolism. The most important natural steroids of this class are cortisol, corticosterone, 11-dehydrocorticosterone, and cortisone.

2. Corticoids that lack oxygen at position 11 have major effects on electrolyte and water metabolism without much action on the metabolism of carbohydrate and protein. 11-Deoxycorticosterone (DOC) and 11-deoxycortisol belong to this class. 11-Deoxycorticosterone was prepared in 1937 from the plant steroid stigmasterol, long before it was known to be present in *trace* amounts in adrenal tissue, and was the first adrenal steroid to be made available commercially.

3. Aldosterone, the most effective adrenocortical steroid in electrolyte metabolism, was finally isolated from the amorphous fraction of adrenal extracts. The distinguishing chemical feature of this steroid is the presence of an aldehyde group at carbon 18 instead of a methyl group. When in solution, the hormone exists in hemiacetal and aldehyde forms.

4. Both androgens and estrogens, as well as progesterone, are elaborated by the adrenal cortex. Since these sex hormones may arise from the

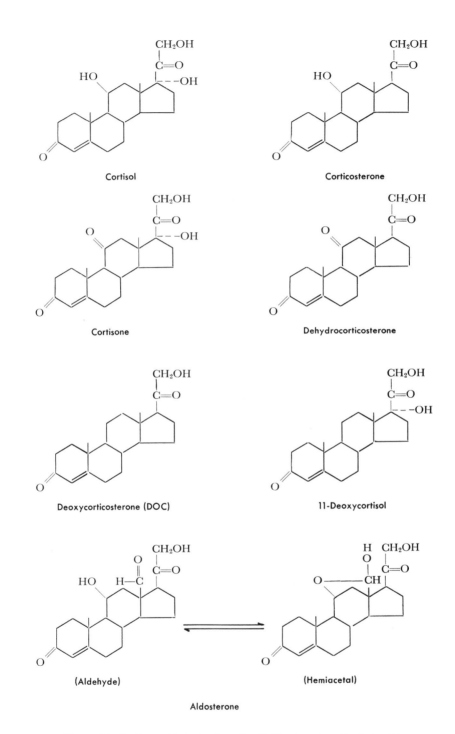

Figure 11–5. Some biologically active C-21 adrenal cortical steroids.

adrenal, there is considerable overlapping between adrenocortical and gonadal functions.

Phyletic Distribution[43, 57, 65, 67]

There is much evidence to support the view that a pituitary-adrenal axis operates in all vertebrates, and that the steroidogenic tissue of the adrenal secretes similar hormones from fishes to mammals (Table 11–1). Either corticosterone or cortisol, or both, have been identified as major adrenal hormones in cyclostomes, elasmobranchs, teleosts, lungfishes, amphibians, reptiles, birds, and mammals. The glucocorticoids must be very ancient molecules since they are secreted by adrenal tissue of cyclostomes, the most primitive living vertebrates. Both cortisol and corticosterone have been found in the peripheral blood of two hagfishes *(Myxine* and *Polistotrema)* and in a freshwater lamprey *(Petromyzon).* If aldosterone is present in the Cyclostomata, it is in very minute concentrations and has not been identified. Aldosterone is secreted by all mammalian adrenals that have been examined, and it is known to occur in low concentrations in many nonmammalian vertebrates. It has been detected in the adrenal venous blood of birds and in the peripheral blood of the salmon. By use of *in vitro* incubation methods, aldosterone has been identified in at least three species of elasmobranchs and in several species of teleosts, amphibians, snakes, lizards, and birds. The principal corticoid of elasmobranchs appears to be 1 α-hydroxycorticosterone, although other corticoids are widely distributed among various sharks and rays.[43] Cortisol is a consistent product of the teleost adrenal, but reptiles and birds appear to secrete a preponderance of corticosterone. The adrenals of the toad *(Bufo marinus)* and bullfrog *(R.*

Table 11–1 THE GENERAL DISTRIBUTION OF CORTICOSTEROID SYNTHESIS AMONG VERTEBRATES.*

CLASS	CORTICOSTEROIDS SYNTHESIZED
Cyclostomata	Cortisol, corticosterone
Chondrichthyes	1α-Hydroxycorticosterone; cortisol, corticosterone, aldosterone
Osteichthyes	Cortisol, cortisone, 11-deoxycortisol
Amphibia ⎫ Reptilia ⎬ Aves ⎭	Corticosterone, aldosterone, 18-hydroxycorticosterone
Mammalia Most Orders	Cortisol, cortisone, corticosterone, 18-hydroxycorticosterone, aldosterone
Rodentia, Lagomorpha	Corticosterone, 18-hydroxycorticosterone, 18-hydroxy-11-deoxycorticosterone, aldosterone

*Modified from Sandor, T.: Gen. Comp. Endocr., Suppl. 2, 1969.

catesbeiana) are known to secrete corticosterone and aldosterone; the salamander *(Amphiuma)* is known to produce both cortisol and corticosterone;
and only cortisol has been identified in the African frog *(Xenopus)*. In general, it appears that there is relatively little difference in the steroid biochemistry of the adrenals of amphibians, reptiles, and birds. Cortisol is the
predominant glucocorticoid in man, monkey, dog, and hamster, whereas
rats, mice, and rabbits secrete mainly corticosterone.[9, 13, 17, 18, 58, 66]

In searching for generalizations about the biochemistry of the adrenal
cortex, it is striking to find such a uniformity of pattern. The existence of the
same or similar corticosteroid hormones in groups which are unrelated
from the point of view of taxonomy or physiology suggests that the evolution of adrenal steroids met with early success. Accordingly, evolutionary
modifications in the function of these corticoids are more striking than are
changes in their molecular structure. This might be suspected, for it is likely
that mutations relative to steroid biochemistry would necessitate many
more base changes than would those pertaining, for example, to alterations
in the structure of peptide hormones. In the evolution of peptide hormones,
mutations could affect the composition of the molecule directly, while those
affecting steroid molecules would be reflected indirectly, through their effects on the composition of enzymes involved in steroid biosynthesis.

Artificial Corticoids

A variety of new compounds have been produced in the laboratory by
modifying the molecular structure of cortisone, cortisol, and deoxycorticosterone (Fig. 11–6). Some of these unnatural substances possess biologic properties and potencies that are quite different from the parent steroids.
9α-Fluoro-, chloro-, bromo-, and iodocortisol acetate have been prepared.
Halogenation at the 9α position not only enhances mineralocorticoid activity, but the glucocorticoid activity as well is about 10 times greater than that
of cortisone acetate. When cortisol is dehydrogenated at positions C-1 and
C-2, the glucocorticoid function is exaggerated, but the sodium-retaining
activity appears to be diminished. Perhaps the most potent corticoid that
has been prepared is 2α-methyl-9α-fluorocortisol acetate. This compound is
60 to 90 times more potent than deoxycorticosterone acetate (DOCA) in
sodium-retaining activity and is about 40 times more active than cortisone
acetate in the liver glycogen deposition test in rats.[63]

Microbial Transformations

Certain bacteria, yeasts, molds, and protozoans are known to possess
enzyme systems that can effect certain oxidative and reductive changes in
the steroid molecule. These enzymic changes are of great interest since
they may be models of those that operate in tissues at the vertebrate level.
In the synthetic manufacture of cortisone and other adrenal steroids, one of
the most difficult operations is the introduction of an oxygen atom at posi-

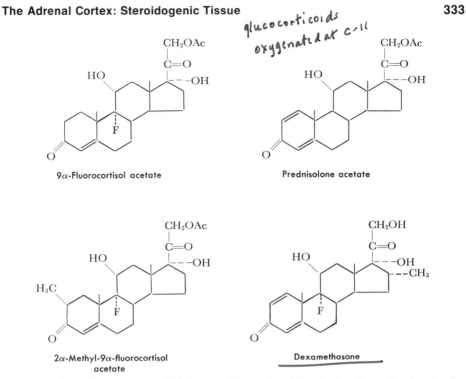

Figure 11–6. Four potent artificial corticoids produced by altering the molecular structure of cortisol.

tion 11. Certain plants provide raw material for the manufacture of progesterone, a compound having some of the required structure of cortisone and cortisol but no 11-oxo-group. When progesterone is used as substrate, certain molds *(e.g., Rhizopus, Aspergillus, Streptomyces)* introduce the 11-hydroxyl group. Much progress has been made in the isolation and culture of pure strains of microorganisms that are capable of effecting specific hydroxylations in steroid molecules.[23]

Assay Methods

In the past, various bioassay procedures were used for the determination of adrenocortical hormones. Usually, they were based upon the ability of the hormone extract to restore various functions in the adrenalectomized animal. The 11-oxysteroids may be bioassayed on the basis of their ability to promote the deposition of glycogen in the liver, to prolong life during exposure to cold, or to improve tolerance to traumatic injury. The abilities of corticoids to reduce the number of circulating eosinophils and to kill the lymphocytes in lymph nodes *in vitro* have also been used as bioassay parameters. Other tests, measuring principally mineralocorticoid activity, are based on the maintenance of life in adrenalectomized subjects, improvement in muscular work performance, and effects on the Na : K ratio of the urine.

The bioassays played an important part in the isolation of the active hormones and still find occasional application; however, they have been surplanted by newer, direct methods and by radioimmunoassays. These newer methods eliminate the basic weakness of bioassays—the problem of indirect effects—and are less laborious, less time consuming, and cheaper in the long run. Methods for steroid extraction have improved, and thin-layer chromatography has allowed for a relatively simple separation of closely related steroids from such tissues as adrenals, gonads, and blood. Quantitative or semiquantitative determinations of such steroids have often employed both colorimetric techniques and ultraviolet absorption. The use of gas chromatography has become a routine procedure in some laboratories and has proved to be a sensitive method for the detection of some steroids. The use of radioactive steroids in conjunction with the various techniques has also found considerable application. Among the newer physical methods, nuclear magnetic resonance (NMR) spectroscopy and mass spectrometric procedures are of value to the steroid chemist, and the use of combined techniques such as gas chromatography—mass spectrometry has become a valuable analytic tool.

Biosynthesis and Metabolism of Adrenal Steroids

The main sequence of biosynthetic steps from acetate through cholesterol and pregnenolone to the adrenocortical and gonadal hormones can be traced. Although much remains to be determined with reference to alternative pathways and the specific enzymes that effect the transformations, this work represents one of the most significant contributions to endocrinology. The important concept has emerged that all of the organs that synthesize steroid hormones, viz., adrenal cortices, testes, ovaries, and placenta, possess the same enzyme systems. Although the enzymes that catalyze particular transformations at particular times may predominate in specific steroid hormone-producing tissues, the others are not necessarily completely absent. It is also significant that the presence, function, and biosynthesis of mammalian-type adrenocortical and gonadal steroid hormone molecules are common to nonmammalian vertebrates, invertebrates, higher and lower plants, and prokaryotes.[67] It appears that little or no evolutionary change has occurred in the metabolism of these steroids. These accomplishments have been made possible largely through the use of radioactive isotopes, combined with chromatography and improved perfusion and in vitro techniques.[20, 35, 36]

Adrenal Corticoids

The biosynthesis of these compounds is illustrated in Figure 11–7, and the pathways are common to all species that have been studied. Acetate and cholesterol are known to be the important precursors, although the possibility exists that cholesterol is not an obligatory intermediate. Preg-

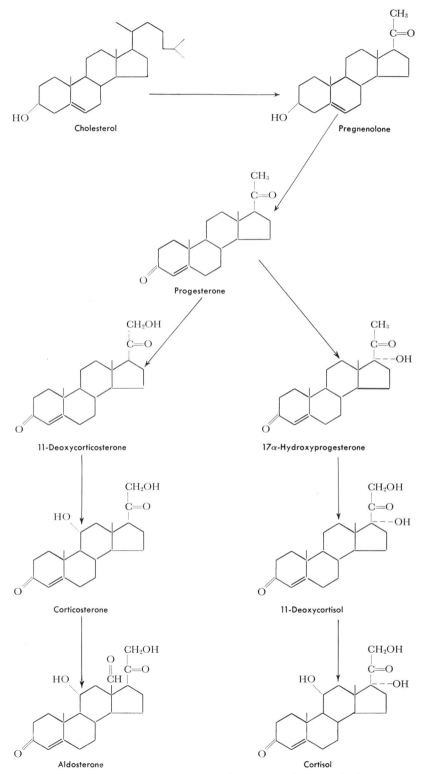

Figure 11–7. Some main pathways of corticosteroid biosynthesis.

nenolone is the first C-21 compound to be produced from cholesterol, and it is oxidized to progesterone. Three enzyme systems, the 11β, 17α, and 21-hydroxylases, catalyze the reactions leading to cortisol and corticosterone. Aldosterone may arise from cholesterol, progesterone, deoxycorticosterone, or corticosterone, hydroxylation being accomplished at carbon atom 18. The conversion of androgens to estrogens involves hydroxylation at carbon 19. A separate hydroxylating system appears to be present for each position, and molecular oxygen and reduced nicotinamide adenine dinucleotide phosphate (NADPH) are used in the hydroxylations.[37, 71]

There are many indications that the pituitary-adrenal axis begins to function before birth. Human fetal adrenals appear to possess the necessary enzyme equipment for the synthesis of cortical steroids. When homogenates of such adrenals are incubated *in vitro* with an NADPH generating system, with progesterone or α-hydroxyprogesterone used as substrate, cortisol is formed.[51, 75, 80]

Adrenal Androgens

The adrenal androgens arise from the C-21 corticoids and also directly from cholesterol (Fig. 11–8). Incubation and perfusion experiments leave no doubt that C-21 steroids can be converted to adrogens by adrenal tissue. When labeled progesterone is perfused through an adrenal, labeled androstenedione and 11β-hydroxyandrostenedione may be isolated from the perfusate. Trace amounts of these two androgens have been detected in human adrenal venous blood. There are reasons for believing that a significant percentage of the total adrenal androgen may be formed directly from cholesterol via pregnenolone. For instance, the adrenal cortices of the human fetus contain androgens before significant amounts of corticoids can be detected. In patients with masculinizing tumors of the adrenal cortices, the output of dehydroepiandrosterone and other androgens is increased tremendously, but the secretion of C-21 steroids may not increase proportionately. On the other hand, in patients with Cushing's syndrome, there is an excessive production of cortisol with no increase in androgens other than those that may arise through the catabolism of C-21 corticoids. In conditions of stress, there is a profound increase in corticoids, but the 17-ketosteroids tend to diminish. These facts suggest that androgens in the adrenal may arise indirectly from corticoids or be synthesized directly from cholesterol.

Catabolism of Adrenal Steroids

The steroid hormones are rapidly catabolized in the organism and are excreted in the urine as conjugates of glucuronic acid, or, in the case of androgens, of sulfuric acid. Few of the steroids are excreted without change. The liver is the main site of steroid hormone catabolism, although

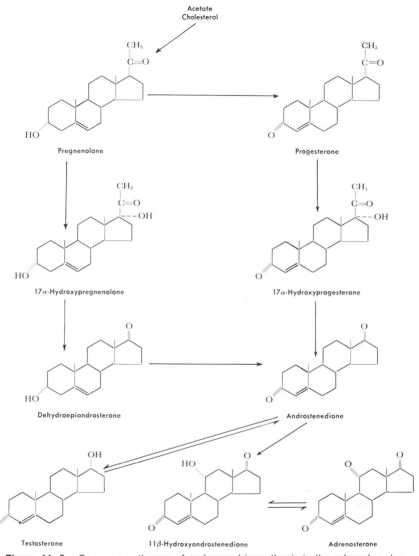

Figure 11–8. Common pathways of androgen biosynthesis in the adrenal cortex.

the kidneys and perhaps other tissues may function in this capacity to some extent. Biologic inactivity of the compound correlates with the loss of the α,β-unsaturated ketone grouping at position 3 and, in some cases, with loss of the α-ketol side chain at carbon 17. Much information is available concerning the catabolic transformations, so that it is possible to predict what hormones the adrenal cortex is secreting from the metabolites that can be isolated from the urine. The secretory behavior of the cortex may be evaluated by measuring the urinary metabolites in the resting subject or after the administration of ACTH.[62]

The 17-ketosteroids of the urine may be determined colorimetrically by the Zimmermann reaction, and this gives an indication of the metabolites that are derived from the adrenocortical and testicular hormones. The total of neutral 17-ketosteroids is about 33 per cent less in normal women than in men. The daily output for women is 5 to 15 mg and that for young men ranges from 10 to 22 mg. The difference is presumably due to the testicular steroids. Complete failure of the adrenal cortices may cause the output to fall to zero in the female and to below 5 mg in the male. Although most of the neutral 17-ketosteroids are derived from adrenal cortical hormones, it must be emphasized that quantitation of these substances as a group is no infallible measure of either testicular or adrenal function. Not all of the ketones that are determined by the Zimmerman reaction are necessarily 17-ketosteroids. For example, 17-ketosteroids appear to rise during pregnancy when large amounts of pregnenolone are being produced; this compound is a C-20 ketone and the Zimmerman reaction does not differentiate it from a 17-ketosteroid.[39]

Enzymatic Defects and Adrenal Androgens

During embryonic life, the adrenal cortices originate in close association with the gonadal primordia. Clinicians have known for a long time that tumorous conditions of the adrenals and gonads may lead to the release of hormones that simulate the action of the other gland. For example, certain hyperplasias and malignant tumors of the adrenal cortices may release large quantities of androgen or estrogen, thus resembling the normal action of the testes and ovaries. Although the older pathologists suggested that "embryonic rests" of these tissues might be carried over from embryonic life and account for these conditions, the theory never received confirmation. In the light of present knowledge, it is more probable that such defects result from alterations in the functioning of enzyme systems that are normally present in all steroid hormone-producing organs.

The adrenogenital syndrome is a human disease characterized by bilateral hypertrophy of the adrenal cortices or by a cortical neoplasm. Tremendous amounts of androgen are secreted, but the production of cortisol remains within normal limits or is slightly decreased. The masculinizing influences depend on the age of onset and the sex of the patient. The adrenal has a limited ability to produce cortisol in response to ACTH injections but a marked ability to produce androgens. Thus, ACTH treatment increases the already high levels of urinary 17-ketosteroids. The production of adrenal androgen may be diminished by the administration of cortisol, this naturally occurring corticoid being a powerful inhibitor of ACTH release by the pituitary. Two different enzymatic deficiencies in the biosynthetic sequence of adrenal cortical steroids have been suggested, either of which may lead to this syndrome. The fundamental adrenal defect in the adrenogenital syndrome seems to be a relative deficiency of either the 21-hydroxylase system or the 11β-hydroxylase system. With these enzymic defects there is a piling up of "unfinished corticoids," such as 17-hydroxyprogesterone and 11-deoxycortisol. Since the adrenal does not add enough cortisol to the circulation to inhibit the pituitary release of ACTH, the adrenal responds to the continuing high titers of ACTH by producing androgens. Several other adrenal diseases have been explained as abnormalities of specific enzyme systems.[4]

REGULATION OF ADRENOCORTICAL SECRETION[85]

The adrenal cortex is the most complex of the steroid-secreting glands, and its complexity is reflected not only by the array of steroids it synthesizes, but by its structural morphology as well. The clearly defined cytologic areas (zona glomerulosa, zona fasciculata, and zona reticularis) are distinguished both by ultrastructural differences and by a distinctive biochemical machinery that allows for the production of given steroids by specific areas of the cortex. The regulation of synthesis and secretion of these various steroid groups is specified by feedback mechanisms that affect the cytophysiology of the adrenal cortex. This can be best understood by a consideration of the relationship between the circulating levels of the various steroid groups and the characteristics of the adrenocortical zones. The alteration of steroid levels can be effected by such procedures as hypophysectomy and sodium deprivation, and by administration of hormones such as ACTH or various steroids.

Effects on the adrenal cortex are usually assessed by various morphologic and physiologic features, and progress is being made in our understanding of ultrastructural differences.[24] Just as with the testis and ovary, the steroid-producing cells of the adrenal cortex are striking in that they contain an extensive endoplasmic reticulum. Many zones containing parallel arrays of granular reticulum are seen, and these are often connected to an extensive network of agranular tubular elements that, together with mitochondria, occupy a large part of the cell. The specific zones can be identified on the basis of the appearance and distribution of the various organelles. These criteria can also be used to determine the physiologic state of the cell. The human fetal adrenal cortex has been studied at the ultrastructural level and its cells appear to be remarkably active (Fig. 11–9). This cytologic picture is consistent with the knowledge that the fetal adrenal possesses a significant capacity for steroid biosynthesis. A more complete knowledge of adrenocortical cytology and ultrastructure will ultimately be of even greater importance as we attempt to learn more about the action of various factors in regulating corticoid synthesis and release from specific cells of the adrenal cortex. Possibly, comparative studies will help in this regard. For example, from a recent study of the ultrastructure of a shark adrenal, it has been concluded that adrenocorticosteroids may be secreted by a holocrine secretory mechanism.[78]

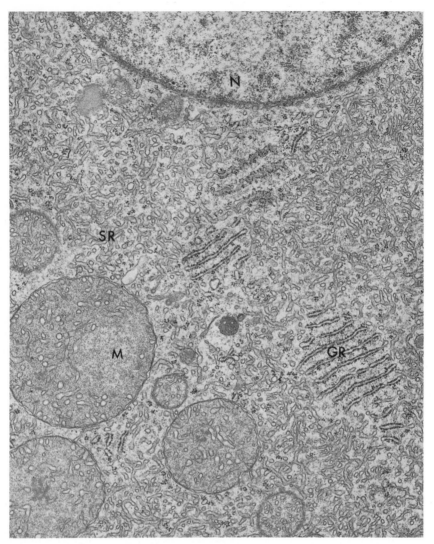

Figure 11–9. Electron micrograph of human fetal adrenal cortex showing typical mito-chondria, with tubular cristae, some granular reticulum, and abundant agranular or smooth reticulum. GR, granular reticulum; M, mitochondrion; N, nucleus; SR, smooth reticulum. (Courtesy of Dr. Scott McNutt, Department of Anatomy, Harvard Medical School.)

Glucocorticoids

x - adrenals → ↑ pituitary ACTH
x - pituitary → ↓ adrenal glucocort.

Adrenalectomy results in an increased release of ACTH by the pituitary, and, in the hypophysectomized animal, the adrenal output of glucocorticoids is reduced to a very low level. The administration of ACTH to intact or hypophysectomized subjects is followed by adrenocortical hypertrophy and a consequent increase in the production of glucocorticoids such as cortisol and corticosterone. The levels of ascorbic acid in the cortex are depleted under conditions of heightened secretory activity. The cholesterol content of the cortex falls after ACTH treatment, whereas the concentration of glucocorticoids in adrenal venous blood and of their metabolites in the urine is strikingly increased. The prolonged administration of glucocorticoids to normal animals causes the adrenal cortices to regress until they are equivalent to the cortices of hypophysectomized animals (Fig. 11–10). The pituitary releases increasing amounts of ACTH when the blood levels of glucocorticoids are low, and diminishes the output as the plasma glucocorticoids are elevated. Certain enzymatic reactions in the cortex may be blocked by such nonsteroidal agents as amphenone and metopyrone (SU 4885), thus preventing the biosynthesis of cortisol and corticosterone, and, in the absence of these steroid inhibitors, the pituitary releases large amounts of ACTH. Insecticides of the DDT type produce a selective necrosis of the dog's adrenal cortex; this reduces the synthesis of steroids and augments the release of ACTH.

In vitro studies have shown that adrenal grafts of the rat, consisting only of regenerated cortex, are capable of secreting corticosterone, deoxycorticosterone, and aldosterone. Under *in vivo* conditions of deliberately imposed stress, the grafts respond to ACTH stimulation, but circulatory failure seems to prevent the grafts from releasing their hormones in normal quantities.[48, 52]

Nonfunctional enlargement of the adrenal cortex follows the administration of estrogens, particularly the synthetic ones, such as stilbestrol and hexestrol. This response is dependent on the integrity of the pituitary. It is probable that the estrogens act in some manner to block the synthesis of corticoids, and as these diminish in the blood, the pituitary releases increased amounts of ACTH to stimulate the cortex.[70, 81]

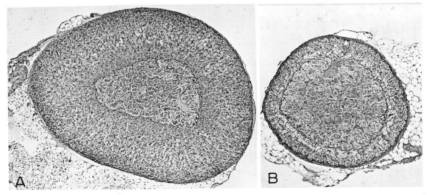

Figure 11–10. Effect of prolonged administration of cortisone on the adrenal cortex of the adult mouse. *A,* Adrenal gland of the normal mouse, showing medullary and cortical components. *B,* Adrenal gland of an adult mouse following the administration of 1 mg. of cortisone daily for 30 days. Note that the cortex has diminished in width until it is structurally equivalent to that of a hypophysectomized animal; the medulla remains normal. The circulating steroid acts by way of the hypothalamus and anterior pituitary to inhibit the production of ACTH, a trophic hormone required for normal functioning of the cortex. Both glands are at the same magnification.

There is general agreement that a negative feedback mechanism operates to control the levels of glucocorticoids in the blood. The concentration of these hormones in the blood depends on how rapidly the adrenal releases them, and on how rapidly they are inactivated and eliminated from the system. Only negligible amounts of active adrenal steroids are lost through the urine and bile, and the liver is the main organ that possesses the enzymatic equipment for their inactivation.

A sexual dimorphism in adrenal size is known to occur in the rat, the females having larger adrenals than the males. A parallel relationship between the capacity of the liver to inactivate adrenal steroids *in vitro* and the size of the adrenals has been found. An enzyme system has been identified in liver homogenates of rats, and the concentration of the enzyme is three to 10 times higher in females than in males. Even the rapid enlargement of the rat's adrenal during estrus is associated with an increase in this liver enzyme. The hepatic and adrenal sex differences in rats may be abolished by castration at an early age. These differences can be reestablished or reversed in young castrates by giving androgens or estrogens. Since the liver of the female rat inactivates corticoids at a high rate, the adenohypophysis must release large amounts of ACTH to stimulate the adrenal cortex to maintain adequate blood levels of corticoids. These results show that the rate of hepatic inactivation of the circulating steroids is an important determinant of ACTH release and adrenocortical secretion rate, and lend support to the feedback hypothesis.[2, 30, 47, 79, 84]

Although ACTH is the main hormone that stimulates adrenocortical secretion, other hormones probably act in conjunction with it. It has been reported that synthetic vasopressin, applied by direct arterial infusion, stimulates the adrenal glands of the dog to secrete cortisol. This seems to be a direct effect of the vasopressin, and not one mediated by the adenohypophysis or any other organ.[38]

Aldosterone

This steroid from the adrenal cortex functions primarily in the regulation of electrolyte and water metabolism. It is by far one of the most potent regulators of electrolyte secretion. Just as with other steroids, this hormone binds to specific protein receptors present in sensitive cells of the kidney and subsequently acts on the nucleus, where it directs transcription of DNA. The RNA thus formed directs translational events leading to the synthesis of proteins which are presumably involved in facilitating sodium entry into these cells. In effect, sodium resorption is thus enhanced.

The factors which control aldosterone synthesis and discharge are highly involved and seem to be somewhat species dependent. Although ACTH appears to exert a trophic influence on the glomerulosa and on aldosterone secretion in the frog, it has little such action in mammals. Even before aldosterone was discovered, it was known that hypophysectomized animals survived quite well without serious impairment of their electrolyte metabolism, whereas adrenalectomized animals died unless additional salt was provided. Histologic studies of adrenals from hypophysectomized animals revealed that most of the adrenocortical involution occurs in the fasciculata-reticularis areas, the glomerulosa appearing unaffected by the absence of ACTH. The postulate that the zona glomerulosa is the source of a salt-regulating hormone, the production of which does not depend entirely upon ACTH, has been amply confirmed, and it is now thought that this effect is attributable to the renin-angiotensin system. ACTH seems to be one factor among many which can stimulate the adrenal to produce and discharge aldosterone.[3, 10, 16]

In the beef adrenal, it is possible to separate the outer capsule and glomerulosa from the underlying fasciculata with considerable accuracy, thus making it possible to test the separate zones for their capacity to produce steroids. When ACTH is incubated with glomerulosa strippings, it does not promote the conversion of cholesterol to aldosterone; if fasciculata-reticularis slices are used, ACTH causes the conversion of cholesterol to cortisol. This indicates that ACTH has no effect, or a very insignificant effect, on aldosterone biogenesis.

When progesterone, deoxycorticosterone, and corticosterone are used as substrates for beef adrenal slices, they are metabolized in radically different ways, depending on whether the adrenal tissue consists of glomerulosa or fasciculata-reticularis. When these steroids are added to glomerulosa, they are converted to aldosterone. Progesterone enhances the production of cortisol only when it is added to fasciculata-reticularis tissue. From these studies, it has been concluded that cortisol is produced almost entirely from the fasciculata-reticularis, aldosterone from the glomerulosa, and corticosterone from both the glomerulosa and the two inner zones of the cortex. It is becoming apparent that specific pathways of corticosteroid biosynthesis occur within different zones of the adrenal cortex, which implies that there is a corresponding zonation of the enzyme systems involved. This would explain how it is possible for cortical cells from different zones to synthesize different kinds of hormones from an identical precursor. Thus, it appears that the glomerulosa is the site of 18-oxygenation, but the fasciculata-reticularis is not; 17-hydroxylase activity occurs in the fasciculata-reticularis, but not in the glomerulosa; and 3β-dehydrogenase and 11- and 21-hydroxylase activities occur in both areas of the gland.[28, 29, 74, 76]

Angiotensin, a potent vasopressor substance produced in the blood under the influence of the kidneys, may be another factor which operates to release aldosterone. Synthetic angiotesin, administered to normal human subjects, releases aldosterone, cortisol, and corticosterone. It has the same effect in dogs deprived of their kidneys and pituitary glands. Minute amounts of angiotensin stimulate aldosterone release from adrenocortical tissue *in vitro*.[27, 55, 61]

Sodium-loading diminishes the release of aldosterone, whereas sodium deprivation increases it. Changes in blood volume also influence the output of this hormone, reduced volumes increasing and increased volumes decreasing its production. In dogs, stretching of the right atrium, but not of the left atrium, causes a marked fall in aldosterone production. Pregnancy and various kinds of stress increase the urinary excretion of aldosterone, and this suggests that central nervous system mechanisms are involved in the regulation of its production. The problem is a very difficult one since so many factors seem to be involved, and final conclusions are not warranted at this time.

The Release of Adrenal Steroids

Almost any kind of stress to which the animal is subjected can cause an outpouring of adrenal cortical hormones. In man and other mammals there are strong indications of a daily rhythm in the release of 11-oxygenated hormones from the adrenal. In male and female mice, the level of eosinophils in the blood is higher at noon than at night, whereas mitotic divisions are more frequent in adrenal cortices at night than at noon. Since these adrenal hormones act to depress the eosinophils, it is probable that the mouse adrenal discharges mostly at night. The levels of 11-oxygenated steroids in the blood of nocturnal mice, as compared with the predominantly diurnal human subject, differ in environmental phase relations. It may be that there are species differences in the manner in which the daily rhythms of hormone release are synchronized.[6, 34]

The adrenals of wild and domesticated Norway rats are strikingly different. The cortices of wild rats not only are larger but contain more lipid, aldehyde, and ketonic carbonyl groups, and have a richer blood supply. When the wild animals are tamed, the adrenals gradually diminish in size. The cortex of the wild rat apparently continues in a state of heightened secretory activity. There are sex differences in the size of the adrenal cortices. For example, the female rat has a larger adrenal than the male, but in the hamster this sexual dimorphism is reversed. The adrenal glands of birds seem to be less reactive to various stimuli than those of laboratory mammals.[17, 26, 56, 83]

Increased population densities, acting to increase the number of aggressive confrontations between individuals, frequently correlate with an augmented production of adrenocortical hormones. The degree of response to changes in population size depends upon the behavioral aggressiveness of the strain or species. The house mouse (Mus musculus) is very aggressive, whereas the deer mouse (Peromyscus maniculatus) is much less so. Population increases have much more effect on the adrenals of the former species than on the latter. The adrenal cortices of the two species respond equally well when subjected to trained fighters of their own species or when exposed to cold. Brief encounters of adult male mice with trained fighters cause increases in the size of the adrenals and elevate the amount of corticosterone in the plasma. This response occurs in the absence of physical injury, indicating that the stimulus is sociopsychologic or "emotional." It has been observed that in growing populations of mice, the most submissive members, no longer offering any resistance, may be completely ignored by dominant individuals, and their adrenals diminish in size and release only small amounts of corticosterone.[5, 12]

Mechanism of ACTH Action

Like that of most peptide hormones, the action of ACTH appears to be mediated by the "second messenger," cyclic AMP.[77] It is thought that the activity of adenylate cyclase at the cell membrane of adrenocortical cells is stimulated by ACTH, leading to an increased conversion of ATP to cyclic AMP. This increased concentration of cyclic AMP within the cell is thought to accelerate the conversion of cholesterol to pregnenolone, a basic and rate-limiting step in adrenal steroidogenesis (Figs. 11–7 and 11–8). The question of how cyclic AMP initiates this basic step in steroidogenesis is as yet unresolved. Since these various biosynthetic steps are enzymatically controlled, it would appear that somewhere in the chain of events, protein synthesis would be involved in order to make available appropriate enzymes. Possibly, either directly or indirectly, the effects of cyclic AMP are mediated through protein synthesis, as is implied from the fact that inhibitors of protein synthesis interfere with the rapid effects of ACTH or cyclic AMP on steroid biosynthesis without altering ACTH effect on adenylate cyclase activities. In an *in vitro* system, it was recently demonstrated that the rapid effects of ACTH and cyclic AMP on steroid biosynthesis in adrenocortical cells are accompanied by rapid protein synthesis, and it was suggested that action of cyclic AMP, the intracellular mediator, is through selective effects on protein synthesis.[33] Resolution of this problem awaits further experimentation; however, it is a challenging thought that may have important implications in interpreting the mechanism of action of other peptide hormones.

PHYSIOLOGY OF THE STEROIDOGENIC ADRENAL

The Effects of Bilateral Adrenalectomy

Bilateral removal of the adrenals produces a series of metabolic disturbances which are identical with those appearing in patients with Addison's disease. If the adrenals have been completely removed and there are no accessory cortical deposits, the animals invariably die within a week or two. The fact that adrenalectomized animals may be maintained indefinitely in normal physiologic condition by the administration of cortical steroids, in the absence of exogenous epinephrine, is direct proof that the cortical portion of the gland is essential for life. The symptoms appearing in untreated animals include extreme muscular weakness, a variable degree of hypoglycemia, gastrointestinal disturbances, hemoconcentration, reduced blood pressure and body temperature, and kidney failure. Growth ceases in young animals, and older ones generally lose weight. Adrenalectomized subjects are unable to tolerate stresses of any type; exposure to trauma, cold, heat, toxins, infections, fasting, forced exercise, etc., are likely to prove fatal. In some mammalian species, the survival period after total adrenalectomy is prolonged by pregnancy and pseudopregnancy. Comparable results are obtained by the administration of progesterone, a hormone of the corpus luteum.

After adrenalectomy, the thymus and lymph nodes tend to become enlarged and the blood lymphocytes are elevated. Regression of these tissues in response to stress does not occur normally. Blood sugar levels tend to be low and the liver is deficient in glycogen. The amount of nitrogen lost from the body during fasting is below normal, suggesting that in cortical deficiency there is a reduced capacity to draw on body protein in order to maintain the blood glucose and liver glycogen.

In the absence of adrenal cortices, there is an excessive loss of sodium, chloride, and bicarbonate through the kidneys, but there is a diminished clearance of potassium. The excretion of sodium is accompanied by a diuresis which leads to hemoconcentration; the loss of bicarbonate decreases the pH of blood, a condition of acidosis. It is well known that life may be prolonged in adrenalectomized subjects or in those with Addison's disease by simply administering large amounts of salt solution. Restricting the consumption of salt precipitates the crisis of adrenal insufficiency. It should be understood, however, that salt therapy merely corrects some of the symptoms, without repairing the basic defects.

Electrolytes and Fluid Shifts

The main action of mineralocorticoids is to regulate the body electrolytes and water. Though traces of deoxycorticosterone, a potent salt-retaining hormone, are found in cortical tissue and in adrenal vein blood, it is probably a precursor of aldosterone, the most important mineralocorticoid. The principal action of aldosterone in mammals is to reduce the amount of sodium lost from the body through the urine. This is accomplished by the enhanced reabsorption of sodium from the glomerular filtrate through the walls of the renal tubules. The reabsorption is an active process since the ions are moved against an electrochemical potential gradient. The role of aldosterone as the principal mineralocorticoid has been demonstrated for several species and it is known to be effective at low concentrations. The administration of aldosterone can maintain the life of adrenalectomized animals not only through its salt-retaining capacity, but also by virtue of its intrinsic glucocorticoid activity. The latter activity is explained by virtue of the fact that aldosterone is oxygenated at carbon 11, as are the glucocorticoids. Although glucocorticoids such as cortisol and corticosterone are potent factors in the regulation of carbohydrate metabolism, they are also capable of enhancing or inhibiting the excretion of water and sodium. The neurohypophysial peptides also exert important influences upon the kidney tubules, and thus influence the osmolarity of the body fluids.

Though other hormones, such as thyroxine, insulin, estrogens, parathyroid hormone, and somatotrophin, are known to affect particular ions or alter the water content of specific tissues, the adrenocortical steroids and neurohypophysial peptides (vasopressin, vasotocin) are most profoundly concerned with salt and water balance of the body. It has been pointed out earlier that these hormones are widely distributed among the vertebrates. Aldosterone, cortisol, and corticosterone are present in all of the major groups, from fishes to man. The neurohypophysial octapeptides emanating from the posterior pituitary have undergone only minor changes in structure during vertebrate evolution. Both the pituitary peptides and the adrenal steroids act upon targets which are essentially epithelial surfaces capable of allowing the transcellular movement of water and osmotic solutes. Such targets include the kidney tubules, gills, skin, gastrointestinal mucosa, urinary bladder, and various types of exocrine glands.

Animals may be divided into two categories with reference to their methods of meeting osmotic stress: (1) The _osmoconformers_ are osmotically labile and change their body fluids in accordance with the medium in which they live, and (2) the _osmoregulators_ are independent of their environments and maintain their body fluids at remarkably constant osmotic concentrations regardless of the medium in which they live. All gradations are found between these two extremes, but the great majority of vertebrates are osmoregulators. The body fluids of vertebrates have about 25 to 33 percent of the salinity of sea water. Although not all osmoregulations are under direct hormonal control, the endocrine system clearly performs an important role in adjusting body fluids in response to environmental changes.[41]

Mammals

These highest of vertebrates have radiated into a variety of ecologic niches; they are found in fresh water, in sea water, and in moist or dry air, and are able to tolerate a wide range of temperatures. By being able to regulate the salt and water concentrations of their body fluids, they have become relatively independent of their environments. Perfection of the kidney tubules, coupled with hormonal and neural controls, permits the mammals to discharge urine which is hyperosmotic to the blood.

Reptiles and Birds

Nasal (supraorbital) glands are present in all birds and are especially well developed in marine species.[45, 68] Their only known function is to serve as osmoregulatory organs. Certain marine species (_e.g.,_ albatross) consume only salt water, and this can be tolerated since the nasal glands secrete a fluid containing high concentrations of salt, principally sodium chloride. Marine birds are known to have larger adrenals than those which are strictly terrestrial. Sea birds are difficult to maintain under laboratory conditions, and the domestic duck has been used as an experimental animal for studies on the nasal glands. The glands of this species are of intermediate size, but they enlarge and secrete hypertonic salt solutions after salt-loading. Forcing the ducks to drink salt water, instead of fresh water, induces hypertrophy of the steroidogenic part of the adrenal gland and causes a concentrated salt solution to drip from the external nares. The urine decreases in volume after salt-loading and contains less sodium and more potassium than when fresh water is consumed. Bilateral adrenalectomy prevents the extrarenal response to salt loads, and the administration of corticosterone or cortisol restores normal excretory patterns in both kidneys and nasal glands.[42] Although it is possible that the nasal glands are partly regulated by parasympathetic innervation, as has been suggested, these experiments on the duck indicate that adrenal steroids and possibly neurohypophysial octapeptides are also involved. Although the exact mechanisms controlling the activation of the nasal glands are unknown, it is probable that the first step is triggered by the increased osmolarity of the blood; this could affect the secretion of the pituitary gland as well as the steroidogenic adrenal. It has also been found that DNA-RNA ratios of the salt gland vary in accordance with saline levels, suggesting that protein synthesis is involved in the development of a sodium transport system.[42] Possibly the induction of this system is glucocorticoid dependent. Since corticosteroids influence the secretion of the nasal glands of the duck, the adrenals probably function naturally in regulating these glands in marine birds.[40, 41]

Marine reptiles, as well as certain terrestrial species, also possess nasal salt glands and can secrete significant quantities of salt extrarenally. No careful studies have been made on reptiles with respect to the possible involvement of hormones in regulation of the nasal glands. Studies on the tropical lizard (Iguana iguana) have shown that secretion of the nasal salt gland is stimulated by the intraperitoneal injection of sodium chloride.[69] Many turtles have a large, bilobed bladder, and large quantities of water are reabsorbed from it. Aldosterone increases the active transport of sodium across the bladder membrane of the tortoise but spirolactone, an aldosterone antagonist, has the reverse effect.[1]

The amount of finished urine eliminated from the cloaca in birds and reptiles is small and may be in the form of a viscous paste of uric acid crystals. There is considerable evidence that large amounts of water, together with sodium and potassium, are reabsorbed from the cloacae of birds and reptiles. Possibly as much as 66 per cent of the net sodium influx of some aquatic turtles occurs through the cloaca. It has been suggested that the appearance of an extrarenal mechanism for the excretion of salt (nasal glands) in these classes is related to their ability to reabsorb water from the cloaca.[69] Relatively little is known about the mechanisms that may be involved in regulating the permeability of cloacal and bladder membranes in reptiles and birds.

Amphibians

Permanently aquatic amphibians are surrounded by a hypotonic medium and actively absorb salts through the kidneys, urinary bladder, gills, skin, and intestinal mucosa in order to maintain the ionic concentration of their body fluids. When not in water, amphibians conserve water by decreasing its evaporative loss through the skin. The neurohypophysial hormones exert antidiuretic effects by reducing the glomerular filtration rate, by increasing the reabsorption of fluid from the kidney tubules and urinary bladder, and by enhancing the uptake of water and salt through the skin.

Excessive hydration may be a threat to amphibians living in hypotonic (freshwater) environments, and it appears that the adrenal steroids may be involved in these adjustments. Adrenalectomy of *Rana temporaria* results in an accumulation of water in the tissues and a loss of sodium.[11] The administration of ACTH or adrenocorticoids to amphibians promotes the uptake of sodium from their freshwater environments. Aldosterone is the only adrenal steroid capable of stimulating active sodium transport by the isolated toad bladder *in vitro*.[14, 15] Cortisol and corticosterone have no effect on such bladder preparations when they are used alone, but they do block the effects of aldosterone. Pretreatment of amphibians with ACTH or adrenal steroids increases sodium influx through the isolated skin. These various studies suggest that the neurohypophysial principles are of especial importance when amphibians are threatened by dehydration, and that the adrenal steroids bring about adjustments which are essential for life in hypotonic environments, in which hydration is a threatening factor.

Fishes[7, 53]

The stenohaline fishes are unable to tolerate salinities differing from their normal environments (freshwater or marine), whereas the euryhaline species can adjust to a variety of salinities. Many teleosts live continuously in fresh water or sea water, whereas others (salmon) return to fresh water to spawn, or, like the eels, breed in the sea and become adults in fresh water. Freshwater fish do not drink water, but water enters osmotically through the gills and perhaps through the skin; since the renal tubules reabsorb salts from the glomerular filtrate, large volumes of dilute urine are excreted. Certain ions are actively taken in through the gills to assist in maintaining the proper osmotic and ionic equilibrium. Marine teleosts drink sea water and excrete large amounts of sodium and chloride through the gills; the urine flow is much reduced.

Osmoregulatory mechanisms are poorly understood among the stenohaline fishes. Most workers have found that hypophysectomy has no effect upon their metabolism of water and electrolytes. The killifish *(Fundulus)* is a euryhaline species and adjusts well to either fresh or sea water. Hypophysectomized killifishes do not live long in fresh water, and the blood chloride falls rapidly; prolactin partially restores their ability to adjust to fresh water. It is known that depletion of neurosecretory material from the preoptic nucleus and neurohypophysis occurs when certain species are exposed to increased salinities. Bioassay procedures have demonstrated that the neurohypophysis is deficient in antidiuretic potency under these conditions. This would seem to indicate that the neurohypophysial hormones are involved in osmoregulation, and indeed, it has been demonstrated that renal and branchial effects occur following the injection of isotocin and arginine vasotocin.[54]

Studies on euryhaline fishes strongly suggest that the adrenal steroids, together with other factors, are involved in the physiologic adjustments which promote the excretion of sodium. Aldosterone reduces the rate of sodium influx by the gills of the eel *(Anguilla anguilla)* in fresh water. The administration of corticosterone, cortisol, or aldosterone to the freshwater trout *(Salmo gairdneri)* reduces the concentration of sodium in the plasma. This over-all effect results from a diminished loss of sodium through the kidneys and an accelerated efflux of this ion through the gills. When untreated trout are transferred to sea water, there is a temporary increase in blood sodium followed by a progressive decline to a level slightly above that of fish in fresh water. The decline is due to the accelerated loss of sodium through the gills. During smoltification (preparation for life in the sea) in salmonid fishes, there is heightened activity of the steroidogenic adrenal, and the animals adjust rapidly to increased salinities. Thyroidal and gonadal hormones also play an important role in initiating smoltification and migration to salt water.[41]

The elasmobranchs are unusual among vertebrates in that their blood osmoconcentration is higher than that of their environment, whether fresh water or sea water. The urine contains large quantities of urea, but is hypoosmotic to the blood. The rectal gland of sharks is an intestinal diverticulum specialized for the excretion of sodium chloride. These glands are much smaller in freshwater species than in species living in marine habitats. The secretion from the rectal gland of *Squalus* is isosmotic with the blood, but contains about twice as much sodium chloride, and practically no urea. There is no information on the functional regulation of the rectal glands.[60]

Carbohydrate Metabolism

The disturbances in carbohydrate metabolism occurring in the adrenalectomized animal are due chiefly to removal of the cortex and are similar in many respects to those that follow hypophysectomy. In the fasted, untreated, adrenalectomized animal, severe depletion of liver glycogen, low blood glucose levels, and decreased intestinal absorption of glucose ensue. Muscle glycogen is lost during the terminal stages of cortical insufficiency. These changes may be prevented by giving sufficient carbohydrate and are largely corrected by the administration of sodium salts. Adrenalectomized animals excrete less nitrogen during fasting than do normal subjects, which suggests a decrease in the rate of formation of glucose from tissue protein (gluconeogenesis). The adrenalectomized animal, like the hypohysectomized animal, utilizes carbohydrate at an accelerated rate. Muscle glycogen is oxidized at an increased rate and this leads to depletion of the liver glycogen stores. In the absence of cortical hormones, the animal cannot replenish liver glycogen by glyconeogenesis from protein. The adrenalectomized animal is known to be very sensitive to the action of insulin. Adrenalectomy, like hypophysectomy, alleviates the symptoms of pancreatic diabetes; blood sugar is lowered, and the urinary excretion of glucose, ketone bodies, and nitrogen decreases. The two fundamental defects in carbohydrate metabolism consequent upon adrenalectomy are (1) excessive oxidation of glucose and (2) decreased gluconeogenesis from body protein.[32, 50, 82]

Although the 11-oxygenated adrenal hormones have some effect on

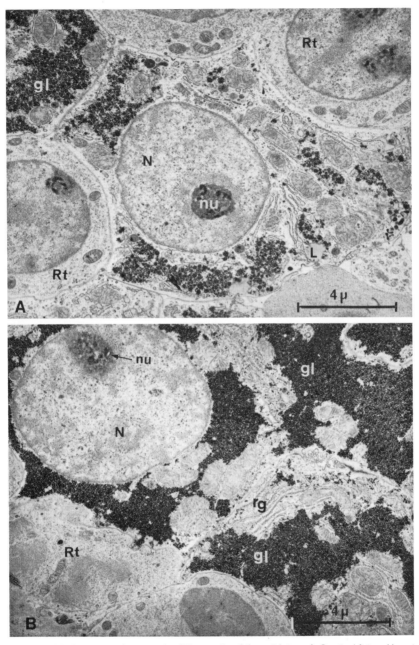

Figure 11–11. Electron micrograph of liver cells of the rat fetus. *A*, Control fetus. Hepatocyte cytoplasm is rich in glycogen (gl) and associated lipid bodies (L). Both the nucleus (N) and the nucleolus (nu) are prominent. Surrounding reticulocytes (Rt) are visible. *B*, Cortisol-injected embryo. Hepatocyte cytoplasm is filled with glycogen. The endoplasmic reticulum (rg) is well ordered. (From Dupouy, J., and A. Jost: Arch. Anat. Micro. Morph. Exp. *58*:183, 1969.)

electrolytes and fluid shifts, they are especially potent in correcting the defects in carbohydrate metabolism that follow adrenalectomy. Cortisol is three to five times more potent in this respect than corticosterone or 11-dehydrocorticosterone; cortisone is two to three times more potent than 11-dehydrocorticosterone and corticosterone. Aldosterone has about 33 per cent of the activity of cortisone in causing liver glycogen deposition, but is about 30 times more effective than DOC in this respect.

The administration of 11-oxygenated corticoids to fasting normal or adrenalectomized animals causes a rise in blood sugar and a striking increase in liver glycogen and total body carbohydrate, but muscle glycogen stores are not appreciably changed. The increased carbohydrate stores are the result of diminished oxidation of glucose and accelerated gluconeogenesis from tissue protein. The latter is indicated by an increased urinary elimination of nitrogen. In adrenalectomized animals, the respiratory quotient (R.Q.) is increased, but the adrenal cortical hormones lower it, indicating that the hormones have an inhibitory effect on glucose utilization. The phosphorylation of glucose to glucose-6-phosphate, catalyzed by hexokinase, is the first reaction in the utilization of glucose, and it appears that the cortical steroids exert an inhibitory influence at this point. There are indications that the corticoids may act at this level by potentiating the inhibitory effect of pituitary somatotrophin on the hexokinase reaction. Both the accelerated gluconeogenesis and diminished utilization of glucose, effected by the 11-oxygenated corticoids, are antagonized by the action of insulin.

When hypophysectomized rodents are made to fast, the liver glycogen is soon exhausted, and the blood sugar drops to low levels. These changes may be prevented by administering adrenal corticoids or they may be restored to normal if the levels are already low. The muscle glycogen stores are not appreciably affected by this treatment.

During normal ontogeny, liver cells of the rat fetus accumulate glycogen. Injection of cortisol into rat fetuses *in utero* leads to an early maturation of hepatocytes and to the accumulation of large stores of glycogen (Fig. 11–11). Glycogen deposits appear in the form of rosettes and are closely associated with the endoplasmic reticulum and with lipid inclusions.[21]

Diabetes, produced by pancreatectomy or alloxan, is aggravated by administering cortical hormones. Insulin convulsions in mice and rats may be prevented by giving 11-oxygenated corticoids, the adrenal hormones acting to provide sugar by stimulating gluconeogenesis.

The cortical steroids exert three main effects on carbohydrate metabolism: They discourage the utilization of carbohydrate, presumably by acting with somatotrophin to inhibit the hexokinase reaction; they promote the formation of glucose from tissue protein; and they cause the deposition of glycogen in the liver.

Protein and Fat Metabolism

The 11-oxygenated steroids cause an increased deposition of hepatic glycogen that is accompanied by an increased elimination of urinary nitrogen and an overall negative nitrogen balance. Although such steroids can influence the nitrogen balance of the body, it has not been determined how this is accomplished; they may diminish the rate of protein synthesis or they may increase the rates of breakdown of tissue proteins and amino acids. Moreover, it seems that the effects of such steroids are differential since the injection of cortisol or corticosterone stimulates protein and nucleic acid synthesis in the liver, but has a catabolic effect in lymphoid tissue. There are suggestions that the adrenal steroids may reduce the rate of protein synthesis by antagonizing the effects of insulin, thus reducing the rate of energy production through the breakdown of glucose. It is also possible that cortical hormones may retard protein synthesis by an effect on the metabolism of nucleic acids.

Studies have been made on the effects of cortical steroids on the mobilization of protein nitrogen from lymphoid tissues (spleen, thymus, lymph nodes) and from liver. The administration of cortical extracts to adrenalectomized mice or of ACTH to hypophysectomized mice leads to a rapid liberation of nitrogen from these tissues when they are tested *in vitro*. Tissues taken from adrenalectomized animals release relatively little protein nitrogen.[31, 49]

The conversion of carbohydrate to fat is markedly increased in the adrenalectomized rat. The 11-oxycorticoids depress the synthesis of fat from carbohydrate, and *in vitro* studies have demonstrated that glucocorticoids have the capacity to increase the output of free fatty acids from adipose tissue.[46] The mechanism of this action is not known. The administration of cortisol or cortisone to rats suppresses the ketosis that occurs during fasting or that is consequent upon cold exposure. Increased ketosis results from the administration of purified somatotrophin or of purified ACTH. The latter hormone has a ketogenic effect even in the absence of the adrenal cortices. It appears that these two pituitary hormones (*i.e.,* STH and ACTH) accelerate the breakdown of fatty acids. Either directly, or indirectly through the adrenal cortex, they act antagonistically to insulin not only in carbohydrate metabolism but in fat metabolism as well. Altogether, it is known that epinephrine, norepinephrine, ACTH, glucagon, and the glucocorticoids are involved in the fat-mobilizing effect and it seems certain that whatever the specific mechanism of glucocorticoid action is, it differs markedly from that of these other hormones.

Miscellaneous Effects

A striking action of 11-oxycorticoids, whether injected or produced endogenously, is to diminish the number of eosinophils (eosinopenia) and lymphocytes (lymphopenia) in the peripheral circulation. Aldosterone is about half as active as cortisone in causing eosinopenia. Deoxycorticosterone does not produce eosinopenia unless very high doses are used.

Although the cortical hormones can fully restore the resistance of adrenalectomized animals to various kinds of stressors, such as toxins, temperature changes, trauma, etc., there is no clear evidence that they can augment the resistance of intact animals to such stresses. In the cold stress test, often used for the bioassay of cortical steroids, the animals are adrenalectomized and are then subjected to low temperatures. Aldosterone and cortisone are about equal in their capacity to enable adrenalectomized animals to tolerate cold; the 11-deoxycorticoids are weak in this respect.

The oxysteroids of the adrenal profoundly influence the inflammatory reactions of the tissues. Local inflammatory responses to irritating substances are reduced or delayed, as are the hypersensitivity reactions to most antigens. The mechanism of the anti-inflammatory response is not yet explained; however, it is possible that it results from localized metabolic stimulation by glucocorticoids. Such cortical hormones also delay the healing of wounds and may reduce the capacity of the tissues to wall off infectious agents. They are known to have important effects on antibody formation. The symptomatic relief provided by cortisol, cortisone, or ACTH may be helpful in certain diseases but distinctly deleterious in other circumstances.

Reproductive functions are arrested during periods of chronic adrenal insufficiency. The failure of lactation that occurs after adrenalectomy is attributable, in part at least, to generalized disturbances in the vascular system, in the distribution of inorganic ions and water, and in the metabolism of carbohydrate, fat, and protein.

Considerable evidence has accumulated indicating that the adrenocortical hormones have important influences on the excitability of the brain and on the metabolism of nervous tissue.

Stress and Disease

It is an established fact that adrenalectomized animals have very little ability to tolerate stressors, such as temperature extremes, prolonged muscular activity, trauma, infections, intoxications, etc. This inability to withstand damaging stimuli may be repaired by the administration of adrenal cortical hormones. Furthermore, when intact animals are stressed, the pituitary-adrenal axis is activated, and a rather stereotyped sequence of reactions occurs in response to an outpouring of secretions from these glands. The response of the organism to nonspecific stress has been called the "General Adaptation Syndrome." The endocrine adjustments that occur during stress must be of utility to the organism in its attempt to maintain homeostasis.

Selye has proposed the hypothesis that the adaptive mechanisms that are called into operation during exposure to nonspecific stress may be detrimental to certain physiological functions and cause disease.[72] For example, the secretion of large amounts of ACTH and anti-inflammatory adrenal steroids during stress may be useful in enabling an organism to survive during the emergency by suppressing excessive inflammatory reactions; but, on the other hand, the same response may be harmful, inasmuch as it permits the spread of infections. By administering pituitary and adrenal hormones to "sensitized" laboratory animals, Selye and his coworkers have been able to induce a variety of pathologic changes, such as hypertension, arthritis, arteriosclerosis, nephrosclerosis, gastrointestinal ulcers, and many others. Most of the work has involved the administration of overdoses of hormones to animals sensitized by unilateral nephrectomy and by a high dietary load of sodium chloride. These pathologic changes have been interpreted as simulating human diseases. According to Selye's concept of "adaptation diseases," maladjustments to stress may play an etiologic role in certain diseases of man. Although an enormous amount of research has been published on the physiologic effects of stress, there is a paucity of evidence showing that diseases can be produced in normal subjects by exposing them to naturally occurring stressors.

The "permissive" action of adrenal cortical hormones has been emphasized by a number of workers.[44] According to this view, the adrenocortical hormones are essential for the full-blown manifestation of certain responses to stress, but they are not direct causative agents of the responses. A number of situations have been studied in which a hormone acts to produce the necessary environment for other biologic substances to exercise the full scope of their functions.

That adaptive mechanisms in response to stress may produce disease by hormonal excesses or imbalances is an interesting concept, but the supporting evidence is largely indirect and not sufficient to establish it as a fact. However, like most unifying concepts it has provoked much thought, speculation, and research. This is a contribution whose value is difficult to assess.

MECHANISM OF ACTION OF ADRENAL STEROIDS

In surveying the multitude of effects attributable to hormones produced by the adrenal cortex, one is struck by their great diversity. On this basis, it seems difficult to establish any general concept that could explain all these effects in terms of one basic mechanism. If, however, there is such a general mechanism of action, it probably relates to protein synthesis effected by the action of the steroid on the genome. Evidence that sex hormones function in this way is quite convincing and it seems a reasonable assumption, in the light of current knowledge, that glucocorticoids and mineralocorticoids also function through the mediation of protein synthesis.

Studies of the mechanism of action of cortisol have revealed that the hormone causes an accumulation of amino acids in the livers of adrenalectomized rats. This stimulation of protein synthesis is paralleled by an increase in liver RNA and leads to the appearance of specific liver enzymes. The administration of actinomycin completely blocks the synthesis of those enzymes induced by cortisol, but does not affect blood-sugar or hepatic glycogen levels, implying that these two hormonal effects are mediated separately. Apparently, the action of cortisol on lymphatic and muscle tissue also operates through different means since the hormone inhibits protein synthesis in these tissues.

Considerable attention has been given to the mechanism of action of aldosterone.[22, 73] Evidence is available from studies on the isolated toad bladder that the stimulation of sodium transport is ultimately mediated by the regulation of gene activity. A period of 60 to 90 minutes is required before the induction of sodium transport is observed, implying that synthetic events are taking place. Both puromycin and actinomycin block the action of aldosterone, and evidence has been obtained that DNA-dependent synthesis of RNA is stimulated by the steroid, leading to the production of proteins. These proteins may be permeases involved in sodium transport. The concept that the hormone acts primarily on the genome is supported by the demonstration of aldosterone receptor sites in the nucleus, allowing for the accumulation of aldosterone on this target.[8]

REFERENCES

1. Bentley, P. J.: Studies on the permeability of the large intestine and urinary bladder of the tortoise (*Testudo graeca*) with special reference to the effects of neuro-hypophysial and adrenocortical hormones. Gen. Comp. Endocr. *2*:323, 1962.
2. Bernstein, D. E.: Autotransplantation of the adrenal of the rat to the portal circulation: Effect of administration of testosterone in male rats. Endocrinology *67*:685, 1960.
3. Blair-West, J. R., Coghlan, J. P., Denton, D. A., Goding, J. R., Wintour, M., and Wright, R. D.: The control of aldosterone secretion. Rec. Progr. Hormone Res. *19*:311, 1963.
4. Bongiovanni, A. M., and Eder, W.: *In vitro* hydroxylation of steroids of whole adrenal homogenates of beef, normal man, and patients with the adrenogenital syndrome. J. Clin. Invest. *37*:1342, 1958.
5. Bronson, F. H., and Eleftheriou, B. E.: Chronic physiological effects of fighting in mice. Gen. Comp. Endocr. *4*:9, 1964.
6. Brown, H. E., and Dougherty, T. F.: The diurnal variation of blood leucocytes in normal and adrenalectomized mice. Endocrinology *58*:365, 1956.
7. Butler, D. G.: Structure and function of the adrenal gland of fishes. Amer. Zool. *13*:839–978, 1973.
8. Cameron, I. L., Tolman, E. L., and Harrington, G. W.: Aldosterone receptor sites in tissues and cells of salamander, chicken, goldfish and mouse. Texas Rep. Biol. Med. *27*:2, 1969.
9. Carstensen, H., Burgers, A. C. J., and Li, C. H.: Demonstration of aldosterone and corticosterone as the principal steroids formed in incubates of adrenals of the American bull frog (*Rana catesbeiana*) and stimulation of their production by mammalian adrenocorticotropin. Gen. Comp. Endocr. *1*:37, 1961.
10. Chester Jones, I.: The role of the adrenal cortex in the control of water and salt-electrolyte balance in vertebrates. Mem. Soc. Endocr. *5*:102, 1956.
11. Chester Jones, I., Phillips, J. G., and Holmes, W. N.: Comparative physiology of the adrenal cortex. *In* A. Gorbman (ed.): Comparative Endocrinology. New York, John Wiley & Sons, 1959, p. 582.
12. Christian, J. J., and Davis, D. E.: Endocrines, behavior, and population. Science *146*:1550, 1964.
13. Cortés, J. M., Péron, F. G., and Dorfman, R. I.: Secretion of 18-hydroxydeoxycorticosterone by the rat adrenal gland. Endocrinology *73*:713, 1963.
14. Crabbé, J.: Stimulation of active sodium transport across the isolated toad bladder after injection of aldosterone to the animal. Endocrinology *69*:673, 1961.
15. Crabbé, J.: Effects of adrenocortical steroids on active sodium transport by the urinary bladder and ventral skin of Amphibia. *In* P. C. Williams (ed.): Hormones and the Kidney. New York, Academic Press, 1963, p. 75.
16. Davis, J. O.: Mechanism regulating the secretion and metabolism of aldosterone in experimental hyperaldosteronism. Rec. Progr. Hormone Res. *17*:293, 1961.
17. deRoos, R.: *In vitro* production of corticoids by chicken adrenals. Endocrinology *67*:719, 1960.
18. deRoos, R.: The corticoids of the avian adrenal gland. Gen. Comp. Endocr. *1*:494, 1961.
19. deRoos, R.: The Physiology of the Avian Interrenal Gland: A Review. *In* C. G. Sibley (ed.): Proc. 13th Internat. Ornithological Congress, Vol. 2, 1963, p. 1041.

20. Dorfman, R. I.: Biosynthesis of adrenocortical steroids. Cancer *10*:741, 1957.
21. Dupouy, J.-P., and Jost, A.: Aspect ultrastructural de l'accumulation anticipée de gly-cogéne dans le foie du foetus de rat soumis au cortisol. Arch. Anat. Micro. Morph. Exp. *58*:183, 1969.
22. Edelman, I. S., and Fimognari, G. M.: On the biochemical mechanism of action of aldoster-one. Rec. Progr. Hormone Res. *24*:1, 1968.
23. Eppstein, S. H., Meister, P. D., Murray, H. C., and Peterson, D. H.: Microbiological transfor-mations of steroids and their applications to the synthesis of hormones. Vitamins Hor-mones *14*:359, 1956.
24. Fawcett, D. W., Long, J. A., and Jones, A. L.: The ultrastructure of endocrine glands. Rec. Progr. Hormone Res. *25*:315, 1969.
25. Fieser, L. F., and Fieser, M.: Steroids. New York, Reinhold Publishing Corp., 1959.
26. Flickinger, D. D.: Adrenal responses of California quail subjected to various physiologic stimuli. Proc. Soc. Exp. Biol. Med. *100*:23, 1959.
27. Ganong, W. F.: The central nervous system and the synthesis and release of adrenocorti-cotropic hormones. *In* A. V. Nalbandov (ed.): Advances in Neuroendocrinology. Urbana, University of Illinois Press, 1963, p. 92.
28. Giroud, C. J. P., Stachenko, J., and Piletta, P.: *In vitro* studies on the functional zonation of the adrenal cortex and of the production of aldosterone. *In* A. F. Muller and C. M. O'Connor (eds.): An International Symposium on Aldosterone. London, J. & A. Churchill, 1958, p. 56.
29. Giroud, C. J. P., Stachenko, J., and Venning, E. H.: Secretion of aldosterone by the zona glomerulosa of rat adrenal glands. Proc. Soc. Exp. Biol. Med. *92*:154, 1956.
30. Glenister, D. W., and Yates, F. E.: Sex difference in the rate of disappearance of corticoste-rone-4-C14 from plasma of intact rats: Further evidence for the influence of hepatic Δ4-steroid hydrogenase activity on adrenal cortical function. Endocrinology *68*:747, 1961.
31. Glenn, E. M., Bowman, B. J., Bayer, R. B., and Meyer, C. E.: Hydrocortisone and some of its effects on intermediary metabolism. Endocrinology *68*:386, 1961.
32. Greengard, O., Weber, G., and Singhal, R. L.: Glycogen deposition in the liver induced by cortisone: Dependence on enzyme synthesis. Science *141*:160, 1963.
33. Grower, M. F., and Bransome, E. D., Jr.: Adenosine 3',5'-monophosphate, adrenocorti-cotropic hormone, and adrenocortical cytosol protein synthesis. Science *168*:483, 1970.
34. Halberg, F., Peterson, R. E., and Silber, R. H.: Phase relations of 24-hour periodicities in blood corticosterone, mitoses in cortical adrenal parenchyma, and total body activity. Endocrinology *64*:222, 1959.
35. Hechter, O., Jacobsen, R. P., Schenker, V., Levy, H., Jeanloz, R. W., Marshall, C. W., and Pincus, G.: Chemical transformation of steroids by adrenal perfusion: Perfusion methods. Endocrinology *52*:679, 1953.
36. Hechter, O., and Pincus, G.: Genesis of the adrenocortical secretion. Physiol. Rev. *34*:459, 1954.
37. Hechter, O., Solomon, M. M., Zaffaroni, A., and Pincus, G.: Transformation of cholesterol and acetate to adrenal cortical hormones. Arch. Biochem. Biophys. *46*:201, 1953.
38. Hilton, J. G., Scian, L. F., Westermann, C. D., and Kruesi, O. R.: Direct stimulation of adreno-cortical secretion by synthetic vasopressin. Proc. Soc. Exp. Biol. Med. *100*:523, 1959.
39. Hirschmann, H., de Courcy, C., Levy, R. P., and Miller, K. L.: Adrenal precursors of urinary 17-ketosteroids. J. Biol. Chem. *235*:PC48, 1960.
40. Holmes, W. N., Phillips, J. G., and Butler, D. G.: The effect of adrenocortical steroids on the renal and extra-renal responses of the domestic duck (*Anas platyrhynchus*) after hyper-tonic saline loading. Endocrinology *69*:483, 1961.
41. Holmes, W. N., Phillips, J. C., and Chester Jones, I.: Adrenocortical factors associated with adaptation of vertebrates to marine environments. Rec. Progr. Hormone Res. *19*:619, 1963.
42. Holmes, W. N., Phillips, J. G., and Wright, A.: The control of extrarenal excretion in the duck (*Anas platyrhynchos*) with special reference to the pituitary-adrenal axis. Gen. Comp. Endocr., Suppl. *2*:358, 1969.
43. Idler, D. R., and Truscott, B.: Production of 1α-hydroxycorticosterone *in vivo* and *in vitro* by elasmobranchs. Gen. Comp. Endocr. Suppl. *2*:325, 1969.
44. Ingle, D. J.: Permissibility of hormone action: A review. Acta Endocr. *17*:172, 1954.
45. Inoue, T.: Nasal salt gland: Independence of salt and water transport. Science *142*:1299, 1963.
46. Jeanrenaud, B., and Renold, A. E.: The effects of glucocorticoids upon adipose tissue *in vitro. In* L. Martini, F. Fraschini, and M. Motta (eds.): Proceedings of the Second Interna-tional Congress on Hormonal Steroids. Amsterdam, Excerpta Medica Foundation, 1967, p. 769.

47. Kitay, J. I.: Pituitary-adrenal function in the rat after gonadectomy and gonadal hormone replacement. Endocrinology 73:253, 1963.
48. Kolthoff, N. J., Macchi, I. A., and Wyman, L. C.: Isotopic determinations of blood volume in intact and regenerated rat adrenals during cold stress. Endocrinology 73:27, 1963.
49. Kostyo, J. L.: In vitro effects of adrenal steroid hormones on amino acid transport in muscle. Endocrinology 76:604, 1965.
50. Landau, B. R., Mahler, R., Ashmore, J., Elwyn, D., Hastings, A. B., and Zottu, S.: Cortisone and the regulation of hepatic gluconeogenesis. Endocrinology 70:47, 1962.
51. Lanman, J. T., and Silverman, L. M.: In vitro steroidogenesis in the human neonatal adrenal gland, including observations on human adult and monkey adrenal glands. Endocrinology 60:433, 1957.
52. Macchi, I. A., and Wyman, L. C.: Qualitative characterization of corticoids produced by adrenal autografts in the rat. Endocrinology 73:20, 1963.
53. Maetz, J.: Observations on the role of the pituitary-interrenal axis in the ion regulation of the eel and other teleosts. Gen. Comp. Endocr., Suppl. 2:229, 1969.
54. Maetz, J., and Rankin, J. C.: Quelques aspects du rôle biologique des hormones neurohypophysaires chez les Poissons. In La spécificité zoologique des hormones hypophysaires et de leurs activités. Paris, Centre National de la Recherche Scientifique, 1969, p. 45.
55. Marieb, N. J., and Mulrow, P. J.: Role of the renin-angiotensin system in the regulation of aldosterone secretion in the rat. Endocrinology 76:657, 1965.
56. Mosier, H. D.: Comparative histological study of the adrenal cortex of the wild and domesticated Norway rat. Endocrinology 60:460, 1957.
57. Nandi, J.: Comparative endocrinology of steroid hormones in vertebrates. Amer. Zool. 7:115, 1967.
58. Nandi, J., and Bern, H. A.: Chromatography of corticosteroids from teleost fishes. Gen. Comp. Endocr. 5:1, 1965.
59. Oertel, G. W., and Eik-Nes, K. B.: Isolation and identification of 11-ketoprogesterone, 11-hydroxyprogesterone and 11-hydroxyandrostenedione in canine adrenal vein blood. Endocrinology 70:39, 1962.
60. Oguri, M.: Rectal glands of marine and fresh-water sharks: Comparative histology. Science 144:1151, 1964.
61. Peart, W. S.: The renin-angiotensin system. Pharmacol. Rev. 17:143, 1965.
62. Pechet, M. M., Hesse, R. H., and Kohler, H.: The metabolism of aldosterone: Isolation and characterization of two new metabolites. J. Amer. Chem. Soc. 82:5251, 1960.
63. Perrine, J. W., Bortle, L., Heyder, E., Partridge, R., Ross, E. K., and Ringler, I.: Adrenal cortical activities of 9α-fluoro-11β,16α,17α-21-tetrahydroxy-1,4-pregnadiene-3,20-dione. Endocrinology 64:437, 1959.
64. Samuels, L. T., and Reich, H.: The chemistry and metabolism of the steroids. Ann. Rev. Biochem. 21:129, 1952.
65. Sandor, T.: A comparative survey of steroids and steroidogenic pathways throughout the vertebrates. Gen. Comp. Endocr., Suppl. 2:285, 1969.
66. Sandor, T., Lamoureux, J., and Lanthier, A.: Adrenocortical function in birds: In vitro biosynthesis of radioactive corticosteroids from pregnenolone-7-H³ and progesterone-4-C¹⁴ by adrenal glands of the domestic duck (Anas platyrhynchos) and the chicken (Gallus domesticus). Endocrinology 73:629, 1963.
67. Sandor, T., Sonea, S., and Mehdi, A. Z.: The possible role of steroids in evolution. Amer. Zool. 15 (Suppl. 1):227–253, 1975.
68. Schmidt-Nielson, K.: The salt-secreting gland of marine birds. Circulation 21:(Part 2):955, 1960.
69. Schmidt-Nielson, K., Borut, A., Lee, P., and Crawford, E., Jr.: Nasal salt excretion and possible function of cloaca in water conservation. Science 142:1300, 1963.
70. Segal, S. J.: Embryology of adrenal hyperplasia following estrogen administration. Anat. Rec. 113:47, 1952.
71. Seltzer, H. S., and Clark, D. A.: Evidence for conversion of corticosterone to aldosterone in man. Proc. Soc. Exp. Biol. Med. 98:674, 1958.
72. Selye, H.: Perspectives in stress research. Perspect. Biol. Med. 2:403, 1959.
73. Sharp, G. W. G., and Leaf, A.: Studies on the mode of action of aldosterone. Rec. Progr. Hormone Res. 22:431, 1966.
74. Sheppard, H., Swenson, R., and Mowles, T. F.: Steroid biosynthesis by rat adrenal: Functional zonation. Endocrinology 73:819, 1963.
75. Solomon, S., Lanman, J. T., Lind, J., and Lieberman, S.: The biosynthesis of Δ⁴-androstenedione and 17α-hydroxyprogesterone from progesterone by surviving human fetal adrenals. J. Biol. Chem. 233:1084, 1958.

76. Stachenko, J., and Giroud, C. J. P.: Functional zonation of the adrenal cortex: Pathways of corticosteroid biogenesis. Site of ACTH action. Endocrinology *64*:730, 1959.

77. Sutherland, E. W., Robison, G. A., and Butcher, R. W.: Some aspects of the biological role of adenosine 3',5'-monophosphate (cyclic AMP). Circulation *37*:279, 1968.

78. Taylor, J. D., Honn, K. V., and Chavin, W.: Adrenocortical ultrastructure in the squaliform elasmobranch (*Ginglymostoma cirratum*): Cell death a postulate for holocrine secretion. Gen. Comp. Endocr. *27*:358, 1975.

79. Urquhart, J., Yates, F. E., and Herbst, A. L.: Hepatic regulation of adrenal cortical function. Endocrinology *64*:816, 1959.

80. Villee, D. B., Engel, L. L., and Villee, C. A.: Steroid hydroxylation in human fetal adrenals. Endocrinology *65*:465, 1959.

81. Vogt, M.: The effects of hexoestrol and of "Amphenone B" on morphology and function of the rat adrenal cortex. Yale J. Biol. Med. *29*:469, 1957.

82. Winternitz, W. W., Dintzis, R., and Long, C. N. H.: Further studies on the adrenal cortex and carbohydrate metabolism. Endocrinology *61*:724, 1957.

83. Woods, J. W.: The effects of acute stress and of ACTH upon ascorbic acid and lipid content of the adrenal glands of wild rats. J. Physiol. *135*:390, 1957.

84. Yates, F. E., Herbst, A. L., and Urquhart, J.: Sex difference in rate of ring A reduction of Δ^4-3-keto-steroids *in vitro* by rat liver. Endocrinology *63*:887, 1958.

85. Yates, F. E., and Urquhart, J.: Contol of plasma concentrations of adrenocortical hormones. Physiol. Rev. *42*:359, 1962.

CHAPTER 12

The Biology of Sex and Reproduction

All groups of living organisms can reproduce in some manner, and the continuity of the species depends upon this capacity. Unlike reproduction, sexual dimorphism is by no means a universal attribute of organisms. Since monoecious, or hermaphroditic, organisms are capable of producing both sperms and eggs, it is obvious that the ability to produce a particular kind of gamete is not dependent upon the differentiation of specific sexual characters. In sexual reproduction, two cells (gametes) fuse to form a new individual (zygote), and the significance of this event is that it promotes genetic diversity.

Many lower organisms form gametes of like size and shape (isogametes), and the fusion of these is suggestive of sexuality. However, the isogametes cannot be designated as "male" or "female" since they are morphologically indistinguishable and, in many instances, seem capable of performing either role. The most basic feature of this cellular union (syngamy) is the succession of haploid and diploid phases. The chromosome number is doubled at fertilization and halved by the meiotic process. Even the behavior of chromosomes during meiosis is suggestive of "sex." Homologous chromosomes of a diploid set make contact with each other and the chromomeres and gene loci are lined up with remarkable precision (conjugation); this is followed by divisions which reduce the number of chromosomes. Polyploidy may occur in certain species, giving rise to more than two full sets of homologous chromosomes. At the chromosomal level, there is some kind of opposing polarity in the molecular patterns and forces which direct their movements, and this may lie at the very core of the "sex" problem. Among bacteria (*Escherichia coli*), a single chromosome passes from one conjugant into the other, and the alignment of the two chromosomes is suggestive of that occurring during meiosis. These facts indicate that reproduction through the fusion of cells is not necessarily dependent upon male-female differentiation. The great majority of vertebrates are dioecious, the anisogametes being proliferated by dimorphic individuals of the species.

SEX DETERMINATION AND ONTOGENETIC
DIFFERENTIATION

In the vertebrates, a sex-determining mechanism is established at fertilization (sex determination), and this directs and controls all of the later ontogenetic processes involved in male-female differentiation of the genital system (postgenetic differentiation). The genetic determination is not final and irrevocable; many external and internal environmental factors may come into operation during the developmental process and modify or completely reverse the genetic constitution of the individual. Germ cells, presumably of identical genetic constitution, may lie close together and differentiate as sperms or ova within the same individual (Figs. 12–1 and 12–2). This is encountered very often among hermaphroditic invertebrates and lower vertebrates, and suggests that male-determining and female-determining territories arise in the body during ontogenesis.

Genotypic sex is established at fertilization and depends upon the "sex" chromosomes which are contributed by the parents. For simplicity, the two major types of sex determination may be called the *mammalian* and *avian* types. The XX-XY type of determination is characteristic of mammals, most frogs, some fishes, and dipterous insects. The whole problem of sex determination in man remains uncertain, but it appears to differ in some

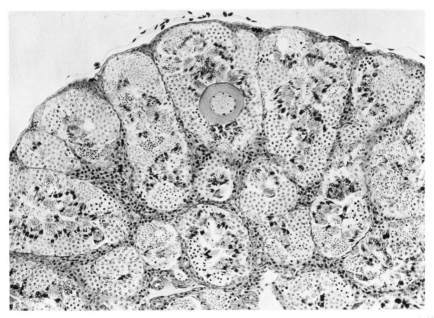

Figure 12–1. Section of an adult frog testis showing an oocyte within one of the seminiferous tubules. It is possible that this egg cell migrated, at an early stage, from the cortex into the medulla and became confined within a seminiferous tubule; it is also possible that an indifferent spermatogonium might have escaped the masculinizing influence of the medulla of the testis and differentiated into an egg instead of a sperm. Genetically, it is not known whether this abortive cell was determined as an egg or a sperm, but it is known that the early germ cells of vertebrates are bipotential. (Courtesy of Robert R. Cardell, Jr.)

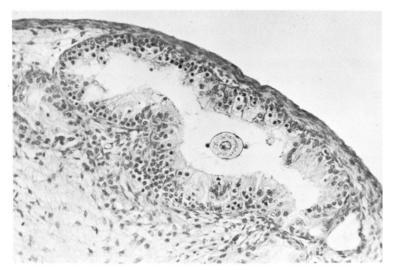

Figure 12–2. An oöcyte within a seminiferous tubule of a testis graft in the rat. A fetal testis and a fetal ovary were transplanted next to each other below the kidney capsule of an adult host; the double graft was removed after 40 days. The early germ cells of the ovary are capable of ameboid movement; at this early stage, many oögonia may migrate from the ovary into the tubules of the contiguous testis graft. (Courtesy of C. D. Turner and H. Asakawa.)

respects from that of *Drosophila,* which has been used so frequently as a model. Improved methods of chromosome identification indicate that the human being has 46 chromosomes, instead of 48, as was believed for many years: There are 22 pairs of autosomes and one pair of sex chromosomes. While the Y chromosome of *Drosophila* is necessary for male fertility, it is essentially inert with reference to the differentiation of phenotypic sex. Recent studies indicate that the Y chromosome is strongly "male determining" in man, in contrast to the same chromosome in *Drosophila.* In mammals and the other groups mentioned, the male is the heterogametic (XY) sex, half of the spermatozoa being X bearers and the other half Y bearers.[43, 51, 53] Fluorescent dyes such as quinacrine dihydrochloride are being used to identify and study Y chromosomes in fixed preparations. Two classes of human spermatozoa can be recognized, presumably those containing an X chromosome and those with a Y chromosome. Studies involving the separation of X- and Y-bearing sperms, or determining their ratio in different individuals, should be facilitated by these methods. The quinacrines may also be useful in following the behavior of chromosomes during the process of spermatogenesis.

In the avian type of determination, the female is the heterogametic sex. The small chromosome, equivalent to the Y in mammals, is designated by the letter W, and X chromosome is designated in these cases as Z. Half of the eggs carry a W chromosome and the other half a Z chromosome; all of the sperms carry a Z chromosome. The homozygous (ZZ) condition produces males, and the heterozygous (ZW) produces females. This is the type of mechanism that operates in birds, most reptiles and salamanders, and in some fishes and insects. In certain species, the inert Y and W chromosomes are absent and the mechanism may be designated XO and ZO. The W chromosome then is not present in birds, and the Y is lost in certain mammals (*e.g.,* Japanese mouse).

Sex mosaics, or gynandromorphs, are infrequently found among vertebrate groups. This condition probably occurs occasionally in man, though it has not been proved by sex chromosome studies. In gynandromorphism, known to result from an abnormality of the sex chromosomes, sharply delimited fractions of the body show male characteristics and the rest female. A frequent cause of this abnormality is the loss of an X (or Z) chromosome from an early cleavage cell derived from an XX (or ZZ) zygote. Other cases apparently result from the parthenogenic development of an ovum followed by the fertilization of an early blastomere.

Early embryos of the mouse, ranging from two-cell stages to morulae, may be brought together *in vitro* and allowed to fuse. Such chimeras arising from two original individuals may be transferred to suitable hosts and are frequently capable of developing to maturity. The indications are that the gonads differentiate normally—either as testes or as ovaries.[55]

There is abundant proof that individuals from many vertebrate species, without changing their chromosomes and genes, may differentiate in a direction opposite to their genotypic sex. Sexual characters, like other somatic characters determined by multiple genes, are subject to extreme variability. When populations are analyzed, some individuals are found to be weighted heavily in the male or in the female direction, with many individual variations between these two extremes. This suggests the existence of a quantitative relationship, or balance, between the set of genes determining maleness and the set determining femaleness.

Sex Chromatin

While studying the structural features of nerve cells in cats, Barr and his associates discovered a characteristic mass of chromatin in the nuclei of such cells from genetic females.[5] The chromatin mass is Feulgen-positive, measures about 1μ in diameter, and usually lies on the inner surface of the nuclear membrane (Fig. 12–3). This sexual dimorphism has been found in man and in numerous other mammals. The Barr test is now widely used in analyzing sex abnormalities in man. Skin biopsies, leukocytes, exfoliate cells from the vagina, or scrapings from the oral or nasal epithelia all provide readily available material for execution of the test. In "intersex" individuals, in whom there is an admixture of male and female characters, knowledge of the genetic sex may be valuable in deciding which direction the hormonal or surgical therapy should take. The genetic sex of very young embryos can be determined long before this would be possible by histologic study of the gonads. The sex chromatin is present even in the gonocytes, or primordial germ cells, before they reach the gonadal primordia.

The general inference is that the presence of sex chromatin is diagnostic of a genetic female (XX) and its absence is diagnostic of a genetic male

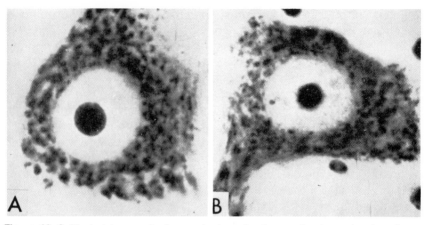

Figure 12–3. Ventral horn cells from spinal cords of normal calves, showing absence of sex chromatin in the normal male *(A)* and the presence of a sex chromatin mass in the nucleus of the cell from a normal female *(B)*. (From K. L. Moore, M. A. Graham, and M. L. Barr: J. Exp. Zool. *135*, 1957.)

(XY). This chromatin body is thought to arise from the fused heteropyknotic portions of two X chromosomes. The presence of a drumstick-like append-age on the nucleus of female polymorphonuclear leukocytes has been found useful in determining genetic sex in man and several other vertebrates.

ANATOMY OF THE REPRODUCTIVE SYSTEM

The *primary* sex characters are the gonads, *i.e.,* testes in the male and ovaries in the female. The higher vertebrates have evolved elaborate sys-tems of ducts and glands for the conveyance of viable germ cells toward the exterior of the organism (Figs. 12–4 and 12–5). These systems of ducts and glands involved in the transmission of gametes or developing zygotes con-stitute the *sex accessories.* The gonads not only proliferate gametes but also secrete hormones that condition the functional state of the accessory sex organs and, to some extent at least, influence the psychobiologic phe-nomena involved in the mating reactions. The proliferation of gametes and the mating reaction are basically rhythmic processes, and it is recognized that both are controlled or conditioned by a wide variety of intrinsic and extrinsic factors.

The *secondary* sex characters are more or less external specializations that are not essential for the proliferation and movement of germ cells but are concerned chiefly with mating and with the birth and nutrition of the young. These characters are more highly developed and diversified in birds than in any other vertebrate class. The ornamental secondary characters in birds, such as the dimorphic differentiation of feathers, head furnishings, and various other types of integumentary derivatives, are physiologically conditioned and serve to bring the sexes together during the reproductive periods. In mammals, the secondary sex characters are less pronounced

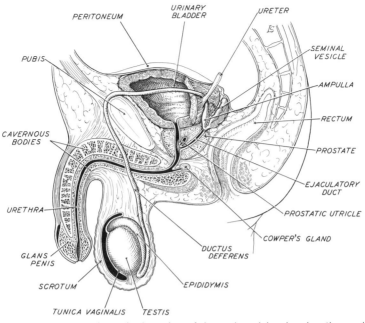

Figure 12–4. Diagrammatic sagittal section of the male pelvis, showing the genital organs and their relations to the bladder and urethra.

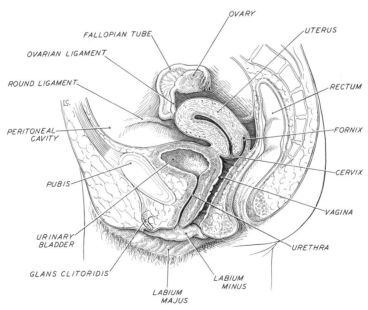

Figure 12–5. Diagrammatic sagittal section of the female pelvis, showing the genital organs and their relations to the bladder and urethra.

than in many of the fishes, amphibians, reptiles, and birds. Among these characters are the differential conditioning of the mammary glands in the two sexes, pelvic modifications for the facilitation of parturition, reddening and swelling of the circumanal "sex skin" during the follicular phase of the menstrual cycle in some primates, and differences in the size and shape of the larynx.

THE VERTEBRATE TESTIS

Mammals

In man and most other mammals, the testes of the adult are lodged in an integumentary pouch, the *scrotum.* Many types of experiments have shown that this organ is an adaptation for regulating the internal temperature of the testes. The spontaneous or experimental retention of the testes in the abdominal cavity in species in which they normally descend into the scrotum is called *cryptorchism* and is associated with profound damage to the seminiferous tubules. In seasonally breeding mammals, the testes ascend through the inguinal canals and remain in the body cavity during the nonbreeding period. Scrota are lacking in a few mammals, *e.g.,* the whale, elephant, seal, and rhinoceros, and the testes remain permanently in the abdominal cavity. There is no scrotum in the armadillo, but the testes descend to the entrance into the inguinal canal. The human testes usually assume scrotal positions during the terminal month of fetal life, and the inguinal canal becomes sealed off shortly after birth.

The stratified lining of the seminiferous tubules constitutes an epithelium from which the spermatozoa are proliferated. The tubule is limited by a thin basement membrane and a small amount of lamellated connective tissue. Contractile epithelial cells have been described in the limiting membrane of the seminiferous tubules of many vertebrates, and these play a role in the release of spermatozoa from the epithelium and their movement into the rete testis.[13] Pressure effects produced by accumulating cells may also be a factor involved in the movement of spermatozoa through the tubules. The *spermatogonia,* lying next to the basement membrane, exhibit a series of mitotic divisions leading to the formation of *primary spermatocytes.* These undergo the first meiotic division and give rise to haploid cells called *secondary spermatocytes.* The latter begin the second meiotic division almost immediately and produce smaller cells which are the *spermatids.* The transformation of spermatids into spermatozoa involves principally cytoplasmic loss and the differentiation of tailpieces. These cells are displaced toward the lumen of the tubule by the appearance of further generations of maturing spermatogonia. Spermatogonial mitoses do not occur at random; groups of cells at comparable stages of development undergo mitosis in unison. Well-defined cellular associations succeed each other in time in any given region of the tubule, and the sequence is repeated indefinitely. Three different processes are distinguishable therefore in the seminiferous epithelium: (1) increase in the number of cells by mitosis, (2) formation of haploid cells by reduction in the number of chromosomes by meiosis, and (3) the production of sperms from spermatids by spermiogenesis.

The sustentacular cells of Sertoli are relatively large elements extending from the basement membrane toward the lumen. They are regarded as supporting cells, which probably provide nourishment for the spermatids with which they are intimately associated. Ultrastructural and chemical studies support the view that they are capable of synthesizing steroid hormones, but it is very unlikely that they release appreciable quantities of such agents into the circulation. In some species, the sperm heads remain embedded in the Sertoli cells for relatively long periods. The release of spermatozoa from the Sertoli cells is termed *spermiation,* a process that is analogous to ovulation in the female.

In immature males, the seminiferous tubules are solid and contain only spermatogonia and undifferentiated cells. The testes of seasonally breeding males involute at the end of the breeding season and become comparable to those of the sexually immature animal. The human testes are almost stationary in growth during the first 10 years of life. Although wide variations are found among individuals, by the age of 12 the tubules have become luminal and the epithelium contains many spermatogonia, Leydig cells, primary and secondary spermatocytes, and spermatids. Spermatogenic function is generally well established by the age of 15. Although there is generally a decrease in spermatogenic activity in aging men, it is known that complete spermatogenesis may continue later than the ninth decade.[52]

The interspaces between the seminiferous tubules are occupied by blood vessels, connective tissue, and the *interstitial cells of Leydig.* The latter cells are of mesenchymal origin and appear singly or in clusters of varying sizes. Both the interstitial cells and the seminiferous tubules (probably Sertoli cells) of the mammalian testis can convert progesterone to androstenedione and testosterone.[22] Testicular estrogen also appears to be derived from the Leydig cells. In aging men, there is generally a decline in androgen secretion, but the production of estrogen is preferentially retained.

Like steroid-secreting cells in general, the Leydig cells possess a very extensive smooth endoplasmic reticulum and some of the enzymes involved in the biosynthesis of steroids reside in these membranes. The smooth reticulum often forms concentric lamellae around lipid droplets, lysosomes, and other organelles. The testicular interstitium is supplied with a very rich system of capillaries, venules, and thin-walled lymphatics. Sensitive histochemical techniques have been developed and used for determining the cellular sites of steroidogenic activity. Since the hydroxysteroid dehydrogenases are essential enzymes for the biosynthesis of steroid hormones, histochemical demonstration of their presence in particular tissues provides circumstantial evidence that the tissue is capable of producing such hormones.[45] Functional activity of the interstitium cannot be determined accurately by Leydig-cell counts or by estimating fluctuations in cell size. Such studies under the light microscope may give a very misleading picture of testicular function. The number appears to vary within normal individuals and also among species. For example, the testes of mature cocks contain fewer Leydig cells than those of younger, growing birds; but there is no evidence that the mature cock secretes less androgen than it did previously. Massive deposits of interstitial cells are present in the testis of the boar, whereas relatively scanty aggregates of such cells occur in normal human and bovine testes.[44]

The testes of the horse, seal, giraffe, and elephant are strikingly enlarged at birth, and shrink greatly during the first few days of postnatal life. The large size of the testis is due to a remarkable proliferation of the interstitial cells, which compose the bulk of the organ. The response must be due to the action of circulating maternal hormones upon the fetus.

The testes of the human infant are also enlarged at birth, owing to the extensive intertubular deposits of Leydig cells. These cells, which develop *in utero*, disappear promptly after birth and do not reappear again until the boy reaches the age of 11 to 13 years. There is normally little evidence of the presence of testicular hormone during childhood. Although small amounts of 17-ketosteroids are present in the urine, these compounds may emanate from the adrenal cortex rather than from the testis. At puberty, the testes secrete effective amounts of androgen, and the accessory sex organs undergo rapid growth and maturation. Secondary sex characters, such as deeper voice, beard, and body hair, begin to appear.

Nonmammalian Vertebrates

The Leydig cells of most mammalian species constitute a permanent secretory unit but, in wild birds, the interstitium becomes exhausted *en masse* at the end of the breeding season. A new crop of Leydig cells promptly begins to differentiate from the intertubular connective tissue cells in preparation for the next season's sexual activities. Special histologic methods are required to distinguish connective tissue cells from young Leydig cells; this appears to account for many of the erroneous statements in the literature that Leydig cells are absent at certain periods of the avian cycle.[38]

The tubules of the anuran testis contain nests of cells which undergo spermatogenesis nonsynchronously. The segmented testes of mature urodeles consist of active lobes filled with sperms, and quiescent lobes from which the next crop of spermatozoa will arise. The testes of teleostean fishes are generally organized into lobules which contain cysts of differentiating germ cells (Figs. 12–6 and 12–7). In some teleosts, urodeles, and turtles, tubule-boundary cells are observed instead of typical interstitial cells of Leydig. Most teleosts possess interstitial cells in the typical vertebrate position,[16, 28] but, in a few species such as the pike *(Esox lucius)*, boundary cells originate in the lobule wall.[39] The boundary cells are homologous to the Leydig cells and apparently have the same endocrine function. They disintegrate after the spermatozoa are shed and are renewed from fibroblasts in the wall of the lobule.

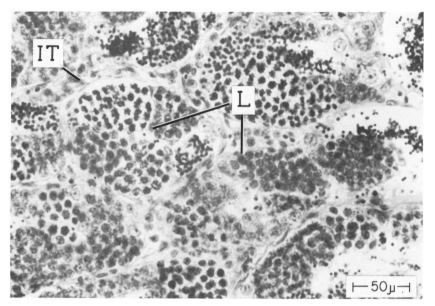

Figure 12–6. Testis of pond specimen of *Tilapia nigra*, showing active spermatogenesis and very little interstitial tissue (IT) between the testis lobules (L). (Courtesy of M. Hyder.)

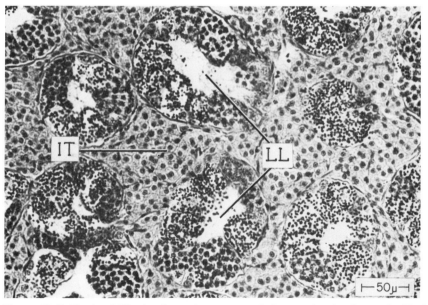

Figure 12–7. Testis of *Tilapia nigra* taken at spermiation or shortly afterwards. Maximal development of the interstitium (IT) occurs in this fish during spermiation and correlates with the time of maximal sexual coloration. Some residual spermatozoa remain in the lobule lumen (LL). (Courtesy of M. Hyder.)

THE VERTEBRATE OVARY

Mammals

The human ovaries are flattened glands lying on the side of the pelvic cavity and are attached by the mesovaria and the ovarian ligaments. The free surface of the organ is covered by a single layer of cuboidal cells, the gonadal epithelium. The gland is roughly divisible into a *cortex,* which extends over the entire surface except at the hilus, and an inner *medulla.* Although these two regions appear to contain distinct structures, there is no sharp line of demarcation between them in the mature organ. *Follicles* and *corpora lutea* in various stages of differentiation and destruction characterize the cortex of the sexually mature individual, whereas the medulla contains the larger blood vessels of the organ. In many species, the stroma is pervaded with epithelioid elements, the interstitial cells, which probably arise from the theca interna of *atretic* follicles or from stromal cells proliferated during early life. Distinct masses of interstitial cells are not present in the human ovary but, in the rabbit, cells of this type fill all the space not occupied by follicles, corpora lutea, rete cords, and blood vessels.

It is important to understand the behavior of germ cells within the developing ovary. The gonocytes that populate the embryonic ovaries undergo a period of vigorous multiplication and then differentiate successively into oögonia and primary oöcytes. The latter cells begin the first reduction division, which has a complicated and protracted prophase. The first meiotic division proceeds to the diplotene stage, which is reached just before or shortly after birth, depending on the species. The meiotic process is arrested at this late prophase stage, while the follicle and the oöcyte itself increase greatly in size. Human oöcytes are held in abeyance from the time of birth until ovulation occurs after the onset of puberty. In adult mammals running estrous cycles, a characteristic number of primary oöcytes complete their first meiotic divisions at each heat period, and release the first polar bodies shortly before ovulation. The haploid secondary oöcytes promptly begin the second meiotic division but remain in metaphase, and do not extrude a second polar body until the oöcyte has been penetrated by a sperm cell. The arrested maturation of the mammalian oöcyte is believed to correlate with an inhibitory action of the granulosa cells, and this restraint is overcome by the preovulatory surge of luteinizing hormone from the anterior pituitary.[20, 36, 40]

During late fetal life, as well as in the postnatal female, clusters of cells arise from the ovarian epithelium. One cell in the cluster enlarges more rapidly than the others and is called the oögonium, whereas the remaining cells constitute the early follicle. After the oögonium enlarges and becomes distinguishable from its neighbors, it is called a *primary oöcyte.* A hemogeneous membrane, the *zona pellucida* appears between the primary oöcyte and the follicular cells. The latter cells increase rapidly, forming many layers, the thecal layers are differentiated, and the follicle assumes a deeper position in the substance of the ovary. The germ cell becomes a mature ovum

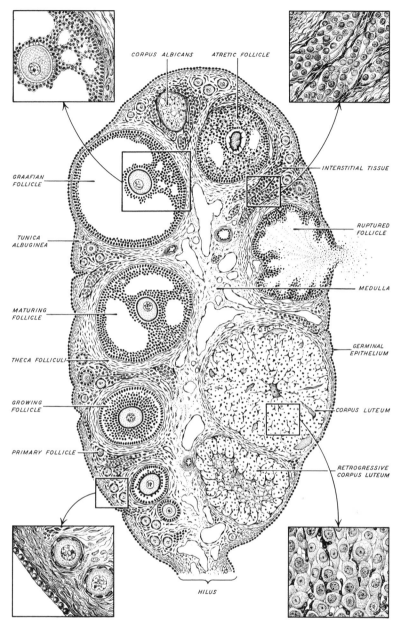

Figure 12–8. Diagram of a composite mammalian ovary. Progressive stages in the differentiation of a graafian follicle are indicated on the left. The mature follicle may become atretic (top) or ovulate and undergo luteinization (right).

after the second polar body is released. The polar bodies are entrapped within the zona pellucida, this membrane remaining with the ovum until its implantation or death. Under the influence of pituitary gonadotrophins, a fluid-filled space, the antrum, appears in the membrana granulosa and the structure becomes a *vesicular* or *graafian* follicle (Fig. 12–8). Although there is general agreement that the vesicular follicle is the main source of ovarian estrogen, the exact cells responsible for its production have not been unequivocally determined. Some workers attribute estrogen production to the cells of the theca interna; others feel that it is a function of the granulosa.[19]

Both ovaries of the human infant may contain as many as 500,000 primary follicles, but there is little likelihood that any additional germ cells can be formed postnatally. It is generally estimated that not more than 400 eggs are ovulated from puberty (age 12 to 15) to menopause (age 40 to 50). This means that there is normally a progressive and rapid rate of follicular degeneration or *atresia.* Follicles at all stages of development are subject to atresia, signs of impending follicular degeneration generally being observed first in the germ cell itself.

In vespertilionid bats, vesicular follicles are known to persist in the ovaries for unusually long periods. Such follicles may be well developed in October, as much as six months before ovulation occurs at the end of hibernation. The cells of the cumulus oöphorus of these long-lived follicles undergo marked hypertrophy and accumulate enormous quantities of glycogen.[60] This cumulus mass surrounds the ovum and is regarded as an adaption that makes possible the long survival of the follicle under conditions of drastically reduced metabolism in the individuals as they hang torpid in hibernation (Fig. 12–9).

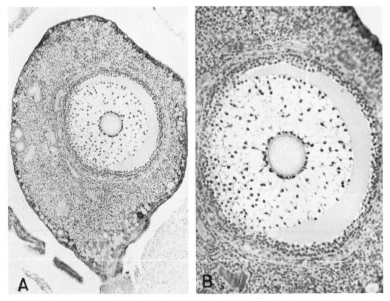

Figure 12–9. An ovarian follicle of the bat *Myotis lucifugus lucifugus* at two levels of magnification. The cumulus cells hypertrophy and accumulate enormous quantities of glycogen, an adaptation which enables the follicle to survive the prolonged period of hibernation. *A,* Lower magnification showing the follicle in relation to the whole ovary; *B,* the same follicle at higher magnification. (From Wimsatt, W. A., and Kallen, F. C.: Anat. Rec. *129*:115, 1957.)

The endocrine aspects of reproduction need to be studied more carefully in the Insectivora, *i.e.,* hedgehogs, shrews, and moles. In the European mole (*Talpa europaea* L.) there is a deposit of interstitial tissue massed separately from the ovigenous part of the ovary, and the former shrinks in size during heat and pregnancy. In the shrews *(e.g., Blarina, Elephantus),* luteinizing granulosa cells obliterate the antrum and push the ovum and its surrounding ball of cumulus cells out of the follicle. It thus appears that in these species preovulatory luteinization is a major factor in freeing the egg from the follicle.

The vesicular follicles of the sow are semitransparent and stand out from the surface of the ovary like a bunch of grapes. The follicles that are about to rupture measure 7 to 10 mm in diameter. Relatively large quantities of liquor folliculi are lost at ovulation, and a slight oozing of blood may occur. The ovaries of the horse are kidney-shaped, the depression being called the "ovulation fossa." It was formerly thought that ovulations occurred only from this fossa, but it is known now that they may occur elsewhere as well. The vesicular follicle of the mare may reach a diameter of 2 inches and contain from 60 to 80 cc of fluid.[2] The ovaries of the newborn seal weigh 32 to 36 gm and those of the mother weigh 25 to 28 gm. Several weeks after birth, the ovaries are fully involuted and weigh only 2 to 4 gm. Ovulation is usually suppressed during pregnancy, but it has been said to occur occasionally in women, cattle, sheep, rats, rabbits, hamsters, cats, and other species.

Another ovarian component of endocrine importance is the *corpus luteum,* a yellow-colored body that typically differentiates from the wall of the postovulatory follicle. Although clotted blood, forming a *corpus hemorrhagicum,* accumulates in the newly ruptured follicles of rodents and certain other mammals, such a structure is not conspicuous in primates. In human ovaries, the collapsed follicle is promptly filled with proliferating cells, which grow inwardly from the theca interna and membrana granulosa. Changes in the follicular wall, signifying impending luteinization, are observable in most species a short time before the follicle actually ruptures. The corpora lutea are an important source of progesterone and, since estrogens can be extracted from luteal tissue, it is probable that they synthesize both types of steroid hormones. During the human menstrual cycle the corpora lutea remain functional for 7 to 11 days but, if pregnancy occurs, functional activity is prolonged for several months. Vesicular follicles sometimes undergo extensive luteinization without having ovulated and give rise to the *corpora atretica,* or pseudolutein bodies.

Reproduction in the armadillo *(Dasypus novemcinctus)* is characterized by a specific polyembryony, which normally results in the formation of identical quadruplets. Only one egg is ovulated during each reproductive cycle. Within the ruptured follicle is formed a single, huge corpus luteum, which accounts for about 90 percent of the volume of this ovary.

It appears that ovulations and the formation of *accessory* corpora lutea are the rule in the pregnant mare, African elephant, Indian antelope (nilgai), and perhaps other mammals. The corpora lutea of pregnancy seem to be very short-lived in the pregnant mare, and begin to regress by the end of the first month.[2] During the second and third months of pregnancy, ovarian activity attains a high peak, and it is probable that ovulations occur and new corpora lutea are formed in order to maintain the gestational requirements. By the end of the sixth month of pregnancy, the mare's ovary contains neither corpora lutea nor large follicles. In the mare and many other species, the placenta acts as an adjunct to the ovary and assumes the function of supplying the hormones that are necessary for the continuation of pregnancy.

Corpora lutea may be considered as adaptations that have made possible the evolution of viviparity. Although they have reached their highest degree of functional specialization in mammals, luteal structures are known to occur in the ovaries of other vertebrate classes. They have been described in both oviparous and ovoviviparous selachians, teleosts, and reptiles.[34, 42] Corpora lutea are present in the ovaries of egg-laying mammals (*e.g.,* duck-billed platypus), and it has been suggested that their secretions may perform a role in lactation and in nursing behavior. In general, it seems probable that the hormones of the corpus luteum are concerned with the retention of embryos in the uterus or with the storage of eggs in the oviduct.

The Avian Ovary

In the great majority of birds, only the left ovary and oviduct are functional. The right ovary is present in the chick embryo and remains macroscopically visible for a short time after hatching, but in the mature bird, it is a rudiment that can be identified only by microscopic procedures. The right rudiment undergoes development if the functional ovary is destroyed by disease or is removed surgically.

The avian ovary differs anatomically from that of mammals in several important respects. The larger avian follicles are not contained within the ovarian stroma. The egg cells that are destined to reach ovulatory size, as well as those that become atretic in the process, are borne on follicular stalks (Fig. 12–10). There is no antrum and no collection of follicular fluid. The egg itself is surrounded by the vitelline membrane, the membrana granulosa, and the theca folliculi; all of these are quite comparable to their mammalian counterparts. The *stigma* (cicatrix), the area that ruptures at ovulation to permit the exit of the egg from the follicle, develops on the follicular wall opposite the stalked attachment. Although the follicular sac is gradually absorbed after ovulation, the calyx and stalk are nondeciduate structures and are retained. Each follicular stalk bears a large number of follicles; these range in size from microscopic structures too small to be seen with the unaided eye to an egg just ready to be ovulated. After ovulation, the abandoned stalk continues to be used by the younger follicles; the largest one dominates and grows to ovulatory size.

Avian ova are among the most rapidly growing structures to be found among higher vertebrates. Tremendous quantities of yolk are accumulated quickly. In the domestic fowl, ova weighing less than 100 mg reach mature size and attain a weight of 18 to 20 g in nine days. A very complicated

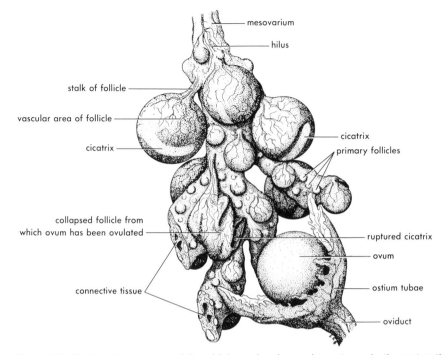

stalk of follicle

vascular area of follicle

cicatrix

collapsed follicle from
which ovum has been ovulated

connective tissue

mesovarium

hilus

cicatrix

primary follicles

ruptured cicatrix

ovum

ostium tubae

oviduct

Figure 12–10. Functional ovary of the chicken, showing various stages in the maturation of the ova. A mature ovum has just been released and is entering the ostium of the oviduct. (From Nelsen, O. E.: Comparative Embryology of the Vertebrates. New York, McGraw-Hill Book Co., 1953.)

vascular supply develops in connection with each growing follicle. This consists of an extensive complex of veins, arranged in three concentric layers in the follicular wall and terminating in a fine meshwork of venules enveloping the growing ovum. In contrast, the arterial supply to the follicle is relatively meager. This venous stasis apparently permits blood to remain in the follicle long enough for the yolk antecedents to be transferred to the egg. The main part of this vascular arrangement is used in succession by other follicles on the same stalk that are awaiting their turn to grow to ovulatory size.[44]

Mammalian species ovulate one or a few eggs at certain periods of the reproductive cycle. In contrast to this, the bird may release eggs from the ovary day after day over protracted periods. Only a single follicle, the largest of the series, responds to the ovulation stimulus but, at the same time, many others accumulate yolk and continue toward maturity.

Corpora lutea are not found in avian ovaries. As in mammals, follicles may become atretic at any stage and these have sometimes been mistakenly described as "avian corpora lutea." There is evidence, however, that both estrogen and progesterone are necessary for the normal integration of the reproductive cycles in birds. Blood from laying hens has progesterone activity, as assayed by the Hooker-Forbes test, and there are indications that progesterone, or a hormone of equivalent effect, is present in the ovarian follicles of such animals. There is also ample evidence that the ovary of the domestic fowl secretes androgen. In the chicken and certain other species, the postovulatory follicle remains visible for a considerable time, and it may well be that it performs some endocrine function. In fowl ovaries, clusters of interstitial cells, similar to those found in the rudimentary gonad, may be present in the vicinity of the theca.

The Amphibian Ovary

The amphibian ovary is a hollow structure; no fluid collects in the growing follicles; and after ovulation, luteal bodies do not typically differentiate in the collapsed follicles. The ovary of the frog is composed of six or seven lobes, which contract separately. Since these spontaneous contractions occur rather constantly in both sexually mature and immature specimens, they do not seem to be associated with ovulation except as this process may be influenced by the circulation of blood.

The ovary is essentially a two-layered pouch with the eggs situated between the two layers. As the eggs leave the ovarian epithelium, they become surrounded by a single layer of follicle cells. The follicles grow and bulge into the cavities of the lobes, but the stalked attachments to the ovarian wall are retained. Outside the follicular cells is a layer of smooth muscle that constitutes the cyst wall. This wall of muscular tissue does not completely enclose the egg but is reflected around the stalk that attaches the follicle to the outer surface of the ovary. The inner epithelial membrane covers the exterior of the follicle and, like the cyst wall, is anchored on all sides of the stalked attachment. Thus, at the stalk there is a region where the egg, together with its surrounding follicle cells, is directly exposed to the outer surface of the ovary. This is the area of ultimate rupture of the follicle. There is no loss of blood at ovulation, apparently owing to the fact that blood vessels are practically absent from the rupture area or stigma. The remaining portion of the follicle is well supplied with blood vessels. Though vascular connections are not essential for the completion of ovulation in frogs and other amphibians, it is noteworthy that the emission of eggs from a lobe of the ovary is retarded by poor circulation. Endocrine mechanisms regulating egg differentiation are quite well understood among the amphibians.[20]

The Fish Ovary

Among viviparous fishes the ovaries are not only structures for the production of ova and hormones, but they are somewhat similar to uteri, inasmuch as they provide shelter and nourishment for the developing young. The eggs may be fertilized within the ovarian follicle and retained there to continue their development; in such cases, ovulation either does not occur, or it is synonymous with the birth of young. In other species, the eggs are ovulated into a special chamber of the ovary, where fertilization occurs and in which the young are retained and nourished. Sperm often live for prolonged periods within the ovaries of such fishes. The teleost fishes are a very versatile group, and one may find among them almost every reproductive device characteristic of the higher vertebrates.

The ovoviviparous elasmobranch, *Squalus acanthias*, has a gestation period of 20 to 22 months. The adult ovary is composed of a germinal epithelium, a connective tissue stroma, and follicles in all stages of development. The entire ovary is invested by an epigonal organ consisting of hematopoietic tissue. Corpora lutea-like structures differentiate within both atretic and postovulatory follicles, the latter persisting for a greater part of the gestation period. Progesterone and estrogens have been detected in ovarian extracts of numerous elasmobranchs. Steroid dehydrogenase has been demonstrated histochemically in the postovulatory "corpora lutea" and this indicates that the tissue is steroidogenic; however, the physiologic significance of such bodies remains to be determined.[34]

THE MALE ACCESSORY SEX ORGANS

The accessory ducts and glands of the male are specializations for the storage of spermatozoa and for their conveyance, in an adequate vehicle, to the exterior at the proper time. These structures in the human male include multiple ductuli efferentes, paired epididymides, vasa deferentia, seminal vesicles, ejaculatory ducts, Cowper's glands, a prostate gland, the urethra with its multiple glands of Littré, and the copulatory organ itself (Fig. 12–4). The urethra of the male serves to convey seminal products as well as urine. There are a large number of anatomic and functional variations among the different mammalian species.

The epididymis is an extremely convoluted tube that, in some domestic animals, measures around 20 feet in length when straightened out. The epididymis is a storage place for spermatozoa, which have been shown to have improved capacity for motility and fertilization after a period of residence in this organ.

The vas deferens ascends through the inguinal canal, arches over the ureter, and continues medially to the base of the urinary bladder, where it receives the duct from the seminal vesicle. It then becomes known as the ejaculatory duct, which courses through the substance of the prostate and enters the prostatic portion of the urethra. The vas deferens contains well-developed muscle layers and is largely responsible for the movement of sperm along the tract. In a number of species, including the human, sperm storage may occur in the proximal end of the vas deferens, as well as in the epididymis. The spermatozoa are believed to be nonmotile in these storage structures but become motile when mixed with the accessory gland secretions. All of these accessory elements depend on androgenic hormones for full functional development and are quite inactive until the advent of puberty.

The seminal fluid, emanating from the accessory glands, is quite variable among mammals, with respect to both volume and chemical composition. It furnishes a vehicle for the conveyance of germ cells and perhaps provides an environment in which they can retain their greatest fertilizing capacity. It appears that the accessory gland secretions may not be absolutely necessary for fertilizing ability: Sperms taken directly from the testis or epididymis have some capacity to fertilize eggs. Sperms become motile when exposed to the air and mixed with any physiologic fluid; motility, however is not necessarily an index of fertilizing capacity. Some species (*e.g.,* cat and dog) have no seminal vesicles. Fertility in the rat and boar is not appreciably affected by removing both the seminal vesicles and prostate.

The semen of rats coagulates promptly upon ejaculation, and this forms a vaginal plug in the female tract after mating. An enzyme contained in the secretion from the coagulating gland causes the semen to harden. This plug often drops out of the vagina during repeated copulations, but it is gradually resorbed if it remains in the vagina. The finding of a vaginal plug is frequently used as a means of obtaining timed copulations. A similar plug is formed in guinea pigs and squirrels, but not in the majority of mammals. Human semen coagulates shortly after ejaculation but soon liquefies, owing to the action of a proteolytic enzyme presumably derived from the prostate.

The male accessory structures of certain passerine birds undergo modifications during the breeding season to form seminal vesicles, or glomera, for the storage of sperms at temperatures lower than those of the body cavity. The glomera arise through the growth and coiling of the vasa deferentia, eventually forming storage organs which protrude from the cloacal wall.[66]

THE FEMALE ACCESSORY SEX ORGANS

The female accessories include the oviducts, or fallopian tubes as they are generally termed in the human subject, the uterus, the vagina, and the external genitalia. The functional status of these organs is conditioned by the ovarian hormones.

Mammals

The oviduct provides a passageway between the ovary and uterus. The ovarian end of this tube is expanded into a funnel, having a fimbriated margin, and is usually closely applied to the ovary. Some of the epithelial cells lining the tube possess cilia that beat inwardly. This, together with the increased activity of the fimbria at the time of ovulation, probably assists in the apprehension of the ovum and in its movement toward the uterus. By removing one ovary and ligating the oviduct on the contralateral side, it has been shown in laboratory animals that some of the eggs that are freed into the body cavity can traverse the patent oviduct. In some species, the oviduct forms a bursa, or periovarial sac, that encapsulates the ovary.[61] In the dog and fox, the bursa contains a slitlike opening through which the ovary may be expressed, but in the rat and mouse, the bursa is completely closed except for a very minute pore.

Fertilization typically occurs in the oviducts. In the human being, this generally occurs in the upper end of the tube, usually within 24 hours after the egg has been freed from the ovary (Fig. 12–5). Secretions from the tubal mucosa are thought to be important in denudation of the ovum and in its penetration by the spermatozoon. The early embryo arrives in the uterus about three days after ovulation and implants in the wall of the uterus about four to six days after arriving there. Experiments on rabbits and rats indicate that the spermatozoa must be exposed to the secretions of the female tract for a certain period before they acquire the capacity to fertilize eggs. This phenomenon is called *capacitation,* and it is not known how extensively it applies to other species.[12]

The primate uterus is a pear-shaped muscular organ suspended in the broad ligament. The uterine wall is composed of a serous covering (perimetrium), a thick mass of interwoven smooth muscle cells (myometrium), and glandular lining (endometrium). The *body,* or corpus uteri, bends forward and rests against the urinary bladder. The *fundus* is the portion of the body that extends cranially above the entrance of the fallopian tubes. The narrow caudal end of the uterus is the *cervix,* which communicates with the vagina by means of the *external os uteri.* The surface of the endometrium is sloughed during each menstruation, but during pregnancy, it becomes highly modified to facilitate implantation of the blastocyst and its subsequent development.

The female accessory organs are derived mostly from the paired Müllerian ducts of the embryo, but the evolutionary tendency has been to produce unpaired structures in the adult. The primitive mammals (*e.g.,* opossum) have two vaginae, two cervices, and two separate and unconnected uterine bodies. The cleft penis of the male marsupial correlates functionally with the existence of paired vaginae in the female. All of the higher mammals have single vaginae. Many gradations may be found between *duplex* and *simplex* types of uteri. In rats and rabbits, each uterus is completely separated from the other and has its own cervix. In such forms as the pig, the cervix has become single and the caudal ends of the uteri have fused a little to produce a small body. In the cow, ewe, dog, cat, etc., the uterine body remains small, but the two uterine horns are separated by a conspicuous septum. Fusion has become more extensive in the mare, giving rise to a large uterine body with small horns. Among primates, the fusion is complete and the horns are absent.

The anatomy of the *cervix* varies among the different species of mammals, but it contains dense fibrous tissue, as well as muscle cells, and functions as a sphincter. The cervical glands produce a large amount of thin, alkaline mucus during the preovulatory period of the primate cycle, and this may favor sperm migration, motility, and longevity. The cervix is kept rather tightly closed at all times except during parturition, when it softens and undergoes marked dilatation. In many species the cervical mucus hardens during pregnancy and forms a plug that seals off the uterus from the vagina. The cervical plug liquefies shortly before parturition. Breaking the seal in cattle apparently exposes the uterus to bacterial invasion and generally leads to the loss of the fetus.

In most mammals, many more eggs are shed than are implanted. An extreme case is the elephant shrew *(Elphantus),* which may release more than a hundred eggs from the ovaries, but only one or two implant in the uterus. The opposite condition is found in the armadillo: Only one egg is shed and fertilized; then it divides and produces identical quadruplets. Furthermore, *delayed implantation* occurs normally in the Texas armadillo. The blastocyst is formed in the tube and then passes into the uterus, where it becomes lodged in a pocket and remains unattached for a period of three or four months. Blastocysts of the grey seal remain in the uterus for about 100 days before becoming implanted.[4] Delayed implantation also occurs in the badger, marten, and roe deer, and probably in bears and mink.

Under certain conditions, delayed implantation occurs in such laboratory mammals as the rat and mouse. These species come into estrus and ovulate after delivering a litter. If copulation is permitted at this postpartum heat, the female carries a litter *in utero* while she is suckling the first litter. However, the gestation period for the second litter appears to be significantly longer than the normal 21 days; the second litter may not be delivered until 30, 40, or even 50 days after the postpartum mating. In these cases the eggs fertilized at the postpartum heat have been found to develop normally in the oviducts, but float free in the uterus without implanting. They eventually implant when the proper endocrine situation prevails and have a gestation period of 21 days, just as in other pregnancies.

A progestational endometrium suitable for the reception of the blastocyst may develop only in localized areas of the endometrium. In mammals that have cotyledonary placentas (*e.g.,* cattle and sheep), no glands are found below the cotyledons, these areas are set aside as special sites for placental attachment. In the giant fruit bat (*Pteropus giganteus* B.), a progestational endometrium develops only in a localized area of one uterus. This asymmetric implantation area appears at the extreme distal end of the uterus and is in close anatomic contact with the single corpus luteum of that ovary. It is possible that progesterone from the corpus luteum is delivered directly to this implantation area, without being distributed by the general circulation. The pregnant females spend much of their time hanging head downward, and it has been suggested that this implantation area may serve the purpose of letting the large fetus rest against the diaphragm, thus preventing strain and injury to the uterus and its attachments.[37]

The human vagina is an unpaired, dilatable tube, approximately 4 inches in length, extending from the caudal end of the uterus to the vestibule. The lining of the vagina is a stratified squamous epithelium devoid of glands; the muscle layers are thin. Before coition the external vaginal orifice is more or less occluded by a membranous *hymen.* This membrane generally becomes perforate during fetal life, but in some instances it may persist until adolescence and interfere with the elimination of menstrual discharge.

In rats, mice, and guinea pigs, the caudal vagina is a solid cord of epithelial cells until ovarian functions become well established during postnatal life. The vaginal introitus in these species is controlled by estrogenic hormones, although it may be influenced by environmental factors such as temperature. In the hamster, however, perforation of the vagina occurs eight to nine days after birth in both intact and ovariectomized females, suggesting that the process may not be under hormonal control in this species. A membrane closes the vagina of the guinea pig during the diestrous periods of the cycle.

The vagina does not provide a satisfactory environment for the survival of spermatozoa. In the human, they die within a few hours, whereas they may remain viable for two or three days in the uterus and fallopian tubes. In bats and certain other species, the spermatozoa may remain viable in the female tract for many months.

The external genitalia of the female consist of the clitoris, the labia majora and minora, and certain glands that open into the vestibule (Figs. 12–5 and 12–14B). The latter groove is bounded laterally by the labia. The clitoris is an erectile organ homologous to the penis; it consists of small cavernous bodies ending in the rudimentary glans clitoridis. The glands of Bartholin, homologous to Cowper's glands in the male, open by ducts into the vestibule.

Birds

At the time of ovulation, the egg cytoplasm contains large stores of proteins, fats, vitamins, and minerals. As it traverses the oviduct, it receives additional supplies of water and protein in the form of an albuminous coating (egg white) and acquires the shell membranes and shell.

In the great majority of birds, only the left oviduct grows to functional size; the right is lost entirely or persists as a rudiment. The avian oviduct is a rather sizable tube extending from the region of the ovary to the cloaca. Craniad to caudad, the main regions are infundibulum, magnum, isthmus, shell gland (uterus), and vagina.

The ovulated egg falls into the body cavity and is fertilized either there or after it is taken up by the funnel-shaped infundibulum. The hen's egg remains in the infundibulum for about 15 minutes and while there acquires the chalazae, the springlike cords that extend through the albumen from the yolk to the poles of the egg. The magnum is the longest portion of the oviduct and contains many large albumen-secreting glands. The next region is the isthmus, the beginning of which is marked externally by the magnum-isthmus junction. The egg spends a little more than an hour here and acquires the shell membranes. The egg is retained longest in the shell gland (about 20 hours), where a porous shell is formed by the deposition of calcium carbonate. After the shell is formed, the egg spends about one minute in the vagina. Here it receives a thin coat of mucus, presumably to seal the pores and thus prevent rapid evaporation of water and to protect against bacterial invasion. The normal interval between ovulation and laying is 25 to 26 hours in the domestic fowl.

When foreign bodies such as glass beads are introduced into the avian oviduct, the various glandular regions deposit their secretions around them just as if they were living ova. The endocrine factors involved in control of

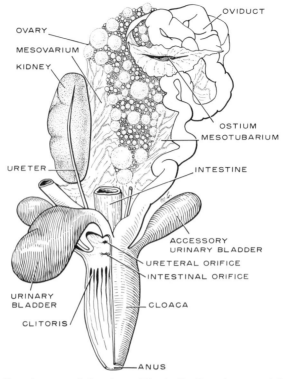

Figure 12–11. Female urogenital system of the turtle, *Pseudemys scripta,* ventral view. The ventral surface of the cloaca has been removed on one side to disclose the various openings into it; the urinary bladder is retracted to the right; only the left ovary is shown.

the avian oviduct are reasonably well known, but the physical mechanisms involved in the deposition of albumen, membranes, and shell are largely obscure. For example, the egg normally traverses the oviduct with the pointed end directed caudad, and this definitive shape becomes apparent shortly after the ovum has entered the magnum and acquired a very meager coating of albumen.

The genital organs of oviparous reptiles are very similar to those of birds (Fig. 12–11). Phylogenetically, reptiles were the first to evolve a *testicular factor* which acts during embryonic life to suppress development of the Müllerian ducts in the male. Birds and mammals employ the same inhibitory factor to produce sexual dimorphism of the Müllerian ducts.[48]

THE SECONDARY SEXUAL CHARACTERS

The secondary sexual characters are physical differences between the sexes that have nothing to do with the production and movement of gametes, but that may serve to bring the sexes together for courtship, to provide for the protection or nutrition of the young, or to facilitate amplexus.[58] In the human species, there are sexual differences in body build, distribution of fat, degree of development of the mammary glands, distribution of hair and pigment, and physical differences in the larynx. It is well established that some of these characters are under the control of hormones. That genetic influences also operate is attested by the fact that there are marked differences in the amount and distribution of body and facial hair among the different ethnic groups. Thus males of the Mongoloid and Caucasian groups are generally very different in this respect. The hormonal control of secondary characters has not been so carefully studied in humans as in birds.

The pattern of control of these sex differences may be very complex and frequently varies from group to group. The immediate expression of the characters may be genetic or hormonal, but it is always basically genetic since the type of regulation is determined by the genetic complex inherent in the species.

In some breeds of sheep, the ram possesses horns, whereas the ewe does not. Orchiectomy suppresses growth of the horns, and they are retained in the same condition as they were at the time of the operation. In breeds in which both sexes have horns, the heavy growth characteristic of the ram is prevented by orchiectomy, ovariectomy having no effect on horn growth. In other breeds, both sexes are hornless, and horns do not develop after gonadectomy.

Antlers are typical secondary sexual characters in Virginia deer that are present in males but not in females. Their development is regulated by a complicated interplay of genetic factors and of hormones from the gonads and hypophysis.

Many birds undergo very striking seasonal and sexual variations in the pigmentation of their bills.[63] The bill pigments are mainly brown and black melanins and red, orange, and yellow carotenoids. The melanins are synthesized by melanophores, located in the basal layer of the epidermis, and the pigments are transferred to epidermal cells which move toward the cornified outer layers of the bill. The carotenoids are derived from food, instead of being synthesized by the bird.

In the English sparrow *(Passer domesticus),* the bills of both sexes are light brown during the nonbreeding season (eclipse) and become jet black as the breeding season begins. Gonadectomy of either sex stops the deposition of melanin and the bills become light ivory in color. Melanin deposition resulting in black bills is reinstated by injecting androgens, but estrogens and progesterone have no effect. It is known that the avian ovary, as well as the testis, is capable of secreting androgens. The bills of male and female starlings *(Sturnus vulgaris)* are bright orange during the breeding season and black during the eclipse. After gonadectomy, the bills of both sexes become black; androgens restore the orange color (carotenoids) of the bills, but estrogens and progesterone do not have this effect.

Plumage changes have been extensively studied in the Brown Leghorn fowl. The cock plumage is generally considered to be the neutral form, the hen plumage requiring estrogen for its differentiation. Orchiectomy has no effect on the plumage, but total ovariectomy causes the appearance of cock plumage. Exogenous androgens also have no effect on the plumage, but estrogens or ovarian transplants induce the "henny" plumage in both sexes.

In the Sebright Bantam, both cocks and hens are normally hen feathered, and both sexes assume the cock plumage following gonadectomy. Treatment of the castrates with either estrogens or androgens induces the reappearance of hen feathering. The failure of cock plumage to develop in normal males of this breed is due to the appearance of a mutant gene which prevents the feather germs from developing cock feathering in response to androgens. Sexual differences in plumage of the English sparrow appear to be determined entirely by genetic factors, and gonadal hormones are without effect.[50]

The breeding plumage of female phalaropes is more ornate than that of males, and this pattern is developed in response to the androgen (testosterone) produced by the ovary. The ovaries of northern phalaropes (Lobipes lobatus) before the breeding season contain a much higher concentration of testosterone than do testes from birds killed during the same period. Estrogen and prolactin are ineffective in inducing nuptial feathers. The high ovarian content of testosterone appears to be related to the brighter plumage of the female and to her more aggressive breeding behavior and pair formation at this season. Only male phalaropes develop brood patches and incubate the eggs.[26, 27, 29]

Many birds in preparation for incubation develop brood patches to supply the necessary warmth for development of the embryos. The ventral abdominal integument becomes defeathered, highly vascularized, edemic and hyperplastic in response to endocrine conditioning. Among passerine birds, the females typically develop patches and incubate the eggs, and it has been shown that estrogen plus prolactin are required for this secondary sex character to develop. In phalaropes, only the male develops a brood patch and incubates the eggs; in these forms, it is androgen instead of estrogen that synergizes with prolactin to produce the brood patch.[30] In California quail (Lophortyx californicus), both sexes incubate and develop patches, and it has been concluded that the patch differentiates in response to high levels of circulating prolactin, which perhaps synergizes with gonadal steroids.[31] The quail seems to be intermediate between most passerine birds and phalaropes with respect to both incubation behavior and the hormonal dependence of the brood patch.

The syrinx is an organ of voice production in birds, and its development is regulated by gonadal hormones. The syrinx of the male duck is asymmetrical and well developed; that of the female is small and symmetrical. Castration of the duck embryo leads to the development of a male type syrinx. It has been shown that ovarian steroids normally operate to inhibit the development of the male type syrinx in females.[64]

The middle foreclaws of the slider turtle (Pseudemys scripta troostii) become modified as secondary characters employed in courtship. Growth of the claws in the juvenile animal may be accelerated by male sex hormone or prevented from developing by removing the testes. The male toad (Bufo arenarum) normally croaks and develops a black callosity on the thumb during the breeding season. Both may be eliminated by castration or reinstated by the administration of testosterone propionate. In these cases, it is obvious that the testicular hormone is the immediate conditioning agent.

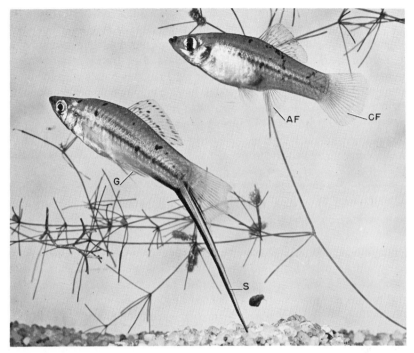

Figure 12–12. Male (left) and female (right) specimens of *Xiphophorus helleri*. Notice that the anal fin (AF) of the female is modified in the male into an intromittent organ, the gonopodium (G): the caudal fin (CF) of the female is modified in the male to form a sword (S). These fin specializations in the male are conditioned by testicular hormones and may be induced in the female by proper treatment with androgens. (Courtesy of James W. Atz, The American Museum of Natural History, New York, N. Y.)

Many kinds of secondary sex characters signaling a state of sexual readiness are found among fishes, and some of these are conditioned by gonadal steroids. Nuptial pigmentation and modifications of the various fins, as well as behavioral patterns, are often very striking. In the swordtail, *Xiphophorus helleri,* the anal fin of the male becomes modified into an intromittent organ (the gonopodium), and the caudal fin develops the characteristic sword (Fig. 12–12). These fin modifications occurring in the male are dependent upon testicular androgens.

AMBISEXUAL ORGANIZATION OF THE AMNIOTE EMBRYO

The Origin of Germ Cells

It is now well established that the gonocytes, or primordial germ cells, originate extragonadally in the vicinity of the yolk-sac entoderm. Gonocytes are first recognizable in very young human embryos near the caudal end of the primitive streak and are seen in the hindgut entoderm in embryos of only a few millimeters in length. In mammals, these early germ cells move through the tissues and reach the genital ridges largely as a consequence of their own ameboid movements, possibly aided by their capacity for histiolytic destruction of cells and membranes that block their way. Living gonocytes of the mouse have been followed from the yolk sac to the genital ridges, and their ameboid movements have been recorded cinematographically.[6] In reptiles and birds, the gonocytes first become segregated in the area pellucida, migrate into the blood islands of the area vasculosa, and are carried to the genital ridge area by the peripheral circulation. Studies on bird embryos indicate that the gonad primordium is the source of a soluble and diffusible agent that acts selectively to attract the gonocytes. It is probable that a similar chemotaxis operates in mammalian embryos. It is generally believed that the gonocytes are unable to differentiate into somatic elements, and those that fail to reach the gonadal primorida degenerate and disappear.[14]

Embryologic studies clearly indicate that the primitive genital ridges are unable to differentiate into anything resembling gonads unless adequate numbers of gonocytes are incorporated into them. Upon arriving at the gonadal blastema, the germ cells lose many of their characteristic features and are difficult to distinguish from nongerminal elements. Many of the germ cells present in the early gonads die off without accomplishing their transformation into oögonia or spermatogonia. Some workers have held that all the gonocytes degenerate after reaching the gonadal primordia, definitive germ cells being derived from later proliferations of the gonadal epithelium. Others have vigorously insisted that some of the gonocytes do survive and give rise to all definitive germ cells of the testis and ovary, thus constituting a continuous germ line, or "Keimbahn." Evidence for the latter point of view has been strengthened by results obtained after the introduction of new techniques and methods.

Embryogenesis of the Gonads and Accessory Sex Organs

The Gonads

The genital ridges first appear as bilateral thickenings along the mesial edges of the mesonephric kidneys. The gonocytes accumulate in the midportions of the ridges, and only these areas contribute to the gonads; the sterile cranial region becomes the suspensory ligament, and the caudal portion contributes to the utero-ovarian ligament. The thickened coelomic epithelium, covering the genital ridge, is at first separated from the underlying mesenchyme by a basement membrane; this soon disappears and cells are actively proliferated from the epithelial surface into the underlying mesenchyme (Fig. 12–13, A, B). This forms a *gonadal blastema* which contains gonocytes and is obviously constructed from mesenchyme and proliferations from the coelomic epithelium. The basement membrane reappears

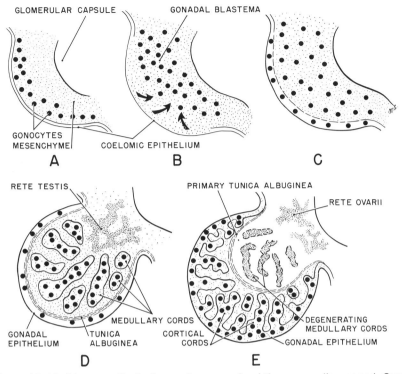

Figure 12–13. Diagrams illustrating embryogenesis of the mammalian gonad. Gonocytes are indicated as blackened circles. *A,* Basement membrane separates coelomic epithelium from underlying mesenchyme. *B,* Basement membrane is lost and coelomic epithelium proliferates actively to form gonad blastema. *C,* Basement membrane is restored and gonocytes are present in the gonadal epithelium. *D,* Medullary cords arise from the gonadal blastema and differentiate into a testis. *E,* Medullary cords regress and cortical proliferations form an ovary. (From Turner, C. D.: Amer. J. Obstet. Gynec., *90*:1208, 1964; modified from figures by R. K. Burns.)

and gonocytes have been incorporated into the epithelial layer (Fig. 12–13, *C*). The medullary (primary) sex cords arise directly from the gonadal blastema; they incorporate gonocytes together with somatic elements. The rete cords arise from the blastema at a deeper level, and a delicate layer of connective tissue forms below the surface epithelium. This is the presumptive tunica albuginea. In the testis (Fig. 12–13, *D*), the medullary cords continue their differentiation; the gonocytes eventually form spermatozoa and the somatic elements within the cords become the sustentacular cells of Sertoli. The interstitial cells of Leydig arise from intertubular elements, and the tunica becomes markedly thickened. The surface epithelium, with its gonocytes, typically disappears early, thus removing all potentiality for cortical development. Cortical (secondary) cords may start to form in the human testis, and in certain other species, but such proliferations are normally abortive.

In ovarian differentiation (Fig. 12–13, *E*), the medullary cords, corresponding to the seminiferous tubules, involute, and a conspicuous system of cortical (secondary) cords arises from the gonadal epithelium. The gonocytes which are entrapped within the cortical cords give rise to ova, whereas the somatic elements of the cords become follicle cells. It is important to note that the somatic elements within the medullary and cortical cords differentiate into Sertoli cells and follicle cells, respectively, and that these constituents of the testis and ovary are homologous. The interstitial cells of the ovary, as well as the thecal layers of the follicles, arise from intertubular components. The medullary part of the ovary may normally undergo considerable development and hypertrophy in some mammalian species, such as the mole, certain shrews, and the fetal ovary of the horse.

The sex-determining mechanism which is established at fertilization directs and controls all of the later ontogenetic processes (postgenetic differentiation) involved in the formation of testes or ovaries and corresponding accessory genitalia. The somatic cells of the embryo, as well as the primordial germ cells, carry sex-determining genes. It appears that the primordial germ cells are dependent upon the somatic components of the early gonad for the special influences that direct their differentiation into sperms or eggs. Gonocytes which lodge in the cortex typically become eggs; those of the medulla become sperms. The cortex and medulla are, of course, genetically determined, and they appear to exert contrasting influences upon the early germ cells. The basic problem is how the sex-determining genes act upon the genital primordia to condition their differentiation into male or female organs.

The Accessory Ducts and Glands

The Wolffian and Müllerian ducts are discrete primordia which temporarily coexist during the ambisexual period of development in all amniotes, regardless of genetic sex (Fig. 12–14, *A*). One type of duct persists normally and gives rise to accessory ducts and glands, whereas the heterologous system disappears except for unimportant vestiges. Though genetic sex is determined at the time of fertilization, regression of the heterologous duct system does not occur until the postgenetic differentiation of the gonad is well advanced.

Neutral Primordia

The urogenital sinus and genital tubercle are neutral primordia which are present in the embryos of both sexes. Whether they differentiate in the male or female direction depends upon whether the gonad becomes a testis or an ovary. Male and female genitalia orginating from primordia of this type are homologous (Fig. 12–14, *B, C*).

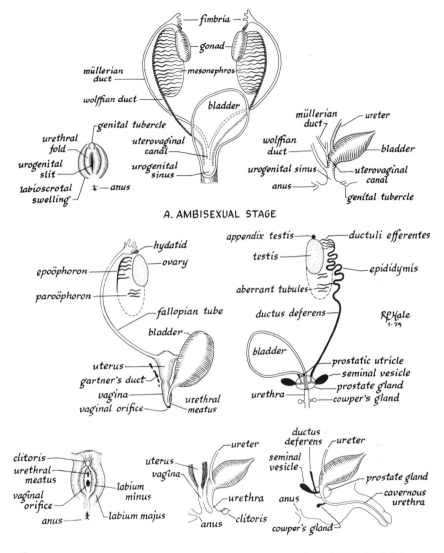

A. AMBISEXUAL STAGE

B. FEMALE DIFFERENTIATION   C. MALE DIFFERENTIATION

Figure 12–14. Embryogenesis of the genital system from Wolffian and Müllerian primordia, urogenital sinus, and genital tubercle. *A,* Ambisexual stage; a sketch of the external genitalia is shown at the left of the main figure; the sketch on the right shows the caudal region from side view. *B,* Female differentiation; below the main figure are sketches of the external genitalia and caudal structures from side view. *C,* Male differentiation; the sketch below the main figure shows a side view of the penis, and the main ducts and glands of the male.

MODIFICATIONS OF POSTGENETIC SEXUAL DEVELOPMENT

Theories of Sexual Differentiation

Hormone Theory

The freemartin of cattle is an intersexed female, always associated *in utero* with a male co-twin. Lillie attempted to account for cattle freemartins on the basis of androgenic hormones arising from the fetal testes of the male co-twin.[35] The condition results only in those cases in which there is an early fusion of the two placentae and a consequent intermingling of blood between the two fetuses. The external genitalia of the freemartin are generally female in type, but the clitoris is often enlarged. Although there are many gradations in severity, the accessory sex organs usually consist of both Wolffian and Müllerian duct derivatives. The gonads are hypoplastic and may contain sterile seminiferous tubules with practically no cortical development; in other instances, both cortical and medullary components may be present to form the equivalent of an ovotestis. Similar anomalies have been reported in sheep, goats, and pigs. Placental fusion may occur in cats, rabbits, marmosets, and human beings without resulting in any sexual anomaly. These negative findings do not necessarily invalidate the hormone theory; they do suggest that the vascular anastomoses must occur at a very early age in order to modify the sexual development of the female fetus. It is also possible that in certain species effective amounts of testicular hormones are absent from the blood at the critical period, or that the masculinizing agents are counterbalanced in some manner by the female recipient. There may also be species variations with respect to the androgen production by the fetal testis. Since pure steroid hormones became available, there have been repeated failures to duplicate the gonadal impairments experimentally.

Theory of Cellular Chimerism

This is the most recent theory advanced as an explanation of freemartinism in cattle. Briefly stated, it is proposed that masculinization of the freemartin ovary and genital ducts may occur through the direct action of XY cells from different tissues that reach the female co-twin via the chorionic vascular anastomoses. Ohno and his collaborators have reported XX cells, possibly primordial germ cells from the freemartin, lodged in the testes of the male co-twin. Though difficult to detect, it is reasonable to suppose that XY cells could be transmitted by the blood in a reverse direction. The report that these XX cells entered meiosis within the testis of the male co-twin encouraged other workers to explore the possibility of germ cell reversal through the fusion of very young mouse embryos.[46, 47, 49]

Corticomedullary Inductor Theory

This concept is based on the fact that the early gonads of vertebrates are composed of discrete primordia (medulla and cortex) which are determined genetically to form testes or ovaries, respectively. There is no transformation of one primordium into the other, but rather a development of one accompanied by the recession of the other. Witschi theorized, largely on the basis of his amphibian studies, that the medulla and cortex might be the source of special substances (medullarin and corticin) which act after the manner of embryonic inductors. According to this view, corticin would have the over-all effect of inhibiting the medulla, and medullarin would inhibit the cortex.[62]

Several facts should be kept in mind with respect to the hypothetical gonadal inductors: (1) There is necessarily much vagueness in the use of the term "inductor"; (2) such materials have never been isolated and chemically identified; and (3) there is no information on the biochemical mechanisms which intervene between the sex genes and the characters they determine. There is no doubt that steroid hormones and gonadal grafts can modify or completely reverse gonadal differentiation in certain vertebrates. It is not known whether steroid hormones act directly, in these instances, as "inductors," or produce their effects secondarily by modifying some kind of an inductor system.

Spontaneous and Experimental Sexual Transformations

Intersexuality occurs spontaneously in all classes of vertebrates, and may be produced experimentally by a variety of procedures, particularly when these are applied during the ambisexual period of development. Hermaphroditism occurs in many of the lower vertebrates, and this may be considered a normal aspect of their life cycles. Experimental procedures that have been ultilized include gonad grafting, administration of hormones, chimerism, surgical ablations, parabiosis, tissue culture, and the creation of various unfavorable states. The literature in this area is voluminous, and space does not permit more than a brief account of current concepts and the description of only a few examples.

Fishes

The gonads of the lamprey and other cyclostomes are unpaired structures extending almost the entire length of the body cavity. The accessory sex organs of the cyclostome are simple (Fig. 12–15). The mature germ cells are freed into the body cavity and are passed through peritoneal funnels and abdominal pores into a urogenital sinus which opens to the exterior. The sinus of the male opens to the outside through a small orifice at the tip of a penis-like structure. Although both ovarian and testicular tissues are general-

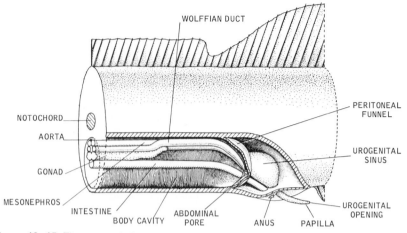

Figure 12–15. The urogenital system of an adult lamprey *(Lampetra planeri)*. Mature germ cells are freed into the body cavity and reach the exterior by passing through abdominal pores and the urogenital sinus. (From a dissection by Dr. S. Ishii.)

ly present in the same gonad, the individuals of most species function either as males or as females throughout their lives.

Reproductive processes are more varied among bony fishes than in any other vertebrate class.[3] Some species function first as males and later as females (protandry); others function first as females and become males later in life (protogyny). *Rivulus marmoratus* is the only teleost definitely known to reproduce regularly by fertilizing its own eggs. Self-fertilization apparently occurs in the ovarian cavity, and nearly all of the young are females.[23] Many gradations are found between species characterized by hermaphroditism and those that are highly gonochoristic.

The developing gonads of cyclostomes and teleosts do not possess cortical and medullary components, and, in this respect, they differ from all other vertebrates. The gonad primordium arises from the coelomic epithelium, without the participation of a mesonephric blastema. Some have argued that this unique character of the gonad primordium might correlate with the relatively high frequency of hermaphroditism in these groups, but this remains uncertain.

The medaka *(Oryzias latipes)* is an oviparous cyprinodont fish in which complete sex reversals have been obtained by the administration of gonadal hormones to genetically analyzed breeds. The newly hatched young have sexually indifferent gonads, and there is no tendency for the juvenile males to undergo a temporary female-like stage of gonadal development. In the medaka, the sex determining mechanism is XX for female and XY for male, the genes for skin color (R = orange-red; r = white) being present in the sex chromosomes (Fig. 12–16).

Through the use of proper mating types, it has been shown that intersexes and complete sex reversals can be produced in *Oryzias* by administering estrone to genetic males (XY). Sex-reversed orange-red males, functioning as females (X^rY^R), were mated with normal orange-red males (X^rY^R)

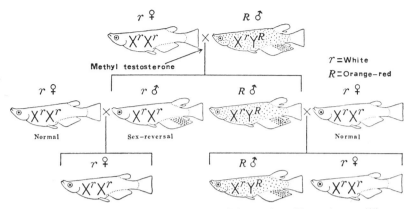

Figure 12–16. Sex reversal in genetic female medaka produced by androgen. When reversed genetic females are mated with normal genetic females, all-female progenies result. (From Yamamoto, T.: J. Exp. Zool. *137*, 1958.)

and progeny testings made on F_1 sons. A single orange-red son among the F_1 offspring was identified as the $Y^R Y^R$ male, which had sired all-male offspring.[68]

When genetic females of *Oryzias* are treated with methyltestosterone, they become completely reversed and develop the sex equipment and reproductive capacity of normal males. Progenies consisting only of females resulted when sex-reversed males of the female genetic constitution ($X^r X^r$) were crossed with normal females ($X^r X^r$), either by natural mating or by artificial fertilization (Fig. 12–16). When excessive amounts of the androgen are given, both genetic males and genetic females differentiate into males with rudimentary testes and later become neuters because of the complete destruction of germ cells.[69, 70]

Studies on *Oryzias* illustrate two important principles: (1) The early gonads, as well as the accessory system, have the ability to differentiate in a direction opposite to their own genetic constitution, and (2) the early germ cells are bipotential and, in spite of their genetic constitution, can become functional eggs or sperms. The breeding experiments show that the genome, or genetic complement, of the germ cells is not altered by the procedures employed in producing the reversal of sex.

The experiments on these fishes indicate that there is a critical period in development during which the hormones are effective. Sex differentiation in genetic males of *Oryzias* has been reversed by injecting estrone or stilbestrol into the eggs, the estrogens apparently being retained until sex differentiation begins.[24]

Amphibians[17]

It is well known that many physiologic alterations, such as nutritional level, disease, and factors in the physical environment, can result in sex reversals in certain animals. Among certain amphibians, low temperatures, prevailing during larval life, have been found to encourage the differentiation of females and higher temperatures to be productive of males. Histologic studies indicate that low temperatures retard the medullary component of the gonad, whereas high temperatures retard or completely destroy the cortex. Thus, at high temperatures the gonads that genetically should become ovaries are gradually changed into testes. Body temperatures may adversely affect the differentiation of gonads from embryonic rats and mice. Overripeness of the amphibian egg before fertilization occurs is harmful to the germ cells. If anuran eggs are inseminated after being retained within the ovisac for an extended time, a high preponderance of males results therefrom. The cortical portion of the gonad is impaired in the young that develop from these "stale" eggs. It is not known whether such environmental factors influence sex differentiation in the human, but they may well do so.

It is apparent from our previous discussion of embryology that sex differentiation is a competitive process between genital primordia. It would be instructive to remove the dominant portion of a gonad surgically and determine how the suppressed portion differentiates, but this can be accomplished only in certain species. The male toad has a cortical deposit, or rudimentary ovary, at the cranial end of each testis. This is called *Bidder's organ.* When the testes are removed, this organ enlarges and slowly develops into a functional ovary capable of producing fertile eggs (Fig. 12–17).

Among amphibians, it is relatively easy to graft gonad primordia and to unite animals parabiotically. When heterosexual combinations are made, one sex is suppressed and partial or complete sex reversals result. The male gonad is typically dominant but, in rapidly differentiating species, the ovary may predominate. In heterosexual combinations, complete functional transformations may result or, if there is incomplete dominance, a prolonged period of intersexuality prevails. Removal of the dominant gonad graft, or separation of the parabionts, may permit the transformed individual to return to the type of sexual development typical for its genetic constitution.

The African frog *Xenopus* has been extensively employed in experiments on sex reversal. When young larvae are raised in aquarium water containing 50 μg of estradiol per liter, the genetic males differentiate completely and permanently as functional females. This exposure to hormone must be made at a critical period of development, and does not need to prevail for more than three days. Exogenous androgenic steroids do not interfere with normal gonadal development in *Xenopus,* but testicular grafts do produce functional sex reversal in female hosts. Complete reversal of the ovaries into testes has been accomplished by Mikamo and Witschi by transplanting testes into the body cavities of larval recipients prior to the onset of gonad differentiation. The females of *Xenopus* are normally heterozygous (ZW) and the males are homozygous (ZZ). When reversed males (ZZ) are mated with normal males (ZZ), they yield only male offspring. Crossing a normal female (ZW) with a reversed female (ZW) gives 25 per cent WW females, 50 percent ZW females, and 25 per cent ZZ males. Only ZW females are produced when an estradiol feminized male (ZZ) is mated with a testis-graft masculinized WW female. Breeding experiments have shown that all three possible chromosome-gene combinations (ZZ, ZW, WW) can develop into either fertile males or fertile females.[10, 11, 41]

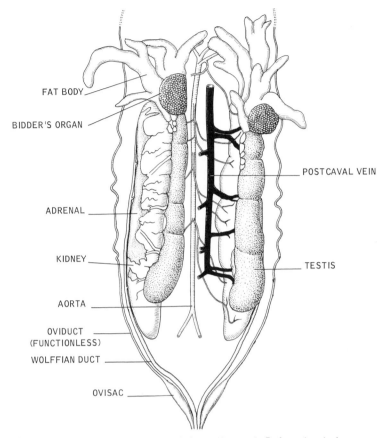

Figure 12–17. The urogenital system of the male toad, *Bufo vulgaris formosus.* (From a dissection by Dr. H. Kobayashi.)

These studies on *Xenopus* are important because they provide unequivocal evidence that the differentiation of primordial germ cells can be reversed without altering their constitution. They clearly indicate that the final "decision" on maleness or femaleness is made at the level of the gonad (postgenetic differentiation), and not at the time of fertilization. Unless environmental factors intervene, sex determination and sex differentiation are harmonious.

Birds

The *in vitro* culture of amphibian and avian gonads by Wolff and his collaborators indicates that gonad differentiation is an autonomous process which can occur quite independently of the whole organism.[65] Among birds, in contrast to mammals, it is the ovary that plays the dominant role in determining genital development.[21, 54] When heterosexual pairs of chick or duck gonads are placed contiguous to each other in culture dishes, the ovary stimulates the testis to proliferate cortical tissue until it becomes an ovotestis. The transformation may go far enough to make it indistinguishable from a normal ovary of the same age. Estradiol benzoate, added to the culture medium, modifies the testis in the same manner as does living ovarian tissue.[14]

The gonocytes do not begin their differentiation as germ cells until they enter the gonad primordia and become associated with the somatic tissue of this organ. The early effect of this tissue on female germ cells has been demonstrated by culturing left gonads from female chick embryos at 4 to 12 days of incubation. Isolated germ cells maintained *in vitro* fail to divide mitotically and never enter the zygotene stage of meiosis. The addition of pieces of 6-day ovarian cortex causes the young germ cells to undergo their normal pattern of differentiation; however, 12-day germ cells fail to respond in this manner when cultured with 12-day pieces of cortex. It is apparent that the follicular cells of the young gonad act very early to influence differentiation of the female germ cells.[15]

Castrations of chick and duck embryos have been accomplished by localized irradiation of the genital ridges as early as the third day of incubation. In castrated male embryos, the Müllerian ducts, instead of regressing as they normally do, continue to develop. In castrated female chicks, the right oviduct, which normally is lost in intact birds, likewise continues to develop. The Wolffian ducts serve as nephric ducts and remain after castration in an undifferentiated state. The genital tubercle of the male duck forms a prominent intromittent organ, whereas it becomes a rudimentary clitoris in the female. The administration of estrogen to young embryos suppresses development of the penis in the male, and, at hatching, it appears equivalent to the clitoris of the female. After castration of early embryos, both sexes develop genital tubercles of the male type. It is apparent that the ovary determines this sexual dimorphism by inhibiting the differentiation of the genital tubercle into a penis.

The exposure of chick embryos to estrogens has profound effects upon the differentiation of male gonads and sex accessory organs. Such steroids convert the left testis into an ovotestis; the epithelium of the right testis can form cortex only to a limited extent and consequently responds less markedly to estrogens. This treatment causes both oviducts of genetic males to persist. The chorioallantoic grafting of ovaries into male embryos produces genital anomalies which are quite comparable to those resulting from treatment with exogenous estrogens. All of the experiments are consistent with the concept that genital differentiation in birds in controlled by factors from the ovary. Enzyme studies indicate that steroid hormone production by the chick gonad begins sometime between days 2 and 6 of incubation. It is likely that such hormones are involved in the differentiation of the gonad itself, in addition to their well-known effects on the differentiation of accessory sex organs.[67]

The right ovary of the chicken remains rudimentary and retains its medullary component. When the left functional ovary is removed from a young bird, the right rudiment may form a testis-like structure or an ovotestis. After sinistral ovariectomy of older chickens, the right rudiment generally develops into a functional ovary.

Mammals

Many degrees of intersexuality appear spontaneously in laboratory and domesticated mammals, and others may be produced experimentally. Some of these are remarkably similar to sexual anomalies known to occur in man. For example, a type of hereditary tubular dysgenesis has been found in King-Holtzmann hybrid rats, and the defect is associated with a color marker which makes it possible to identify the abnormal offspring at birth. Spermatogenesis fails at an early age, and parts of the accessory system are missing. The animals are chromatin negative, and the karyotype is normal. The mutant genes act in some manner to mask the male potential in these rats and, in many respects, the syndrome resembles a type of pseudohermaphroditism occurring in the human male.[1]

After purified androgens and estrogens became available for experimental purposes, many workers tried to simulate the freemartin condition in ambisexual young by introducing the steroids into the maternal circulation. The hormones apparently can traverse the placenta and cause anomalous sexual development of the young *in utero*. Androgens are known to induce female intersexuality when administered in this manner to rats, mice, guinea pigs, hamsters, rabbits, monkeys, and human beings. A wide range of genital defects results from this treatment, with degree of severity depending upon the species, the developmental stage of the embryo, the kind of androgen used, the quantity administered, and the route of administration. When synthetic androgens are administered to the pregnant mother, Wolffian ducts are retained in genetic female embryos, but the Müllerian ducts are not caused to involute. Furthermore, the ovaries of the intersexed young are not conspicuously impaired in structure. The highly modified ovaries of cattle freemartins contain sterile seminiferous tubules, but this anomaly has not been simulated in any mammalian species through the administration of exogenous hormones.

The administration of estrogens to gravid rats and mice produces sexual maldevelopments in both male and female offspring. There is often persistence and hypertrophy of the Müllerian ducts in genetic males, shortening of the anogenital distance, and arrested development of accessory sex glands. The treatment may cause isolated segments of the Wolffian ducts to be retained in genetic females.

A few milligrams of testosterone propionate, administered subcutaneously to the mouse on the twelfth day of pregnancy, are sufficient to masculinize all of the female fetuses, thus resulting in permanent sterility. The female intersexes possess ovaries and derivatives of both Müllerian and Wolffian systems: Oviducts, uteri, and cranial vaginae persist together with epididymides, ducti deferentes, seminal vesicles, prostate lobes, bulbourethral glands, and a clitoris modified in the direction of a penis. The anogenital distance in the newborn females is increased, and they cannot be distinguished externally from normal males in the same litter until penile development and testicular descent occur in the latter. As the intersexed females mature, the perineal region appears somewhat like an empty scrotum, and this is more pronounced if androgen treatment is continued post-natally. The short cranial vagina opens by a minute orifice into the urethra, the caudal vagina being absent. The uteri become extremely distended with fluid, and this usually causes death by the end of the second month.[56]

The young of the opossum are born in a very immature state, after a brief gestation period of about 13 days, and complete their development in the marsupial pouch. The young are sexually undifferentiated at birth, and hormones may be administered directly while they are within the marsupium and attached to nipples of the mammary glands. Burns was able to induce cortical development in the testes of neonatal opossums by giving minute amounts of estradiol from the day of birth. The testes continued to proliferate cortex until they became ovotestes, or, in some cases, until they were equivalent to normal ovaries of the same age. The gonocytes present in the proliferating cortex of the testis differentiated as oöcytes, and early follicles were observed in some cases. This is the only report of gonadal reversal in a mammalian species being accomplished through the administration of steroid hormones.[7, 8, 9]

Ovotestes have been produced in mice by homotransplanting fetal ovaries (11½ days) next to fetal testes of the same age, below the kidney capsules of adult castrated hosts. Large areas of the modified ovaries consisted of dilated seminiferous tubules, which contained Sertoli cells and early stages of spermatogenesis. It is believed that the young testis is the source of an agent which masculinizes the fetal ovary; it acts over short distances, and its chemical identity is obscure. Attempts to duplicate the effects of these testicular grafts by administering exogenous androgens have not been successful.[56, 57]

There remains much controversy related to the possibility of sex reversal in the germ cells of mammals. Many studies have employed mouse chimeras composed of male and female cell lines (XY and XX cells), and relatively few of these individuals develop as females. Differentiation of the gonad is complicated by the fact that it is influenced by the presence of XX and XY types of somatic cells. There is not sufficient evidence to conclude that reversal of mammalian germ cells is impossible, though genetic control of gonadogenesis appears more rigid than in submammalian groups.

Studies on mammalian fetuses, gonadectomized during the ambisexual stage, indicate that normal differentiation of the male accessory ducts and glands depends upon the presence of a testis; it cannot occur in the absence of gonads or in the presence of an ovary.[33] In genetic male rabbit fetuses, orchiectomized in utero at the fetal age of 19 days, when the Müllerian and Wolffian systems are still sexually indifferent, the Wolffian ducts degenerate and no ducti deferentes or seminal vesicles are formed. The Müllerian ducts persist and differentiate into oviducts, uterine horns, and a large segment of the vagina; the urogenital sinus and external genitalia become of the female type. Female organogenesis progresses normally after the fetal ovaries are removed. Thus, in the absence of the gonads, both genetic males and genetic females acquire the female type of accessory system. It appears that the fetal testis exerts two effects: (1) stimulation of the masculine differentiation of the Wolffian ducts, urogenital sinus, and genital tubercle, and (2) an inhibitory influence leading to the rapid loss of the Müllerian ducts. Similar results have been obtained in mice and rats following removal of fetal gonads.[59]

There are many advantages in being able to excise genital complexes and culture them apart from the body. In this way, it is possible to observe the organs differentiating on culture media which are known to be free from hormones arising from other endocrine glands of the mother or fetus, such as the adrenal cortices, placenta, and pituitary gland. Moreover, the genital complex is removed from the influence of the liver, an organ known to inactivate steroid hormones. Under these circumstances, the effects exerted by endogenous gonadal hormones or exogenous hormones added to the culture are known to be direct rather than mediated through other glands.

Rat fetuses at 17 days of age are in the ambisexual stage, and the genital tracts may be removed *in toto* and allowed to develop on a proper culture medium. The explanted tracts may be observed under different experimental conditions: with both gonads present; with one gonad absent; with both gonads absent; with gonads of the opposite sex; or with both gonads absent and exogenous hormones added to the medium (Fig. 12–18). In this figure, A and B are male and female tracts at 17 days, the age of explantation. When male tracts are cultured for 4 days, the Müllerian ducts disappear except for vestiges, whereas the Wolffian ducts persist and seminal vesicles begin to arise from their caudal ends (A1). In the absence of both testes (A2), the Wolffian ducts regress and seminal vesicles do not form. The addition of testosterone micropellets to the culture medium substitutes for a testis; the gonadless male tracts develop normally as in A1. One testis

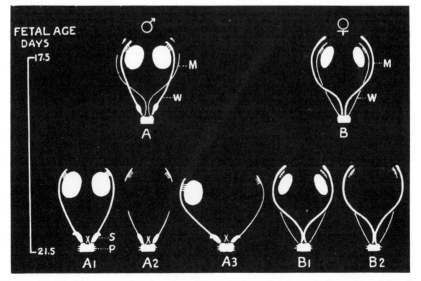

Figure 12–18. Diagrams showing the differentiation of rat genitalia cultured *in vitro*. M, Müllerian ducts; P, prostrate gland; S, seminal vesicle; W, Wolffian duct. (From Price, D., and Pannabecker, R.: *In* Watterson [ed.]: Endocrines in Development. Chicago, University of Chicago Press, 1958.)

can promote normal differentiation of the male tract: When one testis is removed, and the two sides of the tract are widely separated (A3), the side of the tract possessing the testis develops normally, but the contralateral side tends to regress. Removal of the ovaries (B2) has no effect on the Müllerian ducts; they persist as in B1, and the Wolffian ducts regress. These experiments show that the Wolffian ducts depend upon androgens from the testis for their maintenance and development, whereas loss of the Müllerian ducts is due to another testicular factor.[18, 32, 33, 48]

PATTERNS OF REPRODUCTIVE BEHAVIOR

Vertebrates fall into two categories: those that breed continuously throughout the year (continuous breeders) and those that restrict reproductive events to a particular season (seasonal breeders). There is a tendency for animals in the wild to reproduce in those seasons during which environmental factors such as food supply, temperatures, and shelter are most propitious for the pregnant or incubating mother and for survival of the young. Domestic animals are removed from many of the natural environmental exigencies, thus making it possible for the breeding periods to be prolonged or even for the animals to become continuous breeders.

The wild Norway rat is anatomically and physiologically very different from its domesticated prototype. The laboratory rat reproduces continuously, whereas the wild rat is definitely more seasonal, the high peak of reproductive efficiency extending from December through June. Reproduction may occur sporadically at other periods, but estrous cycles are irregular and the litters are small. Gonadectomy greatly reduces the spontaneous running activity of laboratory rats but has little effect on the activity of wild Norways. The adrenal cortices are much heavier in the wild rat than in the laboratory rat. It has been suggested that during the process of domestication the gonads of the domesticated rat have taken over the control of certain functions that are largely controlled by the adrenal in the wild Norway rat.

Wild cattle show a definite tendency to reproduce during the fall, spring, and early summer, but domesticated forms may conceive at any time. Horses of the North American continent usually breed during the spring and early summer, and although they may conceive at other periods, the heats become irregular and unpredictable. Domestic rabbits are continuous breeders, but, under North American climatic conditions, the wild form shows a low point of reproductive activity during the summer months. Among domesticated chickens, there are annual variations in the rates of egg production, and the high and low levels of fecundity correlate with daily light periods and other environmental conditions. In man there are variations in reproductive proficiency that correlate with the latitude.

Among seasonal breeders, the gonads of both sexes may involute and become practically quiescent during the nonbreeding periods; in other species, the male may retain reproductive competence at all seasons, with only the female becoming sexually impotent at certain periods.

The seasonal release of eggs or embryos is the most prevalent reproductive pattern among the fishes but, under laboratory conditions, successive broods may be produced throughout the year.[25] In some species, the period of sexual inactivity is very brief or does not exist at all, the production of eggs being almost as continuous as the production of spermatozoa. *Oryzias latipes* may ovulate and spawn every day for prolonged periods, but the process eventually becomes irregular. At the other extreme are some fishes *(e.g.,* genus *Oncorhynchus)* in whom the gonads become mature only once during a lifetime, death being an inevitable consequence of spawning.

A seasonal wave of reproductive activity occurs in the majority of amphibians, mating and oviposition taking place during the spring. In some of the Urodela, pairing occurs in the early autumn and ovulation does not take place until spring. In these cases, the sperm are stored during the winter in the receptaculum of the female. Most reptiles are seasonal breeders, though certain tropical species extend their reproductive activities throughout the year, without any evidence of a seasonal rhythm.

In the tropics, apparently both continuous and seasonal patterns are found among birds. Though most domestic birds are continuous breeders, the turkey and goose retain their seasonal rhythmicity even in captivity. Migratory birds provide the clearest example of seasonally breeding forms. The breeding season is a very labile characteristic of animals, as is shown by removing eggs from the nests of birds as they are laid, without giving the parent a chance to incubate them. The sparrow generally lays three to five eggs and then incubates them, but if the eggs are removed daily, the female can be induced to lay 50 to 80 eggs. Broodiness is linked with cessation of egg production and does not appear unless a characteristic number of eggs is in the nest.

The common breeds of sheep confine their reproductive periods to the autumn or winter months, but this can be modified by genetic selection. The Merinos and Dorset Horn breeds have prolonged breeding seasons, and at least two strains have been produced that are continuous breeders. This provides another example of the lability of reproductive rhythms.

The Estrous Cycle

In most vertebrates, with the exception of the primates, sexual receptivity is restricted to recurring periods called *estrus.* During heat, or estrus, the female is physiologically and psychologically conditioned to receive the male, and structural changes occur in the female sex accessories. *Monestrous* animals complete a single estrous cycle annually, a long anestrous period separating the heats. *Polyestrous* forms complete two or more cycles annually if not interrupted by pregnancy.

Ovulation is the dominant event in the estrous cycle and usually occurs during estrus, but in a few species *(e.g.,* cow) it occurs shortly after the end of estrus. In most mammalian species, ovulation occurs *spontaneously* and is ushered in by a short period of very rapid follicular growth; in other species (*e.g.,* rabbit, cat, ferret) ovulations do not occur spontaneously but are *induced* by the act of coitus or some comparable stimulation of the uterine cervix. The induced ovulators generally remain in continous heat, the ovary being characterized by large follicles for long periods, and preovulatory growth of the follicles and ovulation occur after coitus. In the latter animals, there are occasional diestrous intervals during which the female is not receptive to the male; these periods correlate with massive atresia of the vesicular follicles. Careful studies of vaginal smears and histology of the reproductive tract of the rabbit suggest that there is a latent tendency for cyclic alterations to occur at four- to six-day intervals.

Ovulation is dependent upon the release of gonadotrophins from the anterior pituitary, and there is much evidence that this release is mediated by a hypothalamic mechanism. Possibly in all forms the central nervous system is involved in the ovulatory process. In many fishes, amphibians, reptiles, and birds it is very probable that courtship encounters have a bearing upon ovulation and that it would not occur in their absence. Among induced ovulators, the intensity and duration of coitus is also variable. In the rabbit, squirrel, and cat, coitus is relatively brief, but in the ferret it is protracted and violent. Copulations must be repeated frequently in the short-tailed shrew to induce the release of eggs from the ovary, approximately 20 copulations in one day being necessary to cause ovulation. Mechanical (glass rod) stimulation of the cervices of the estrous rabbit generally does not produce ovulation unless the threshold of pituitary activation is lowered by giving exogenous progesterone. It thus appears that the act of coitus has an effect which is not completely duplicated by the artificial means. These observations suggest that ovulation is consummated by a neurohumoral or neurohormonal stimulation of the anterior hypophysis.

Some domestic animals, particularly cows and mares, occasionally exhibit so-called *quiet heat.* These animals may show all the anatomic and physiologic alterations of typical estrus, including ovulation, but sexual receptivity is lacking. It may be that such animals are not receiving sufficient estrogen or that there is not a proper balance between estrogen and progesterone to bring them into psychologic heat.

The Menstrual Cycle

The menstrual cycle, characteristic of primates, is fundamentally comparable to the estrous cycle, but there are two important differences: In primates there are no unequivocal peaks of heightened sexual receptivity, and the breakdown of the endometrium at the end of the cycle is accompanied by a loss of blood. The primate cycle is approximately 28 days in length, and ovulation ordinarily occurs about midway between the two menstrual periods. Anovulatory cycles are frequent in otherwise normal women. In most estrous mammals, excepting the mouse and rat, the uterus thickens appreciably under the influence of ovarian hormones, and deterioration and sloughing of the uterine lining occur at the end of the cycle. These changes are quite comparable to those that occur in the primate uterus. Although estrous mammals do not menstruate, the lining of the uterus is periodically lost and renewed. In ewes, cows, and swine, large plaques of tissue are often peeled off from the lining of the uterus during the end of the luteal phase or the beginning of the follicular phase. All mammalian uteri respond in much the same manner to the presence of ovarian hormones, or to their absence.

REFERENCES

1. Allison, J. E., Stanley, A. J., and Gumbreck, L. G.: Idiograms from rats exhibiting anomalous conditions associated with the reproductive organs. Amer. Zool. 4:401, 1964.
2. Amoroso, E. C., Hancock, J. L., and Rowlands, I. W.: Ovarian activity in the pregnant mare. Nature 161:355, 1948.
3. Atz, J. W.: Intersexuality in fishes. In C. N. Armstrong and A. J. Marshall (eds.): Intersexuality in Vertebrates Including Man. New York, Academic Press, 1964, p. 145.
4. Backhouse, K. M., and Hewer, H. R.: Features of reproduction in the grey seal. Med. Biol. Illustration 14:144, 1964.
5. Barr, M. L.: Sex chromatin and phenotype in man. Science 130:679, 1959.
6. Blandau, R. J., White, B. J., and Rumery, R. E.: Observations on the movements of the living primordial germ cells in the mouse. Fertil. Steril. 14:482, 1963.
7. Burns, R. K.: Experimental reversal of sex in the gonads of the opossum, Didelphys virginiana. Proc. Nat. Acad. Sci. 41:669, 1955.
8. Burns, R. K.: Urogenital system. In B. H. Willier, P. A. Weiss, and V. Hamburger (eds.): Analysis of Development. Philadelphia, W. B. Saunders Co., 1955, p. 462.
9. Burns, R. K.: Role of hormones in the differentiation of sex. In W. C. Young (ed.): Sex and Internal Secretions, Vol. 1. Baltimore, The Williams & Wilkins Co., 1961, p. 76.
10. Chang, C. Y., and Witschi, E.: Breeding of sex-reversed males of Xenopus laevis Daudin. Proc. Soc. Exp. Biol. Med. 89:150, 1955.
11. Chang, C. Y., and Witschi, E.: Genetic control and hormonal reversal of sex differentiation in Xenopus. Proc. Soc. Exp. Biol. Med. 93:140, 1956.
12. Chang, M. C.: Capacitation of rabbit spermatozoa in the uterus with special reference to the reproductive phases of the female. Endocrinology 63:619, 1958.
13. Clermont, Y.: Contractile elements in the limiting membrane of the seminiferous tubules of the rat. Exp. Cell. Res. 15:438, 1958.
14. Dubois, R., and Croisille, Y.: Germ-cell line and sexual differentiation in birds. Phil. Trans. Roy. Soc. Lond. B, 259:73, 1970.
15. Erickson, G. F.: The control of the differentiation of female embryonic germ cells in the birds. Devel. Biol. 36:113, 1974.
16. Follenius, E.: Cytologie et cytophysiologie des cellules interstitielles de l'epinoche: Gasterosteus aculeatus L. Gen. Comp. Endocr. 11:198, 1968.
17. Foote, C. L.: Intersexuality in amphibians. In C. N. Armstrong and A. J. Marshall (eds.): Intersexuality in Vertebrates Including Man. New York, Academic Press, 1964, p. 233.
18. Forsberg, J. G., Jacobsohn, D., and Norgren, A.: Development of the urinogenital tract in male offspring of rats injected during pregnancy with a substance with antiandrogenic properties (cyproterone). Z. Anat. Entwicklung. 126:320, 1968.
19. Franchi, L. L., Mandl, A. M., and Zuckerman, S.: The development of the ovary and the process of oogenesis. In S. Zuckerman (ed.): The Ovary, Vol. 1. New York, Academic Press, 1962, p. 1.
20. Gallien, L.: Sequential endocrine activities controlling oogenesis. A general survey. Amer. Zool. 15(Suppl. 1):197, 1975.
21. Gardner, W. A., Jr., Wood, H. A., Jr., and Taber, E.: Demonstration of a nonestrogenic gonadal inhibitor produced by the ovary of the brown leghorn. Gen. Comp. Endocr., 4:673, 1964.
22. Hall, P. F., Irby, D. C., and de Kretser, D. M.: Conversion of cholesterol to androgens by rat testes: Comparison of interstitial cells and seminiferous tubules. Endocrinology 84:488, 1969.
23. Harrington, R. W., Jr.: Twenty-four-hour rhythms of internal self-fertilization and of oviposition by hermaphrodites of Rivulus marmoratus, a cyprinodontid fish. Physiol. Zool. 36: 325, 1963.

24. Hishida, T.: Reversal of sex-differentiation in genetic males of the medaka *(Oryzias latipes)* by injecting estrone-16-C^{14} and diethylstilbestrol (monoethly-1-C^{14}) into the egg. Embryologia, *8*:234, 1964.
25. Hoar, W. S.: Reproduction in teleost fish. Mem. Soc. Endocr., No. 4, p. 5, 1955.
26. Höhn, E. O.: Gonadal hormone concentrations in northern phalaropes in relation to nuptial plumage. Canadian J. Zool. *48*:400, 1970.
27. Höhn, E. O., and Cheng, S. C.: Gonadal hormones in Wilson's phalarope *(Steganopus tricolor)* and other birds in relation to plumage and sex behavior. Gen. Comp. Endocr. *8*:1, 1967.
28. Hyder, M.: Histological studies on the testes of pond specimens of *Tilapia nigra* (Gunther) (Pisces: Cichlidae) and their implications of the pituitary-testis relationship. Gen. Comp. Endocr. *14*:198, 1970.
29. Johns, J. E.: Testosterone-induced nuptial feathers in phalaropes. Condor *66*:449, 1964.
30. Johns, J. E., and Pfeiffer, E. W.: Testosterone-induced incubation patches of phalarope birds. Science *140*:1225, 1963.
31. Jones, R. E.: Hormonal control of incubation patch development in the California quail *Lophortyx californicus*. Gen. Comp. Endocr. *13*:1, 1969.
32. Josso, N.: *In vitro* synthesis of müllerian-inhibiting hormone by seminiferous tubules isolated from calf fetal testis. Endocrinology *93*:829, 1973.
33. Jost, A.: Hormonal factors in the sex differentiation of the mammalian foetus. Phil. Trans. Roy. Soc. Lond. B. *259*:119, 1970.
34. Lance, V., and Callard, I. P.: A histochemical study of ovarian function in the ovoviviparous elasmobranch, *Squalus acanthias*. Gen. Comp. Endocr. *13*:255, 1969.
35. Lillie, F. R.: The free-martin: A Study of the action of sex hormones in the fetal life of cattle. J. Exp. Zool. *23*:371, 1917.
36. Linder, H. R., Tsafriri, A., Lieberman, M. E., Zor, U., Koch, Y., Bauminger, S., and Barnea, A.: Gonadotropin action on cultured graffian follicles: induction of maturation division of the mammalian oocyte and differentiation of the luteal cell. Rec. Progr. Horm. Res. *30*:79, 1974.
37. Marshall, A. J.: The unilateral endometrial reaction in the giant fruit-bat *(Pteropus giganteus* Brünnich). J. Endocr. *9*:42, 1953.
38. Marshall, A. J., and Coombs, C. J. F.: Lipoid changes in the gonads of wild birds: Their possible bearing on hormone production, sexual display and the breeding season. Nature *169*:261, 1952.
39. Marshall, A. J., and Lofts, B.: The Leydig-cell homologue in certain teleost fishes. Nature *177*:704, 1956.
40. Masui, Y., and Markert, C.: Cytoplasmic control of nuclear behavior during meiotic maturation of frog oocytes. J. Exp. Zool. *177*:129, 1971.
41. Mikamo, K., and Witschi, E.: Masculinization and breeding of the WW *Xenopus*. Experientia *20*:622, 1964.
42. Miller, M. R.: The seasonal histological changes occurring in the ovary, corpus luteum, and testis of the viviparous lizard, *Xantusia vigilis*. Univ. Calif. Pub. Zool. *47*:197, 1948.
43. Moore, J. G., Van Campenhout, J. L., and Brandkamp, W. W.: Chromosome analysis in abnormal sexual differentiation and gonadal dysfunction. Int. J. Fertil. *9*:469, 1964.
44. Nalbandov, A. V.: Reproductive Physiology, 2nd ed. San Francisco, W. H. Freeman & Company, 1964.
45. Nandi, J.: Comparative endocrinology of steroid hormones in vertebrates. Amer. Zool. *7*: 115, 1967.
46. Ohno, S.: Regulatory genetics of sex differentiation. *In* A. G. Motulsky and W. Lenz (eds): Birth Defects. Amsterdam, Excerpta Medica, 1974, p. 148.
47. Ohno, S.: The problem of the bovine freemartin. J. Reprod. Fert. Suppl. *7*:53, 1969.
48. Price, D., Zaaijer, J. J. P., Ortiz, E., and Brinkmann, A. O.: Current views on embryonic sex differentiation in reptiles, birds, and mammals. Am. Zool., *15*(Suppl.1):173, 1975.
49. Price, D.: Mammalian conception, sex differentiation, and hermaphroditism as viewed in historical perspective. Amer. Zool. *12*:179, 1972.
50. Ralph, C. L.: The control of color in birds. Amer. Zool. *9*:521, 1969.
51. Russell, L. B.: Genetics of mammalian sex chromosomes. Science *133*:1795, 1961.
52. Segal, S. J., and Nelson, W. O.: Initiation and maintenance of testicular function. *In* C. W. Lloyd (ed.): Endocrinology of Reproduction. New York, Academic Press, 1959, p. 107.
53. Sohval, A. R.: Chromosomes and sex chromatin in normal and anomalous sexual development. Physiol. Rev. *43*:306, 1963.
54. Taber, E.: Intersexuality in birds. *In* C. N. Armstrong and A. J. Marshall (eds.): Intersexuality in Vertebrates Including Man. New York, Academic Press, 1964, p. 285.

55. Tarkowski, A. K.: Germ cells in natural and experimental chimeras in mammals. Phil. Trans. Roy. Soc. Lond. B. *259*:107, 1970.
56. Turner, C. D.: Experimental reversal of germ cells. Embryologia *10*:206, 1969.
57. Turner, C. D., and Asakawa, H.: Experimental reversal of germ cells in ovaries of fetal mice. Science *143*:1344, 1964.
58. Vandenbergh, J. G.: Hormonal basis of sex skin in male Rhesus monkeys. Gen. Comp. Endocr. *5*:31, 1965.
59. Wells, L. J.: Effect of fetal endocrines on fetal growth. *In* Gestation, 3rd Conf. New York, Josiah Macy Jr. Foundation, 1957, p. 187.
60. Wimsatt, W. A., and Kallen, F. C.: The unique maturation response of the graafian follicles of hibernating vespertilionid bats and the question of its significance. Anat. Rec. *129*:115, 1957.
61. Wimsatt, W. A., and Waldo, C. M.: The normal occurrence of a peritoneal opening in the bursa ovarii of the mouse. Anat. Rec. *93*:47, 1945.
62. Witschi, E.: The inductor theory of sex differentiation. J. Fac. Sci., Hokkaido University, Series VI, Zoology, *13*:428, 1957.
63. Witschi, E.: Sex and secondary sexual characters. *In* A. J. Marshall (ed.): Biology and Comparative Physiology of Birds, Vol. 2. New York, Academic Press, 1961, p. 115.
64. Wolff, E.: Endocrine function of the gonad in developing vertebrates. *In* A. Gorbman (ed.): Comparative Endocrinology. New York, John Wiley & Sons, 1959, p. 568.
65. Wolff, E., and Haffen, K.: Sur l'intersexualité expérimentale des gonades embryonnaires de canard cultivées *in vitro*. Arch. Anat. Micr. Morph. Exper. *41*:184, 1952.
66. Wolfson, A.: The ejaculate and the nature of coition in some passerine birds. Ibis *102*:124, 1960.
67. Woods, J. E., and Weeks, R. L.: Ontogenesis of the pituitary-gonadal axis in the chick embryo. Gen. Comp. Endocr. *13*:242, 1969.
68. Yamamoto, T.: A further study on induction of functional sex reversal in genotypic males of the medaka *(Oryzias latipes)* and progenies of sex reversals. Genetics *44*:739, 1959.
69. Yamamoto, T.: Effects of 17α-hydroxyprogesterone and androstenedione upon sex differentiation in the medaka, *Oryzias latipes*. Gen. Comp. Endocr. *10*:8, 1968.
70. Yamamoto, T.: Sex differentiation. *In* W. S. Hoar and D. J. Randall (eds.): Fish Physiology, Vol. 3. New York, Academic Press, 1969.

CHAPTER 13

Endocrinology of the Testis

The testis performs two functions that are to a large extent complementary: the proliferation of spermatozoa and the secretion of steroid hormones. The hormones determine the physiologic state of the accessory ducts and glands and usually condition the appearance of the secondary sex characters. Phylogenetically, the older function of the gonad seems to be the proliferation of gametes. In the protochordates (*e.g.,* amphioxus) accessory sex organs are absent; the ripe gonads free the germ cells into the atrial cavity, and these are conveyed to the exterior by the water leaving the atriopore. It is not certain that the gonads of protochordates secrete sex hormones. The genital system of the cyclostome is poorly developed, and the urinary ducts are not employed for the conveyance of genital products, as in teleost fishes and higher forms. In aquatic vertebrates, such as fishes and amphibians, the gonadal hormones become indispensable adjuncts for reproduction. In general, the accessory sex mechanism increases in complexity with the advent of terrestrial or aerial life, and the hormones of the gonads assume even broader functions than in the lower aquatic species.

STRUCTURE OF THE TESTIS

The testis is composed of seminiferous tubules and the interstitial cells of Leydig which are present in the angular spaces between the tubules. The interstitium contains abundant blood and lymphatic vessels, but the tubules are completely avascular. This means that all components of the tubular epithelium have to be nourished and maintained by the diffusion of essential agents provided by the circulation. The youngest germ cells (spermatogonia) rest on the inner surface of a basement membrane and are covered by the bases of the huge somatic elements called Sertoli cells. The tunica propria, or tubular wall, also contains smooth muscle-like (myoid) cells, bundles of collagen-like fibers, and an outer layer of endothelial cells lining the extensive lymphatic spaces present in the interstitium. The lumina of the tubules contain fluid in which spermatozoa are typically suspended. This fluid is actively secreted by seminiferous tubules and by the rete testis and is discharged by efferent ductules into the epididymis. The secretion can be collected by cannulating the tubule or the rete testis, and biochemical analyses show that its composition is unlike that of blood plasma or testicular lymph.

The Sertoli cells, together with the peritubular myoid cells, constitute a blood-testis barrier somewhat comparable to the blood-brain barrier (Fig.

13-1). Many substances such as proteins or dyes present in blood or testicular lymph spaces are prevented by specialized junctions from entering the tubular fluid. The spermatogonia occupy the *basal compartment* and can be exposed to essential hormones when the myoid junctions are open. The other germinal cells move luminally between contiguous Sertoli cells, the most advanced stages becoming embedded in the cytoplasm along the luminal edges of the Sertoli cells. Special junctional complexes arise between the cell membranes of adjacent Sertoli cells. These junctions mark the beginning of the *adluminal compartment,* containing spermatocytes and spermatids, and serve to further regulate the composition of the tubular fluid (Fig. 13-1). Certain substances, such as particular steroids, do cross this blood-testis barrier when the junctions permit and may be expelled through the rete testis fluid.[21, 83]

Two essential processes are involved in the transformation of spermatogonia into spermatozoa: (1) reduction of the number of chromosomes (meiotic divisions), and (2) the transformation of haploid cells into spermatozoa (spermiogenesis). As the spermatids transform into spermatozoa they lose cytoplasm and are temporarily confined to the Sertoli cells. They are found in rather discrete aggregations, all cells of the group having originated from a single spermatogonium. In man, as in other mammals, intercellular bridges tend to persist between dividing germ cells and give rise to clones which involve large numbers of cells. Since the cells derived from a spermatogonium remain together and differentiate synchronously, cellular associations of fixed composition appear along the length of the seminiferous tubule.[76, 80]

Radioautographic techniques have been employed in several mammalian species in attempts to determine the time required for the completion of spermatogenesis. Thymidine-H³, a specific precursor of deoxyribonucleic

Figure 13-1. Diagrammatic section through a mammalian seminiferous tubule showing a Sertoli cell and a mobile population of differentiating germ cells. Features of the blood-testis barrier, as determined by electron microscopy, are indicated. The tubule is covered by a tunica propria, and the contractile cells (myoid layer) provide a primary barrier against the entrance of substances from the interstitial blood vessels and lymphatic spaces. Most of the myoid cell junctions are closed by a tight apposition of membranes (A), but some may be open as indicated at B. Substances entering through the myoid layer have access to the intercellular spaces between Sertoli cells and spermatogonia (see arrows). The specialized junctions between adjacent Sertoli cells are usually tightly closed (stars), and these form the

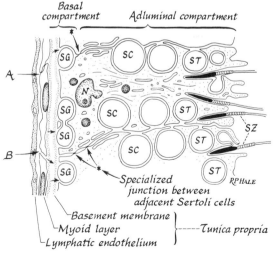

most efficient component of the blood-testis barrier. They divide the tubular epithelium into two compartments: a *basal* one containing spermatogonia (SG) and early preleptotine spermatocytes, and an *adluminal* one containing spermatocytes (SC), spermatids (ST), and spermatozoa (SZ). N, nucleus of Sertoli cell. (Based on figures by Dym, M., and Fawcett, D. W., 1970.[21])

acid (DNA), is an excellent tracer substance since it is incorporated into the nuclei of spermatogonia preparing for mitosis and into spermatocytes preparing for meiosis. By preserving the testes at different intervals after injection of the radioactive tracer, it is possible to determine how rapidly the labeled germ cells develop. Germ cells which are in the process of synthesizing DNA may also be labeled with P^{32}. Spermatogenesis in the mouse extends over a period of four cycles and requires about 33.5 days for completion. Four cycles are also identifiable in rats, and the duration of spermatogenesis in the Sherman strain has been estimated as 48 days. Sprague-Dawley rats have slightly longer cycles and require about 51.6 days to complete the process. Studies on testicular biopsies of the human testis, taken at frequent intervals after the intratesticular administration of thymidine-H^3, indicate that there are 4.6 cycles, each cycle of the epithelium lasting 16 days. These studies on man indicate that it requires about 74 days for a spermatogonium to transform into functional spermatozoa.[37, 38] The indications are that the rate of germ-cell development is constant for given species and strains of mammals, and that this rate cannot be accelerated by hormones such as gonadotrophins and androgens. Cytologic observations suggest that germ cells must move forward in their differentiation; if unfavorable environments make it impossible for them to pursue their differentiation at the normal rate, they degenerate and are eliminated from the system. Although hormones do not accelerate the *rate* of germ-cell differentiation, they must contribute to the creation of favorable environments for their transformation into spermatozoa.[12]

Sites of Steroidogenesis Within the Testis

Leydig cells are often difficult to distinguish from intertubular connective-tissue elements, and variations in size and number cannot be quantitated with much accuracy. Consequently, the evidence obtained by observing seasonal changes and breeding behavior is largely indirect and circumstantial. Information derived from histochemical tests and ultrastructural studies leave no doubt that the cells of Leydig are an important source of steroid hormones. These cells are characterized by an extensive smooth endoplasmic reticulum, a prominent Golgi complex, the presence of lipid droplets, and numerous lysosomes. The smooth reticulum is in the form of branching and anastomosing tubules, and several of the enzymes involved in steroidogenesis are known to be associated with it. The lipid droplets tend to diminish when steroid secretion is maximal, and to increase during periods of relative inactivity. In the guinea pig, and to a lesser extent in other species, annulate lamellae are frequently found around lipid droplets, lysosomes, and other organelles (Fig. 13–2). The concentric lamellae arise from the smooth reticulum and consist of flattened sacs or cisternae. Unlike cells that secrete proteins, the steroid-secreting cells contain no granules or vacuoles of stored secretory product, and the granular (rough) reticulum is comparatively meager.

Studies on the fine structure of Sertoli cells are consistent with the view that such cells are steroidogenic. Human Sertoli cells possess an elaborate

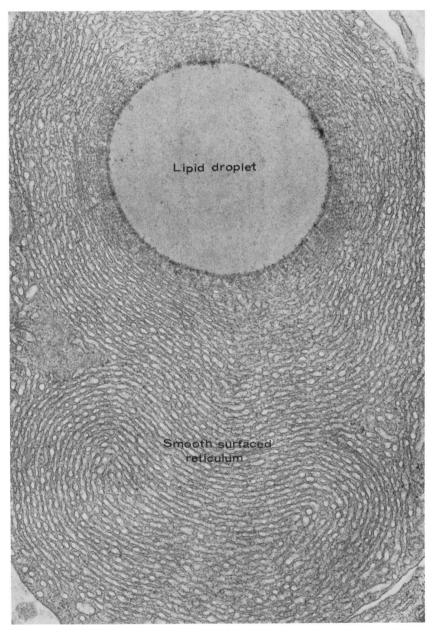

Figure 13-2. Electron micrograph of a field of cytoplasm from a Leydig cell of the guinea pig testis. The extensive, smooth endoplasmic reticulum often takes the form of concentric systems of fenestrated cisternae in this species. (From Fawcett, D. W., Long, J. A., and Jones, A. L.: Rec. Progr. Horm. Res. *25*, 1969.)

smooth reticulum, lipid droplets, annulate lamellae that partially envelop lipid droplets, prominent Golgi bodies, and abundant mitochondria. The organelles and inclusions, probably concerned with steroidogenesis, tend to be concentrated toward the base of the cells, in the vicinity of the nucleus. As each generation of spermatids attains maturity, the spermatids discharge small units of cytoplasm (the residual bodies) and, in the rat, these are found to contain lipid droplets, ribosomes and a few other organelles. The residual bodies are phagocytosed by the Sertoli cells, and this markedly increases their content of lipid. The Sertoli cells contain the most abundant lipid shortly after the release of sperm and before the spermatocytes have completed the maturation divisions. The over-all cycle of events within the Sertoli cell is repeated each time a new generation of spermatids differentiates into spermatozoa. It has been proposed that the residual bodies, which are engulfed by the Sertoli cells, serve as a source of precursor materials that may be utilized by these cells in the biosynthesis of specific steroids for the support of each new wave of spermatogenic activity.[45] This concept can be doubted since it has been shown that isolated tubules of the rat do not contain the enzymes necessary for the conversion of cholesterol to pregnenolone and progesterone.[34] It is probable that the testis tubule relies upon an extratubular source of testosterone for the support of spermatogenesis.

Histochemical procedures applied to the gonads of the domestic fowl and rat indicate that androgens are synthesized by the interstitial cells of Leydig, as well as by the Sertoli cells and certain germinal cells within the tubules.[92] The testes of the rat lack septa, and the interstitial tissue is very loosely attached to the seminiferous tubules. It is possible, by using a dissecting microscope, to pull out the tubules from the interstitial tissue. Tubules can be obtained which are virtually free of interstitial cells, the latter remaining in a coherent web of connective tissue. The biosynthetic competence of these two testicular components may be tested by incubating them separately with a labeled androgen precursor. Both tubular and interstitial-cell fractions are capable of transforming progesterone to 17-hydroxyprogesterone, androstenedione, and testosterone, but the interstitial tissue is much more efficient in this respect than the seminiferous tubules. Germinal elements of the scrotal testis may be eliminated or greatly reduced by irradiation or the application of heat, leaving the Sertoli cells intact. Isolated tubules from such testes, practically denuded of germ cells, continue to be capable of producing androgenic steroids. Enriched preparations of Sertoli cells or spermatocytes may be prepared from isolated seminiferous tubules for *in vitro* studies.[10]

CHEMISTRY OF THE ANDROGENS

Androgens are masculinizing compounds that are produced chiefly by the testis under normal conditions. They also arise from the adrenal cortices and ovaries and are very probably present in the placenta. Such compounds are found in the urine of males, females, and castrates; androsterone is the principal androgen of human urine and was isolated in 1931. A yield of 15 mg of crystalline androsterone was obtained from 15,000 liters of normal male urine. Testosterone was isolated from testicular tissue in 1935. It is probable that androgenic steroids perform significant roles in the reproductive processes of all vertebrates. A significant portion of the androgen present in the mammalian organism arises from the adrenal cortex. These compounds are formed from adrenocortical steroids such as cortisol and are released into the blood as biologically active material. Certain types of ovarian and testicular tumors may produce and release tremendous amounts of androgen.

It is certain that a number of organs possess the necessary enzymatic equipment to produce androgenic steroids. It is reasonably well established that all of the steroid hormones, whether adrenocortical, testicular, or ovarian, are produced by biosynthetic pathways common to all these organs. Thus, the endocrine differences between testis, ovary, and adrenal cortex are quantitative rather than qualitative. This accounts for the fact that the adrenal cortex, for example, may function abnormally and liberate an excess of gonadal steroids.

The common pathways employed by different organs in the synthesis and degradation of steroids account for the interconvertibility of these compounds. *Proandrogens* are compounds which are not androgenic when applied locally, but acquire androgenic activity during their metabolism within the organism. 17α-Hydroxyprogesterone produces no growth of the chick's comb when applied by inunction, but when it is given orally, a pronounced growth of the comb occurs. Cortisone and cortisol are adrenal glucocorticoids and are not androgenic, but the organism may convert them into androgens such as 11-hydroxyandrosterone, adrenosterone, 11-ketoandrosterone, and 11β-hydroxyandrostenedione. 17-Hydroxyprogesterone and 11-deoxycortisol may also serve as proandrogens and yield androsterone and androstenedione.

Testosterone and androstenedione are the main circulating androgens of testicular origin. Sensitive and reliable procedures are available for determining the quantity of testosterone in the blood plasma. The plasma of normal men contains about 0.5 μg of testosterone per 100 ml of plasma; in normal women, the value is about 0.1 μg per 100 ml of plasma. Certain estrogens, particularly estradiol-17-β and estrone, have been identified in extracts of normal human testis as well as in blood from the spermatic vein. The total estrogen content of male urine is the equivalent of about 40 I.U. of estrone per day; this is less than one-tenth the quantity excreted by women at the time of ovulation.[22, 23, 49, 89]

When steroids are administered orally or intraperitoneally, they enter the portal veins and are carried to the liver, where they are promptly inactivated. Greater activity is generally observed following subcutaneous or intramuscular administrations; the compounds are released slowly from the site of injection and are absorbed into the systemic circulation, thus avoiding liver inactivation.[55]

Much evidence has accumulated since 1965 indicating that *dihydrotestosterone* (5α-androstan-17β-ol-3-one), a metabolite of testosterone, is

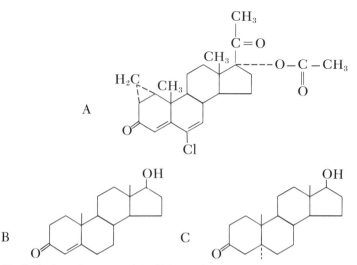

Figure 13-3. *A,* Cyproterone acetate (1,2α-methylene-6-chloro-Δ$^{4, 6}$-pregnadiene-17α-ol-3,20-dione-17α-acetate), a synthetic steroid having potent antiandrogenic effects. The compound has progestational activity, but is neither androgenic nor estrogenic. *B,* Testosterone, the chief circulating hormone of testicular origin. *C,* 5α-dihydrotestosterone, a potent metabolite of testosterone formed in certain androgen-responsive tissues.

formed in many androgen-responsive tissues, in which it probably serves as the "active form" of the hormone (Fig. 13-3, *B* and *C*).[4, 24, 90] The common metabolites of testosterone, such as epitestosterone, androstanediol, androstenedione, etiocholanolone, and androsterone, have much weaker androgenic actions than testosterone. In certain bioassay systems, DHT is a much more potent androgen than testosterone itself (Table 13-1). Some androgen targets, such as prostate, seminal vesicle, epididymis, preputial gland, kidney, penis, and certain hypothalamic neurons, preferentially metabolize testosterone to DHT and retain it in their cell nuclei. Sertoli cells and spermatocytes of the rat have the capacity to metabolize testosterone to 5α-reduced products, particularly DHT and 5α-androstane-3α, 17β-diol. Prostatic tissue is known to contain a number of hydroxysteroid dehydrogenases, as well as a NADPH-dependent testosterone 5α-reductase, an enzyme that converts testosterone to DHT. The conversion of DHT to testosterone cannot be reversed by the tissues. It appears that not all androgen-sensitive tissues readily metabolize testosterone to DHT in this way. For example, some muscles, such as the levator ani of rodents, are known to be very sensitive to androgens but, after the injection of labeled testosterone, very little DHT accumulates in them. Since androgens are essential for spermatogenesis, the testis must be regarded as a target acted upon by its own hormones. However, organs such as muscles do not respond to androgens with the same promptness as the various male accessory glands and ducts. It is possible that the manner in which testosterone acts at the cellular level may not be the same in all tissues. The hypothesis that DHT rather than testosterone itself acts on targets has some merit, but should be accepted cautiously until more is known.[14, 17, 84]

Table 13-1 RELATIVE ANDROGENIC AND ANABOLIC ACTIVITIES OF SOME REPRESENTATIVE ANDROSTANES AND ANDROSTENES*

EXPERIMENTAL ANIMALS	CHICK COMB‡	VENTRAL PROSTATE	RAT SEMINAL VESICLE	LEVATOR ANI MUSCLE	RAT EXORBITAL LACRIMAL GLAND
Testosterone†	100	100	100	100	100
5α-Dihydrotestosterone	228	268	158	152	74
17α-Methyltestosterone	300 (231)	103	100	108	162
17α-Methyl-5α-dihydrotestosterone	480	254	78	107	—
Androst-4-ene-3, 17-dione	121 (262)	39	17	22	14
5α-Androstane-3, 17-dione	115 (182)	33	13	11	—
5α-Androstane-3α, 17β-diol	75	34	24	30	238
Androst-4-ene-3β, 17β-diol	(76)	124	133	95	—
5α-Androstane-3β, 17β-diol	2	—	10	—	5
Androst-4-en-3-on-17α-ol	—	8	2	3	—
5α-Androstan-3α-ol-17-one	115 (238)	53	8	10	46
19-Nortestosterone	(86)	—	10	180	52
19-Nordihydrotestosterone	118	—	—	—	—
17α-Methyl-19-nortestosterone	—	25	25	60	81
Testosterone propionate	(380)	161	146	187	195
5α-Androstan-17β-ol	128 (227)	—	—	—	5

*From Liao, S., and Fang, S.: Vitamins Hormones 27:17, 1969.

†Testosterone as 100. Rat tests are by injection; comb test by inunction.

‡For comb test, relative activity numbers without parentheses are from Dorfman et al.; with parentheses are from Ofner et al.

For purposes of terminology, the androgens may be regarded as derivatives of androstane; they contain 19 carbon atoms and possess methyl groups at C-10 and C-13. Biologic activity is altered by making relatively small additions or substitutions at the various carbon positions. The natural androgens vary greatly in their potencies even when bioassayed by the same end points; they also differ in their capacities to stimulate different end points. For example, testosterone and androstenedione possess a high degree of androgenicity when tested by the ordinary fowl and mammalian parameters, but they have little capacity to maintain spermatogenesis in the testis of the hypophysectomized rat. Pregnenolone, on the other hand, is not androgenic by the usual tests, but it is extremely potent in maintaining testicular weight and spermatogenesis in the hypophysectomized rat. Biochemists have tried, with some measure of success, to produce steroid compounds with mild or no masculinizing actions but with marked protein anabolic actions.

Several interrelated routes to the biosynthesis of androgens have been demonstrated, and some of these are shown in Fig. 13-4. The degradation products of the steroid hormones are not salvaged by the organism and used again for the synthesis of new compounds. Hence there is little or no feedback, and the level of hormones in the blood depends upon the availability of precursors and the capacity of the cells to produce new hormones. It has been shown that androgens may be synthesized from acetate, and that cholesterol is not an obligatory intermediate. Since acetate is a precur-

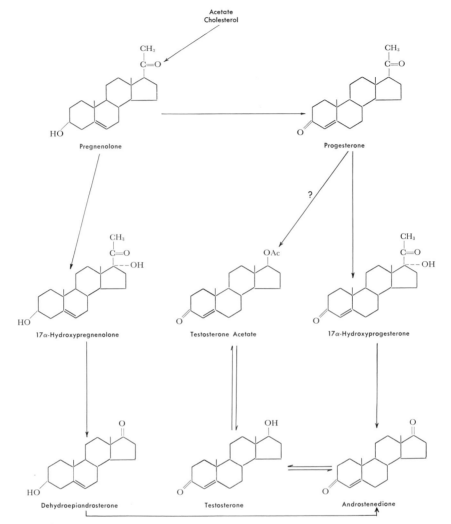

Figure 13–4. Probable pathways of androgen biosynthesis in the gonads.

sor to cholesterol, however, it should not be concluded that the organism never uses the latter as a precursor for the androgens.[17]

Testosterone in the circulation is bound to the blood proteins and hence does not normally filter through the kidney glomeruli. It is not stored in the body but is quickly utilized, or degraded into relatively inactive androgens, which are excreted through the urine or through the bile and feces. The androgens of the urine are present as water-soluble sulfates and glucuronides and are not biologically active.

The testis of the stallion contains large quantities of estrogenic material, and the urine contains high titers of estrogen metabolites. After removal of the testes, the urinary estrogens diminish to very low levels. The administration of chorionic gonadotrophin to adult men stimulates the testes and increases the output of both androgen and estrogen. When testosterone and other androgens are administered to human subjects, there is an accelerated excretion of estrogenic material, which has been identified as estrone, estradiol, and estriol. Slices of human ovaries, incubated with C^{14}-labeled testosterone, release labeled estradiol-17β. The *in vitro* conversion of testosterone to estrogens can also be accomplished by the placenta. Testosterone and related 19-carbon compounds apparently serve as precursors for testicular estrogens, as they do in the ovary and adrenal cortex.

Urinary 17-Ketosteroids

The common bioassay methods for androgens include growth of the capon's comb, enlargement of various muscles, increased weight of the ventral prostate or seminal vesicles of the castrated rat, or increase in quantities of fructose and citric acid in the sex accessories of the castrated mammal after treatment with such compounds. Several chemical methods are available for assessing the levels of androgens in the organism and, in clinical work, these are more practical than the biologic tests. The determination of neutral 17-ketosteroids in the urine is commonly practiced. These are the catabolic end products of the androgens formed by the testes and the adrenal cortices.

These 17-ketosteroids (*e.g.,* androsterone) have a keto group at position 17 of the steroid nucleus. Because of this feature, they give characteristic color reactions with *m*-dinitrobenzene (Zimmermann reaction) and antimony trichloride (Pincus reaction). Since estrone, an ovarian hormone, contains a phenolic ring, it is acidic, but it may be removed from the neutral fraction by washing with alkali. The neutral 17-ketosteroids, freed of estrone, represent the androgens produced by the adrenal cortex and the testis. During the first two years of life, children excrete only small amounts of 17-ketosteroids, and there are no significant sexual differences in normal subjects before puberty. Normal adult women excrete 5 to 15 mg daily, and the amount may increase during late pregnancy. The values for normal adult men, during the reproductive years, usually range from 7 to 20 mg daily. Very high values are obtained in diseases characterized by adrenal or testicular hyperplasia. Hypofunctions of the anterior hypophysis, testes, or adrenal cortices produce low 17-ketosteroid values.

Experiments with Antiandrogens

Antiandrogens are substances that act upon target sites to prevent androgens from expressing their activity. These have been used experimentally to explore the physiologic significance of androgens at all stages of the life cycle, and it is probable that they will prove useful in the treatment of androgen-dependent clinical conditions. Cyproterone and cyproterone acetate (CTA) are steroids synthesized from hydroxyprogesterone and are among the most potent antiandrogens; CTA is a strong progestogen, whereas cyproterone is not (Fig. 13–3, *A*). Neither compound is estrogenic.

Antiandrogens apparently act competitively at the receptor sites on the target tissues to block the action of androgenic steroids. Cyproterone acetate has been shown to suppress the uptake of radioactive androgens by rat ventral prostate, and to diminish the retention of dihydrotestosterone by the prostate cell nuclei. *In vitro* studies indicate that CTA antagonizes the formation of a specific dihydrotestosterone-receptor protein in the prostate cell.[16, 27]

Androgens, which act through a feedback system to control the release of pituitary gonadotrophins, are essential for the differentiation and maintenance of male accessories and secondary sex characters. They are involved in the prenatal morphogenesis of the genital tract, the maturation of pathways within the central nervous system, and, in addition, play a very essential role in the initiation and maintenance of spermatogenesis. All these actions can be prevented by CTA and similar compounds, though large doses may have to be employed over prolonged periods. Male accessory glands and ducts are caused to regress and, after administration of large doses, a castrate condition prevails in these organs. Antiandrogens delay the closure of epiphyseal junctions in young animals without affecting the ultimate length of the bones. Spermiogenesis is diminished, and this may result in the loss of fertility. Such agents prevent the stimulating effect of androgens on the chick comb and, in mammals, block the actions of androgens on sebaceous and salivary glands. In fetal and neonatal rats, CTA inhibits almost completely the organizing action of testosterone upon accessory sex organs, mammary glands, and certain areas of the brain that regulate gonadotrophin secretion and sexual behavior.

Studies on fetal castration, destruction of gonads by irradiation, and organ culture of genital tracts indicate that mammary glands and external genitalia undergo feminine organogenesis unless a functioning testis is present. Nipple formation in rats and mice is suppressed by the administration of androgens. Male fetuses develop nipples following treatment with CTA, and differentiation of the genital tubercle corresponds to that of a clitoris.

Male pseudohermaphroditism may be induced in various mammalian species by administering antiandrogens to pregnant mothers when the fetuses are in the ambisexual stage of development. The direction of gonadal differentiation is not impaired. There are species differences in the extent of modification of the internal genital structures, and *complete* feminine differentiation is not induced. For example, the Müllerian ducts of male fetuses exposed to CTA generally regress as they normally do, and hence such feminized males have no uterus. Male accessory glands are not formed and, in rabbits and dogs receiving high doses of antiandrogens, the deferent ducts and epididymides fail to develop. The external genitalia may be highly feminized, and the situation simulates the spontaneous human defect known as the "androgen insensitivity syndrome" or "testicular feminization." Through the proper treatment of genetic male rats with CTA and estrogen, the formation of a patent vagina may be induced from the urogenital sinus (Fig. 13–5). These genetic male rats receiving antiandrogen early in life develop the female (cyclic) type of hypothalamic-pituitary system; they

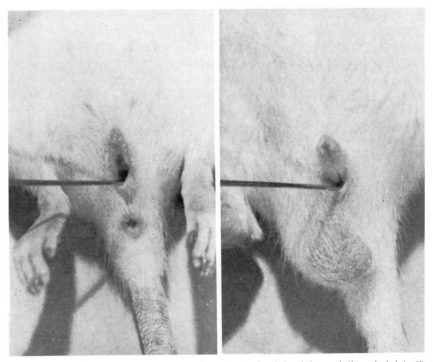

Figure 13–5. External genitalia of genetic male rats feminized through the administration of cyproterone acetate. Observe the patent vagina (indicated by probe) and the clitoris-like penis. In *B,* the anus is obscured by the scrotum; treatment with estrogen caused the testes of *A* to ascend into the body cavity. The mother of these animals received 10 mg of cyproterone acetate per day from the thirteenth to the twenty-second day of gestation; the newborn rats received 0.3 mg of the antiandrogenic agent per day for 3 weeks. These animals had also received 1 mg estradiol daily for 1 week. (From Neumann, F., Elger, W., and Kramer, M.: Endocrinol. *78:*628, 1966.)

behave like females toward other males and appear to be regarded as females by the other animals.[61, 62]

Mechanism of Action of Androgens

It appears that androgens follow the same pattern of action upon target cells as do other steroid hormones. The first step is the entrance of androgens into the cell cytoplasm, where they become bound to a specific receptor protein. This steroid-receptor complex is transported to the nucleus, where it binds to "acceptor" sites on the genome. The activation of specific genes is thought to allow the transcription of new species of mRNA, which code for the synthesis of particular proteins in the cytoplasm.[42, 48, 86]

Binding proteins have been found in the cytosol of a great variety of mammalian tissues upon which androgens are known to exert major effects. Growth of the mouse kidney is enhanced by androgens, and this is accomplished by a marked increase in RNA, principally in the microsomal fraction.[43, 77] The treatment of orchiectomized guinea pigs with testosterone causes a rapid increase in RNA of both temporal and masseter muscles; the weight and amounts of RNA and DNA of the oblique and gastrocnemius muscles undergo little change after castration or the injection of androgen. Androgen-receptor complexes within the seminiferous epithelium of the rat have been identified. Testosterone and 5α-dihydrotestosterone are tightly bound to receptors within the testis tubules and are similar to those of the prostate and epididymis. The cytoplasmic androgen-receptor complexes are translocated to the nuclei, where they mediate the stimulus for spermatogenesis.[26, 73, 91]

The head appendages of the cock were employed early for the identification and bioassay of male hormone, and androgen binding proteins have recently been studied in the comb, wattles, and ear lobes as well as in other tissues (with the exception of blood). Dihydrotestosterone binding was found in the cytosol of head furnishings, lung, skin, bone marrow, breast muscle, liver, and other tissues.[19]

The clinical features of testicular feminization (androgen insensitivity syndrome) can now be attributed to the inability of target tissues to respond to androgens. Genetic models of rats and mice displaying male pseudohermaphroditism have yielded information that makes it likely that the human disorder results from a genetically determined defect of the cytosol androgen receptors. Inherited defects in the vet rat (vestigial testes) and in tfm (feminizing testis) rats and mice lead to male pseudohermaphroditism by impairing androgen-dependent differentiation during critical embryonic periods. The vet rat has a defect in Leydig cell maturation that practically prevents the biosynthesis of testosterone, whereas the tfm animals are insensitive to androgens because of a lack of androgen receptors in the cytosol of many tissues. The obligatory nature of androgen receptors is well illustrated by studies on the tfm animals, in which defects cannot be repaired by the administration of exogenous androgens.[6, 79]

TESTICULAR PHYSIOLOGY

The androgens are essential for the control of secondary sex characters of the male and for the functional competence of the accessory reproductive ducts and glands. The most profound metabolic action of these steroids is the promotion of protein anabolism. At the human level, androgens are involved in the control of hair patterns, voice changes, skeletal configurations, and the regulation of sebaceous-gland activity.[81] Androgens also exert effects upon the germinal epithelium of the testis tubules and thus influence sperm production; chemistry of the seminal fluid is determined through their actions upon the accessory glands.

Spermatogenesis: Hormonal Dependence

An important function of androgens is to facilitate spermatogenesis within the testis tubule. Testosterone is synthesized by the cells of Leydig, under the influence of luteinizing hormone (LH or ICSH), and diffuses into the tubule where it is the principal stimulus for germ cell differentiation. The level of testosterone in the testicular lymph that bathes the exterior of the testis tubule is about the same as that present in spermatic venous blood. The concentration of testosterone in the tubular fluid of the rat is much higher than that of the peripheral circulation. Though the various cellular elements within the tubule can metabolize androgens in various ways, they cannot synthesize steroids from cholesterol, and it is not known to what extent the tubules can supply their own androgens; it is certain that they depend heavily upon the influx of testosterone from the interstitium. The formation of germ cells is an extremely complex process and is influenced by many agents that must be derived from the circulation, such as pituitary gonadotrophins (LH and FSH), epinephrine, insulin, fatty acids, proteins, and glucose.[18, 70, 78]

Spermatogenesis in the male rat may be maintained or restored following hypophysectomy by the prompt administration of testosterone or 5α-dihydrotestosterone alone or LH acting via the cells of Leydig. Complete repair of the germinal epithelium requires the synergistic action of follicle stimulating hormone (FSH) and either LH or androgen. The testes of rats quickly become aspermic under continuous treatment with estrogens; miotic activity continues, but the meiotic divisions are not completed. Sperm proliferation in these testes can be restored by giving FSH or by using relatively large doses of androgen. Fluorescence-labeled FSH accumulates mostly in the Sertoli cells, whereas labeled LH accumulates largely in the Leydig cells.[8, 53, 59]

There is the possibility that some of the steroids produced within the seminiferous tubules or within the ductus deferens and epididymis may be added to the semen. Appreciable quantities of dehydroepiandrosterone have been found in human, bull, and stallion semen. It has been reported that some of the epithelial cells lining the ductus deferens and epididymis of the mouse and rat can synthesize sterols and that the biosynthetic activity is androgen dependent. There are indications that compounds beyond cholesterol may be produced: The rabbit's epididymis *in vitro* can convert pregnenolone to dehydroepiandrosterone. It is probable that the sterols and steroids added to the sperm within the male tract may have important effects on sperm metabolism or on the membrane changes associated with maturation. *In vitro* experiments have shown that the submaxillary glands of male rats have the necessary enzymes to synthesize cholesterol from acetate, and to convert the cholesterol to pregnenolone and dehydroepiandrosterone. The significance of this is not known.[35, 40, 71]

Androgen Binding Protein

An androgen binding protein (ABP) secreted by the Sertoli cells has been identified in intact rats. This protein has a high affinity for testosterone and dihydrotestosterone, and serves to retain the androgens within the tubular compartment of the testis, where germ cell proliferation is occurring.

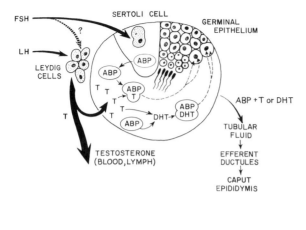

Figure 13–6. The actions of pituitary gonadotrophins on the mammalian testis. FSH stimulates the Sertoli cells to produce an androgen-binding protein (ABP) for transporting androgen (testosterone, T, or 5α-dihydrotestosterone, DHT) to the proliferating germ cells lining the testis tubules. ABP leaves the testis through the efferent duct fluid, thus conveying bound androgen to the caput epididymis where it may be involved in the metabolic processes required for sperm maturation. (Based on studies by French, F. S., Nayfeh, S. N., Ritzen, E. M., and Hansson, V.[31])

The ABP is secreted into the tubular fluid and is finally concentrated in the caput epididymis (Fig. 13–6). Testicular lymph around the exterior of the tubules does not contain ABP. The Sertoli cells, properly stimulated by FSH, seem to be the exclusive source of ABP, since it continues to be formed in normal amounts in rats completely deprived of germ cells by gamma irradiation or nitrofurazone treatment. There is a complete loss of ABP from testis and epididymis following hypophysectomy; it is restored in both sites following the administration of FSH. This effect is not obtained by the treatment of hypophysectomized rats with androgen, LH, prolactin, growth hormone, TSH, or estrogen. The epididymis is an important androgen target, and it appears that the organ receives androgen from the rete testis fluid and via the blood supply.[31, 32, 82]

A Spermatogonial Chalone

Evidence has been published indicating that the mitotic rate of spermatogonial stem cells of the rat is influenced by locally-secreted agents known as chalones. There are normally two classes of spermatogonial stem cells in the rat: the A^0 cells constitute the quiescent, reserve type, whereas the A_1–A_4 cells proliferate actively to renew the epithelium. It is possible that the proliferating cells produce a mitotic inhibitory substance which prevents the A^0 spermatogonia from dividing. Following X-irradiation (300 r) of the testis, most of the dividing A_1–A_4 cells are killed, whereas the reserve A^0 spermatogonia dramatically restore the population within a few days and then return to their dormant condition. A testicular extract from normal rats was given to animals that had been irradiated eleven days previously. The incorporation of thymidine-H^3 into testicular DNA was diminished by more than half, and similar extracts from liver lacked this effect. Autoradiography revealed that the mitotic rate decreased only in A-type spermatogonia, no effect being found in the intermediate B-type spermatogonia or in the spermatocytes. These studies showed that the testis extract specifically inhibited the proliferation of the A spermatogonia during the repair phase of these cells following irradiation, and the active agent was considered to be a chalone.[13]

Chalones have been studied in epidermis and associated structures, hemopoietic tissues, granulocytes, and liver. A chalone is thought to act upon the same tissue that produced it; the agent is thought to be non-cytotoxic and tissue-specific though not species-specific.

Inhibin and Spermatogenesis

The name "inhibin" was applied to an inhibitory product of the mammalian testis many years ago; its identity was not established and, lacking confirmation, most investigators regarded it skeptically or theorized that it might alter mitotic rates in the testis and exert various kinds of feed-back actions on gonadotrophins. In case such a compound is produced by the testis epithelium, it could gain access to the circulation following the movement of rete testis fluid into the epididymis. Many workers believe that impaired spermatogenesis activates a mechanism for controlling the production and release of FSH from the adenohypophysis.[75]

Regulation of Male Accessory Organs

The accessory system of male ducts and glands are, morphologically and physiologically, dependent upon the production of androgens (Figs. 13–7 and 13–8). In the prepuberal animal, as in seasonal breeders during the anestrus, all of these structures are small and relatively nonfunctional. Castration of the adult functional male likewise causes these organs to involute until they approximate the same structures of juvenile animals. Androgens completely restore all of these organs in the castrate or cause them to surpass the normal conditions. Since the degree of restoration of the accessory glands is, within limits, proportional to the amounts of androgen administered, these end organs have been employed for the bioassay of androgens. Secondary sex characters such as the capon's comb may also be used for the assay of androgens (Fig. 13–9). When testosterone is applied to the capon's comb by inunction, the amount required to produce a significant enlargement of the comb is about one-hundredth the amount required by injection.

Structural Changes

Androgens have been shown to prolong the life of epididymal spermatozoa in the castrated guinea pig, and this provides a sensitive mammalian test. If the epididymis is surgically disconnected from the testis, some of the spermatozoa stored in the epididymis, when diluted with saline solution, are capable of motility for a period of 65 to 70 days after epididymal section. In the bilaterally castrated animal, the epididymal sperms usually lose their capacity for motility within 30 days after removing the source of male sex hormone.[68]

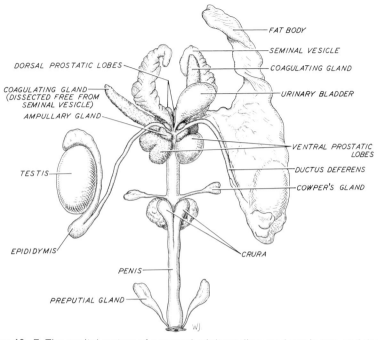

Figure 13–7. The genital system of a normal adult rat dissected out *in toto* and drawn from ventral view. The urinary bladder was pulled slightly toward the animal's left. The fat body was removed on the right side, and the coagulating gland dissected free from the seminal vesicle. The membranous covering was removed from the right lobe of the ventral prostate. The coagulating glands may be regarded as anterior prostatic lobes.

In the guinea pig, as in the rat, the male ejaculate hardens rapidly after emission from the male, and this is responsible for the copulation plug that forms within the vagina of the female. The hardening is due to the action of a prostatic enzyme upon the secretion of the seminal vesicles. An alternating current of 30 volts delivered to the head of the guinea pig elicits an ejaculation from the genital tract, feces and urine not being voided. The ejacu-

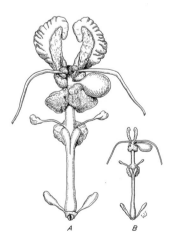

Figure 13–8. The effect of male sex hormone upon the genital tract of the castrated rat. Both littermate animals were bilaterally orchiectomized at 30 days of age and autopsied six months later. *A,* This animal received daily injections of testosterone propionate for 20 days before autopsy. *B,* This castrated littermate received no replacement therapy. It is apparent that male sex hormone builds up the accessory organs of the castrate until they approximate the normal. Both tracts were dissected *in toto* and drawn to scale from ventral view. See Figure 13–7 for identification of parts.

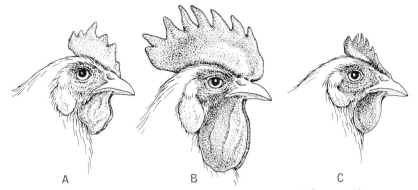

Figure 13–9. *A*, White Leghorn capon; *B*, normal cock; *C*, normal hen.

late hardens within a few minutes after leaving the male tract, and its firm, rubbery consistency permits it to be weighed with ease and accuracy. After castration, the seminal vesicles and prostate become atrophic, and a coagulable ejaculation cannot be obtained. The administration of androgens rehabilitates the accessory glands and coagulable ejaculates are obtainable within a few days.[20]

The ventral lobes of the rat's prostate shrink markedly in gross size after castration.[36] Histologically, the epithelial cells decrease in height from tall columnar in the normal animal to low cuboidal in the castrate. Within four or five days after removal of the testes, the characteristic light areas disappear from the luminal ends of these cells. The light areas occupy approximately the same position in the cells as the Golgi bodies. After castration, the Golgi bodies in these secretory cells are reduced quickly. The administration of androgen to the castrate rat restores the light areas and the Golgi bodies, and increases the height of the epithelial cells (Fig. 13–10).

After castration, the seminal vesicles diminish in size and lose their ability to secrete normally. By two or three days after castration, the epithelial cells have lost the secretory granules normally present in the distal ends of these cells. Within 20 days, they have changed from a tall columnar to a low cuboidal shape. Both macroscopic and microscopic features are brought back to normal by the administration of androgens.

Since the production of androgen by the testis depends on pituitary gonadotrophin, the sex accessories of the hypophysectomized animal are equivalent to those of the castrate (Fig. 13–11). Using hypophysectomized-orchiectomized rats, it is possible to administer adrenocorticotrophin and stimulate the adrenal cortices to produce enough androgen to partially restore the male accessory organs. Somatotrophin facilitates this response to ACTH by producing general improvement of the secretory epithelium and connective tissue stroma of the accessory glands. Ovaries or adrenals, implanted directly into the seminal vesicles of castrated rats, produce local androgenic effects on the seminal vesicle epithelium. These observations suggest that androgens, like other hormones, do not normally produce their effects in isolation but act in concert with other hormones present in the organism.

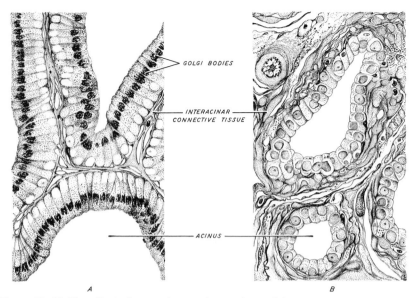

GOLGI BODIES

INTERACINAR CONNECTIVE TISSUE

ACINUS

A   B

Figure 13–10. The effect of castration on the cytology of the ventral prostatic lobes of the adult rat. *A*, Normal gland. The secretory cells lining the acini are high columnar in shape and have conspicuous Golgi bodies (blackened filaments in the supranuclear ends of the cells). *B*, The ventral prostate from a littermate who had been orchiectomized six months previously. Notice the shrinkage of the acini, diminished height of the epithelial cells, and absence of the Golgi bodies. Both tissues were prepared according to the technique of Mann-Kopsch and drawn to scale.

Most of the androgen tests described above require killing the animal and making histologic observations. Androgenic activity may be assessed more quickly and conveniently by determining changes in the secretory capacity of the male accessory glands, as reflected by changes in the chemical composition of the seminal plasma.

Chemical Changes

The seminal plasma originates almost entirely from the accessory sex glands, the prostate and seminal vesicles generally being involved to the greatest extent. There is a close interdependence between the chemical composition of the seminal plasma and the quantity of androgen present in the organism. In most mammals, fructose is the only sugar present in the semen, although glucose may be present in the semen of cocks and rabbits. The sugar is an important source of energy for the spermatozoa and its rate of breakdown (fructolysis) correlates with the number of motile sperms present in the semen. The fructose arises through the enzymatic conversion of blood glucose to fructose in the accessory organs. In pancreatic diabetes, both blood glucose and seminal fructose are increased and both can be reduced by the administration of insulin.

The semen contains several dephosphorylating enzymes that are pro-

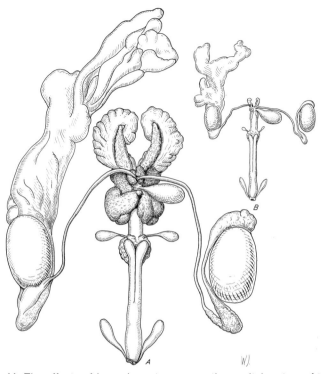

Figure 13–11. The effects of hypophysectomy upon the genital system of the male rat. *A,* Genital tract from a normal male rat 7 months of age. *B,* Genital tract from a littermate male who was hypophysectomized when 30 days old and autopsied at 7 months of age. Observe the juvenile condition of the tract from the hypophysectomized littermate. Both tracts were dissected *in toto* and drawn to scale from ventral view. See Figure 13–7 for identification of parts.

duced by the accessory glands. Human semen and prostatic tissue contain much acid phosphatase and small amounts of alkaline phosphatase. In bull semen, the proportions are reversed. The level of the enzyme in the human prostate is low in children but increases markedly at puberty. Like fructose, the level of these enzymes in the seminal plasma depends on the androgen titers of the blood.

Citric acid occurs in the semen of many species. In the bull, stallion, boar, and ram, most of the fructose and citric acid are produced by the seminal vesicles. In the rat, citric acid is formed by the ventral prostate and seminal vesicle, but most of the fructose arises in the dorsal prostate and coagulating glands.[47, 65]

The functional state of the male accessory sex organs may be accurately evaluated by determining the fructose, citric acid, and phosphatase activity of the seminal plasma. These chemical methods for assessing androgen production are especially useful in following progressive changes that may result from age, nutritional states, etc. By these methods, androgen production may be determined in the living animal, at desired intervals, and over extended periods. There are, however, many factors other than male sex hormone that can influence the presence of these materials in the semen. Frequency of ejaculation, sexual excitation, storage capacity of the glands, nutritional state, the level of blood glucose, and other factors, may cause marked variations.

The Protein Anabolic Action of Androgens

The most profound general metabolic action of androgens is the promotion of protein anabolism. Testosterone or similar androgens decrease the urinary loss of nitrogen without increasing the nonprotein nitrogen of the blood, and produce at least a temporary increase in body weight. This suggests that the hormone causes a true storage of nitrogen in the form of tissue protein. In the dog, androgens have been reported to increase the synthesis of proteins and decrease the rate of catabolism of amino acids. Testosterone or methyltestosterone, administered to orchiectomized men whose diet and exercise are controlled, produces nitrogen retention and progressive gains in weight. The protein anabolic response to androgens may be materially altered by the state of the protein stores at the time the treatments are begun. When the androgen treatment is withdrawn, the level of urinary nitrogen increases and, for a limited time, surpasses that of the untreated castrate. Androgens produce nitrogen retention less effectively in normal males than in hypogonadal or castrated subjects. Since androgens increase the protein matrix of bone, they have been used in the clinical treatment of certain skeletal defects.

The male accessories of starved and fed animals respond to equivalent extents when androgens are given, and it therefore appears that these sexual structures accumulate protein in advance of other tissues, such as skeletal muscles. In general, however, the quantity of nitrogen retained is too great to be accounted for by an effect on the sex accessories alone; body muscles, bones, kidneys, and other tissues are generally increased, owing to protein accumulation. Experiments have clearly shown that androgens can induce protein anabolic effects in animals deprived of their gonads, pituitary, pancreas, or adrenals.

Testosterone has no significant effect on the body length of the hypophysectomized rat unless somatotrophin is given jointly with it. Although androgens increase the body weights of young hypophysectomized rats, most of this gain is accounted for by the increased mass of the genital complex, apparently consequent upon protein retention.

Castration has a variable effect on the skeletal muscles: Some cease growing immediately, others continue to grow at a reduced rate, and certain ones show no significant effect. Androgens also selectively stimulate certain muscles (myotrophic effect) more than others. The masticating muscles of the guinea pig undergo the greatest atrophy after castration, and these are the ones that increase most after androgen injections. In several species of frogs and toads, the muscles of the forelimb, associated with the clasping reflex of the male, show seasonal fluctuations. These muscles atrophy after castration, and can be returned to a breeding condition by testicular grafts or the injection of testosterone.[58] The levator ani muscles of the rat respond similarly. It is significant, however, that such hormones cannot stimulate any of the castration-atrophied muscles to exceed normal proportions by increasing the dosage or prolonging the treatment. It is interesting to note that testosterone and methyltestosterone, both equally potent in stimulating the male accessory organs, promote the growth of different muscles in the guinea pig.

The changes in body weight produced by testosterone vary with the species and also depend on the nutritional status of the animals. Growth is markedly inhibited in young chicks by large doses of this hormone, whereas it produces little effect on the male guinea pig. In normal and castrated young rats, low doses of androgen produce increases in body weight, but continued treatment, especially with higher doses, prevents body weight gains. The initial stimulation is very brief in the intact rat, but is more marked and prolonged in castrated animals. The loss of body weight in the rat, after excessive androgen, may result from reduced food intake and an accelerated utilization of body fat. These metabolic adjustments probably represent fat-catabolic, as well as protein-anabolic, effects of the androgen.

Although androgens can suppress testicular functions through the pituitary, a direct supportive effect on the seminiferous tubules has been demonstrated. The androgens differ in their capacity to maintain spermatogenesis in hypophysectomized animals. They can maintain the testicular tubules of hypophysectomized rats fed protein-free diets, but the hormones are less effective in this respect if the animals are given no protein prior to hypophysectomy. When rats are deprived of dietary protein for one month, the seminal vesicles shrink in size and the gonadotrophin content of the pituitary is reduced, but it requires prolonged protein deprivation to reduce the protein stores of the testis. The role of androgen in the spermatogenic function of the testis remains obscure, but it may correlate in some manner with the protein-anabolic action of these steroids.

After the administration of androgen, the volume of urine diminishes and the loss of sodium, chloride, potassium, and inorganic phosphorus, as well as nitrogen, is reduced. There is no conspicuous increase in any of these materials in the blood plasma. The retention of nitrogen, potassium, and phosphorus is probably related to the increased anabolism of tissue protein. The protein concentration of the plasma generally remains normal. The capacity of the androgens to promote retention of sodium and chloride resembles that of the adrenal cortical steroids; however, androgens are much weaker in this respect than the adrenal steroids and are unable to maintain the lives of adrenalectomized animals.

THE REGULATION OF TESTICULAR FUNCTIONS

Pituitary Gonadotrophins

The production of spermatozoa is known to be under the influence of pituitary hormones and of androgens derived from the testis itself. Within a few days after hypophysectomy, the epithelial lining of the seminiferous tubules becomes disorganized and spermatozoa are not produced thereafter (Figs. 13–12 and 13–13). The testes decrease in size, become soft, and regress into the abdominal cavity in certain species. The testicular alterations are not attributable to the movement of the gonad out of the scrotum since the experimental retention of the testis in the scrotum does not prevent the impairments. Furthermore, the testes do not become intra-abdominal until several weeks after the removal of the hypophysis. The accessory sex organs become quite atrophic following removal of the pituitary, and this indicates that the cells of Leydig secrete little, if any, androgen.

Testicular tissue from neonatal rats has been maintained *in vitro* for long periods. The seminiferous tubules retain their configurations and Sertoli

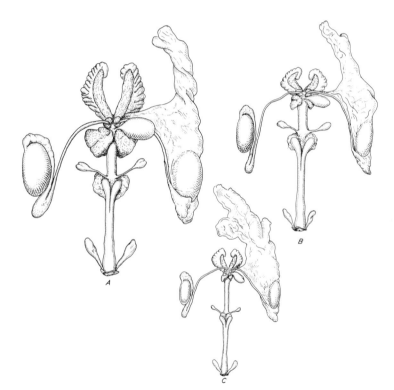

Figure 13–12. The hypophyseal regulation of the endocrine function of the testis. *A,* Genital system of a normal adult rat. *B,* Genital tract of a littermate male who had been hypophysectomized 30 days previously. In the absence of the hypophyseal gonadotrophins the testes shrink and do not secrete sufficient male sex hormone to maintain the sex accessories. Compare the sizes of the testes and accessory glands in this animal with corresponding organs of the normal littermate *(A).* *C,* Genital complex of a third littermate, who had received heavy doses of estrogen at frequent intervals for 6 months. Note the pronounced atrophy of the testes and sex accessories. Large amounts of estrogens or androgens, injected for long periods, apparently injure the adenohypophysis to such an extent that it becomes unable to release sufficient gonadotrophin to maintain the gonads. The result of such treatment is an impaired genital system which simulates that present in an animal that has been deprived of its hypophysis for an extended period. The three tracts were dissected *in toto* and drawn to scale from ventral view. See Figure 13–7 for identification of the genital organs.

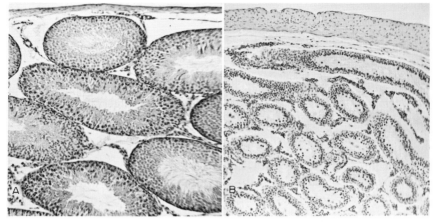

Figure 13–13. The effects of hypophysectomy upon the testis of the rat. *A,* Testis of a normal adult rat. *B,* Testis of a rat hypophysectomized at 4 months of age and sacrificed 6 months later. Observe atrophy of the seminiferous tubules and thickening of the tunica albuginea (tunica albuginea is at the top of each figure). The testes shrink markedly in size after removal of the pituitary gland, and this is reflected in the thickening of the tunica and the decreasing in size of the seminiferous tubules. Both figures are of the same magnification.

cells persist, but the primordial germ cells do not go far in their differentiation toward spermatozoa. The interstitial cells of Leydig do not differentiate under these circumstances. The addition of follicle-stimulating hormone (FSH) or human chorionic gonadotrophin (HCG) to the culture medium does not stimulate the primordial germ cells to undergo maturational changes; these hormones do cause the nongerminal elements of the tubules to assume the morphologic characteristics of mature Sertoli cells. Early germ cells in these cultures can advance to the stage of primary spermatocytes, in the absence of gonadotrophins, if vitamins A, E, and C are added.[80]

Some residual spermatogenesis occurs in the tubules of hypophysectomized rats, all adenohypophysial hormones being absent. A few spermatogonia divide to give rise to primary and secondary spermatocytes, and the latter form a few spermatids. The spermatids never give rise to spermatozoa in the untreated hypophysectomized animal. The prompt injection of appropriate gonadotrophins or of androgens into hypophysectomized subjects prevents degeneration of the germ cells. These hormones have some capacity to restore the seminiferous epithelium and the interstitial tissue, if hypophysectomy has not prevailed too long. After prolonged posthypophysectomy regression of the testis, some of the tubules apparently lose their ability to respond to these hormones. Restoration of the Leydig cells is generally possible if the replacement therapy is continued for sufficient periods. Though testosterone alone can restore spermatogenesis to a limited extent in adult rats at 70 days after hypophysectomy, the androgen is much more effective if pituitary growth hormone (STH) is given in conjunction with it.

The hypophysis of the male liberates the same gonadotrophins as those of the female, *i.e.,* follicle-stimulating hormone (FSH), luteinizing hormone (LH or ICSH), and prolactin. In some domestic mammals, coitus may increase the release of LH and result in an elevated level of circulating testosterone. Current research indicates that FSH, LH, and androgens are all involved in the normal development and function of the testis. The action of LH is to stimulate the cells of Leydig to produce androgen, and the latter hormone acts directly upon the germinal epithelium. Although purified LH alone is effective in maintaining spermatogenesis for relatively short periods in hypophysectomized rats and mice, if given immediately after the operation, definitive experiments show that both LH and FSH are required for sperm production over long periods.[44, 51, 52, 85]

Leydig cell stimulation has been produced in the immature hypophysectomized rat by injecting ovine or human LH (ICSH) directly into the testis. With low doses (0.025 μg), the effect was localized; that is, it did not spread to the contralateral testis. The intratesticular injection of FSH in adult hypophysectomized rats does not stimulate or maintain either the Leydig cells or the germinal cells, but it does induce secretory hypertrophy of the Sertoli cells.[59, 78]

Control of the Spermatogenic Cycle

Recent studies indicate that it is necessary to distinguish two aspects of the spermatogenic process, namely, the *rate* at which it progresses and the *yield* in terms of the number of spermatozoa produced per spermatogonial stem cell. Studies employing the technique of autoradiography indicate that the time required for the spermatogonia to differentiate into spermatozoa is a biologic constant, varying with the species and strain, but which is not altered by hormones and other factors. On the other hand, observations on many species of vertebrates leave no doubt that the number of spermatozoa produced is dependent upon pituitary gonadotrophins, androgens, nutritional factors, temperatures, light, etc.

It is well known that spermatogenesis in rams is influenced by photoperiods and temperatures. Short periods of daily illumination increase the output of pituitary gonadotrophin and increase the number of spermatozoa produced by the testis; long daily photoperiods have the reverse effect. Ortavant labeled the germ cells with P[32] and found that the time required for the completion of spermatogenesis was the same in animals exposed to long days and those exposed to short days. He concluded that gonadotrophins have no effect on the rate of spermatogenesis, but increase the yield of spermatozoa from the seminiferous epithelium.[64]

Studies on the rat have shown that the duration of the cycle of the seminiferous epithelium is the same in normal animals, hypophysectomized animals, hypophysectomized animals receiving testosterone, and hypophysectomized animals receiving chorionic gonadotrophin. Furthermore, the rates of spermatogenesis in human subjects receiving norethandrolone (known to depress sperm formation) and in those receiving chorionic gonadotrophin (known to promote sperm formation) were found to be identical with that of normal men. These observations indicate that differentiating germ cells die and are removed if their tissue environment becomes unfa-

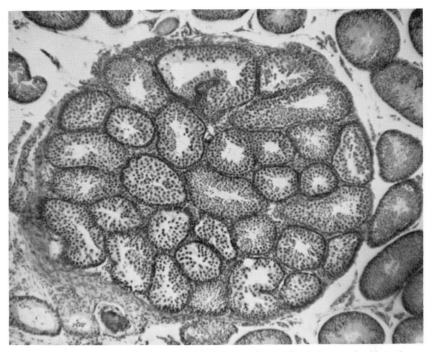

Figure 13–14. The testis of a 11-day-old mouse embryo after being grafted into the scrotal testis of an adult host for 30 days. The tubules of the graft are approximately the same size as those of the host testis. Interstitial tissue is well developed and most of the tubules contain many spermatids. Mature spermatozoa appear in such grafts after about 35 days. (Courtesy of H. Asakawa, Duquesne University.)

vorable; in other words, they cannot stop their differentiation at any stage of the cycle and resume from that point when the milieu becomes favorable. Maximal sperm counts mean that a high percentage of the derivatives of the spermatogonial stem cells have had environments favorable to their progressive differentiation. The stem cells may persist for long periods in the tubules, without differentiating.[37]

Experiments on the intratesticular transplantation of embryonic testes of the mouse have shown that the early germ cells are capable of beginning the spermatogenic process about seven days earlier than they normally do (Fig. 13–14). In normal mice of this strain, advanced spermatids (stage 16 of Oakberg[63]) appear in the normal scrotal testes 35 days after birth. If testes are removed from embryos on the eleventh day of gestation (seven days before parturition) and transplanted into the scrotal testis of a normal host, late spermatids appear in the grafts 33 to 35 days later. The time required for the completion of spermatogenesis apparently is not shortened but, under the favorable adult environment, the primordial germ cells are stimulated to begin the process earlier than they would in the normally developing individual.[5]

Cryptorchism, Scrotum and Pampiniform Plexus

In the human species, the testes normally descend into the scrotum shortly before birth and remain permanently in that position. Scrotal sacs are absent in all vertebrates below mammals, the testes remaining abdominal throughout life. Though most mammals have scrota, the rhinoceros, seal, elephant, and whale are notable exceptions. In most rodents, the inguinal canals remain open, and the testes occupy the scrota only during the breeding season. Although typical scrotal sacs are not present in the Insectivora and the Chiroptera, the testes distend the caudal abdominal wall during the breeding season and assume positions close to the exterior of the body.

In man and domesticated mammals it is not uncommon for the testes to be retained in the abdominal cavity rather than to descend normally into the scrotum. This condition is called cryptorchism (Greek *kryptos,* hidden; *orchis,* testis); when it occurs bilaterally, complete sterility results. Cryptorchism in the human being may result from obstruction of the inguinal canals and possibly from certain hypophysial dysfunctions. Laboratory rodents in whom the inguinal canals remain open have been used extensively as subjects for experimental testing of the effects of confining one or both testes to the abdominal cavity. It is a simple surgical procedure to open the abdomen of the rat or guinea pig, lift the testes from the scrotum into the abdominal cavity, section the gubernaculum, and ligate the inguinal canals in such a manner that the gonad cannot push back into the scrotum.

After the testis of the adult rat has been surgically confined to the abdominal cavity, a rapid decrease in size and turgidity of the organ ensues (Fig. 13–15). Histologically, severe disorganization of the seminiferous tubules becomes apparent within a week after the operation. The germinal epithelium deteriorates quickly, and the seminiferous tubules shrink in diameter. After one or two months, practically all germinal elements of the tubule have been lost, and little remains except a single layer of Sertoli-like cells next to the basement membrane of the tubule. The most highly differentiated cells disappear first, the order being spermatozoa, spermatids, spermatocytes, and lastly spermatogonia. If all the spermatogonia have not degenerated, replacement of the cryptorchid testis into the scrotum permits the germinal epithelium to recover and again proliferate spermatozoa. Similar results are obtained in the guinea pig and other mammals in which the testes normally occupy scrotal sacs.

The capacity of the cryptorchid testis to renew spermatogenesis after being returned to a scrotal position is directly related to the number of tubules still possessing spermatogonia. In the rat, irreparable damage to all tubules occurs within seven months; hence such testes cannot again proliferate sperms even though they are replaced in the scrotum. It appears that in the rat irreparable damage occurs more slowly than in other mammalian species that have been studied. Investigators do not agree as to how long the human testis can remain in ectopic positions without irreparable damage to the seminiferous epithelium.

An extensive sequence of experiments demonstrates that cryptorchism

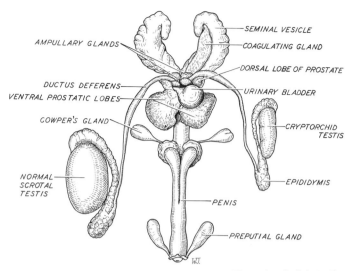

Figure 13–15. Unilateral cryptorchism in the adult rat. The animal's left testis was confined within the abdominal cavity for 6 months, whereas the right testis was permitted to occupy its normal scrotal position. Note the shrunken condition of the cryptorchid testis as compared with the scrotal testis. Spermatozoa were absent from the left epididymis, but were abundantly present in the right epididymis. The accessory sex organs are normal. The tract was dissected *in toto* and drawn from ventral view.

impairs testicular functions because the temperature of the abdomen is higher than that of the scrotum. Simultaneous measurements indicate the temperature of the abdomen is approximately 4° C. higher than that of the scrotum. Insulation of the scrotum of the ram by encasing the organ with nonconductive materials elevates the temperature of the scrotum and produces testicular damage that is in all respects similar to that prevailing during cryptorchism. The same effect is produced by the artificial application of warmth to the exterior of the normal scrotum. A convincing experiment has been performed with the dog. Both testes were confined to the abdomen. Immediately after the operation one abdominal testis was artificially cooled by circulating water of a known temperature through a system of coils. The uncooled testis showed typical heat effects, whereas the other did not. Febrile conditions in man and other mammals contribute to testicular impairment, one of the factors involved being the high temperatures to which the testes are subjected. Testicular homotransplants persisting in the anterior chamber of the eye and in the scrotum are capable of proliferating spermatozoa since the temperatures of these two sites are relatively lower than that of most other parts of the mammalian body. These considerations convincingly demonstrate that the scrotum is a thermoregulator for the testis and is indispensable for sperm proliferation in the majority of mammals.

The effect of high body temperature on the cells of Leydig and their ability to secrete androgens has not been clarified to the satisfaction of most workers. Studies on the rat indicate that artificial cryptorchism results in a temporary increase in androgen production, as evidenced by changes in the accessory reproductive organs; this is followed by a fall in androgen secretion which continues at a fairly constant level. It has been shown that temperature is an important factor in determining the rate of incorporation of acetate-1-C^{14} into testosterone-C^{14} by slices of rabbit testis *in vitro.* Both androgen biosynthesis and lysine incorporation were significantly lower at 40° C. than at 38° C., temperatures which are comparable to those of the abdomen and scrotum, respectively, of the rabbit. There are numerous reports in recent literature indicating that nonscrotal temperatures impair certain enzyme systems of the mammalian testis. It is beginning to appear that the interstitial cells of Leydig share with the germinal epithelium a dependence upon lower temperatures for maximal activity.[11, 25, 41]

The pampiniform plexus is a second mechanism which operates in mammals to keep the temperatures of the testis lower than those of the body cavity. This is a plexus of veins from the testis and epididymis, forming part of the spermatic cord. The plexus is supplied by the spermatic artery, and the venous blood empties into the spermatic vein. The plexus functions to cool the blood from the body before it enters the testis and also to warm the blood from the testis before it is returned to the systemic circulation. The cellular and biochemical mechanisms employed in temperature regulation by the pampiniform plexus are obscure, and little is known about its importance in mammals other than the ram and rat.

Minute amounts of cadmium, administered to the male rat, produce testicular impairments which are exactly the same as those resulting from cryptorchism. The initial effect of cadmium is upon the cells that line the blood vessels of the pampiniform plexus; other blood vessels seem not to be vulnerable to its actions. Since the damaged plexus cannot cool the blood before it enters the testis, the seminiferous tubules promptly become permanently aspermic and the cells of Leydig are probably impaired. Male rats may be protected from cadmium by pretreating them with zinc, or by giving the zinc simultaneously with the cadmium. The latter metal is without effect in female rats since they do not develop a pampiniform plexus.

Vasectomy and Testicular Function

It has long been known that ligation of the pancreatic duct causes the acinar portion of the organ to degenerate more rapidly than the islets of Langerhans. Without adequate experimental evidence, many workers have assumed that ligation or section of the excurrent ducts of the testis would destroy the germinal epithelium and halt the proliferation of spermatozoa.

The experimental evidence indicates that vasectomy does not destroy completely the gametogenic function of the testis, and there are no quantitative studies indicating that the operation results in any actual hypertrophy of the cells of Leydig. The testis of the dog may proliferate mature spermatozoa for as long as five years after the closure of the excurrent passages. Vasoligation in laboratory rodents, *e.g.,* rats, rabbits, and guinea pigs, does not preclude the proliferation of mature germ cells. Since the sperms cannot be passed to the exterior, they degenerate and are resorbed. Histologic examination of testes subjected to vasoligation for long periods has shown that some of the seminiferous tubules contain cells in all stages of spermatogenesis. A certain percentage of the seminiferous tubules degenerate, and it is probable that the tubules alternately degenerate and repair.

It has been reported that vasectomy of the bull results in the loss of certain amino acids from the semen, and that they may be restored by the administration of testosterone; they disappear from the semen again after the androgen injections are discontinued. Extremely high levels of fructose and citric acid are said to appear in the ejaculates of bulls and rams after vasoligation. The semen of the vasectomized animal would be more concentrated than normal, owing to the absence of spermatozoa and fluids from the testis and epididymis, but the reduced volume of the semen after vasoligation is said to be too small to account for the higher levels of fructose in it. Prolonged studies on vasectomized bulls have shown that seminal fructose reaches a high level about one year after vasoligation and, concomitant with the rise in fructose, libido and aggressiveness are increased. The administration of exogenous androgen to the bull does not produce these striking changes in fructose levels and sex drive. Variations in libido occur in human subjects after vasectomy, but since so many psychic factors are involved, it is difficult to evaluate the reported changes.[60]

We must conclude that vasectomy is an effective method of sterilizing the male and that it does not completely prevent spermatogenesis, but its effect, if any, on the endocrine functions of the testis remains obscure.

Castration

Prepuberal castration of the human male prevents the functional differentiation of the accessory sex ducts and glands and also the appearance of certain secondary sexual characters. The larynx remains small and the voice high-pitched. Hair fails to appear on the face and body, but its abundance on the scalp is not modified. The penis remains infantile, and sexual libido is usually suppressed. Frequently, but not invariably, castration of the prepuberal human male seems to retard the closure of the epiphyses. This may result in an enlargement of the stature, especially a disproportioned lengthening of the paired appendages. As to a tendency toward obesity, there seems to be extreme individual variation among eunuchoid human beings; some become obese, whereas others remain lean. Contrary to popular belief, mental attitudes, initiative, and industry are variable among human castrates.

Castration of human males after the attainment of sexual maturity produces regression of all accessory sex organs of reproduction. The urinary excretion of 17-ketosteroids is generally reduced to about one-half the normal value, although it may remain within normal limits. Mental processes are not modified so extensively as in the prepuberal castrate. Clinical literature indicates that orchiectomized males may retain sexual libido for long periods. Male rats castrated during adulthood may copulate with estrous females for eight months or longer after the withdrawal of male sex hormone.

Nutrition and Testicular Functions

It is a well-established fact that malnutrition has an adverse effect on the reproductive organs of both sexes.[46] Inanition, vitamin deficiencies, caloric restriction, or insufficient quantities of specific food substances such as proteins are capable of impairing testicular functions. Hypofunctioning of the Leydig cells is indicated by atrophy of the accessory sex organs, which is followed by disorganization of the seminiferous epithelium and the cessation of spermatogenesis. Inadequate diets may impair the endocrine function of the testis without producing any appreciable defects in the seminiferous tubules. Vitamin B deficiency in the rat causes the male accessory organs to involute until they resemble those of castrated or hypophysectomized animals. This accessory gland atrophy can be repaired by the administration of either androgen or pituitary gonadotrophins. Since the gonads respond to exogenous gonadotrophins and the sex accessories respond to androgen, it becomes apparent that the primary defect is in the release of pituitary gonadotrophins. Various types of underfeeding produce the same general syndrome in man and experimental animals as vitamin B deficiency. For example, if dietary proteins are inadequate to maintain a normal nitrogen balance, the male accessories atrophy as in vitamin deficiency, and their repair is effected by small doses of gonadotrophins. This syndrome resulting from undernutrition is related to diminished pituitary gonadotrophins in the circulation and is often called pseudohypophysectomy.

In chronically undernourished rats, the levels of fructose in the coagulating glands and of citric acid in the seminal vesicles fall until they are quite comparable to those prevailing in total castrates. Both constituents of the accessory gland secretions may be raised to normal levels by exogenous androgen or gonadotrophins. It seems reasonably certain that the primary lesion is in the hypophysial mechanism that is needed for the normal functioning of the testis. In some species, such as the bull, the testicular effects of underfeeding develop more slowly than in the rat; recovery is also slower.

Gonadal functions may be impaired by diets deficient in proteins or specific amino acids. Chronic starvation or protein-free diets prevent testicular maturation in young rats. Diets lacking only protein are less effective than starvation in abolishing spermatogenesis in the adult rat. Diets containing 6 per cent casein are not adequate for body growth in the young rat, but such diets do permit some degree of spermatogenesis. This suggests that the reproductive system may be given some priority when dietary intake of proteins is limited. Many types of experiments indicate that adequate nutrition is especially important in the young animal for proper gonadal maturation, and it is not improbable that some types of adult infertility are consequences of malnutrition during fetal or prepuberal periods.[46]

THE BIOLOGY OF SPERMATOZOA

The spermatozoa of different species show extraordinary diversity of shape and structure (Fig. 13–16). Many of the finer structural details of

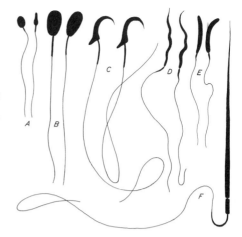

Figure 13–16. Spermatozoa from different species of vertebrates. *A*, Human; *B*, sheep; *C*, rat; *D*, chicken; *E*, frog; *F*, salamander (*Ambystoma*). All are drawn to scale from stained smears.

these cells have been revealed by electron microscopic studies. The axial filament extends the entire length of the midpiece and tail. It consists of a number of fine fibers that are probably the contractile elements of the cell, responsible for the whiplike undulations of the tail. The axial filament of the mammalian sperm cell is surrounded by an axial sheath; the enzymes responsible for sperm motility are probably located in the midpiece region of this sheath. The cytoplasmic sheath contains lipoprotein and forms a protective capsule surrounding the midpiece and tail. The sperm nucleus is present in the head and a caplike structure, called the *acrosome,* fits over the anterior part of the head. The spermatozoa are mature haploid cells and do not undergo mitotic divisions, though various types of morphologically abnormal spermatozoa may be observed.

Cytochemical tests indicate the presence of abundant glycogen in the Sertoli cells and spermatogonia, progressively less in the primary and secondary spermatocytes and spermatids, and practically none in the mature spermatozoa. In mammals at least, the ripening of the spermatozoa continues during their storage in the epididymis. The spermatozoa in the epididymis are immotile but are capable of long survival. The development of motility coincides with their movement along the male tract at ejaculation and with their mixing with the seminal plasma.

Though the spermatozoa possess meager intracellular reserves of nutrients, they can metabolize a wide range of extracellular substrates which are present in seminal plasma and in the secretions of the female reproductive tract. The semen, consisting of spermatozoa and seminal plasma, is somewhat similar to a suspension of motile microorganisms existing in a nutrient medium. Much progress has been made in the biochemical elucidation of sperm cell metabolism.[67, 93]

The Biochemistry of Semen[54]

Although some fluid accompanies the spermatozoa as they move through the testis and epididymis, most of the seminal plasma is derived from the seminal vesicles, prostate, and Cowper's glands. In the epididymis, the sperms are immotile at a pH of around 7. The seminal plasma is approximately isotonic and generally has a pH of 7 or slightly above. The quiescence of the epididymal sperms seems to correlate better with the lack of carbohydrate, low oxygen tension, and crowding than it does with hydrogen ion concentration. The spermatozoa of most species tolerate alkalinity better than acidity; increasing the pH to 8 or higher may enhance motility, but excessive acidity renders the spermatozoa immotile. Most workers agree that pH 7, or slightly higher, is optimum for motility and survival of the sperm cells of most species.

As already mentioned, the accessory gland products contain fructose and citric acid. Fructose occurs in the semen of virtually all mammals, but its concentration varies with the volume of semen ejaculated. Cock semen contains no fructose; that of the rabbit contains both glucose and fructose.

Although there are many species variations, calcium, sodium, magnesium, potassium, phosphate, and chloride ions are present in the seminal plasma. Human seminal fluid contains about 14 mg per 100 ml of zinc, a higher concentration than is found in any other human tissue. The calcium content of human semen is several times higher than that of the blood. Heavy metals and calcium have been found to reduce the viability of mammalian spermatozoa. Spermatozoa of the ram and bull rapidly become immotile in the absence of potassium. It may be that one function of citric acid in the seminal fluid is to combine with calcium and thus prevent the precipitation of insoluble calcium salts.

Polypeptides and proteins of low molecular weight are present in mammalian semen. The proteins present in human seminal plasma are atypical inasmuch as they are not coagulated by heat and pass through cellulose membranes. Free amino acids are also present; some of these probably arise through the breakdown of proteins after the semen is ejaculated. Bull semen contains five free amino acids: glutamic acid, alanine, glycine, serine, and aspartic acid. These disappear after castration and, with the exception of glutamic acid, are restored in part by exogenous androgens. Since glutamic acid comes mainly from the testis and epididymis, it is absent in castrated and vasectomized bulls. There are suggestions that the seminal amino acids may protect the spermatozoa by combining with heavy metals, which may become toxic or, in the case of proteins, by preventing agglutination and the loss of intracellular material as the spermatozoa are diluted. The mammalian prostate releases an antiagglutinic factor, containing sugar, sulfuric acid residues, and a vitamin E derivative, and this acts to prevent the clumping of sperm heads.

Most mammalian semens contain ascorbic acid and traces of B vitamins. The seminal vesicles of the boar produce high concentrations of inositol, and smaller amounts are found in other species. There is no evidence that inositol is utilized by mammalian semen.

Human semen coagulates at first but later liquefies again, the liquefaction being brought about by one of the proteolytic enzymes contained in the prostatic secretion. This secretion is rich in acid phosphatase, its natural substrate (phosphorylcholine) being contributed by the seminal vesicles.

Seminal fluids of the bull and ram, on the other hand, contain little acid phosphatase but high amounts of the alkaline enzyme.

Hyaluronidase is another enzyme present in semen, but its functional role is far from clear. This enzyme is actually contained within the sperm cell, but it is very quickly released into the seminal plasma; thus it is not a product of the accessory glands. Because of its ability to depolymerize hyaluronic acid, it was thought that it might perform a role in facilitating penetration of the ovum by the sperm. This hypothesis has not received much experimental support.

Prostaglandins are a group of chemically related 20-carbon hydroxy fatty acids, and these seem to occur rather ubiquitously in mammalian tissues (see Chapter 16). Thirteen varieties have been isolated from human seminal plasma. They have potent oxytocic effects and have been used to induce labor in women at or near term. There seems to be a correlation between total prostaglandin concentration of human semen and the degree of fertility. Though the prostaglandins produce a broad spectrum of pharmacologic actions, their physiologic significance remains unknown.[9, 69]

Human semen contains high concentrations of choline and spermine, the latter apparently occurring only in the human species. Both of these substances can be easily detected chemically, and they form the basis of various tests employed in medicolegal investigations.

Sperm Metabolism

Mammalian spermatozoa are capable of metabolizing a wide range of materials, such as various sugars, organic acids, and alcohols, found in the seminal plasma, in the fluids of the female tract, or in the artificial media in which they are stored. Under anaerobic conditions, the spermatozoa rely upon the metabolism of carbohydrate as the chief source of energy. When sperms are incubated anaerobically, the fructose concentration of the seminal plasma decreases and lactic acid accumulates. Additional energy is obtained under aerobic conditions by the oxidation of lactic acid to carbon dioxide and water.

The first phase of fructolysis involves the enzymatic conversion of phosphotriose to phosphoglyceric acid, and the simultaneous reduction of nicotinamide adenine dinucleotide (NAD) to NADH. The oxidation of phosphotriose is coupled with the esterification of inorganic phosphate and the synthesis of ATP. The conversion of phosphoglyceric acid to phosphopyruvic acid results in the production of pyruvic acid and ATP. In the second oxidoreduction, NADH is oxidized to NAD and pyruvic acid is reduced to lactic acid (Fig. 13–17).

The cardinal link between carbohydrate metabolism and sperm motility is ATP. The breakdown of ATP apparently provides the energy for the contraction of the sperm fibrils, the replenishment of ATP being dependent on the normal metabolism of fructose. The ATP content of spermatozoa correlates closely with their motility. For example, if spermatozoa are maintained under anaerobic conditions and without a glycolyzable sugar, motility be-

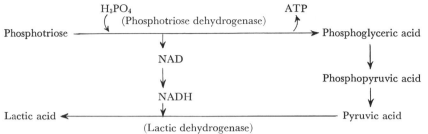

Figure 13–17. Fructolysis in semen. Adapted from Mann, T.: The Biochemistry of Semen and of the Male Reproductive Tract. New York, John Wiley & Sons, 1964.

comes very low. Motility is restored by adding fructose or some other glycolyzable sugar. The highest motility results when oxygen and fructose are present together.

It is not clear why mammalian spermatozoa normally utilize fructose anaerobically, whereas other tissues employ glucose instead of fructose. This special sugar for the sperm cells is localized in the accessory glands and is dependent upon androgen control. It is an arrangement that enables the spermatozoa to derive their energy from fructose without competing with other tissues for glucose, which is so widely distributed within the organism.

Sperm Capacitation and Decapacitation

Mammalian spermatozoa leaving the testis for the epididymis are immotile and incapable of fertilization. A process of maturation or "ripening" normally occurs in the epididymis but, in several mammalian species, the sperm do not achieve the ability to fertilize ova until they have undergone further change within the female tract. This process is called *capacitation* and takes place in the uterus and oviducts. According to current views, the sperm are released in the female tract (capacitated) from a *decapacitation factor* (DF) that is present in seminal plasma. Capacitated sperm taken from the female tract may again be rendered incapable of fertilizing eggs by treating them with DF from seminal fluid. This DF has been partially purified; it binds to the sperm and is not removed by simple washing of the cells.

During fertilization of rabbit and human ova, the sperm must penetrate the corona radiata, the zona pellucida, and finally the vitelline membrane. Hyaluronidase, an enzyme occurring in association with sperm acrosomes, was formerly thought to facilitate sperm entry by dispersing the cells of the cumulus and corona, but this has not been confirmed. A corona-penetrating enzyme (CPE) has recently been obtained from acrosomal extracts of ejaculated rabbit and human sperm. The CPE enables sperm to penetrate the corona cells surrounding rabbit ova; electron microscopy reveals that the sperm pass through the intercellular material rather than penetrate the corona cells themselves. Seminal plasma and partially purified decapacitation factor inhibit CPE activity, but uterine fluids do not.[1, 2, 7, 88]

The In Vitro Storage of Spermatozoa

Artificial insemination is widely practiced in the breeding of domestic animals. This procedure involves the collection of viable spermatozoa, the retention of these cells *in vitro,* and the proper introduction of them into the female tract. The optimal temperature for the storage of most sperms is approximately 12° C.; body temperature is most favorable for maximal motility. Human spermatozoa are unique inasmuch as they survive freezing to very low temperatures moderately well.[39] Human spermatozoa have survived and shown motility after freezing in liquid nitrogen at −195° C.; some have survived after existing in a frozen state for 70 days. Diluents containing glycerol or other polyalcohols offer some protection for bull, goat, horse, and rabbit sperms against the harmful effects of freezing, but the rate of thawing must be slow.

Sperm survive best when they are stored in an isotonic medium of about neutral pH that contains fructose or glucose as a source of energy. Under anaerobic conditions, fructolysis produces large quantities of lactic acid, so it is necessary that the diluent contain a satisfactory buffer. In the presence of oxygen some of the lactic acid can be oxidized and buffer is not so much needed. The phosphate content of the diluent has a marked effect on the amount of lactic acid that can be oxidized. Calcium and high levels of phosphate are harmful to sperm motility. Potassium, on the other hand, promotes motility and glycolysis of washed ram and bull sperms. The egg yolk–citrate medium has been found moderately satisfactory for artificial insemination procedures, although more complex physiologic diluents might give better results.

Experience indicates that mammalian spermatozoa survive best if they are stored at as high a concentration as possible; in other words, dilution has a harmful effect on the germ cells. Small numbers of sperm do not survive well, even when stored in large quantities of an isotonic diluent containing glycolyzable sugars. The depression occurring during storage at low cell concentration seems to be due largely to the loss of substances from the sperms, though little is known about the nature of these substances. It is known, however, that materials of high molecular weight, such as proteins and starch, protect against the dilution effect. Egg yolk is commonly used for this purpose, and the active constituent is probably a lipoprotein.

It is desirable to store semen at a low temperature in order to retard bacterial growth, but if it is cooled to temperatures below 10° C., the temperatures must be reduced slowly in order to avoid cold shock. This causes a rapid reduction of ATP and the loss of intracellular proteins into the medium. Egg yolk and other materials provide some protection against cold shock. It is a common practice to add antibiotics to the diluent because of the harmful effect of bacteria on the sperms and the possibility of spreading genital infections.

There is presently much interest revolving around the inhibition of conception through the use of antibodies.[29] Isoimmunization of female mammals with sperm can produce sterility, and the use of antibody-treated semen in artificial insemination generally results in a failure of conception.

Rabbits do not conceive when inseminated with nonagglutinating, univalent, antibody-treated semen. The motility of such sperm is not visibly affected, but it is thought that the univalent antibody blocks some sperm antigen that has an important role in penetration of the cervical mucus. The treated sperm, installed in the vagina, fail to pass into the uterus and oviducts in normal numbers.[56]

ENVIRONMENT AND SEXUAL PERIODICITY

A wealth of information indicates that various external environmental agencies intervene to adjust reproductive activities to particular seasons of the year. The precise factors that operate appear to vary with the species, and in perhaps all species a multitude of coordinated physical and social factors are involved. It is widely held that the environment acts through the intermediation of the hypothalamus and the anterior pituitary gland, the latter serving as a liaison organ between the nervous system and the target glands, which are regulated by its trophic hormones. The main gap in our knowledge is how the nervous impulses impinging on the hypothalamus trigger the release of pituitary trophic hormones. A few typical examples will now be mentioned to illustrate the manner in which some environmental situations affect breeding states.[3, 66, 87]

Food

The African weaver-finch *(Quelea quelea)* has reproduced so successfully in its native habitat that it is considered a major pest because of its damage to small grain crops. The breeding colonies may consist of more than a million birds. The male uses fresh green grass to construct a perpendicular nest-ring upon which he displays himself in nuptial plumage. Copulation occurs on or near this ring, and the nest is completed by weaving additional green grass into it. The young are fed on insects for the first five days of life and then on green grass seeds. Vast quantities of insects and green grass are necessary for successful reproduction, and breeding sites are frequently abandoned if these requirements are not met. Breeding in this species occurs only after a rainy period. It is probable that environmental conditions prevailing after rainfall, operating in conjunction with the internal sexual rhythm, are the critical factors determining the time of reproduction in this species.[15]

Light

There is overwhelming evidence that light is an important environmental stimulus influencing reproductive rhythms. The onset of the breeding season is controlled in some species by increasing light periods, whereas in other species diminishing periods of light constitute the effective stimulus.

It has been known for many years that egg production in domestic hens may be encouraged by subjecting the animals to increasing periods of light. Rowan in 1926 was the first to show that lengthening the day by providing additional illumination would bring the involuted gonads of the junco into a breeding state.[72] He thought that the increased exercise or activity of the birds incident to increased daily photoperiods was the essential stimulus that induced gonadal recrudescence, but this hypothesis has not been confirmed.

The ferret is sexually dormant during autumn and winter, the long anestrus extending from August to March. Ferrets do not breed during this period, but they can be brought into breeding condition by keeping them in artificial light for a few hours after sunset each day. The female is more easily controlled in this way than the male. The ferret does not respond to increasing photoperiods if it is blind or if either the hypophysis or gonads are removed. The chain of reactions involved seems to be: Transmission of impulses along the optic nerve to the brain (probably hypothalamus); stimulation of the adenohypophysis to release gonadotrophins and perhaps other hormones; activation of the gonads by the pituitary gonadotrophins; stimulation of the accessory sex organs; and the induction of psychologic heat by the gonadal hormones.

In some species, the onset of the breeding season may be hastened by *diminishing* the daily amounts of light and ended by *increasing* the photoperiods. Sheep, for example, start to breed earlier if the amount of light normally available in the spring is reduced. The majority of birds and many mammals (*e.g.,* horse, ferret) tend to have breeding periods in the spring (long-day breeders), whereas other mammals (*e.g.,* deer, sheep) breed during the fall (short-day breeders). Again, in the guinea pig, ground squirrel, rabbit, and cow, light periods seem to be without effect on reproductive processes.

Female rats receiving additional rations of light remain in heat, or estrus, for several weeks instead of for the normal period of 14 hours. Young female rats kept in continuous light from birth attain sexual maturity about a week earlier than normal; constant darkness from the time of birth delays the onset of sexual maturity by two or three weeks. The gestation period of the American marten is about nine months; but implantation is delayed for seven months. Increasing photoperiods hasten the implantation of the blastocysts, and the young are born about four months earlier than usual.

Long photoperiods cause pronounced testicular growth in domestic ducks, but this does not occur after hypophysectomy or after the pathway from the hypothalamus to the pituitary is experimentally blocked. On the other hand, the domestic fowl, parakeet, and house sparrow can attain sexual maturity when kept in complete darkness.

The foregoing examples are sufficient to indicate that light has a pronounced effect upon the production of pituitary gonadotrophins in birds and mammals. There is general agreement now that the effects of light and other environmental stimuli on gonadal activities are mediated by the central nervous system (hypothalamus), the hypophysial portal veins, and the adenohypophysis.[28]

The Mode of Action of Light

Since Rowan's interpretation was published many workers have felt that the effects of light on reproductive phenomena might result secondarily from metabolic alterations consequent upon lengthened periods of wakefulness and physical exercise. However, egg production in domestic hens can be increased by subjecting them to 20-second shocks of intense light at 4:00 A.M. and 4:45 A.M., while the birds are sleeping. Since the birds remain on the roosts and show little if any activity after these shocks, it would seem that increased exercise does not explain the phenomenon.

During midwinter, the gonads of white-crowned sparrows *(Zonotrichia)* are small and inactive. When the animals are caged and subjected to elevated environmental temperatures, they develop periods of nocturnal activity. This provides a convenient and natural way to increase physical activity without lengthening the daily photoperiod. Increasing the daily activity in this species, without an accompanying increase in light, does not produce gonadal recrudescence. Although exercise may be an essential element in certain species, or a factor of some importance in maintaining reproductive behavior once it is begun, a direct action of light *per se* upon the central nervous system seems to provide a more adequate explanation than the wakefulness-activity hypothesis.

Extensive studies on the duck have shown that gonadal recrudescence, even after removal of the eyes, can be achieved by focusing light directly on the pituitary, hypothalamus, or rhinencephalon. By stereotactically implanting small, light-sensitive, photovoltaic cells into the hypothalamic regions of sheep, dogs, rabbits, and rats, it has been shown that sunlight can penetrate deeply into the mammalian brain.[33] This observation indicates that the capacity of light to penetrate the brain directly must be taken into account when studying the effects of light upon the hypothalami and pituitary glands of vertebrates.

Exposure of female rats to constant light causes them to enter periods of prolonged estrus, as is indicated by large numbers of keratinized scales in the vaginal smear, and this response normally depends in large measure upon the eyes as light receptors. If rats are blinded and small glass fibers are implanted into regions of the hypothalamus, with the opposite ends of the fibers projecting above the skull surface, exposure to light induces constant estrus. It thus appears that light falling directly upon hypothalamic neurons can evoke the release of pituitary gonadotrophins which produce functional changes in the gonads. Light appears to act upon the same areas of the hypothalamus which have been shown to respond to implanted sex steroids and to influence the estrous cycle and behavior of the rat.[50]

The *pineal gland* may possibly be involved in the mediation of the gonadal changes effected by continuous light or darkness in the rat. The theory is that melatonin, or some other product of the pineal gland, exerts an inhibitory effect upon gonad functions. The isolation and characterization of a gonadotrophin-inhibiting substance from the bovine pineal gland has been reported (see Chapter 16).

Temperature

It is well known that breeding efficiency among cattle declines during the hot summer months and also that the yields of both milk and butter fat are usually reduced during these periods. In the male ground squirrel, testicular involution is correlated with rising summer temperatures and testicular reactivation with the falling temperatures of autumn and winter. Males of this species remain in a constant breeding condition when maintained at 40° F. for one year, the anestrous phase of the normal cycle not appearing. Light appears not to be important in the ground squirrel, and neither light nor temperature seems to have decisive effects in the male prairie dog.

Social Impact

Most people are aware that many species of birds and mammals, although perfectly healthy and in a comfortable environment, fail to exhibit seasonal reproductive changes and never produce young in captivity. Something seems to be lacking in the psychologic atmosphere that is essential for activation of the pituitary gland and the initiation of reproductive functions.

Certain sea birds nest in colonies, and studies have indicated that the total number of birds present in the colony is an important factor in reproductive efficiency. Within limits, the larger colonies produce more eggs and hatch more young: The period of egg laying becomes more prolonged if the size of the colony is reduced; if it becomes too small, there is no reproductive success. In certain species, a small colony may arrive at the breeding ground but neither produce eggs nor rear any young, and this may continue for several years until the colony has increased its numbers by immigration to an essential minimum.

Many species of seal practice a harem system on the breeding grounds; a male takes over a number of females and guards them against the attention of rival males. In these carnivores there is typically a postpartum estrus during which copulations are permitted. It is probable that this social arrangement is an important factor in providing the necessary psychologic stimulus for reproduction and the maintenance of adequate numbers.

After surgical removal of the olfactory bulbs of mature mice, the ovaries and uteri become significantly smaller than those of the controls. Corpora lutea are absent or atrophic and the vagina remains small. In males similarly operated, the testes appear normal but the accessory sex glands are smaller and lighter than usual. The estrous cycle of the female is modified by the presence of a male or his excreta.

A very rigid social hierarchy is established in male chickens as they become sexually mature. Studies have shown that the weights of the adrenal glands of cocks correlate reciprocally with social rank. The testes of subordinate grouped cocks gain weight more slowly than do those of dominant grouped males; furthermore, the onset of spermatogenesis is delayed, and degenerative changes occur in the testis tubules. These studies show that grouping and social position are important factors in conditioning the production of pituitary gonadotrophins and hence fertility in male birds. Extensive observations of this type have been made on mammalian species.[30]

The Refractory Period

Although light, temperature, rainfall, food supply, social impact, and other environmental factors are important in conditioning seasonal periodicity, it should be pointed out that the reproductive state cannot be prolonged indefinitely even by the most favorable external environment. Neither can another sexual cycle be reinstated immediately after the close of one. This is referred to as the *refractory period.*[57]

The factors responsible for the onset of this period are largely obscure. It may be that the pituitary gland becomes exhausted and cannot supply the necessary gonadotrophins, or that the gonads no longer possess the necessary structure to respond to the gonadotrophins. As mentioned earlier, the cells of Leydig in the bird's testis become exhausted at the end of the reproductive period, and another generation of such cells must be regenerated from connective tissue elements. It may be that the onset of the refractory period in the case of the male bird coincides with the interval required to build up another generation of Leydig cells. In certain fishes, each spawning period is followed by a rapid collapse of the ovary, and the postspawning refractoriness probably correlates with an inability of the gonad to respond to pituitary stimulation.[74]

REFERENCES

1. Abney, T. O., and Williams, W. L.: Inhibition of sperm capacitation by intrauterine deposition of seminal plasma decapacitation factor. Biol. Reprod. 2:14, 1970.
2. Adams, C. E., and Chang, M. C.: Capacitation of rabbit spermatozoa in the fallopian tube and in the uterus. J. Exp. Zool. *151*:159, 1962.
3. Amoroso, E. C., and Matthews, L. H.: The effect of external stimuli on the breeding-cycle of birds and mammals. Brit. Med. Bull. *11*:87, 1955.
4. Anderson, K. M., and Liao, S.: Selective retention of dihydrotestosterone by prostatic nuclei. Nature *219*:277, 1968.
5. Asakawa, H.: Precocious spermatogenesis in intratesticular homotransplants of fetal mouse testes. Amer. Zool. *3*:493, 1963.
6. Bardin, C. W., Bullock, L. P., Sherins, R. J., Mowszowicz, I., and Blackburn, W. R.: Androgen metabolism and mechanism of action in male pseudohermaphroditism: a study of testicular feminization. Rec. Progr. Horm. Res. *29*:65, 1973.
7. Bedford, J. M.: Maturation of the fertilizing ability of mammalian spermatozoa in the male and female reproductive tract. Biol. Reprod. *11*:346, 1974.
8. Boccabella, A. V.: Reinitiation and restoration of spermatogenesis with testosterone propionate and other hormones after a long-term post-hypophysectomy regression period. Endocrinology *72*:787, 1963.
9. Bygdeman, M.: Prostaglandins in human seminal fluid and their correlation to fertility. Int. J. Fertil. *14*:228, 1969.
10. Christensen, A. K., and Mason, N. R.: Comparative ability of seminiferous tubules and interstitial tissue of rat testes to synthesize androgens from progesterone-4-^{14}C *in vitro*. Endocrinology 76:646, 1965.
11. Clegg, E. J.: Some effects of artificial cryptorchidism on the accessory reproductive organs of the rat. J. Endocr. *20*:210, 1960.

12. Clermont, Y.: Kinetics of spermatogenesis in mammals; seminiferous epithelium cycle and spermatogonial renewal. Physiol. Rev. *52*:198, 1972.

13. Clermont, Y., and Mauger, A.: Existence of a spermatogonial chalone in the rat testis. Cell. Tissue Kinet. *7*:165, 1974.

14. Davis, J. R.: Metabolic aspects of spermatogenesis. Biol. Reprod. *1*:93, 1969.

15. Disney, H. J. de S., and Marshall, A. J.: A contribution to the breeding biology of the weaver-finch *Quelea quelea* (Linnaeus) in East Africa. Proc. Zool. Soc. London *127*:379, 1956.

16. Dorfman, R. I.: Biological activity of antiandrogens. Brit. J. Derm. *82*(Suppl. 6):3, 1970.

17. Dorfman, R. I., Forchielli, E., and Gut, M.: Androgen biosynthesis and related studies. Rec. Progr. Horm. Res. *19*:251, 1963.

18. Dorrington, J. H., and Fritz, I. B.: Cellular localization of 5α-reductase and 3α-hydroxysteroid dehydrogenase in the seminiferous tubule of the rat testis. Endocrinology *96*:879, 1975.

19. Dube, J. Y., and Tremblay, R. R.: Androgen binding proteins in cock's tissues: properties of ear lobe protein and determination of binding sites in head appendages and other tissues. Endocrinology *95*:1105, 1974.

20. Dugal, L. P., and Dunnigan, J.: Les poids de l'éctro-éjaculat chez le coyaye soumis à une exposition chronique au froid. Canadian J. Biochem. Physiol. *40*:407, 1962.

21. Dym, M., and Fawcett, D. W.: The blood-testis barrier in the rat and the physiological compartmentation of the seminiferous epithelium. Biol. Reprod. *3*:308, 1970.

22. Eik-Nes, K. B. (ed.): The Androgens of the Testis. New York, Marcel Dekker, 1970.

23. Ellis, LeG. C., and Berliner, D. L.: Sequential biotransformation of 5-pregnenolone-7α-^{3}H and progesterone-4-^{14}C into androgens by mouse testes. Endocrinology *76*:591, 1965.

24. Ewing, L., Brown, B., Irby, D. C., and Jardine, I.: Testosterone and 5α-reduced androgen secretion by rabbit testes-epididymides perfused *in vitro*. Endocrinology *96*:610, 1975.

25. Ewing, L. L., and Schanbacher, L. M.: Early effects of experimental cryptorchidism on the activity of selected enzymes in rat testes. Endocrinology *87*:129, 1970.

26. Fang, S., Anderson, K. M., and Liao, S.: Receptor proteins for androgens. J. Biol. Chem. *244*:6584, 1969.

27. Fang, S., and Liao, S.: Antagonistic action of anti-androgens on the formation of a specific dihydrotestosterone-receptor protein complex in rat ventral prostate. Molecular Pharmacol. *5*:428, 1969.

28. Farner, D. A.: Photoperiodic controls in the secretion of gonadotropins in birds. Amer. Zool., 15(Suppl. 1):117, 1975.

29. Fjällbrant, B.: Sperm antibodies and sterility in men. Acta Obstet. Gynec. Scand. *47*(Suppl. 4):1, 1968.

30. Flickinger, G. L.: Effect of grouping on adrenals and gonads of chickens. Gen. Comp. Endocr. *1*:332, 1961.

31. French, F. S., Nayfeh, S. N., Ritzen, E. M., and Hansson, V.: FSH and a testicular androgen-binding protein in the maintenance of spermatogenesis. Research in Reprod. *6*:2, 1974.

32. French, F. S., and Ritzen, E. M.: A high-affinity androgen-binding protein (ABP) in rat testis: evidence for secretion into efferent duct fluid and absorption by epididymis. Endocrinology *93*:88, 1973.

33. Ganong, W. F., Shepherd, M. D., Wall, J. R., Van Brunt, E. E., and Clegg, M. T.: Penetration of light into the brain of mammals. Endocrinology *72:962, 1963*.

34. Hall, P. F., Irby, D. C., and de Kretser, D. M.: Conversion of cholesterol to androgens by rat testes: Comparison of interstitial cells and seminiferous tubules. Endocrinology *84*:488, 1969.

35. Hamilton, D. W., Jones, A. K., and Fawcett, D. W.: Cholesterol biosynthesis in the mouse epididymis and ductus deferens: a biochemical and morphological study. Biol. Reprod. *1*:167, 1969.

36. Harkin, J. C.: An electron microscopic study of the castration changes in the rat prostate. Endocrinology *60*:185, 1957.

37. Heller, C. G., and Clermont, Y.: Kinetics of the germinal epithelium in man. Rec. Progr. Horm. Res. *20*:545, 1964.

38. Heller, C. G., and Clermont, Y.: Spermatogenesis in man: an estimation of its duration. Science *140*:184, 1963.

39. Hoagland, H., and Pincus, G.: Revival of mammalian sperm after immersion in liquid nitrogen. J. Gen. Physiol. *25*:337, 1942.

40. Inano, H., Machino, A., and Tamaoki, B.-I.: *In vitro* metabolism of steroid hormones by cell-free homogenates of epididymides of adult rats. Endocrinology *84*:997, 1969.

41. Inano, H., and Tamaoki, B.-I.: Effect of bilateral cryptorchidism on testicular enzymes related to androgen formation. Endocrinology *83*:1074, 1968.

42. Karlson, P. (ed.): Mechanisms of Hormone Action. New York, Academic Press, 1965.

43. Kochakian, C. D.: Intracellular regulation of nucleic acids of mouse kidney by androgens. Gen. Comp. Endocr. *13*:146, 1969.
44. Kuehl, F. A., Jr., Patanelli, D. J., Tarnoff, J., and Humes, J. L.: Testicular adenyl cyclase: Stimulation by the pituitary gonadotrophins. Biol. Reprod. *2*:154, 1970.
45. Lacy, D., and Pettitt, A. J.: Sites of hormone production in the mammalian testis, and their significance in the control of male fertility. Brit. Med. Bull. *26*:87, 1970.
46. Leathem, J. H.: Nutritional effects on endocrine secretions. *In* W. C. Young (ed.): Sex and Internal Secretions, Vol. 1. Baltimore, The Williams & Wilkins Co., 1961, p. 666.
47. Levey, H. A., and Szego, C. M.: The effect of androgens on fructose production by the sex accessories of male guinea pigs and rats. Endocrinology *56*:404, 1955.
48. Liao, S., Barton, R. W., and Lin, A. H.: Differential synthesis of ribonucleic acid in prostatic nuclei: Evidence for selective gene transcription induced by androgens. Proc. Nat. Acad. Sci. *55*:1593, 1966.
49. Liao, S., and Fang, S.: Receptor-proteins for androgens and the mode of action of androgens on gene transcription in ventral prostate. Vitamins Hormones *27*:17, 1969.
50. Lisk, R. D., and Kannwischer, L. R.: Light: Evidence for its direct effect on hypothalamic neurons. Science *146*:272, 1964.
51. Lostroh, A. J.: Effect of follicle-stimulating hormone and interstitial cell-stimulating hormone on spermatogenesis in Long-Evans rats hypophysectomized for six months. Acta Endocr. (Kobenhavn) *43*:592, 1963.
52. Lostroh, A. J.: Regulation of FSH and ICSH (LH) of reproductive function in the immature male rat. Endocrinology *85*:438, 1969.
53. Mancini, R. E., Costra, A., and Seiguer, A. C.: Histologic localization of follicle-stimulating and luteinizing hormones in the rat testis. J. Histochem. Cytochem. *15*:516, 1967.
54. Mann, T.: The Biochemistry of Semen and of the Male Reproductive Tract. New York, John Wiley & Sons, 1964.
55. Meli, A.: Route of administration as a factor influencing the biological activity of certain androgens and their corresponding 3-cyclopentyl enol ethers. Endocrinology *72*:715, 1963.
56. Metz, C. B., and Anika, J.: Failure of conception in rabbits inseminated with nonagglutinating, univalent, antibody-treated semen. Biol. Reprod. *2*:284, 1970.
57. Miller, A. H.: The occurrence and maintenance of the refractory period in crowned sparrows. Condor *56*:13, 1954.
58. Muller, E. R. A., Galavazi, G., and Szirmai, J. A.: Effect of castration and testosterone treatment on fiber width of the flexor carpi radialis muscle in the male frog (*Rana temporaria* L.). Gen. Comp. Endocr. *13*:275, 1969.
59. Murphy, H. D.: Sertoli cell stimulation following intratesticular injections of FSH in the hypophysectomized rat. Proc. Soc. Exp. Biol. Med. *118*:1202, 1965.
60. Neaves, W. B.: The rat testis after vasectomy. J. Reprod. Fertil. *40*:39, 1974.
61. Neumann, F., von Berswordt-Wallrabe, R., Elger, W., Steinbeck, H., Hahn, J. D., and Kramer, M.: Aspects of androgen-dependent events as studied by antiandrogens. Rec. Progr. Horm. Res. *26*:337, 1970.
62. Neumann, F., Elger, W., and Kramer, M.: Development of a vagina in male rats by inhibiting androgen receptors with an antiandrogen during the critical phase of organogenesis. Endocrinology *78*:628, 1966.
63. Oakberg, E. F.: A description of spermiogenesis in the mouse and its use in analysis of the cycle of the seminiferous epithelium and germ cell renewal. Amer. J. Anat. *99*:391, 1956.
64. Ortavant, R., Courot, M., and Hochereau, M. T.: Spermatogenesis and morphology of the spermatozoon. *In* H. H. Cole and P. T. Cupps (eds.): Reproduction in Domestic Animals. New York, Academic Press, 1969, p. 251.
65. Ortiz, E., Price, D., Williams-Ashman, H. G., and Banks, J.: The influence of androgens on the male accessory reproductive glands of the guinea pig; Studies on growth, histological structure and fructose and citric acid secretion. Endocrinology *59*:479, 1956.
66. Parkes, A. S., and Bruce, H. M.: Olfactory stimuli in mammalian reproduction. Science *134*:1049, 1961.
67. Peterson, R. N., and Freund, M.: Glycolysis by washed suspensions of human spermatozoa. Biol. Reprod. *1*:238, 1969.
68. Podestá, E. J., Calandra, R. S., Rivarola, M. A., and Blaquier, J. A.: The effect of castration and testosterone replacement on specific proteins and androgen levels of the rat epididymis. Endocrinology *95*:399, 1975.
69. Ramwell, P. W., Shaw, J. E., Clarke, G. B., Grostic, M. F., Kaiser, D. G., and Pike, J. E.: Prostaglandins. *In* Progress in the Chemistry of Fats and other Lipids, Vol. 9 (Part 2). New York, Pergamon Press, 1968, p.231.
70. Roosen-Runge, E. C.: Comparative aspects of spermatogenesis. Biol. Reprod. *1*:24, 1969.

71. Rosner, J. M., Macome, J. C., and Cardinali, D. P.: *In vitro* biosynthesis of sterols and sterroids by rat submaxillary glands. Endocrinology *85*:1000, 1969.
72. Rowan, W.: Experiments in bird migration. Manipulation of the reproductive cycle: Seasonal histological changes in the gonads. Proc. Boston Soc. Nat. Hist. *39*:151, 1929.
73. Sar, M., Liao, S., and Stumpf, W. E.: Nuclear concentration of androgens in rat seminal vesicles and prostate demonstrated by dry-mount autoradiography. Endocrinology *86*: 1008, 1970.
74. Sehgal, A., and Sundararaj, B. I.: Effects of various photoperiodic regimens on the ovary of the catfish, *Heteropneustes fossilis* (Bloch), during the spawning and postspawning periods. Biol. Reprod. *2*:425, 1970.
75. Setchell, B. P.: Testicular blood supply, lymphatic drainage and secretion of fluid. *In* A. D. Johnson, W. R. Gomes, and N. L. Vandemark (eds.): The Testis, Vol. 1. New York, Academic Press, 1970, p. 101.
76. Setchell, B. P., Duggan, M. C., and Evans, R. W.: Effect of gonadotrophins on fluid secretion and sperm production by the rat and hamster testis. J. Endocr. *56*:27, 1973.
77. Shaw, C. R., and Koen, A. L.: Hormone-induced esterase in mouse kidney. Science *140*:70, 1963.
78. Squire, P. G., Johnston, R. E., and Lyons, W. R.: Intratesticular injections of interstitial cell-stimulating hormones in hypophysectomized rats. Internat. J. Fertil. *8*:531, 1963.
79. Stanley, A. J., Gumbreck, L. G., Allison, J. E., and Easley, R. B.: Male pseudohermaphroditism in the laboratory Norway rat. Rec. Prog. Horm. Res. *29*:43, 1973.
80. Steinberger, E.: Hormonal control of mammalian spermatogenesis. Physiol. Rev. *51*:1, 1971.
81. Strauss, J. S., and Pochi, P. E.: The human sebaceous gland: Its regulation by steroid hormones and its use as an end organ for assaying androgenicity *in vivo*. Rec. Progr. Horm. Res. *19*:385, 1963.
82. Tindall, D. J., Hansson, V., Sar, M., Stumpf, W. E., French, F. S., and Nayfeh, S. N.: Further studies on the accumulation and binding of androgen in rat epididymis. Endocrinology *95*:1119, 1974.
83. Tindall, D. J., Vitale, R., and Means, A. R.: Androgen binding protein as a biochemical marker of formation of the blood-testis barrier. Endocrinology *97*:636, 1975.
84. Tveter, K. J., and Aakvaag, A.: Uptake and metabolism *in vivo* of testosterone-1,2-^{3}H by accessory sex organs of male rats; influence of some hormonal compounds. Endocrinology *85*:683, 1969.
85. Van Rees, G. P.: Influence of steroid sex hormones on the FSH-release by hypophyses *in vitro*. Acta Endocr. *36*:485, 1961.
86. Villee, C. A.: Hormonal expression through genetic mechanisms. Amer. Zool. *7*:109, 1967.
87. Whitten, W. K.: The effect of removal of the olfactory bulbs on the gonads of mice. J. Endocr. *14*:160, 1956.
88. Williams, W. L., Abney, T. O., Chernoff, H. N., Dukelow, W. R., and Pinsker, M. C.: Biochemistry and physiology of decapacitation factor. J. Reprod. Fertil., Suppl. 2, 11, 1967.
89. Williams-Ashman, H. G., and Reddi, A. H.: Actions of vertebrate sex hormones. Ann. Rev. Physiol. *33*:31, 1971.
90. Williams-Ashman, H. G., and Reddi, A. H.: Androgenic regulation of tissue growth and function. *In* G. Litwak (ed.): Biochemical Actions of Hormones, Vol. 2. New York, Academic Press, 1972, p. 257.
91. Wilson, J. D., and Gloyna, R. E.: The intranuclear metabolism of testosterone in the accessory organs of reproduction. Rec. Progr. Horm. Res. *26*:309, 1970.
92. Woods, J. E., and Domm, L. V.: A histochemical identification of the androgen-producing cells in the gonads of the domestic fowl and albino rat. Gen. Comp. Endocr. *7*:559, 1966.
93. Zaneveld, L. J. D., and Williams, W. L.: A sperm enzyme that disperses the corona radiata and its inhibition by the decapacitation factor. Biol. Reprod. *2*:363, 1970.

CHAPTER 14

Endocrinology of the Ovary

The ovary functions chiefly in the production of mature eggs and in the elaboration of hormones that regulate the reproductive tract and secondary sex characters, condition the mating reactions, and exert other metabolic effects. Neither the gametogenic nor endocrine functions are continuous processes; they fluctuate rhythmically during the life of the individual. The periodic changes in the female tract are determined by cyclic variations in the pituitary gland and ovaries. The intervals are called *estrous cycles* in subprimate species and *menstrual cycles* in man and other primates. Although both kinds of cycles are regulated by the same or similar pituitary and ovarian hormones, they differ in important details and will be discussed later.

Another type of cycle corresponds to the life span of the individual: The period of prepuberal development is followed by a period of sexually active life, after which the ovaries grow old and reproduction gradually ceases. Menopausal symptoms generally occur in women between the ages of 40 and 50 years, the ovaries involute, and the menstrual cycles gradually cease. Egg production in birds gradually diminishes with age and ceases entirely in the aged animal. Studies on a variety of species indicate that the mammalian ovary usually cannot increase its store of oocytes after the age of puberty. There are some exceptions to this general rule, and it may well be that oogenesis ceases in some species earlier than in others. Generally speaking, however, the mammalian ovary is a transient structure and has little capacity for replenishing the supply of oocytes after the age of puberty. The ovary becomes senescent much earlier than the testis, and no hormones are known that can restore its capacity to proliferate germ cells.

Although reproductive functions and behavioral patterns are clearly influenced by endocrine secretions, it must not be assumed that these are the only factors involved. The secretion of certain interacting hormones is mediated, at least in part, by the nervous system, and the whole reproductive mechanism may be stimulated or inhibited by factors arising in the external environment. Nutritional factors can be extremely important conditioning agents. For example, the onset of puberty in mice is delayed by reducing the caloric intake, but such animals live longer than well-fed controls. These females develop reproductive competence after being given full caloric intake and may bear young at a time when their littermate controls are infertile or already dead.[69]

HISTOLOGY OF THE MAMMALIAN OVARY

In addition to the surface epithelium, the three functional subunits of the ovary are the follicle, corpus luteum, and stroma. The primary follicle consists of an oocyte surrounded by a single layer of flattened epithelial cells. These follicles lack a connective tissue or thecal investment and are most numerous immediately beneath the tunica albuginea (Fig. 14–1). Occasionally, more than one oocyte may be present in a primordial follicle; these may result from the division of a single germ cell, or more probably, from the failure of early germ cells to become separated as they are invested by nongerminal elements. As the follicles mature, they move away from the tunica and assume a deeper position in the stroma. The egg increases in size, and the follicular cells proliferate mitotically. The squamous cells of the primary follicle first turn into a single layer of columnar epithelium but, as proliferation continues, this becomes a stratified epithelium. When the cell membrane of the ovum has transformed into a zona pellucida, and the follicular investment has become multilayered, it is designated a secondary follicle.

The growing follicle is soon encapsulated by a sheath of tissue derived from the stroma. This is the theca, which promptly becomes divided into a well-vascularized theca interna and a theca externa, which is composed of connective tissue. The theca interna is separated from the granulosa layer by a thin membrana propria. Blood vessels and lymphatics penetrate the theca externa and form a rather extensive plexus of fine vessels in the theca interna. These blood vessels do not penetrate the membrana propria; thus

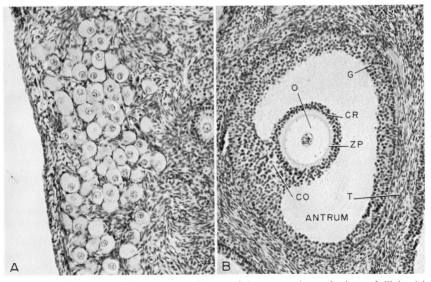

Figure 14–1. Ovarian follicles from an adult cat. *A,* Large numbers of primary follicles (single layer of flattened cells around the oöcyte) near the edge of the ovary. *B,* A graafian follicle located more deeply in the same ovary. CO, cumulus oöphorus; CR, corona radiata; G, granulosa; O, ovum; T, thecal layers; ZP, zona pellucida. Both photographs are of the same magnification.

the cells comprising the granulosa are without direct blood supply until after ovulation. Cavities appear in the multilayered granulosa, and these coalesce to form a fluid-filled antrum. After establishment of the antrum, the follicle is said to be vesicular or graafian. The granulosa cells surrounding the ovum are destined to become the corona radiata, and those which attach it to the wall of the antrum are the cumulus oophorus. The cumulus is generally found on the wall of the antrum opposite to the surface which will rupture at ovulation. In many species, the corona cells remain around the egg after it is ovulated, but in others, the eggs are ovulated without it (Fig. 14–1).

After ovulation, the collapsed follicle transforms into a new endocrine structure, the corpus luteum. The histogenesis of the corpus luteum seems to vary among different species, but, in the human being and many other mammals, it appears to be derived from proliferations of both the granulosa and theca interna. There is no doubt that the cells of the theca interna perform important roles before, during, and immediately after ovulation.

Atresia is a degenerative process whereby eggs are lost from the ovary other than through ovulation. It has been estimated that 99.9 per cent of the 500,000 oocytes present in the human ovaries at birth are destined to be lost by atresia at some stage of their development. The earliest signs of retrogression appear in the ovum itself and then spread to other components of the follicle. The ova in atretic follicles may give off polar bodies and undergo mitotic or amitotic divisions, thus producing several cells within the zona pellucida. Some workers have considered this to be an attempt of the egg to undergo parthenogenetic development. The incidence of atresia may be affected by age, season, nutrition, stage of the reproductive cycle, pregnancy and lactation, hypophysectomy, unilateral ovariectomy, exogenous hormones, and impairments of the blood supply to the ovaries.

Corpora lutea atretica are commonly seen in certain species during pregnancy, pseudopregnancy, and lactation. In these cases, the theca interna and granulosa begin to form thick layers of lutein tissue before ovulation has occurred; the egg may survive for some time near the center of what appears to be a well-formed corpus luteum (Fig. 14–2). It is probable that not all of the copora lutea which contain oocytes are the consequences of atresia; an egg may fail to escape from its antrum at ovulation and be trapped within the center of a normal corpus luteum.

Atresia may also be associated with the formation of enlarged, cystic follicles. The ovum degenerates and the antrum is distended with liquor folliculi. The antrum of cystic follicles is generally lined by a single layer of granulosa cells, or the granulosal lining may practically disappear, the enlarged follicle being supported by heavy thecal tissue. Hemorrhagic cysts result from ruptured blood vessels and the extravasation of blood into the antrum. Follicles of this type are frequently found in unmated rabbits; these become dark brown and are eventually resorbed.

The stroma of the ovary contains connective tissue and variable numbers of interstitial cells. These take the form of cords or irregular clusters of large polyhedral cells. Various interpretations have been expressed as to the origin of these cells. Some have maintained that they originate directly

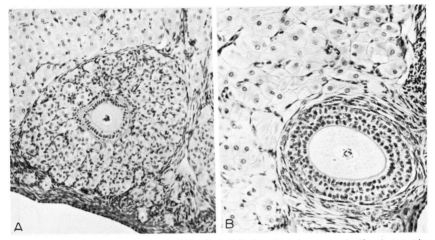

Figure 14–2. Ovary of the adult rabbit. *A*, A follicle which became atretic at an early age. Notice that the granulosa consists of s single layer of columnar cells, indicating that it is quite young, and that thecal tissue is not present immediately exterior to the granulosa. The follicle is completely surrounded by lutein tissue, and hence could never ovulate. This appears to be a case of precocious luteinization; it is probable that the theca interna of this follicle began to proliferate lutein tissue at a very early age, resulting in a structure which has the appearance of a small corpus luteum. This animal was never sexually receptive and was more than five years of age when killed. *B*, An apparently normal multilaminar follicle from the same ovary. Notice the large volume of interstitial tissue in the rabbit's ovary.

from connective tissue cells; others feel that they arise, in part at least, from the theca interna of atretic follicles. In some mammals (*e.g.,* rabbit), the interstitial tissue is very conspicuous and occupies nearly all of the space not taken up by follicles and corpora lutea (Fig. 14–2). Recent evidence indicates that the interstitial cells of the ovary may be capable of producing both androgens and estrogens, and hence constitute an endocrine tissue. *In vitro* studies of human stromal tissue have demonstrated that it can synthesize radioactive steroids from acetate-1-C^{14}. This study showed that the greatest incorporation of radioactivity was in three androgens (androstenedione, dehydroepiandrosterone, and testosterone), and lesser amounts were incorporated into two estrogens (estradiol-17β and estrone).

CYSTIC FOLLICLES OF THE OVARY

It frequently happens that ovarian follicles enlarge beyond the stage of ovulation and remain permanently or for long periods in the ovaries (Fig. 14–3). Cysts are often encountered among women and domesticated and laboratory mammals and are a common cause of abnormal reproductive cycles and sterility. These are the consequences of endocrine imbalances— often impairments in the release of pituitary gonadotrophins—but the specific causes and methods of prevention and treatment remain to be worked out. The multiple cysts of swine ovaries may attain a diameter of 10 cm., and

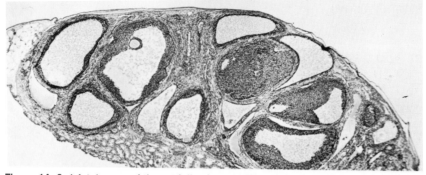

Figure 14–3. A fetal ovary of the rat following persistence in the kidney of a normal male rat for 60 days. The male pituitary does not release FSH and LH cyclically, as does the female's; consequently, the graft consists of vesicular and cystic follicles. Ovulation does not occur, and corpora lutea are seldom found. Notice that the cystic follicles have lost their ova, and, in some cases, the granulosa is reduced to a single layer of flattened cells. Kidney tissue is present below the graft, at the lower left.

are associated with a long history of sterility. These cysts secrete less estrogen than normal follicles; the estrous cycles are abnormal and the animals tend to remain in anestrus for exceptionally long periods. Smaller cysts often show patches of lutein tissue in their walls, and bioassays indicate that they produce progesterone. After prolonged distention with fluid, all components of the follicle degenerate. In cattle, but not in other species, cystic ovaries are often associated with intense psychologic heat (nymphomania), enlargement of the clitoris, and other signs of masculinization. This syndrome is poorly understood, but experimental observations indicate that it is *not* due to an excessive production of estrogen by the cystic follicles, as is often assumed. Hypertrophy of the adrenal cortices has been reported in cattle with cystic ovaries and nymphomania, and this suggests that glands other than the ovaries may be involved. Some amelioration of the symptoms, during early stages of the disease, may be obtained by the administration of gonadotrophins which exert LH actions.

Polycystic ovaries may be induced in rats by giving human chorionic gonadotrophin (HCG) after inducing a state of hypothyroidism. The animals are fed thiouracil (0.5 per cent) in a 20 per cent casein diet for 10 days, and then given HCG (10 I.U. daily) for 20 days. Ovaries weighing 800 to 1000 mg. may result from this dual treatment; neither hypothyroidism nor HCG alone is capable of producing cysts. Once formed, the ovarian cysts do not regress even though the hypothyroidism is corrected and the HCG injections are discontinued. An antiestrogen, ethamoxytriphetol (MER-25), prevents this type of cyst formation when it is administered together with the HCG. The tremendous increase in ovarian weight is due to increased lutein tissue and the retention of fluid in the cysts. Histologically, the large cysts are lined with a simple squamous epithelium, and granulosa cells and lutein tissue are absent. *In vitro* studies on the capacity of this type of cystic ovary to synthesize steroids have demonstrated that they produce excessive progestogens (20α-hydroxypregn-4-en-3-one), but subnormal quantities of estrogens.[7, 33]

It is well known that a single injection of testosterone to 5-day-old rats impairs the hypothalamus and prevents the pituitary gland from secreting adequate quantities of LH.[3, 4, 30, 66] When the treated animals mature, they remain in constant vaginal estrus, and, histologically, the ovaries lack corpora lutea but contain many enlarged follicles (polyvesicular or polycystic) which do not ovulate. Consequently, the animals are permanently sterile. Progesterone, administered in conjunction with the androgen, protects the neonatal rat against this type of steroid-induced sterility.[31] *In vitro* tests show that the ovaries of these androgen-sterilized rats produce several times more testosterone, estrone, and estradiol than do the ovaries of untreated controls.[71] Analyses of human and bovine cystic ovaries, using both *in vivo* and *in vitro* tests, suggest that there may be an enzymatic defect which prevents the normal conversion of androgens (C-19 intermediates) into estrogens, the result being an excessive accumulation of androgens.

BIOCHEMISTRY OF THE OVARIAN HORMONES

The ovary elaborates estrogens, progestogens (a general term for any substance producing progestational changes in the uterus), androgens, and a nonsteroid hormone called relaxin. Most workers agree that the mature ovarian follicle is an important source of estrogen, but the exact component of the follicle that produces it has never been unequivocally settled; most of the evidence implicates either the membrana granulosa or theca interna as the source. The corpus luteum elaborates both estrogenic and progestational steroids. The cellular source of relaxin and ovarian androgens remains unknown. These hormones stimulate growth and differentiation of the female reproductive tract and associated structures and also exert a multitude of systemic effects.

We have emphasized that steroid hormones are produced by testes, ovaries, adrenal cortices, and placenta, and that the same general route of biosynthesis seems to be employed by all of these organs. In the presence of enzymes from these various tissues, a common precursor such as pregnenolone can be converted into any one of the known steroid hormones. Although there is some relationship between biologic activity and chemical configuration of the molecule, it is known that a particular steroid hormone may exert multiple actions. There is no hard and fast dividing line between estrogens, androgens, progestogens, and adrenal corticoids. Some degree of functional overlap is often observed when the dosage of a particular steroid is increased to unphysiologic levels. Thus, steroids generally regarded as "estrogens" because they stimulate the female accessories may also be "androgens" because they stimulate the male tract. Some hormones thought of primarily as adrenal corticoids may be "progestogens," since they have slight ability to produce progestational changes in the endometrium. While progesterone is a natural progestogen, it can stimulate the prostates and seminal vesicles of castrated animals. Women who receive massive doses of natural or synthetic progestogens during pregnancy sometimes give birth to mildly masculinized female infants. An appreciable degree of steroid hormone interconversion may occur within the system after purified hormones are administered.

The Estrogens

The predominant natural estrogens of the human are estradiol-17β, estrone, and estriol. Several other estrogens, representing estrogen metabolites, have been isolated in significant amounts from normal urine. All of the estrogens contain eighteen carbon atoms and, for terminological purposes, may be considered as derivatives of the theoretical parent substance, "estrane." They are characterized by the aromatic nature of ring A (three double bonds), the absence of a methyl group at C-10, and the presence of a phenolic hydroxyl group at C-3.

Estrogens are present in various animal tissues, such as ovaries, testes, adrenals, and placentae, and small amounts have even been found in spermatozoa. Estrogenic activity has been demonstrated in about 50 species of plants. The subterranean clover of Western Australia was found to contain sufficient estrogen to affect the reproductive performance of grazing sheep adversely.[5] In recent years, estrogen and estrogen-metabolizing systems have been found in various invertebrate species, and their role in evolution has been the subject of discussion.[51]

It appears that the human ovary elaborates only estradiol-17β and estrone; estriol is thought to be a degradation product of the former steroids in nonpregnant women. During human pregnancy both estriol and 16-epiestriol are probably produced by the placenta. Estriol has been believed characteristic of the human species and is found primarily in the urine. In the cow, as in numerous other mammalian species, the placenta seems to be the principal source of estrogens during pregnancy. Estrone, estradiol-17β, and estradiol-17α have been isolated from bovine placental extracts. A

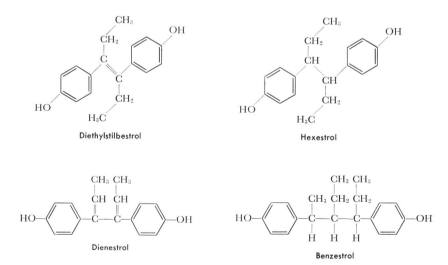

Figure 14–4. Some synthetic estrogens

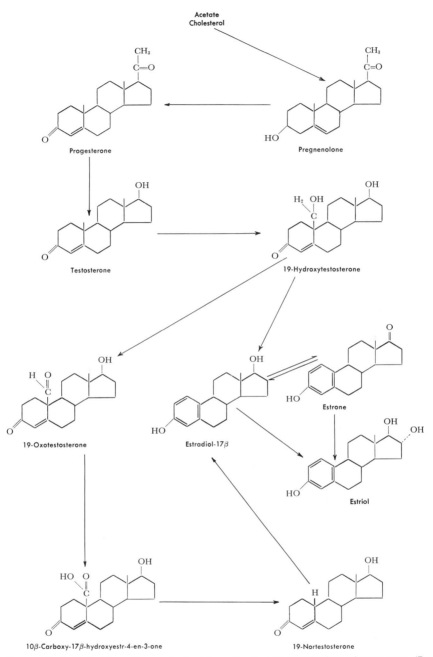

Figure 14–5. Probable pathways in the biosynthesis and metabolism of estrogens. (Based on Dorfman, R. I.: Obstet. Gynec. Survey *18*:65, 1963.)

large group of nonsteroidal estrogens have been produced synthetically and used for clinical purposes (Fig. 14–4). They possess the same biologic characteristics as the naturally occurring estrogens; diethylstilbestrol and hexestrol are examples.

It has been established that both acetate and cholesterol may serve as precursors for the synthesis of estrogens. It is interesting that estrogens in the ovaries, testes, adrenal cortices, and placenta arise from androgens. The biosynthetic pathway proceeds through the 19-hydroxylated intermediates of androstenedione and testosterone. This is followed by elimination of the C-19 side chain and the aromatization of the A ring (Fig. 14–5). Estradiol-17β and estrone are interconvertible, and estriol is the predominant urinary end product of estrogen metabolism.

The circulating estrogens are bound to plasma proteins, and the binding process is accomplished in the liver. It has been proposed that the liver performs a dual role in estrogen metabolism, inactivating these steroids and also exerting an "activating" influence through the formation of estroproteins. About 50 per cent of the blood estrogen is conjugated with glucuronide or sulfate. This conjugation occurs in the liver and the excreted compounds in the urine are in this form. An enterohepatic circulation occurs, and some animals (rat, dog) excrete estrogen mainly through the feces. Ligation of the bile duct may lead to an increased excretion of metabolites through the urine.

Estrogens in human urine increase twice during the menstrual cycle: The first coincides with ovulation and the rise in basal body temperature; the second occurs during the luteal phase of the cycle. Pregnancy urine is very rich in estrogen, which appears to be produced by the placenta. This is indicated by the fact that ovariectomy of the pregnant woman or pregnant mare does not cause the urinary estrogens to disappear. The type of estrogen in the urine during pregnancy varies with the species: Human pregnancy urine contains mostly estriol, whereas that of the mare is mostly estrone. Equilin and equilenin are weak estrogens that have been found only in the pregnant mare. Ring B of these compounds is either partially or totally converted to the aromatic form. During human pregnancy, urine levels of all the estrogens increase rapidly. Just before parturition, estrone and estradiol have increased a hundredfold and estriol a thousandfold. The estrone and estradiol are usually excreted in a constant ratio of about 3:1. The urinary estrogens diminish rapidly after parturition and the loss of the placenta.

The vaginal cornification technique has been used extensively for the bioassay of estrogens. The test material is administered systemically to the ovariectomized rodents, the full-blown estrous reaction being indicated by vaginal smears that contain mostly cornified epithelial cells (Fig. 14–12). A more sensitive bioassay is to introduce the test material directly into the vagina, care being taken not to traumatize the vaginal mucosa. The most sensitive and accurate method is based on the fact that estrogens cause a striking increase in uterine weight when administered to ovariectomized animals. Six hours after the subcutaneous injection of a dose of estrogen to a castrated rat, the uterus increases in weight by imbibition of water; another weight increase occurs 21 to 30 hours after the single injection, owing to hypertrophy and hyperplasia of the uterine tissues.[2]

Physicochemical procedures are available for the determination of estrogenic potency, but they require a rather high degree of sample purity. Although bioassay and chemical techniques are often too laborious and expensive to be applicable for routine use, the development of radioimmu-noassay procedures for estrogenic hormones has been a great convenience and aid to clinical diagnosis. Estrogenic activity can usually be satisfactorily assessed by proper examination of the exfoliated cells of the patient's va-gina. The Greenstein method of staining vaginal smears and endometrial biopsies has been found suitable for office practice and the clinical labora-tory.[21]

The Mechanism of Action of Estrogens

The current hypothesis receiving greatest experimental support is that estrogens act to regulate the expression of particular genes within the cells employed as targets.[67] Biochemical studies on the uterus and other tissues responsive to estrogens indicate that the steroid stimulates the synthesis of messenger RNA, protein, and DNA (see Chapter 2). It is probable that estra-diol enters the cell and becomes associated with an extranuclear receptor protein; one such protein has been called "estrophilin." Following a tem-perature-dependent mechanism, the estradiol-estrophilin complex is trans-located to the nucleus. In the course of this translocation, the steroid-binding component of estrophilin undergoes an alteration called receptor trans-formation or activation. This alteration of the receptor protein can be identi-fied by an increase in its sedimentation rate, by its acquisition of an ability to bind to isolated nuclei and to chromatin, and by its capacity to stimulate RNA synthesis in isolated nuclei of estrogen-dependent tissues. Possible ef-fects of the estradiol-estrophilin complex on gene transcription include in-fluences on the binding of RNA polymerase to DNA and chromatin, the initi-ation of transcription and of RNA synthesis, and influence on the growth and size distribution of RNA chains. Mechanisms involving the influences of the steroid-receptor complex on the synthesis of specific messenger RNA sequences are currently under study.

Among the early changes observed in the uterus of the castrated rat fol-lowing the administration of estradiol is increased vascularity and water content. This suggests permeability changes in the cells and could well re-sult from the action of a biogenic amine like histamine.[65] Estradiol in-creases the content of cyclic AMP in the rat uterus, but the significance of this is unknown.[63]

The distribution of radioactively labeled estrogens in target and nontar-get tissues has been carefully determined both by autoradiography and by scintillation counting, and the nuclear retention of the steroid is indicative of a genomic effect. H^3-estradiol binds strongly within the nuclei of the uter-us, vagina, and oviducts of the rat, within the nuclei of tissues associated with the feedback control of sexual functions (such as the anterior pituitary and the neurons concentrated in circumscribed areas of the brain), and in nuclei of the granulosa cells of the ovary and interstitial cells of the testis. No appreciable radioactivity is observed in such nontarget tissues as the liver and diaphragm.[60] A relatively small amount of labeled estrogen accu-mulates in the cytoplasm of target cells.

Studies with the dry-mount autoradiographic technique show that estradiol is selectively concentrated and retained both by anterior pituitary cells and by neurons in certain areas of the brain (see Chapter 3).[58, 62] These structures, in addition to the female sex accessories, must be regarded as estrogen targets, and estrogen receptors would be expected to exist in them. The estradiol-concentrating neurons of the diencephalon and amygdala appear to be associated with the regulation of gonadotrophin secretion and sex behavior, in accordance with information derived from experiments on lesioning, electric stimulation, and hormone implantation. The topographic distribution of estrogen-binding neurons appears to be identical in male and female rats, and this suggests the presence of estrogen-neuron systems within the brain.[59] Autoradiographic data also indicate the presence of androgen-binding neurons in the brains of both sexes. The estrogen-neurons are not restricted to a hypothetical "center" in the hypothalamus or the preoptic region, but occur in widely different areas of the brain. The location of such neurons in definable anatomic areas supports the concept of an endocrine amygdaloid-hypothalamic-adenohypophysial axis.[59, 61]

The Progestogens

These compounds have varied actions upon the female reproductive organs and, under physiologic conditions, often act synergistically with estrogens. The progestogens and estrogens are also capable of inhibiting the actions of each other and, under these conditions, are considered to act antagonistically. These steroids are of special importance in preparing the uterus for the implantation of blastocysts, in maintaining pregnancy, and in regulating the accessory organs during the reproductive cycle. Progesterone is present in the ovary, the testis, the adrenal cortex, and the placenta; in addition to being an intermediate in the biosynthesis of other steroid hormones, it is an important hormone in its own right. The progestogens are C-21 steroids, having the basic structure of the pregnane nucleus. Compared with the estrogens, it may be noted that ring A of the progesterone molecule is more saturated, a methyl group is present at C-10, and a two-carbon side chain is present on C-17. At least two steroids, in addition to progesterone, are known to occur naturally in mammals and to have progestational effects. These are 20α-hydroxypregn-4-en-3-one and 20β-hydroxypregn-4-en-3-one (Fig. 14–6). These are present in ovarian follicles, corpora lutea, placenta, and blood. A variety of progestogens that are highly potent and orally effective have been produced synthetically.

The principal urinary metabolites of the progestogens are pregnanediol and pregnanetriol, and these are eliminated chiefly as glucuronides. It was formerly supposed that the synthesis of progesterone by the system could be precisely gauged by the quantities of pregnanediol excreted in the urine, but it is now known that this metabolite may also be derived from deoxycorticosterone of the adrenal cortex. Nevertheless, pregnanediol determinations are useful in studying the progesterone output in abnormalities of

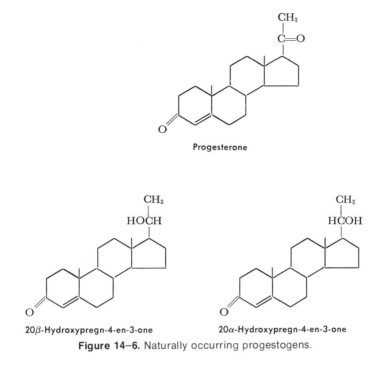

Progesterone

20β-Hydroxypregn-4-en-3-one   20α-Hydroxypregn-4-en-3-one

Figure 14–6. Naturally occurring progestogens.

menstruation and pregnancy. Pregnanetriol is the urinary metabolite of 17α-hydroxyprogesterone, and may be derived to a minor extent from 11-deoxycortisol and 17α-hydroxypregnenolone.

The bioassays for progesterone are complicated by the fact that the responding tissues require preliminary or auxiliary treatment with estrogen. Decidual responses and progestational changes in the endometrium are used as end points in certain tests. Chemical and physicochemical procedures are available for quantitative determinations of the hormone in body fluids.

Ovarian Androgens

In view of the evidence indicating that testosterone is an intermediate in the biosynthesis of estrogen, it is not surprising to find that ovaries secrete androgens. The ovaries of certain avian species may contain abundant androgen; at the time of the prenuptial molt, the amount of androgen in phalarope ovaries exceeds that normally present in the testis.[13, 29] Ovarian extracts have long been known to produce androgenic effects when tested on laboratory rodents, but it has been difficult to determine whether the activity is due to progesterone or to some definitive androgen characteristic of the testis. Ovarian homografts persisting in the ears of orchiectomized mice and rats prevent atrophy of the seminal vesicles and prostates (Fig. 14–7). Cer-

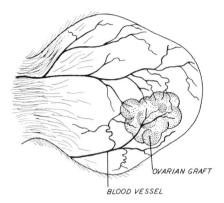

Figure 14-7. An ovarian homograft persisting in the ear of an orchiectomized male rat. Such ovarian grafts become capable of secreting enough androgen to maintain secretion in the male accessory glands. Thus the two ovarian grafts in the ears provide an endocrine substitute for the intact testes of the host. (The graft and blood vessels were sketched from the transilluminated ear.)

OVARIAN GRAFT

BLOOD VESSEL

tain cells have been described in the hilus of the human ovary that are similar to testicular Leydig cells, and these are thought to secrete androgen.

In vitro studies on human polycystic ovaries have suggested that there may be enzymatic defects in the synthesis of estrogens. These defects could accelerate the production of androgen precursors and result in the virilization which is frequently seen in patients with polycystic ovaries. Although there is no doubt that pathologic ovaries may release tremendous amounts of androgen, there is no absolute proof that the normal mammalian ovary secretes significant amounts of such steroids.

Relaxin

This is a water-soluble hormone present in the ovaries, placentae, and uteri of various mammalian species during pregnancy. Various peptides having relaxin activity have been isolated from aqueous ovarian extracts and partially purified. Relaxin was discovered at about the same time as the ovarian steroids, but it bears no structural relationship to them whatever. Although its role in human physiology is not clear, it is apparently a hormone of pregnancy and has not been found in the blood of men or nonpregnant women. Substances having relaxin-like activity have been obtained from the ovaries of elasmobranchs and from the testes of birds. Relaxin levels in the blood reach a high peak during the terminal stages of human pregnancy and disappear within one day after delivery.

The bioassay of relaxin is made difficult because of its functional interrelationship with estrogens and progestogens. Three bioassay methods have been commonly used: (1) manual palpation or x-ray photographs of the innominate bones of the estrogen-primed guinea pig after relaxin injections; (2) measurement of the length of the interpubic ligament in mice by means of a transilluminating device and ocular micrometer; (3) inhibition of motility in mouse uterine segments *in vitro*. Radioimmunoassay procedures for relaxin have now become available, and because they allow for a higher degree of precision than the commonly used bioassay procedures, their use has allowed for the accurate detection of plasma relaxin levels throughout pregnancy and at parturition.[56]

ENDOCRINE CONTROL OF THE OVARY

The ovary is not an autonomous organ; its functional capacity is influenced by a wide variety of external stimuli which are funneled into the central nervous system and then "translated" into chemical messengers which act directly upon it. Perhaps all endocrine glands have at least a modulating influence upon the production of gametes and hormones by the gonads. The ovary, like the testis, is most profoundly regulated by the pituitary gonadotrophins, namely, follicle-stimulating hormone (FSH) and luteinizing hormone (LH).

Anterior Hypophysis

Hypophysectomy of adult mammals causes prompt deterioration of the ovary and female accessory reproductive organs. The animals become irresponsive to many environmental stimuli, and the reproductive cycles are terminated. Young ovarian follicles start to differentiate, but become atretic before ovulation and luteinization occur. Total hypophysectomy of the laying hen causes rapid regression of the ovary, the oviduct, and comb. Oviposition, however, continues after the posterior lobe alone is removed.[41]

The growth and development of ovarian follicles of mammals depend upon FSH, but LH is required for their final maturation. The latter gonadotrophin acts upon the FSH-primed follicle to promote preovulatory growth and the secretion of estrogen. Further release of LH results in ovulation and the transformation of the emptied follicle into a corpus luteum. FSH and LH are both necessary for the production of estrogen by the maturing follicle. It is probable that the circulating estrogen, acting via the hypothalamus, serves to suppress the release of FSH and to facilitate the release of LH. Purified LH alone, administered to hypophysectomized subjects, has no conspicuous effect upon the ovarian follicles. The progestogens of the blood also appear to condition the release of gonadotrophins through effects on the hypothalamus.

Some workers have considered prolactin to be a gonadotrophin since it seems to be necessary for the maintenance of corpora lutea and for the secretion of progestogens by these structures in rats and mice. Thus, prolactin is sometimes called "luteotrophin" because of its action in these species. However, prolactin is not *luteotrophic* in the majority of mammals. In fact, the administration of prolactin to many species of adult birds and mammals causes regression of the testes and ovaries, thus exerting what could be considered an antigonadotrophic effect. Studies on the *in vitro* synthesis of progesterone by human and bovine corpora lutea indicate that LH is the only pituitary hormone capable of stimulating this steroid pathway. Prolactin is completely inert in these systems. A large body of evidence supports the view that prolactin does not stimulate progesterone synthesis by corpora lutea in women, monkeys, sows, ewes, rabbits, and guinea pigs.[52]

Ovarian Hormones

Large amounts of estrogen, given to intact animals, inhibit the gonads by altering the release of pituitary gonadotrophins. Permanent sterility may be produced in neonatal rats of either sex by the administration of exogenous estrogens. For example, if female rats are given estrogen from the day of birth until they are 30 days old, the mature animals remain in a state of persistent diestrus and are permanently sterile. The ovaries contain only small follicles; corpora lutea are absent and the uteri remain threadlike and are equivalent to those of animals ovariectomized during prepuberal life.[66]

In addition to systemic effects by way of the pituitary, there are indications that estrogens can exert direct, local effects upon the ovary.[6] When immature hypophysectomized rats are given a single large dose of estrogen, ovarian weights are increased by the third day and many follicles have advanced to the antrum stage. These follicles show thecal hypertrophy and active proliferation of the granulosa. If estradiol or stilbestrol is applied directly to one ovary of the immature rat, leaving the contralateral ovary untreated, the treated ovary increases in weight due to follicular growth and luteinization. It was formerly thought that hormones could not act directly upon the glands that produce them, but there are strong indications that androgens affect the testis directly and that estrogens exert some direct influences upon the ovaries.

Luteolytic Effects of the Uterus

Progesterone is essential for the development of mammalian blastocysts in the fallopian tubes and for the production of a progestational endometrium in which they can implant. A functional corpus luteum is always necessary during early stages of gestation, and this extension of progesterone secretion beyond the luteal phase of the cycle depends upon a signal derived from the embryo within the uterus. It is quite clear from studies on pregnancy and pseudopregnancy that stimuli originating in the uterus do influence ovarian functions. There is currently much interest in elucidating the factors involved in the maintenance and regression of the corpus luteum, and many species differences have become evident.[40] There are two general schools of thought: one school holds that the corpus luteum is maintained solely by pituitary gonadotrophins and that regression is a consequence of their withdrawal; the other believes that the endometrium produces a specific luteolytic factor (luteolysin) which acts on the ovary to cause luteal involution, thus counteracting the effects of any pituitary luteotrophins that may be present.[25, 36, 49]

Removal of the uterus (hysterectomy) in certain mammals markedly prolongs the functional life of the corpora lutea, just as would occur during pregnancy and pseudopregnancy. Total hysterectomy of the guinea pig, for instance, causes the corpora lutea to persist and secrete progesterone for a period approximately equal to that of normal gestation. Subtotal hysterectomy results in more limited maintenance. Similar results have been reported for the sow, sheep, and cow, but the effect is not observed in primates. After unilateral hysterectomy of swine and guinea pigs, the cycles are lengthened and striking histologic asymmetry develops in the ovaries. The corpora lutea are maintained in the ovary on the operated side, whereas they undergo usual regression on the unoperated side. Removal of the ovary on the operated side (with persistent corpora) permits the contralateral ovary to become cyclic and to undergo ovulation and subsequent luteinization.[14] These experiments might suggest that the uterus exerts a direct inhibitory effect on the corpora lutea, mediated locally, but they do not rule out the possibility that neural and hormonal mechanisms of a systemic nature are also operating.

If young corpora lutea are maintained *in vitro* and provided with proper substrates, they can synthesize progesterone. Their capacity to produce this steroid is greatly increased by adding LH to the medium. When corpora lutea of the sow are maintained *in vitro* and scrapings from the uterine lining (in early luteal phase) are added to the medium, the production of progesterone is significantly enhanced. Endometrial scrapings taken during the end of the luteal phase have an inhibitory effect on steroidogenesis.[1]

Hypophysectomy of hysterectomized animals, removing all endogenous pituitary gonadotrophins, does not prevent the persistence of existent corpora lutea. This indicates that the uterus has an ovarian effect which is not mediated through the pituitary gland. Denervation of the sow's uterus does not prevent the occurrence of estrous cycles. Autotransplanted uteri or pieces of the endometrium into totally hysterectomized guinea pigs prevent the persistence of corpora lutea. This is evidence that the uterine stimulus is not neural.

Attempts to isolate a luteolytic substance have not yielded convincing results. Since a synthetic prostaglandin ($F^2\alpha$) is found to depress the corpora lutea of the rat, it has been postulated that the uterus may possess natural prostaglandins that have luteolytic actions.[22, 43] A protein substance having luteolytic activity has been extracted from bovine endometrium.[35]

The Pineal Gland

Data have accumulated during recent years suggesting that the mammalian pineal gland exerts important actions in regulating photoperiodic influences on the gonads.[48] It is too early to make final evaluation of these studies, but the theory is that the pineal gland serves as a kind of transducer in the mediation of environmental stimuli.[74] Light perceived by the retina is believed to set up impulses which travel through unknown pathways to the superior cervical ganglia and then to the pineal gland. The discharge of impulses in this end organ alters the rate of synthesis and release of melatonin, a blood-borne agent which is regarded as a hormone. The site of melatonin action is not known; it might act directly on the gonad or indirectly through the central nervous system and anterior hypophysis.[37, 46]

The role of melatonin as a pineal hormone active in reproductive events has been challenged (see Chapter 16). Varying results obtained from work on the physiology of this indole in different species are not always compatible, and several laboratories support the view that a peptide, not melatonin, is the active pineal principle. It seems clear that the pineal is somehow involved in reproductive physiology, probably in an inhibitory role; however, its precise function or functions have not yet been elucidated.

BIOLOGIC EFFECTS OF THE OVARIAN HORMONES

The estrogens act directly, or in cooperation with other hormones, to produce a great variety of effects on specific target organs and on the chemistry of the body as a whole. Some of these actions will be discussed more specifically in this chapter in connection with the estrous and menstrual cycles, and in Chapter 15 in connection with pregnancy and lactation. Scarcely a tissue in the organism remains unaffected by estrogens, and no attempt is made to discuss all of their actions.

The Effects of Estrogens

Carcinogenesis

Perhaps the most general effect of the estrogens is to promote tissue growth. This is most pronounced in the accessory sex tissues, but it occurs in other tissues as well. By stimulating cell divisions in the deeper layers of the skin, estrogens cause a more rapid replacement of the outer cornified layers. There is some evidence that the estrogens may be potentially dangerous inasmuch as they may encourage the formation of cancer in certain individuals. This may correlate with the concept that a continued high rate of cell division is one factor predisposing a tissue to become cancerous.

Among the many carcinogenic hydrocarbons that have been studied, 1, 2-benzpyrene, 1, 2, 5, 6-dibenzanthracene, and methylcholanthrene are representative. These compounds typically produce epitheliomas when applied to the skins of susceptible rodents and sarcomas when administered subcutaneously. Some of the synthetic carcinogens are chemically related to the estrogens and initiate estrous changes in test animals. That cancer in experimental animals may follow treatment with estrogens has been proved under special circumstances. The estrogens are the only steroid hormones that have been shown to be carcinogenic.

The Vagina

Ovariectomy causes a marked involution of the vagina. The vaginal lining becomes thin and mitotic divisions are seldom encountered. The administration of estrogen to the castrate causes rapid growth of the vagina, as is indicated by the many mitotic figures in the epithelium and cornification of

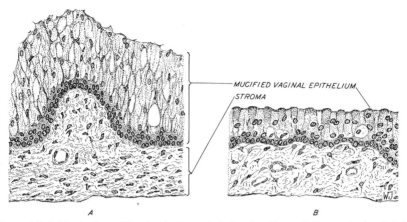

Figure 14–8. Vaginal mucification in the rat. *A,* Section through the vaginal wall taken on the seventeenth day of a normal pregnancy. *B,* Milder degree of mucification in a pseudopregnant rat.

the superficial layers. Characteristic changes take place in the vaginal epithelium of the rodent during pregnancy and pseudopregnancy (Fig. 14–8). Growth of the vaginal epithelium occurs during the follicular phase of the menstrual cycle, accompanied by the deposition of glycogen and mucopolysaccharides in this tissue. The vaginal smear of the estrous rodent contains large numbers of cornified epithelial cells with degenerate nuclei. Similar epithelial cells are exfoliated into the human vagina and are a reliable index of estrogenic action.

The Uterus

A striking effect of estrogens is the promotion of uterine growth. The frequency of endometrial mitoses during the follicular phase of the primate cycle can be correlated with the action of estrogens. Moreover, it is certain that estrogens have an effect on the tonicity of the uterine muscles. The uterus of the rat is highly contractile during estrus, whereas that of the untreated castrate is practically quiescent.

The uterus of the castrated rodent is an excellent target organ for determining the metabolic effects of estrogens (Fig. 14–9). Many experiments have been designed to determine the sequence of the biochemical changes in the uterus of the castrated rodent after the administration of estrogen. The end effect of estrogen treatment is increased weight and growth (hypertrophy and hyperplasia) of all uterine tissues, but these effects are preceded by various alterations in tissue composition and enzymatic activity. An early change in the uterus, occurring within an hour or so after estrogen administration, is an increased blood supply (hyperemia), associated with increased permeability of the uterine capillaries.[65] The hyperemia is accompanied by an augmented uptake of water and electrolytes by the uterine tissues. Within four hours, both aerobic and anaerobic glycolyses are

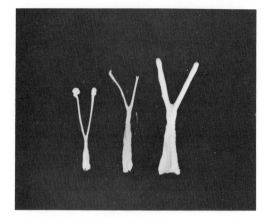

Figure 14–9. Photographs of female tracts of the rat dissected out *in toto. Left,* Tract from a normal animal killed at 20 days of age; *middle,* tract from an animal which was oöphorectomized at 18 days of age and autopsied six months later; *right,* a littermate control which was castrated at 18 days of age and killed six months later after receiving estrogen for 10 days before autopsy.

elevated. The weight of the uterus reaches a peak four to six hours after administration of the estrogen, but this is due almost entirely to the imbibition of water by the tissues.

The dry weight of the estrogen-treated uterus begins to increase by 12 hours, and there is a second wave of water imbibition occuring 20 to 24 hours after the injection. At this time, there is an accelerated incorporation of radioactivity from C^{14}-amino acids into the uterine tissues.[64] This second weight increase is correlated with cellular proliferation and the accumulation of uterine solids. The first increase in uterine weight can be prevented by administering adrenocorticotrophic hormone (ACTH) concurrently with the estrogen. Cortisol and cortisone have the same effect as ACTH. It is thus apparent that certain adrenal steroids antagonize the effects of estrogen on the uterus, possibly by counteracting the effect of estrogen on capillary permeability.

The ribonucleic acid (RNA) content of the uterus rises between 6 and 24 hours after the initial estrogen treatment, and in its wake there is accumulation of protein. Respiration, as well as glycolysis, is substantially increased by 20 hours. No increase in deoxyribonucleic acid (DNA) occurs during the first 24 hours but, if the hormonal stimulus is repeated, increases do occur between 40 and 72 hours. During the first six hours, there is an increase in phosphorylase *a* owing to the conversion of inactive phosphorylase *b* to *a,* but total phosphorylase remains practically unchanged. The total phosphorylase content of the uterus has increased substantially by 24 hours after the hormone stimulus, and by 48 hours the total phosphorylase has increased about 146 per cent, more phosphorylase *a* being formed. Correlated with these enzymic changes, a single injection of estrogen produces the highest concentration of uterine glycogen about 46 hours later.

There has been much interest in trying to account for the simultaneous occurrence of two or more estrogens within the body of an individual. Although no conclusive answer has been found, it is probable that the effects observed after the administration of a steroid hormone are not due solely to that compound but result also from the metabolites that may be formed from it within the system. Some estrogens are more effective than others in promoting the imbibition of fluid into the uterus; others are especially active in promoting true tissue growth. Estriol is the most effective natural estrogen in encouraging the uptake of water by the uterus after a single injection. It is especially effective in this respect when given in saline rather than oil; the activity of estrone and estradiol does not seem to be so dependent on the type of vehicle. For promoting the uptake of water by the rat uterus, the order of effectiveness is: estriol→estradiol-17β→estrone.[26]

In the normal organism the uterine response probably depends upon the combined actions of several estrogens working in concert; some are particularly effective in promoting specific regulations, and the action of one may be limited by that of another. Regulation of the female tract during the estrous and menstrual cycles, and during pregnancy, involves a multitude of intricate endocrine adjustments. The abundance of estriol in pregnant women and of equilin and equilenin in the pregnant mare strongly suggests that they are hormones of pregnancy and probably perform special roles during the course of gestation.

The Mammary Gland

The ovarian hormones are essential for the anatomic preparation of the mammary glands for milk secretion. There are many species variations in the effects of estrogen and progesterone on mammary development. In some species, estrogen alone produces only a lengthening and branching of the duct system; if given in large doses and over long periods, it may also induce the differentiation of mammary alveoli. In many species, progesterone alone produces only alveolar growth without having much effect on the duct system. As a general rule, the mammary glands require pretreatment with estrogen before the progestogens are effective.

Sexual Receptivity or Heat

In mammals exhibiting an estrous cycle, sexual receptivity typically coincides with estrus, a period during which the ovaries are secreting large amounts of estrogen. The ovarian hormones probably act through the central nervous system (hypothalamus) to condition the psychic manifestations such as increased spontaneous activity, lordosis, sexual receptivity, etc. Ovulation is the most important event of the female cycle, but it may occur without any manifestation of sexual receptivity. On the other hand, sexual receptivity may be induced at almost any period of the estrous cycle by giving exogenous estrogens, but this does not mean that ovulation has occurred. Ovulation is a consequence of the effects of pituitary gonadotrophins, whereas heat is the result of ovarian hormones acting upon the nervous system.

Full mating behavior generally depends upon both estrogen and progesterone. Estrogen injections alone induce sexual receptivity in the rat, but smaller quantities of estrogen are required if the female is pretreated with small amounts of progesterone. Psychic heat in the guinea pig, sheep, and many other species requires a trace of progesterone together with the estrogen.

The Effects of Relaxin

Marked *pelvic relaxation* occurs during late pregnancy in a number of mammals, including the human subject. At this time there is a separation of the symphysis pubis and, in some species, a loosening of the sacroiliac union. The pelvic bones become less rigid and the birth canal is enlarged, thus facilitating parturition. These pelvic modifications are brought about by relaxin operating in conjunction with other hormones, especially estrogens. The connective tissue of the symphysis increases in vascularity, and this is followed by the imbibition of water, disaggregation of the fibers, and depolymerization of the mucoproteins in the ground substance.

The mechanisms of softening and relaxation of the reproductive structures in preparation for parturition are complex phenomena and involve more than an effect of relaxin on connective tissue polymers. Some have postulated that estrogens act on the symphysis to convert cartilage into connective tissue, after which relaxin acts to depolymerize the connective tissue ground substance. More recent studies indicate that the biochemical mechanisms are quite involved and probably cannot be accounted for by such a simple hypothesis. In the guinea pig, without prior estrogen priming, relaxin has been found to stimulate the incorporation of glycine into the proteins of the symphysial connective tissue. This protein anabolic effect of relaxin is probably independent of the relaxation process.[23]

Relaxin exerts profound effects on the morphology, physiology, and biochemistry of the uterus. In ovariectomized, estrogen-primed rats, relaxin increases the glycogen concentration and water content of the uterus, as well as the dry weight and total nitrogen. Relaxin promotes water imbibition by the rat uterus, and this response does not require pretreatment with estrogen. Like estradiol, relaxin produces a high peak of water imbibition at six hours, but no secondary peak occurs later. Additive effects on water content of the uterus are obtained when both estradiol and relaxin are administered. Relaxin inhibits uterine motility both *in vivo* and *in vitro*. It also potentiates the action of progesterone in causing progestational proliferation in the rabbit uterus.

A marked dilatation of the uterine cervix of the sow occurs after relaxin administration.[76] As with the relaxation of the pubic symphysis of the guinea pig, the response requires pretreatment with estrogen. The dilatation and softening of the cervix facilitate parturition; they involve depolymerization of the ground substance and increased water content of the connective tissue. Relaxin also increases cervical dilatability in the spayed estrogen-primed rat. There are indications that relaxin may be useful in conditioning the uterine cervix of women prior to the induction of labor.

THE REPRODUCTIVE CYCLES

The cyclic alterations of the reproductive system are regulated by hormones from the anterior pituitary-gonadal axis. The hypothalamic portion of the brain appears to be the source of factors which pass through the portal veins to the adenohypophysis where they act to promote the differential release of hormones. Hypothalamic activity is conditioned to a large extent by external environmental stimuli and by the levels of steroid hormones in the circulation. The accessory sex organs and most of the secondary sex characters, as well as breeding behavior, are under the direct control of the gonadal hormones and the latter, in turn, is conditioned by the pituitary gonadotrophins.

The Estrous Cycle

The structural aspects of the estrous cycle have been very carefully determined for the common laboratory rodents and domestic mammals.[34] The effects of pituitary gonadotrophins on the ovaries and the effects of ovarian hormones on the accessory genitalia are fairly well established. The manner in which the various hormones interact to determine the cyclic events remains poorly understood. The gonadal and hypophysial hormones are most directly involved, but there is no doubt that the adrenal, thyroid, and other glands concerned with general metabolism exert indirect though important influences.[55]

Laboratory rats, mice, hamsters, and guinea pigs are polyestrous species that repeat their cycles throughout the year without much variation, unless interrupted by pregnancy or pseudopregnancy. Although ovulation is

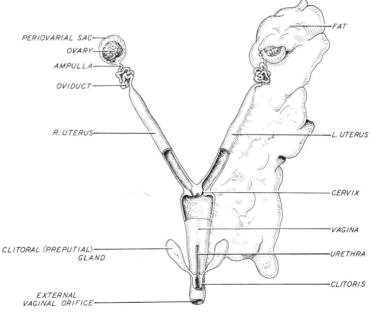

Figure 14–10. Female genital tract of a normal rat dissected out *in toto* and drawn from ventral view. The fat is removed from the right side. Portions of the uterine and vaginal walls are cut away in order to expose the cervices.

governed by a hypothalamic-pituitary mechanism whose final link to the pars distalis is neurohormonal, the process is "spontaneous" in these species. It is not dependent upon mating or some overt nervous stimulation as in reflexly ovulating species such as the rabbit. Eggs are normally released from the ovaries of these species during heat (estrus). Since the rat is used so extensively for the study of reproductive processes, its system will be described as exemplifying a simple estrous cycle (Fig. 14–10).

Rats

The estrous cycle of the rat is completed in four to five days, although the timing of the cycle may be influenced by exteroceptive factors such as light, temperature, nutritional status, and social relationships. In species having such short cycles, the ovaries contain follicles in various stages of formation, as well as corpora lutea of several past estrous cycles. The cycle is roughly divisible into four stages:

1. Estrus. This is the period of heat, and copulation is permitted only at this time. This condition lasts from 9 to 15 hours and is characterized by a high rate of running activity. Under the influence of follicle-stimulating hormone (FSH), a dozen or more ovarian follicles grow rapidly; estrus is thus a period of heightened estrogen secretion. Behavioral changes include quivering of the ears and lordosis, or arching the back in response to handling or to approaches by the male. The uteri undergo progressive enlargement and become distended owing to the accumulation of luminal fluid (Fig. 14–11). Many mitoses occur in the vaginal mucosa and, as new cells accumulate, the superficial layers become squamous and cornified. The latter cells are exfoliated into the vaginal lumen, and their presence in *vaginal smears* is indicative of estrus (Fig. 14–12). During late estrus, there are

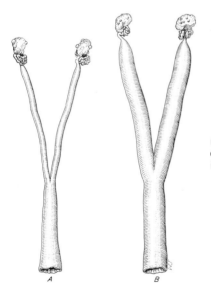

Figure 14–11. Normal female genitalia of adult rats dissected out *in toto* during diestrus *(A)* and proestrus *(B)*. Compare the sizes of the uteri and vaginas in the two instances. (The drawings are to scale.)

A   B

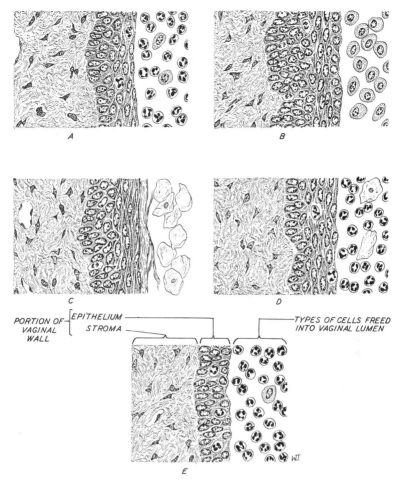

Figure 14–12. Sections through the vaginal wall of the rat during different stages of the estrous cycle, showing the corresponding types of cells which appear in smears obtained from the vaginal lumen. *A,* Diestrus; *B,* proestrus; *C,* estrus; *D,* metestrus; *E,* adult animal which had been oöphorectomized for six months.

cheesy masses of cornified cells with degenerate nuclei present in the vaginal lumen, but few if any leukocytes are found during estrus. Ovulation occurs during estrus and is preceded by histologic changes in the follicle suggestive of early luteinization. Much of the luminal fluid in the uteri is lost before ovulation.

2. Metestrus. This occurs shortly after ovulation and is intermediate between estrus and diestrus. The period lasts for 10 to 14 hours and mating is usually not permitted. The ovaries contain corpora lutea and small follicles, and the uteri have diminished in vascularity and contractility. Many leukocytes appear in the vaginal lumen along with a few cornified cells.

3. Diestrus. This lasts 60 to 70 hours, during which functional regression of the corpora lutea occurs. The uteri are small, anemic, and only slightly contractile. The vaginal mucosa is thin, and leukocytes migrate through it, giving a vaginal smear consisting almost entirely of these cells (Fig. 14–12).

4. Proestrus. This heralds the next heat and is characterized by functional involution of the corpora lutea and preovulatory swelling of the follicles. Fluid collects in the uteri and they become highly contractile. The vaginal smear is dominated by nucleated epithelial cells, which occur singly or in sheets.

In case pregnancy occurs, the cycles are interrupted for the duration of gestation, which lasts for 20 to 22 days in the rat. The animal comes into estrus at the end of pregnancy, but the cycles are again delayed until the termination of lactation.[28]

Pseudopregnancy may be induced in many laboratory mammals by procedures that prolong the secretory function of the corpora lutea of ovulation, thus holding in abeyance the onset of the next estrus. In mammals such as rats and mice, which have short estrous cycles, the luteal phase of the ovary is so abbreviated that the uteri do not undergo the extensive progestational changes generally associated wth progesterone action. Pseudopregnancy in rats and mice may be induced by stimulating the cervix of the estrous animal with a glass rod or other mechanical means, by electrical stimulation, or by mating with a sterile male. The condition has also been produced in rodents by stimulation of the nipples, by adrenalectomy, by irritating the nasal mucosa with silver nitrate, and by experimentally manipulating the steroid hormone balance of the organism. The onset of the next estrus is delayed for about 13 days; the corpora lutea remain functional during this time, and the endometrial changes simulate those of normal pregnancy. Except for the fact that there are no developing young in the uteri, the endocrine balance is very similar to true pregnancy. Stimulation of the cervix at estrus by mechanical or electrical means does not result in pseudopregnancy if the animals are under deep anesthesia when these procedures are applied. Neither do they become pseudopregnant after the nerve supply to the uterus is destroyed. These facts indicate that neural mechanisms are involved. It is probable that cervical stimulation elicits afferent nerve impulses that reach the hypothalamus and promote the release of agents that are conveyed via the hypophysial portal venules to the anterior pituitary. The latter organ then discharges hormones that are essential for prolonging the functional life of the corpora lutea. These neuroendocrine adjustments cause the corpora lutea of the last ovulation to persist and function well beyond the time when they would ordinarily have regressed.

In most species, pseudopregnancy lasts for about half the length of time required for a normal pregnancy. The pseudopregnant state may be prolonged by administering estrogens or by traumatizing the uterus to produce deciduomas. The latter are growths that develop in the estrogen-progesterone–conditioned uterus in response to trauma and represent an attempt of the uterus to form the maternal placenta in the absence of implanting blastocysts (Fig. 14–13). The corpora lutea of pseudopregnancy maintain the uterus in a state capable of receiving blastocysts, and conspicuous proliferation of the mammary glands occurs. The mammary glands of the pseudopregnant bitch may actually lactate. Nest building and retrieving of foster young are often noted in pseudopregnant rats and mice.

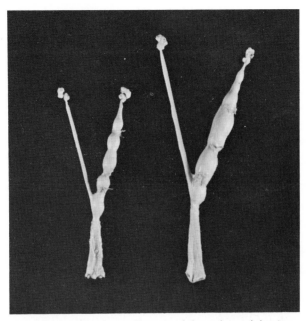

Figure 14–13. Deciduomas in the rat. Trauma of the guinea pig's uterus during the luteal phase of the normal cycle results in the formation of the maternal aspect of the placenta (deciduoma). In the rat, however, the luteal phase is short, and pseudopregnant animals are used for producing the same reaction. Pseudopregnancy in the rat is induced by mechanical stimulation of the cervix at estrus; two or three days later, the uterus is traumatized by sutures or other procedures. The tract on the left was removed three days after uterine trauma; the one on the right was removed four days after trauma. Only the left uteri were traumatized. The deciduomas are the swellings around the sutures.

Endocrine Regulation of the Cycle. Although the reproductive cycles are governed by the interplay of pituitary and gonadal hormones, the picture is far from complete and only a general outline can be given here. According to current concepts, a feedback mechanism operates whereby the pituitary release of FSH and LH is controlled by the levels of estrogen and progesterone in the circulation. It is not known what factors are originally responsible for the activation of the pituitary-ovarian axis, but it has been postulated that very low levels of estrogens, coming from the immature follicles or extragonadal sources, may stimulate the pituitary to augment its release of FSH. Significant production of estrogen by the follicle apparently requires both FSH and LH. When the level of estrogen in the blood becomes high, indicating that the ovarian follicles are full-grown, it acts to prevent a greater release of FSH by the hypophysis and to promote an augmented release of LH. Under the influence of rising titers of LH, preovulatory swelling ensues and definite lutein changes occur in the walls of the mature follicles. The preovulatory follicle undoubtedly secretes some progesterone as well as large quantities of estrogens. Ovulation occurs while LH is in ascendancy, and there is an immediate fall in the circulating estrogens after ovulation. The ruptured follicle becomes transformed into a corpus luteum, which becomes functional under the influence of prolactin. The discharge of LH from the anterior lobe seems to be inhibited by rising titers of progesterone.

The corpora lutea remain functional for only a short period unless pregnancy or pseudopregnancy supervenes, but the ovaries of cyclic rats always contain several sets of corpora lutea in different stages of disintegration. Changes in the ovaries must be regarded as resulting from the interaction of the gonadotrophins and changes in the sex accessories as consequences of the interaction of the various ovarian hormones.

There is ample evidence that in many mammalian species the secretion of progesterone by the follicle begins before ovulation has occurred, during the period of preovulatory swelling. Even in species that ovulate spontaneously, it is an interesting fact that sexual receptivity precedes ovulation. In the cow ovulation is spontaneous, but it does not occur until 13 to 15 hours after the end of heat. The secretion of progesterone by the ovarian follicles of the rat, guinea pig, and perhaps other species probably coincides with the onset of sexual receptivity.

The uteri of the rat become quite small and anemic during diestrus, indicating that while the corpora lutea persist they secrete progesterone only for a brief time in the reproductive cycle. When pregnancy or pseudopregnancy follows a period of estrus, the corpora lutea remain functional much longer, probably owing to the action of prolactin. The progestational changes in rats and mice are much less extensive than those that occur in the uteri of such forms as the rabbit. However, the progestational uteri, conditioned by estrogen plus progesterone, are equally sensitive to implanting blastocysts or to endometrial trauma.

Dogs

Another type of estrous cycle is illustrated by the dog. Ovulation is spontaneous, and there are generally two estrous periods per year; in smaller breeds, they may occur more frequently. Proestrus lasts for about 10 days, and this is followed by estrus, which lasts from six to 10 days. Ovulation typically occurs during early estrus, and copulations may be permitted for six to eight days thereafter. Loss of blood occurs through the vagina during proestrus and not infrequently extends throughout estrus. This blood arises from the uterus by diapedesis, rather than through disintegration of the endometrial surface, and is in no way comparable to menstruation. Each estrus is followed by a functional luteal phase lasting approximately 60 days: a fertile mating leads to pregnancy; an infertile mating, or no mating, is followed by pseudopregnancy. During pseudopregnancy, the reproductive tract and mammary glands are developed much as in normal pregnancy. A brief period of milk secretion may be noted, even though the animal is not pregnant.

Rabbits

Certain species, such as rabbits, ferrets, cats, etc., are often called "induced ovulators" because eggs are not released from the ovaries except

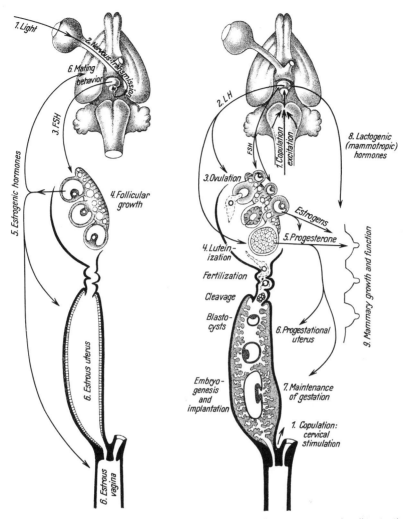

Figure 14–14. Reproduction in the rabbit. Left: Reaction sequences leading to the estrus condition. Right: Reaction sequences following mating. (From Witschi, E.: *Development of Vertebrates,* W. B. Saunders, Co., 1956.)

after coitus or some comparable cervical stimulation. Although there may be slight fluctuations in the degree of sexual receptivity, the adult nonpregnant domestic rabbit is in a constant state of estrus. On the other hand, the ovaries of wild rabbits are inactive in winter, but enlarge in spring following the perception of increasing day length. The sequence of endocrine events in this case is represented in the first diagram of Figure 14–14. In both wild and domestic rabbits, cervical stimulation occurring during mating elicits the chain of events indicated in the second diagram of Figure 14–14. The ovaries contain follicles in all stages of development and atresia, but corpora lutea of ovulation are absent. Full development (progestational proliferation) of the uterus, characteristic of pregnancy and pseudopregnancy, requires both estrogen and progesterone.[9] Pseudopregnancy, lasting about 18 days, may be induced by sterile matings. Although estrous cats may be caused to ovulate by stimulating the cervices with a glass rod, this procedure is generally ineffective in the rabbit unless the animals are given special hormone treatments. The duration of pregnancy in the rabbit is 31 to 32 days. Comparable mechanisms operate in both spontaneous and induced ovulators: Rupture of the follicles is conditioned by the action of ovarian steroids and also by a discharge from sex centers in the hypothalamus. Coital stimulation does not induce ovulation in the hypophysectomized animal. If the pituitary is removed within 1 hour after coitus, or the pituitary stalk is sectioned during this time, ovulations do not occur. Ovulations proceed normally if the pituitary is removed later than one hour after the mating stimulus. The mechanism of ovulation is discussed later in this chapter.

The Menstrual Cycle

Menstrual cycles are characteristic of primates and do not occur in other vertebrate groups. The length of the cycle is highly variable, though 28 days is generally regarded as typical for women. The cycle in the chimpanzee requires about 35 days. Both estrous and menstrual cycles are regulated by the same interplay of pituitary and ovarian hormones, and the effects of the ovarian hormones on the reproductive tract are comparable in most respects. The chief differences between the two types of cycles are the presence of a menstrual phase in primates and the spreading of sexual receptivity throughout the cycle, rather than the limitation of it to a definite period. During the menstrual phase the superficial layers of the endometrium are sloughed with accompanying bleeding; this type of bleeding does not occur in nonprimates. Spiral arteries are absent from the uteri of estrous mammals but are present in primates with the exception of the New World monkeys. The latter animals menstruate, but the loss of blood is greatly reduced.

The menstrual phase, lasting four to seven days, is regarded as the beginning of the primate cycle. This arrangement is sanctioned because menstruation is the easiest period of the cycle to recognize and because it corresponds with the formation of new follicles in the ovaries (Fig. 14–15). However, if the uterus alone is considered, menstruation represents the terminal event: with subsidence of the corpus luteum and a consequent deficiency of ovarian hormones, the endometrium cannot maintain itself and hence regresses and the surface disintegrates.

Four phases of the menstrual cycle are usually distinguished: the menstrual, proliferative (follicular), ovulatory, and progestational (luteal). The *proliferative phase* is conditioned by estrogen and extends from the end of menstruation to ovulation, the latter occurring near the middle of the cycle. At the end of menstrual disintegration, the endometrium is thin and poorly vascularized, and only the basal parts of the endometrial glands remain. The endometrium thickens as the estrogen titers rise, and the glandular and vascular patterns are restored.

No conspicuous changes occur in the endometrium during the *ovulatory process.* Cyclic variations in the body temperature of the human female

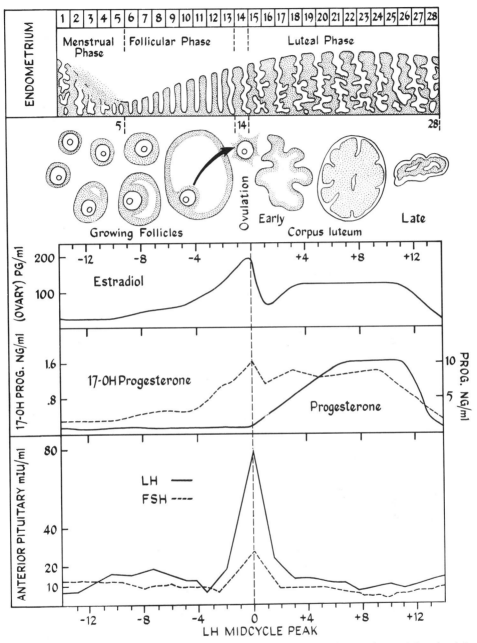

Figure 14–15. Diagram showing changes in the endometrium, the ovaries, and the circulating ovarian hormones during the menstrual cycle.

correlate with menstrual changes. A distinct rise in basal body temperature occurs at ovulation and remains high until the onset of the next menstrual period. The changing titers of hormones during the menstrual cycle apparently account for the temperature fluctuations.

During the *progestational phase* the uterus is under the influence of both estrogens and progestogens, and the endometrium differentiates into a tissue that can fulfill the requirements of an embryo ready to implant. The stroma becomes highly vascularized and edematous, the mucosa is thicker, and the glands develop corkscrew and serrate features. The progestational endometrium, normally requiring both estrogens and progesterone, is the only type of structure in which blastocysts can readily implant and develop normally. If implantation has not occurred, the corpus luteum diminishes in function, and degenerative changes are observable in the endometrium. Predecidual cells form solid sheaths below the surface epithelium, leukocytes invade the tissue, necrotic changes occur in the stroma, and the uterine glands involute. With menstruation, the outer portion of the endometrium is lost, and there is bleeding into the uterine cavity.

Endocrine Interactions

At the beginning of menstruation the inhibitory influence of the corpus luteum on the pituitary is removed and FSH is secreted in increasing amounts. This stimulates the growth of the young follicles and, as they grow, they release increasing quantities of estrogens. The high estrogen content of the blood causes the pituitary to diminish its production of FSH and increase the output of LH. Ovulation occurs when the balance between FSH and LH has swung sufficiently in favor of the latter hormone. There is evidence that small amounts of progesterone are produced by the preovulatory follicle, and this hormone may be involved in the ovulatory process, perhaps through its action on the brain or the anterior hypophysis. After ovulation, the corpus luteum begins to form in the ruptured follicle under the influence of LH.

Gonadotrophins activate the corpus luteum and cause it to secrete progesterone and small amounts of estrogen. If a fertilized egg is not produced, functional degeneration of the corpus luteum begins eight to 10 days after ovulation. The onset of menstrual bleeding correlates with the withdrawal of progesterone and, to a lesser extent, of estrogen from the circulation (Fig. 14–15). The factors immediately involved in the breakdown of the endometrial blood vessels with subsequent bleeding remain largely unknown.

If the egg is fertilized, the pituitary continues to release luteinizing hormone, and the corpus luteum increases in size and augments its output of hormones. Secretory competence of the corpus luteum diminishes slowly after the fourth month of pregnancy, although it remains structurally intact until the end of pregnancy. The placenta, rather than the ovary, is the principal source of progesterone and estrogen during the latter half of pregnancy. Removal of the ovaries after midpregnancy neither terminates pregnancy nor diminishes the levels of the two types of steroid hormones in the circulation.

Oral Contraception

Use of the interactions of estrogen, progesterone, and the gonadotrophins has found important applications in the development of the anti-ovulation oral contraception pill. Such pills employ synthetic estrogens and progestogens which simulate the anti-LH activity of the normal steroids during the menstrual cycle. Thus, ovulation is prevented through the action of these compounds in the inhibition of LH secretion. The usual scheme for oral contraception employs a "combination pill" which contains both an estrogen and a progestogen. A second scheme involves a sequential regimen of estrogen followed by progestogen. The sequential scheme more closely resembles the hormonal sequence of a normal menstrual cycle, but has the disadvantage of employing two different pills. In either scheme menstruation is induced by cessation of steroid intake and is terminated by the resumption of steroid ingestion. Thus, the patterns of hormone secretion in the normal menstrual cycle are mimicked. The use of such steroids in regimens of this type has noteworthy side effects, and they are under constant scrutiny because of possible carcinogenic activity.

The Mechanism of Ovulation

Ovulation has been observed and studied in a variety of mammals, birds, and amphibians. The indications are that the process is initiated by a neural mechanism in the hypothalamus that releases pituitary gonadotrophins at the proper time. The ovulation-inducing hormone (OIH) is thought to be principally LH, but the exact manner in which it brings about rupture of the ovarian follicle is not understood. The administration of a combination of highly purified FSH and LH to immature rats 7 to 100 days after hypophysectomy induces ovulation and the formation of corpora lutea. Neither hormone is effective when given alone, and this is strong evidence that both FSH and LH are involved in ovulation and luteinization.[11, 57] All of the available evidence indicates that the pituitary starts to release OIH very quickly, in a matter of minutes, after application of the neurogenic stimulus. Furthermore, it seems that OIH does not need to act on the ovarian follicle for long periods. It probably acts on the follicular wall rather quickly, producing subtle changes that remain microscopically hidden until just before rupture. If the frog is pretreated with pituitary gonadotrophins, the excised ovaries ovulate in the absence of vascular and nervous connections. The ovarian follicle of the hen, previously subjected to pituitary gonadotrophins, ovulates normally even after the stalk that attaches it to the ovary is sectioned or clamped off in such a manner as to eliminate nervous and vascular supplies.

It does not appear likely that increased intrafollicular tension, arising through the accumulation of fluid in the antrum, is the immediate cause of rupture of the mammalian follicle. Ovarian cysts occur commonly in pathologic ovaries, and in these follicles there is a tremendous increase in liquor folliculi, yet they do not rupture. In all species that have been studied, ovulation is found to occur as a slow oozing rather than as an explosive process. The preovulatory follicles of swine, cattle, and sheep lose follicular fluid before any break in the follicular wall can be detected. In certain species of bats, there is a tremendous hypertrophy of the cumulus oöphorus and, just before ovulation, the antrum is reduced to a mere slit.

Since the fimbriated ends of the oviducts become very active at the time of ovulation, it was formerly believed that they might promote ovulation by a massaging action on the ovaries. It has been shown that ovulations occur normally in the pig, fowl, and other species after surgical removal of the oviducts. Ovulation in several species may be accomplished when the ovaries are maintained *in vitro*. The modern view is that certain hypothalamic areas signal the anterior hypophysis in some manner and promote the release of OIH, which initiates a series of changes in the follicular wall leading to its eventual rupture.

Ovulation in Mammals

Ovulation in mammals appears to depend upon a neural stimulus that leads to a brief surge of pituitary gonadotrophin. The use of radioimmunoassay techniques in the rat indicates that there is a marked and comparatively brief rise in both LH and FSH just before ovulation. In the rat, the surge of OIH is controlled by a biologic clock having a circadian rhythm, but it is not known whether this is true for other mammals as well. Much interest is presently focused on the high catecholamine content of the median eminence and on the possible role of these neural products in the discharge of *releasing factors* which control the pituitary gonadotrophins.[12, 50, 54]

Induced ovulators, such as the rabbit, ferret, cat, and mink, require coitus or some comparable stimulus for ovulation to occur (Fig. 14–14). There are strong indications that participation in coitus leads to a reflexive stimulation of the pituitary gland and a consequent discharge of OIH. The rabbit hypophysis releases enough OIH within 1 hour after coitus to cause ovulation. A similar neural mechanism appears to be involved in the rat when it is induced to become pseudopregnant by artificial stimulation of the cervices. Although this species ovulates spontaneously, the corpora lutea of ovulation do not remain functional in the absence of pregnancy unless a cervical stimulus is applied before the corpora lutea become nonfunctional. Segregated female rats of certain strains show a tendency to exhibit persistent estrus. If such females accept coitus or receive small injections of progesterone, ovulation and the recurrence of cycles may follow. These procedures apparently act directly or indirectly via the nervous system to cause the pituitary release of OIH.

Direct electrical stimulation of the pituitary gland of the anesthetized rabbit does not induce ovulation unless there are indications that the stimulus has spread to the hypothalamic region. Lower voltages applied directly to the hypothalamus do induce ovulation. Stimulation of the hypothalamus of the unanesthetized rabbit, for only 3 minutes by the remote control method, results in ovulation; similar stimuli applied directly to the anterior pituitary for periods up to 7 hours do not result in ovulation. These and other studies make it apparent that the hypothalamic portion of the brain is intimately involved in the pituitary release of OIH.[24, 53]

Very careful studies have been made of inbred strains of rats kept under strictly controlled environments.[18, 27] Some strains ovulate at four-day intervals and others at five-day intervals. Under these controlled conditions ovulations occur between 1 and 2 A.M. The five-day cycle may be shortened to four days by injecting estrogen on the second day or progesterone on the third day of diestrus. In other words, these treatments advance the time of ovulation by 24 hours. The capacity of progesterone to cause early ovulation can be blocked by the administration of either dibenamine (antiadrenergic) or atropine (anticholinergic). A study of the effects of atropine blockade at intervals after the administration of progesterone on the third day of diestrus has shown that pituitary release of OIH does not occur until 2 P.M. no matter how early the progesterone is administered. Furthermore, ovulation in normal cyclic animals may be blocked by dibenamine or atropine if administered before 2 P.M. on the day of proestrus. If the drugs are administered after 4 P.M. on this day, ovulations occur as usual early the next morning. The conclusion is that in rats, under controlled conditions, the release of pituitary OIH is triggered by a neurohumoral mechanism on the day of proestrus between 2 and 4 P.M., 10 to 12 hours before ovulation occurs.

If the rats are kept under moderate barbiturate anesthesia during the critical hours (2 to 4 P.M.) on the day of proestrus, ovulation is prevented and activation of the pituitary is delayed for a full day. The graafian follicles persist when this treatment is applied for several days at the same hours, but, if the anesthesia is withheld until 4 P.M. on any day, ovulations will occur during the night. The follicles that are prevented from ovulating by barbiturate anesthesia for several days undergo atresia about two days before the beginning of the next proestrus.

It is possible to surgically remove ova ("ovectomy") from the mature follicles of rabbits and pigs. Follicles deprived of their ova promptly luteinize and form a structure histologically indistinguishable from the corpus luteum; this remains functional for only 4 days and then degenerates. When only one follicle in an ovary is ovectomized, it luteinizes but neighboring vesicular follicles are not induced to do so. This indicates that the follicles possess considerable autonomy. It also suggests that the ova of mature follicles may be the source of an agent, presumably freed into the liquor folliculi, which prevents the granulosa from undergoing luteinization. Individual follicles of the estrous rabbit can be induced to ovulate by injecting into them minute amounts of LH. The treated follicle ovulates 10 hours later and forms a corpus luteum which persists for the full period of pseudopregnancy. Here again, untreated follicles in the same ovary do not respond.[40]

In both the rat and rabbit, ovulations occur about 10 hours after the anterior pituitary releases OIH. It thus appears that in both spontaneous ovulators (rat) and induced ovulators (rabbit) the ovulatory process involves the action of ovarian hormones and the release of transmitter substances from certain neurons in the hypothalamus. In the rabbit, the hypothalamic area is apparently stimulated by the act of copulation or, in some instances, by psychic stimuli without actual mating. In the rat, on the other hand, the hypothalamic center either discharges at a particular time of the day because of its own inherent rhythmicity or is regulated by some nervous mechanism that has diurnal rhythm.

In summary, most workers who have studied ovulation in mammals feel that a neuroendocrine mechanism is involved in species that ovulate spontaneously (rat), as well as in those that ovulate reflexively (rabbit). Current concepts may be summarized as follows: (1) Ovulation is controlled by both the hypothalamus and the pituitary gland; hence the mechanism is both neural and hormonal. The final link to the adenohypophysis involves neurohormonal agents which travel via the hypophysial portal vessels, causing the pituitary to release OIH. (2) The hypothalamus contains one or more centers that are stimulated or inhibited by circulating estrogens and progestogens, as well as by afferent nerve impulses of various kinds. (3) The ovarian steroids may influence the ovulatory process by modifying thresholds in the nervous system. (4) Some, if not all, mammalian species possess potential mechanisms which subserve both reflexive and spontaneous ovulation.

Ovulation in Birds

The domestic fowl is a very suitable form for studying the ovulatory process.[16] The hen's ovary produces eggs in clutches, and a single egg is oviposited at daily intervals. Under conditions of natural illumination, ovulation usually occurs in the morning and seldom takes place after 3 P.M. It requires 25 to 26 hours for the egg to traverse the oviduct, most of this time being spent in the shell gland. Ovulation of the next egg occurs 30 to 60 minutes after the previous one is laid. Since the time required for egg formation is greater than 24 hours, oviposition will occur a little later each day. When this lag brings the time of oviposition to late afternoon, laying is held in abeyance for several days, after which ovulations begin anew from the early morning.

Multiple steroid hormones are required for the functional development of the avian oviduct. Full development of the magnum, the region of the oviduct that secretes the albumin around the ovum, can be produced by giving estrogen followed by either androgen or progesterone. Estrogen alone induces differentiation of the cells which synthesize egg white proteins, such as ovalbumin and lysozyme; progesterone then effectively induces the secretion of another protein, avidin, from a different cell type.[32] When the organ has been built up by the proper steroid hormones, the actual secretion of albumin occurs in response to any foreign body in the oviduct. Ovulation does not generally occur while there is an egg in any part of the oviduct. The presence of an irritant in the magnum, such as a loop of thread, completely prevents ovulation in the great majority of laying hens. It is probable that the suture in the magnum neurogenically inhibits the release of ovulating hormone from the hen's anterior pituitary, and ovulation of the next ovum in the series cannot occur.

For hens to lay 365 eggs in a year, as they sometimes do, a rather vigorous metabolism of calcium must be required. The shell gland differs from the

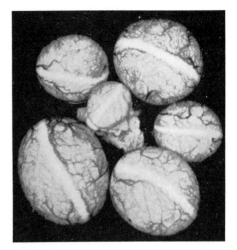

Figure 14–16. Mature follicles of the domestic fowl, treated to show the stigma, or cicatrix. (From Fraps, R. M.: *In* J. Hammond, (ed.): Progress in Physiology of Farm Animals, vol. 2. London, Butterworth & Co., 1955.)

other parts of the oviduct inasmuch as estrogen alone is sufficient for its development. Hypercalcemia and lipemia are characteristic of laying hens and may be produced in males or nonlaying females by the administration of estrogens. The medullary bone of laying birds undergoes sequences of deposition and destruction that correlate with the storage and liberation of calcium. Laying soon ceases when calcium is withheld from the diet. It is not known how estrogen acts to promote both the deposition of calcium in bone and its withdrawl from bone.

The process of ovulation in the bird is easily observed. During the period of rapid growth, the future site of follicular rupture, the stigma, may be observed as a light band extending across the hemisphere opposite to the stalked attachment (Fig. 14–16). Just before rupture of the follicle, the stigma appears to widen owing to the blurring of blood vessels that extend into it. Rupture usually begins at one pole of the stigma and extends rapidly to the opposite pole, freeing the ovum almost immediately. The ruptured follicle, or calyx, persists and, together with the most mature follicle, performs a role in the timing of oviposition. If the calyx is surgically removed, the egg that originated from it is held in the shell gland for an abnormally long period.

The pituitary principle responsible for ovulation in birds is believed to be LH, or a gonadotrophin similar to it, and this is released some 6 to 8 hours before the next ovulation. The administration of mammalian LH to intact laying hens hastens the release of the mature follicle destined to ovulate next, but this treatment never provokes the ovulation of any of the smaller follicles in the ovary. Ovulation does not occur in the laying hen if the pituitary is removed 10 hours before the expected event. If a laying hen is hypophysectomized and injected promptly with LH, not only the largest follicle but also several of the smaller ones are ovulated and passed into the oviduct. Since this cannot be duplicated in animals with intact hypophyses, it appears that the pituitary is the source of a substance which inhibits the ovulation of immature ova. If the hypophysectomized hen is first given FSH, immediately after the operation, the subsequent administration of LH causes only the largest follicle to ovulate. Thus, it appears that FSH inhibits the ovulation of all follicles except the one which is largest and most mature.[41, 42]

Ovulation and Vitellogenesis in Amphibians[17]

The homoimplantation of pituitary glands in various species of amphibians causes ovulation in the female and spermiation in the male. These two processes are quite comparable since the sustentacular cells (Sertoli cells) of the testis are homologous with the granulosa cells of the ovary. Spermiation may also be induced in *Bufo, Xenopus,* and certain common frogs by small amounts of pregnancy urine, a reaction that is frequently used as a test for pregnancy. Ovulation may also be induced by human pregnancy urine, but it is a much less sensitive reaction than spermiation.

Generally, amphibians are seasonal breeders whose annual cycles are regulated by the perception of external cues leading to the production or release of gonadotrophic hormones. Most of the evidence suggests that luteinizing hormone (LH) is the chief ovulation hormone, but FSH and ACTH, as well as gonadal hormones, probably cooperate with it in the intact animal (Fig. 14–17). Hypophysectomized frogs and toads do not ovulate, though they may be caused to do so by homoimplanting pituitaries into the coelomic cavity or under the skin shortly after the pituitary is removed. Some workers have found that hypophysectomy has a sensitizing effect, a smaller dose of pituitary extract being required to bring about ovulation than is required in intact animals. This effect is probably explained by the

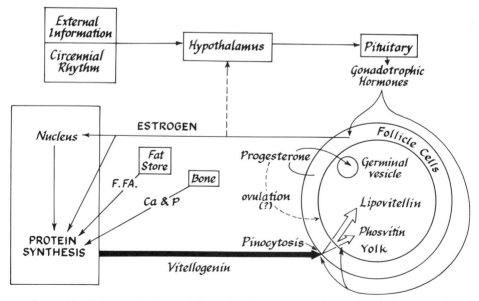

Figure 14–17. General scheme of the major relationships between the pituitary gonadotrophins and the amphibian ovary in the seasonal events of vitellogenesis and ovulation. (Modified from Follett *et al.,* 1968, and Redshaw, 1972.)

escape of hypophysial hormones into the circulation during surgical manipulation of the hypophysis. Ovulation may be induced in nonbreeding *Rana temporaria* merely by exposing the hypophysis and crushing it *in situ.* This indicates that the pituitary contains sufficient LH during the nonbreeding season but does not release it. On the other hand, newer evidence indicates that pituitary LH levels are high only during or near the breeding season. It is striking that pieces of ovaries from mature animals ovulate *in vitro* when treated with dilute suspensions of pituitary tissue.

Ovulation has been observed to occur in the following manner. It is a dual process involving rupture of the follicle and emergence of the egg. Follicular rupture is not a cataclysmic process but is completed in approximately 1 minute at laboratory temperatures. Under similar conditions the emergence of the egg requires from 4 to 10 minutes. The initial break in the follicular wall is small at first, but rapidly enlarges until the whole rupture area is involved. After rupture, there is no leakage of follicular fluid, as in mammals. There is no preovulatory growth or any other visible change within the follicle that can be regarded as signifying an impending rupture. After the rupture area has given way, the smooth musculature of the cyst wall contracts and gradually squeezes the egg through the relatively small opening. After the egg has been discharged, the follicle closes and the original rupture lines are drawn together. The follicle cells lying next to the vitelline membrane do not escape with the ovum but remain within the collapsed follicle. Around the postovulatory follicle may be observed an accumulation of spindle-shaped cells, presumably relaxed smooth muscle cells derived from the cyst wall of the follicle.

In sexually inactive frogs slitting of the rupture area by a lancet leads only to incomplete ovulation; the follicular muscles are able to force the egg only partially through the aperture. Electrical and mechanical stimuli applied directly to the musculature of the follicle do not cause a breaking away of the rupture area. However, after rupture has occurred, the application of these stimuli does cause the egg to emerge more rapidly than normally. Escape of the egg through the open rupture area is clearly due to the hormonal activation of the smooth musculature in the wall of the follicle itself. The breaking of the rupture area is likewise conditioned by hormonal agents.

The ovulation of frogs' eggs *in vitro* in response to pituitary extracts may be enhanced by addition of certain steroids, including androgens, progestogens, and adrenal corticoids. Some of the nonestrogenic steroids induce ovulation *in vitro* in the absence of pituitary factors. Progesterone is one of the most effective steroids tested. It has been suggested that in amphibians the pituitary gonadotrophins may stimulate the ovaries to produce steroidal hormones, the latter acting directly on the ovarian follicles to induce ovulation.[73]

In vitro observations on *Rana pipiens* indicate that pituitary gonadotrophins act on the follicle cells of ripe oocytes, causing such cells to secrete a progesterone-like hormone which provokes the maturation divisions in the enclosed oocytes. In anurans, the maturation division occurs just before ovulation and, after ovulation, the eggs receive a protective coat of jelly from the oviducal glands.[38] It has been reported in the toad that a progesto-gen (probably progesterone) is released by the ovarian follicle about 12 hours before ovulation, and this hormone appears to evoke both oocyte maturation and jelly release from the oviducts.[68] It appears that progesterone does not act directly in inducing oocyte maturation, but does so through the production of a cytoplasmic maturation promoting factor (MPF).[39] Apparently, progesterone acts at the cell surface to induce the formation of MPF, for *in ovo* injection of progesterone fails to bring about maturation. Whether or not the events of egg maturation and ovulation are interrelated but separate actions of progesterone is not yet clear; however, there is some evidence that the two processes may be temporally dissociated.[19]

In addition to their roles in oocyte maturation and ovulation, pituitary gonadotrophins play a dual role in vitellogenesis (Fig. 14–17). They first activate the follicle cells to produce estrogen, which promotes the elaboration of vitellogenin by the liver.[70] At the level of the oocyte, gonadotrophins stimulate the uptake of vitellogenin by a process of micropinocytosis. Once in the oocyte, lipovitellin is converted to the yolk proteins lipovitellin and phosvitin, which are subsequently incorporated into the yolk platelets.

The Progestogens and Decidual Reactions

The classic experiments of Loeb demonstrated that decidual responses in the uterus could be elicited experimentally only after luteinization of the ovary. Loeb's work provided the first experimental evidence that the corpora lutea perform a secretory function. He permitted estrous guinea pigs to copulate with vasectomized males. Several days later, when implantation would have occurred normally, glass beads were inserted into the uteri. He observed that overgrowths of uterine cells occurred around the beads and recognized that the beads, by simulating implanting blastocysts, had induced the uterus to begin the differentiation of the maternal portion of the placenta. These tumorous responses of the progestational endometrium to trauma are called *deciduomas* or placentomas (Fig. 14–18). In the guinea pig the luteal phase of the normal cycle is long enough to permit the production of deciduomas without bringing the animal into a state of pseudo-pregnancy.

It is interesting to note that in animals with normal cycles the period when deciduomas can be elicited corresponds to the time when nidation of the blastocysts would occur. The reaction results also from traumatization of the uterus during early pregnancy and the first half of lactation. In the intact animal the essential requisite is the production of traumatic injury to a uterus that has been acted upon first by estrogen and subsequently by progesterone. Extremely large doses of progesterone administered to the ovariectomized animal sensitize the uterus for the production of deciduomas, but much smaller amounts of the luteal hormone are effective in this respect if pretreatment with estrogen is made. Endometrial proliferations have been produced in the monkey by mechanically traumatizing the progestational uterus at the proper time. These traumatic responses in the pri-

mate differ from Loeb's decidual reactions inasmuch as the growths originate from the epithelium rather than from the stroma.

Though it is impossible to produce deciduomas during the normal four-
or five-day cycle of the rat, it becomes possible to do so when the functional lives of the corpora lutea are prolonged by pseudopregnancy resulting from either sterile copulation or mechanical stimulation of the cervices,
or from the application of suckling stimuli to the nipples. Although pseudopregnancy in the rat normally lasts about 13 days, it can be extended to the
length of a normal pregnancy (20 to 22 days) by inducing deciduomas in the
uterus. Furthermore, the extended length of the pseudopregnancy is proportional to the number of deciduomas induced in the uteri.

After traumatization of the endometrium, the first reaction is the proliferation of decidual cells in the subepithelial region of the stroma. These
cells grow and multiply rapidly and soon form a tumorous growth that practically occludes the uterine lumen and distends its walls. The deciduoma-
tous cells lying next to the mesometrium become packed with glycogen
granules. The storage of glycogen invariably occurs in the decidual cells
that occupy the mesometrial side of the uterus, irrespective of the site of the
trauma. The position of these glycogen-storing cells corresponds to that of
similar cells that appear below the fetal placenta during normal pregnancies. In rodents the placentae invariably form on the mesometrial side of the
uterus, and this site seems to be determined by factors operating in the
uterus rather than in the implanting blastocysts. The deciduomas attain
maximal differentiation about five days after uterine trauma; after this they
undergo necrosis and gradually disappear. The glandular cells at the point
of mesometrial attachment are the last to disappear.

During the involution of each deciduoma a *metrial gland* develops on
the mesometrial side of the uterus (Fig. 14–18). The gland consists of large
cells of epithelial appearance arranged in thick sheaths around certain
blood vessels in this area of the uterus. In most mammals these cells appear
to be scattered throughout the uterine tissue, but in the rat they form a cir-

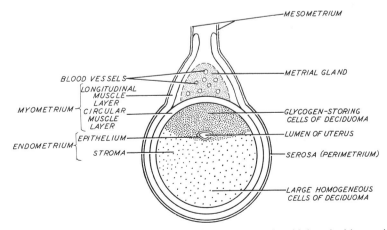

Figure 14–18. Diagrammatic section through a rat uterus in which a deciduoma has been
caused to differentiate.

cumscribed, macroscopically visible organ that seems to be glandular in nature. This structure develops below the insertion of each placenta during normal pregnancy and at the mesometrial edge of each deteriorating decid-uoma. It has been suggested that the protein granules of the metrial gland may be related to the presence of relaxin.[72]

A problem of great importance is how uterine trauma or blastocysts in the lumen of the uterus signal the anterior hypophysis to release the neces-sary hormones for prolonging the secretory function of the corpora lutea. Experiments on sheep have shown that blastocysts fail to implant normally after surgical section of the uterine nerves or partial resection of the pitui-tary stalk. After either operation the estrous cycles remain normal in length; ovulation and fertilization occur normally, but most of the blastocysts do not implant. Sectioning the uterine nerves interrupts the nervous connec-tion between the uterus and pituitary, and partial resection of the pituitary stalk interrupts the connection between the hypothalamus and pituitary. Under these conditions, it appears that the pituitary gland does not contin-ue to release gonadotrophin and maintain functional corpora lutea. Conse-quently, the progesterone titers fall too early and the uterus involutes before the blastocysts can implant.

GONADAL HORMONES AND SEXUAL BEHAVIOR IN MAMMALS

There is a vast amount of information indicating that hormones perform important roles in determining and regulating the patterns of sexual behav-ior.[45, 75] It is important to recognize that the gonads begin to secrete hor-mones during early stages of development, though maximal production of hormones and the release of mature germ cells occur much later. Since behavior relates to the nervous system, the implication is that hormones in-fluence neural tissues, and there is ample documentation of this concept. We have repeatedly emphasized that the relationship between the nervous and endocrine systems is one of reciprocity. The problem of reproductive behavior is extremely complex and may be influenced by a multitude of fac-tors, such as genetic constitution, social contacts, the kinds of hormones present, and the age at which they act. Only a few salient aspects can be considered here, and the discussion will be limited to mammals.

Gonadal Hormones and the Control of Neural Function

Adult Mammals

The production and release of ovarian and testicular steroids are deter-mined by the pituitary gonadotrophins. The gonadal steroids in the blood-stream operate through a feedback mechanism to adjust the kinds and amounts of gonadotrophins released by the anterior pituitary. The circulating steroids act upon the hypothalamus, and this portion of the brain regulates pituitary functions through the production of neurohormonal releasing factors. This seems to be a stabilizing and self-balancing system which makes it possible for environmental stimuli and various neural factors to affect gonadal functions. The gonadal hormones, and perhaps others, appear to act directly upon the central nervous system to initiate the behavioral responses characteristic of the species during the breeding periods. In certain species, the gonads of both sexes are quiescent for long periods of time, during which reproductive behavior is entirely absent. In polyestrous forms, there are recurring periods of heat or sexual receptiveness in the female, the male being in a state of sexual readiness at all times.

Reproductive processes in the female are definitely rhythmic, whereas testicular functions lack this high degree of cyclicity. The female hypothalamus is rhythmic and this causes a rhythmic ripening of the ovarian follicles (FSH secretion), ovulation, and luteinization (LH secretion). The hypothalamus of the male, on the other hand, maintains a steady state output of FSH and LH which keeps the testis functional at all times, thus making it possible for environmental stimuli to elicit sexual behavior at any time.

The beginning of heat in such animals as the rat and guinea pig coincides with preovulatory growth of the graafian follicle, when large amounts of estrogen and some progesterone are being secreted. There can be no doubt that the change from diestrous to estrous behavior is due to the action of these hormones on the nervous system. The females of infraprimate mammals are never sexually receptive after castration or hypophysectomy, though they may be brought into heat by the administration of estrogen and progesterone. Males generally do not copulate if castrated during prepuberal life; copulations may continue for weeks or months in certain mammals following removal of the adult testes. Though exogenous gonadal hormones have an effect on the strength of the sex drive in adult mammals, including man, they do not determine the direction it will take or the means by which it is expressed.

Fetal or Neonatal Mammals

Since there is a difference in the release of gonadotrophins by adult male and female pituitaries, it follows that the hypothalami must be different. One could speak of a "male" brain and a "female" brain, thinking largely in terms of the hypothalamus. Current studies indicate that there is a critical period in development during which the undifferentiated hypothalamus is sensitive to the gonadal hormones in the circulation. In animals with long gestation periods (guinea pig, monkey), this period of hypothalamic sensitivity ensues in the fetus; in species having relatively short gestation periods (rat and mouse), the sensitive period is not ended until about 8 days after birth. Briefly stated, the indications are that the immature hypothalamus differentiates in the male direction when it is exposed to the influence of a testis or to exogenous androgens; if an ovary is present, or if gonads are absent, during this critical period, the hypothalamus differentiates into the female type.[8, 19, 44, 75]

We mentioned earlier that if rabbit and mouse fetuses are gonadecto-mized while the reproductive tracts are undifferentiated, female genital or-gans develop regardless of genotypic sex. This indicates that secretions of the fetal testis are essential for the differentiation of male genitalia, whereas the female genitalia develop independently of the ovarian hormones. This concept seems to be applicable to the differentiation of neural tissues which mediate mating behavior. It has been shown that the administration of testosterone to pregnant guinea pigs and monkeys, while the neural and genital tissues of the genetic female fetuses are immature, results in inter-sexuality. Objective studies on female intersexes of this type have shown that there is a permanent suppression of the capacity to display female behavior and an intensification of the capacity to display male behavior.

If male rats are castrated at birth, while the hypothalamus is still undif-ferentiated, they display feminine mating behavior as adults.[10, 20] Two crite-ria have been employed in assessing male and female type hypothalami: First, the type of sexual behavior displayed by the adult and, secondly, the type of ovarian development. The latter reflects the pattern of release of the pituitary gonadotrophins. If female rats are given a single dose of testoster-one before the eighth day after birth, the adult ovaries contain only vesicu-lar follicles and these do not ovulate or luteinize. This indicates that the hypothalamus is not releasing FSH and LH cyclically and hence is of the male type. Ovarian grafts, persisting in male hosts, typically contain vesicu-lar follicles which do not ovulate or form corpora lutea. Studies of the adult sexual behavior of these androgen-sterilized female rats reveal that they are incapable of female mating behavior, but show marked patterns of male behavior.

These various studies suggest that androgens, acting during fetal or neonatal life, have an organizing effect on the neural tissues, which mediate mating behavior after the attainment of adulthood. In the adult, both ovarian and testicular hormones serve to activate a pattern which is latent within the central nervous system. In other words, the presence or the absence of androgens exerts a fundamental influence upon the brain during ontogene-sis, and this determines whether the sexual reactions brought to expression by the gonadal hormones of the adult will be masculine or feminine in char-acter. Once the definitive organization of the hypothalamus has been ac-complished, it cannot be changed by gonadal hormones or by any other procedure.

REFERENCES

1. Anderson, L. L., Bland, K. P., and Melampy, R. M.: Comparative aspects of uterine-luteal relationships. Rec. Progr. Horm. Res. 25:57, 1969.
2. Astwood, E. B.: A six-hour assay for the quantitative determination of estrogen. Endocri-nology 23:25, 1938.
3. Barraclough, C. A.: Production of anovulatory, sterile rats by single injections of testoster-one propionate. Endocrinology 68:62, 1961.
4. Barraclough, C. A., and Haller, E. W.: Positive and negative feedback effects of estrogen on pituitary LH synthesis and release in normal and androgen-sterilized female rats. Endo-crinology 86:542, 1970.

5. Biggers, J. D., and Curnow, D. H.: Oestrogenic activity of subterranean clover. Biochem. J. *58*:278, 1954.
6. Bradbury, J. T.: Direct action of estrogen on the ovary of the immature rat. Endocrinology *68*:115, 1961.
7. Callard, G. V., and Leathem, J. H.: *In vitro* synthesis of steroids by experimentally induced cystic ovaries. Proc. Soc. Exp. Biol. Med. *118*:996, 1965.
8. Clemens, L. G., Hiroi, M., and Gorski, R. A.: Induction and facilitation of female mating behavior in rats treated neonatally with low doses of testosterone propionate. Endocrinology *84*:1430, 1969.
9. Falk, R. J., and Bradin, C. W.: Uptake of tritiated progesterone by the uterus of the ovariectomized guinea pig. Endocrinology *86*:1059, 1970.
10. Feder, H. H., and Whalen, R. E.: Feminine behavior in neonatally castrated and estrogen-treated male rats. Science *147*:306, 1965.
11. Ferin, M., Tempone, A., Zimmering, P. E., and Vande Wiele, R. L.: Effect of antibodies to 17β-estradiol and progesterone on the estrous cycle of the rat. Endocrinology *85*:1070, 1969.
12. Ferrando, G., and Nalbandov, A. V.: Direct effect on the ovary of the adrenergic blocking drug dibenzyline. Endocrinology *85*:38, 1969.
13. Fevold, H. R., and Pfeiffer, E. W.: Androgen production *in vitro* by phalarope gonadal tissue homogenates. Gen. Comp. Endocrinol. *10*:26, 1968.
14. Fischer, T. V.: Local uterine inhibition of the corpus luteum in the guinea pig. Anat. Rec. *151*:350, 1965.
15. Follett, B. K., Nicholls, T. J., and Redshaw, M. R.: The vitellogenic response in the South African clawed toad (*Xenopus laevis* Daudin). J. Cell. Physiol. Suppl. 1. *72*:91, 1968.
16. Fraps, R. M.: Twenty-four hour periodicity in the mechanism of pituitary gonadotrophin release for follicular maturation and ovulation in the chicken. Endocrinology *77*:5, 1965.
17. Gallien, L.: Sequential endocrine activities controlling oogenesis. A general survey. Amer. Zool. *15*(Suppl. 1):197, 1975.
18. Goldman, B. D., Kamberi, I. A., Siiteri, P. K., and Porter, J. C.: Temporal relationship of progestin secretion, LH release and ovulation in rats. Endocrinology *85*:1137, 1969.
19. Gorski, R. A., and Wagner, J. W.: Gonadal activity and sexual differentiation of the hypothalamus. Endocrinology *76*:226, 1965.
20. Grady, K. L., and Phoenix, G. H.: Hormonal determinants of mating behavior; the display of feminine behavior by adult male rats castrated neonatally. Amer. Zool. *3*:482, 1963.
21. Greenstein, J. S.: A new diagnostic method of staining vaginal smears and endometrial biopsies for office practice and clinical laboratory. Internat. J. Fertil. *9*:493, 1964.
22. Gutknecht, G. D., Cornette, J. C., and Pharriss, B. B.: Antifertility properties of prostaglandin F2$_\alpha$. Biol. Reprod. *1*:367, 1969.
23. Hall, K.: Relaxin: A review. J. Reprod. Fertil. *1*:368, 1960.
24. Harris, G. W., and Naftolin, F.: The hypothalamus and control of ovulation. Brit. Med. Bull. *26*:3, 1970.
25. Hawk, H. W., and Bolt, D. J.: Luteolytic effect of estradiol-17β when administered after mid-cycle in the ewe. Biol. Reprod. *2*:275, 1970.
26. Hisaw, F. L., Jr.: Comparative effectiveness of estrogens on fluid imbibition and growth of the rat's uterus. Endocrinology *64*:276, 1959.
27. Hoffmann, J. C.: Light and reproduction in the rat: Effect of lighting schedule on ovulation blockade. Biol. Reprod. *1*:185, 1969.
28. Hoffmann, J. C., and Schwartz, N. B.: Timing of post-partum ovulation in the rat. Endocrinology *76*:620, 1965.
29. Höhn, E. O.: Gonadal hormone concentrations in northern phalaropes in relation to nuptial plumage. Canad. J. Zool. *48*:400, 1970.
30. Johnson, D. C.: Sexual differentiation of gonadotropin patterns. Amer. Zool. *12*:193, 1972.
31. Kincl, F. A., and Maqueo, M.: Prevention by progesterone of steroid-induced sterility in neonatal male and female rats. Endocrinology *77*:859, 1965.
32. Kissel, J. H., Rosenfeld, M. G., Chase, L. R., and O'Malley, B. W.: Response of chick oviduct adenyl cyclase to steroid hormones. Endocrinology *86*:1019, 1970.
33. Leathem, J. H.: Biochemistry of cystic ovaries. Ciba Found. Colloq. Endocrinol. *12*:173, 1958.
34. Long, J. A., and Evans, H. M.: The estrous cycle of the rat and its associated phenomena. Mem. Univ. Calif. *6*:1, 1922.
35. Lukaszewaska, J. H., and Hansel, W.: Extraction and partial purification of luteolytic activity from bovine endometrial tissue. Endocrinology *86*:261, 1970.
36. Macdonald, G. J., Tashjian, A. H., Jr., and Greep, R. O.: Influence of exogenous gonadotropins, antibody formation, and hysterectomy on the duration of luteal function in hypophysectomized rats. Biol. Reprod. *2*:202, 1970.

37. Machado, C. R. S., Machado, A. B. M., and Wragg, L. E.: Circadian serotonin rhythm control: Sympathetic and nonsympathetic pathways in rat pineals of different ages. Endocrinology *85*:846, 1969.

38. Masui, Y.: Relative roles of the pituitary, follicle cells, and progesterone in the induction of oocyte maturation in *Rana pipiens*. J. Exp. Zool. *166*:365, 1967.

39. Masui, Y., and Markert, C.: Cytoplasmic control of nuclear behavior during meiotic maturation of frog oocytes. J. Exp. Zool. *177*:129, 1971.

40. Nalbandov, A. V.: Comparative aspects of corpus luteum function. Biol. Reprod. *2*:7, 1970.

41. Opel, H.: Oviposition in chickens after removal of the posterior lobe of the pituitary by an improved method. Endocrinology *76*:673, 1965.

42. Opel, H., and Nalbandov, A. V.: Ovulability of ovarian follicles in the hypophysectomized hen. Endocrinology *69*:1029, 1961.

43. Pharriss, B. B., and Wyngarden, L. J.: The effect of prostaglandin F2$_\alpha$ on the progestogen content of ovaries from pseudopregnant rats. Proc. Soc. Exp. Biol. Med. *130*:92, 1969.

44. Phoenix, C. H.: Hypothalamic regulation of sexual behavior in male guinea pigs. J. Comp. Physiol. Psychol. *54*:72, 1961.

45. Phoenix, C. H., Goy, R. W., and Resko, J. A.: Psychological differentiation as a function of androgenic stimulation. *In* M. Diamond (ed.): Perspectives in Reproduction and Sexual Behavior. Bloomington, Indiana University Press, 1968, p. 33.

46. Quay, W. B.: Circadian rhythm in rat pineal serotonin and its modifications by estrous cycle and photoperiod. Gen. Comp. Endocrinol. *3*:473, 1963.

47. Redshaw, M. R.: The hormonal control of the amphibian ovary. Amer. Zool. *12*:289, 1972.

48. Reiter, R. J., and Fraschini, F.: Endocrine aspects of the mammalian pineal gland: A review. Neuroendocrinology *5*:219, 1969.

49. Rowson, L. E. A.: The evidence for luteolysin. Brit. Med. Bull. *26*:14, 1970.

50. Rubinstein, L., and Sawyer, C. H.: Role of catecholamines in stimulating the release of pituitary ovulating hormone(s) in rats. Endocrinology *86*:988, 1970.

51. Sandor, T., Sorin, S., and Mehdi, A. Z.: The possible role of steroids in evolution. Amer. Zool. *15*(Suppl. 1):227, 1975.

52. Savard, K., Marsh, J. M., and Rice, B. F.: Gonadotropins and ovarian steroidogenesis. Rec. Progr. Horm. Res. *21*:285, 1965.

53. Sawyer, C. H.: Nervous control of ovulation. *In* C. W. Lloyd (ed.): Endocrinology of Reproduction. New York, Academic Press, 1959, p. 1.

54. Schneider, H. P. G., and McCann, S. M.: Mono- and indolamines and control of LH secretion. Endocrinology *86*:1127, 1970.

55. Schwartz, N. B., and Ely, C. A.: Comparison of effects on hypophysectomy, antiserum to ovine LH, and ovariectomy on estrogen secretion during the rat estrous cycle. Endocrinology *86*:1420, 1970.

56. Sherwood, O. D., Chang, C. C., Bevier, G. W., and Dzuik, P. J.: Radioimmunoassay of plasma relaxin levels throughout pregnancy and at parturition in the pig. Endocrinology *97*:834, 1975.

57. Smith, E. R., Weick, R. F., and Davidson, J. M.: Influence of intracerebral progesterone on the reproductive system of female rats. Endocrinology *85*:1129, 1969.

58. Stumpf, W. E.: Hypophyseotropic neurons in the brain: Topography of estradiol concentrating neurons. *In* C. H. Sawyer and R. A. Gorski (eds.): Steroid Hormones and Brain Function. UCLA Forum Med. Sci. No. 15. Los Angeles, University of California Press, 1971.

59. Stumpf, W. E.: Estrogen-neurons and estrogen-neuron systems in the periventricular brain. Amer. J. Anat. *129*:207, 1970.

60. Stumpf, W. E.: Nuclear concentration of ³H-estradiol in target tissues. Dry-mount autoradiography of vagina, oviduct, ovary, testis, mammary tumor, liver and adrenal. Endocrinology *85*:31, 1969.

61. Stumpf, W. E.: Estradiol-concentrating neurons. Topography in the hypothalamus by dry-mount autoradiography. Science *162*:1001, 1968.

62. Stumpf, W. E.: Cellular and subcellular ³H-estradiol localization in the pituitary by autoradiography. Z. Zellforsch. *92*:23, 1968.

63. Szego, C. M., and Davis, J. S.: Adenosine 3',5'-monophosphate in rat uterus: Acute elevation by estrogen. Proc. Nat. Acad. Sci. *58*:1711, 1967.

64. Szego, C. M., and Lawson, D. A.: Influence of histamine on uterine metabolism: Stimulation of incorporation of radioactivity from amino acids into protein, lipid and purines. Endocrinology *74*:372, 1964.

65. Szego, C. M., and Sloan, S. H.: The influence of histamine and serotonin in producing early uterine growth in the rat. Gen. Comp. Endocrinol. *1*:295, 1961.

66. Takewaki, K., and Kawashima, S.: Some effects of neonatal administration of androgen or estrogen in female rats. Gunma Symposia on Endocrinol. *4*:195, 1967.
67. Talwar, G. P.: Mechanism of action of estrogens. Gen. Comp. Endocrinol. Suppl. *2*:123, 1969.
68. Thornton, V. F., and Evennett, P. J.: Endocrine control of oocyte maturation and oviducal jelly release in the toad, *Bufo bufo* (L). Gen. Comp. Endocrinol. *13*:268, 1969.
69. Visscher, M. B., King, J. T., and Lee, Y. C. P.: Further studies on influence of age and diet upon reproductive senescence in strain A female mice. Amer. J. Physiol. *170*:72, 1952.
70. Wallace, R. A., and Bergink, E. W.: Amphibian vitellogenin: Properties, hormonal regulation of hepatic synthesis and ovarian uptake, and conversion to yolk proteins. Amer. Zool. *14*:1159, 1974.
71. Weisz, J., and Lloyd, C. W.: Estrogen and androgen production *in vitro* from 7-³H-progesterone by normal and polycystic rat ovaries. Endocrinology *77*:735, 1965.
72. Wislocki, G. B., Weiss, L. P., Burgos, M. H., and Ellis, R. A.: The cytology, histochemistry and electron microscopy of the granular cells of the metrial gland of the gravid rat. J. Anat. *91*:131, 1957.
73. Wright, P. A.: Induction of ovulation *in vitro* in *Rana pipiens* with steroids. Gen. Comp. Endocrinol. *1*:20, 1961.
74. Wurtman, R. J., and Anton-Tay, F.: The mammalian pineal as a neuroendocrine transducer. Rec. Prog. Horm. Res. *25*:493, 1969.
75. Young, W. C., Goy, R. W., and Phoenix, C. H.: Hormones and sexual behavior. Science *143*:212, 1964.
76. Zarrow, M. X., Neher, G. M., Sikes, D., Brennan, D. M., and Bullard, J. F.: Dilatation of the uterine cervix of the sow following treatment with relaxin. Amer. J. Obstet. Gynec. *72*:260, 1956.

CHAPTER 15

The Hormones of Pregnancy and Lactation

The hormones that are most directly involved in pregnancy and lactation originate from the pituitary gland, the ovary, the placenta, and probably, in certain species, from the uterine endometrium. Like many other physiologic processes, these events involve a whole train of balanced forces and cannot be accounted for on the basis of hormones acting in isolation. Other endocrine glands, whose products are more directly concerned with systemic metabolism, exert indirect but important influences on pregnancy, parturition, and lactation.

THE EVOLUTION OF VIVIPARITY

With the evolutionary movement of organisms from aqueous to terrestrial habitats, many changes have occurred in the nature of the egg and in the structure and function of the genital system. Although widely separated taxonomic groups have exploited different devices for retaining the developing young on or within the body of a parent, there are suggestions that endocrine mechanisms have played an important role in making these adaptations possible. Evolutionary innovations are difficult to prove, and no unifying concept has emerged that accounts for all the facts. Although many specific exceptions can be found, the following evolutionary trends seem to be apparent: (1) a reduction in the number of eggs produced; (2) a closer association of the sexes and internal fertilization; (3) the addition of reserve food materials to the egg and compression of the larval stages into the embryonic period; (4) retention of embryos within the female tract and parental protection of the young; (5) reduction in size of the egg and the development of a placenta; and (6) endocrine regulation of the mammary glands for early nutrition of the newborn.[3, 9, 35, 41]

The most primitive method of sexual reproduction is that of discharging innumerable gametes into the surrounding water, fertilization occurring without any participation of the parents. Such eggs generally contain little yolk and are largely devoid of protective coverings. A closer association between the sexes became established, and in many fishes and amphibians the spermatozoa are discharged in close proximity to the eggs. Among salamanders, males discharge packets of sperms in structures called spermatophores, which the females take up through their cloacas and store in their reproductive tracts. Thus fertilization is internal, but there is no copulation. With the production of fewer eggs, various kinds of mechanisms have arisen to assure the survival of the embryos. One finds among teleost fishes many kinds of parental care, nest building, and brooding. Male pipefishes and sea horses, for example, have specialized brood pouches on the ventral body wall. In other species, either the males or the females take up the fertilized eggs and incubate them in their mouths. In the primitive ovoviviparous condition the eggs contained tremendous quantities of yolk and they were retained within the oviducts to provide greater protection and more uniform environments for development.

The zygotes of most salamanders and of a few reptiles only begin to cleave before leaving the female tract. The eggs of birds are in the early gastrula stage when they leave the oviduct, but reptilian eggs may be retained much longer. Almost all amphibians are oviparous and return to water for breeding, but there are a few exceptions. Adaptive viviparity has been described in a small toad, *Nectophrynoides occidentalis,* which breeds in arid mountainous environments. After a gestation period of nine months, the young are born in a fully metamorphosed condition and do not require an aqueous habitat. Parturition is accomplished by inflation of the lung sacs and contraction of thoracic muscles, but delivery cannot occur unless the animal finds suitable mechanical support in the environment.[27]

The oviducts secrete a great variety of materials for the protection and nutrition of the eggs. The aquatic eggs of fishes and amphibians are provided with jelly envelopes, membranes, and shells. In reptiles and birds, the albuminous covering of the egg contains large quantities of water, which are absorbed by the yolk before or after laying. In ovoviviparous selachians, with no intimate apposition of fetal and maternal vascular structures, the secretory products of the uterus provide an important source of nourishment. The viviparous selachians develop circulatory structures as an additional source of nourishment to supplement a reduced supply of yolk in the egg.

Corpora lutea have been identified in the ovaries of a number of vertebrates, and they are not invariably associated with viviparity.[20] They have been found in oviparous and ovoviviparous selachians, teleosts, amphibians, and reptiles, as well as in the oviparous monotremes and all higher mammals. They correlate with the retention of eggs in the oviducts in ovipara and with the retention of embryos in the uteri in the vivipara. The luteal structures of certain teleost fishes have been shown to release progesterone-like agents that control the growth of the ovipositor. The ovaries of some ovoviviparous snakes appear to contain progesterone, and similar materials are found in the blood plasma.[8] Elevated levels of progesterone have also been found recently in the blood of pregnant *Nectophrynoides,* the viviparous toad mentioned previously. It is clear that progesterone is not exclusively a mammalian hormone, and this is another indication that there have been evolutionary changes in steroid hormone emphasis rather than changes in the types of hormones.

The monotremes *(Ornithorhynchus, Echidna)* are the only mammals that lay eggs. The eggs are relatively small but contain enough nutriment to support development up to an advanced stage, though not to the level of self-sufficiency. In all other mammals, methods of uterine feeding have been perfected and the size of the egg is radically reduced. Mammalian eggs are typically fertilized in the oviducts and undergo early development while retained there. The cleaving eggs of many species are coated with albuminous secretions from the oviducts, but the nutritional requirements are met largely by the limited stores contained within the developing egg. During oviducal development, lasting from 4 to 10 days, the bulk of the embryo shrinks rapidly indicating that there has not been any appreciable absorption of materials from the fluids of the oviduct. The embryotroph elaborated by the uterine glands is of great importance in many species for nourishment of the blastocyst before the placenta has been established. It is probable that in the Artiodactyla and Perissodactyla the uterine secretions are an important source of nourishment for the embryo and fetus, from the beginning to the end of pregnancy. In cases of delayed implantation, the uterine secretions apparently maintain the blastocysts for weeks or months.

The first step toward viviparity in mammals has been the retention of embryos within the uterus, nothing more than a primitive yolk-sac placenta being established. The gestation period of the opossum *(Didelphis virginiana)* is only 12 or 13 days, the young being born as soon as the metamorphic changes have been completed. The luteal phase of the estrous cycle is prolonged and parturition correlates with the involution of the corpora lutea. Pregnancy may be terminated at any stage by removal of the ovaries, which suggests that in this species pregnancy does not involve any hormones other than those that regulate the estrous cycle. Extraovarian mechanisms operate in higher mammals and produce hormones that make it possible for embryos to be retained in the uterus for periods longer than the limits of the estrous cycle.[2, 34]

In the final analysis, it is apparent that we cannot yet visualize a unifying theme for the evolution of the various mechanisms by which different vertebrate groups have achieved viviparity. It is obvious, however, that mechanisms of mammalian viviparity are far more complex and are far more consistent than those of lower vertebrates. Probably mammalian viviparity evolved separately from that of lower vertebrates, and its success has been based upon the utilization, at first, of hormones of the hypophysial-gonadal axis. Viviparity or ovoviviparity of lower vertebrates is a much more passive process and probably relatively more easily achieved in an evolutionary sense. Thus, in closely related taxonomic groups (especially elasmobranchs), some genera utilize viviparity while others remain oviparous.[12] Much more information about the endocrinology of gestation of lower vertebrates is needed before we can make any significant advancements in our total understanding of the evolution of viviparity.

HORMONES IN PREGNANCY AND PARTURITION

The Hypophysis

We have seen that the anterior pituitary gonadotrophins are essential for the periodic release of eggs from the ovary and for the secretion of ovarian hormones that build up the type of uterus most suitable for the reception of the blastocysts. After the animal has become pregnant, the effects of hypophysectomy vary with the species and in accordance with the stage of gestation at which the operation is performed. In the rabbit, cat, and dog, hypophysectomy produces abortion regardless of at which stage of pregnancy it is performed. In other species, such as the mouse, rat, guinea pig, and monkey, hypophysectomy at approximately midterm or later may not interrupt gestation or interfere appreciably with delivery. Lactation fails to occur or is of short duration. The gestation period of the dogfish *(Mustelus canis)* is 10 months, and hypophysectomy during the first 5 months does

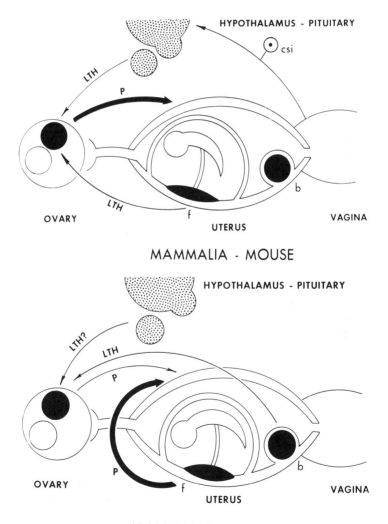

MAMMALIA - MOUSE

MAMMALIA - MAN

Figure 15–1. Diagrammatic representation of gestation in two mammals, the mouse and man. *Open circle in ovary,* mature follicle; *solid circle,* corpus luteum; LTH, pituitary or placental lactogen; P, progestin; *csi,* coital sensory impulse; *b,* early embryo or blastocyst; *f,* late embryo or fetus. (From Browning, H. C., Gen. & Comp. Endocrinol., Suppl. 2:42, 1969).

not interfere with embryonic development, the absorption of yolk, or the establishment of the yolk-sac placenta. The pituitary gland is necessary for the maintenance of normal gestation in viviparous snakes.

The physiology of mammalian gestation is best known, and diverse aspects are represented by the mouse and by man (Fig. 15–1). A fundamental difference between the two relates to the fact that during later fetal stages, progesterone is entirely of luteal origin in the mouse, while in man it originates from the placenta. During earlier fetal stages, the corpus luteum of the mouse is maintained by the action of prolactin of hypophysial origin, while in man, luteal stimulation is provided primarily by chorionic gonadotrophin. In the mouse, release of hypophysial prolactin during gestation results from a coital sensory stimulus. Similarly, rats may be hypophysectomized at midpregnancy and carried to term by the administration of estrogen and progesterone. Since the ovaries of the rat are indispensable throughout the course of pregnancy, it appears that the maintenance of pregnancy after hypophysectomy depends upon the continued function of the corpora lutea brought about by a luteotrophic principle (prolactin), which must be of extra-hypophysial origin. The corpora lutea appear to be the main source of progesterone in the rat. Extracts possessing luteotrophic action have been prepared from the rat's placenta. There is circumstantial evidence indicating that in certain mammalian species the placenta functions as an adjunct to the anterior hypophysis and takes over the production of gonadotrophins, which are necessary for the maintenance of gestation.[25, 33, 51]

Studies suggest that maintenance of the copora lutea of the pregnant rabbit is a function of estrogenic hormones rather than a direct consequence of gonadotrophin action. The corpora lutea of hypophysectomized rabbits may be maintained by the administration of either estrogens or gonadotrophins.[30] It may be that in this species the gonadotrophins do not act directly on the corpora lutea to cause the continued release of progesterone, but prolong luteal secretion by encouraging the production of estrogens. It is probable that the gonadal hormones *per se* have more important direct actions on the gonads than is commonly supposed. It is well known that estrogens have considerable ability to promote growth of the ovarian follicles of hypophysectomized rats. There are apparently many species variations in the relative importance of estrogens and pituitary gonadotrophins in maintaining luteal function.

The Ovary

Full differentiation of the endometrium requires both estrogen and progesterone, and removal of the ovaries while the developing zygotes are in the tubes invariably prevents implantation of the blastocysts and placentation.[11] If pregnant females are ovariectomized while the blastocysts are floating free in the uterine lumen, the blastocysts generally die. However, if the armadillo is bilaterally ovariectomized at about the middle of the four-month period of delayed implantation, implantation occurs about 30 days later and is indistinguishable from normal implantation.[10] Hence, in this species some nonovarian tissue can assume the function of maintaining the uterus. As with the pituitary gland, the ovary is more essential for the maintenance of pregnancy in some species than in others. The ovaries are indispensable at practically all stages for the maintenance of pregnancy in the opossum, mouse, rat, rabbit, golden hamster, 13-lined ground squirrel, goat, and viviparous snakes. In women, monkeys, and mares, ovariectomy during the early months of pregnancy usually does not cause abortion. In the guinea pig, cat, dog, and ewe, the ovaries may be dispensed with during the second half of gestation. The ovaries are not essential during the terminal stages of pregnancy in cows and pigs. Failure of implantation or abortion in castrated animals may be prevented by the administration of progesterone. There is ample evidence that the placenta performs endocrine functions during pregnancy, being capable of secreting gonadotrophins, prolactins, and steroids of the ovarian type in certain species.[22, 55]

In a variety of mammals, the quantity of estrogen excreted through the kidneys is increased strikingly during pregnancy. The total estrogen in the urine of pregnant women increases gradually after the first week, reaches a peak shortly before parturition and drops abruptly a few days after the birth of young (Fig. 15–2). The increased quantities of estrogen in the urine are not the result of a diminished renal threshold because after the second month of pregnancy, such compounds are present in the blood in greater amounts than at any other time. Nonpregnant women excrete about 300 M.U. (mouse units) of estrogen per day, whereas during pregnancy the level rises to 20,000 M.U. per day. It is noteworthy that over 99 per cent of the urinary estrogen is in the form of estriol glucuronide and that such conjugated estrogens have little physiologic potency. The total amount of conjugated estrogen begins to fall shortly before parturition, whereas the amount

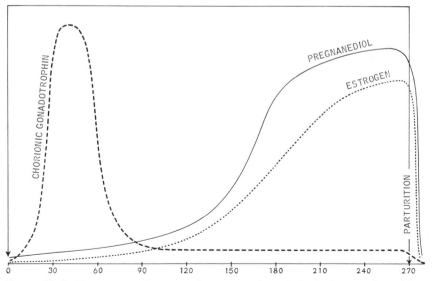

Figure 15–2. Diagram showing the urinary excretion of chorionic gonadotrophin, total estrogen, and pregnanediol during human pregnancy.

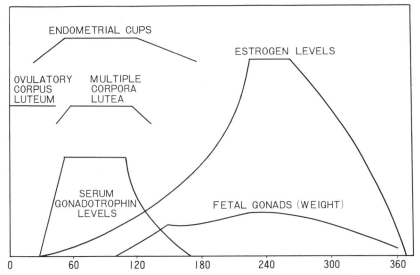

Figure 15–3. Sequence of events during gestation in the mare. Note that the ovulatory corpus luteum wanes and accessory corpora lutea are formed when the serum gonadotrophin levels rise. Urinary estrogens reach a high peak at about 220 days and fall before parturition (After Amoroso, E. C.: Brit. Med. Bull, *11,* 1955.)

of unconjugated, physiologically active estrogen undergoes a relative increase at this time. This would seem to suggest that estrogen performs some role during parturition that it does not exercise during the preceding months of pregnancy.

The nonpregnant mare excretes around 2,000 M.U. of estrogen daily, but during pregnancy it exceeds one million mouse units per day. Estradiol and estrone are found during the estrous cycle of the mare, but during pregnancy at least three additional steroids appear—equilin, equilenin, and dehydroequilenin, the first two being the most abundant. The abundance of estriol in pregnant women and of equilin and equilenin in pregnant mares supports the concept that these are estrogens of pregnancy and that they probably perform some role peculiar to gestation. Bilateral ovariectomy of pregnant women, monkeys, and mares does not abolish the high excretion of estrogens. The excretion rate of estrogens in pregnant monkeys is not altered by removing the ovaries and fetus, but it falls to nonpregnant levels after removal of the placenta. The development and regression of the fetal gonads of the horse correlate with the rise and fall of the maternal estrogens (Fig. 15–3).

Small amounts of progesterone are thought to be secreted by the preovulatory follicle and the titers rise markedly during the course of pregnancy. Pregnanediol excretion in pregnant women rises progressively after the second or third month and falls precipitously after loss of the placenta (Fig. 15–2). The indications are that the corpus luteum of the human ovary produces progesterone during early pregnancy, whereas an additional supply is secreted by the placenta after the second month. Apparently, maternal cholesterol is the major precursor of placental progesterone.[53] The source of the progesterone during pregnancy apparently varies with the species. Since ovariectomy of the ewe around midgestation neither causes abortion nor prevents the rise of blood progesterone, it is clear that the placenta is the major source of the hormone. On the other hand, if the ovaries of the pregnant rabbit are removed seven days before expected delivery, the levels of blood progesterone fall very promptly, and this is followed by abortion. The ovaries of the rabbit seem to be the main, if not the exclusive, source of progesterone.

Progesterone disappears very rapidly from the blood stream, and its excretory metabolites seem to vary with the species. Sodium pregnanediol glucuronidate is the chief urinary catabolic product in the human subject. The feces of pregnant cows contain large amounts of androgen, but very insignificant amounts are found in the feces of bulls and nonpregnant animals. It is probable that the placental progesterone of the pregnant cow is converted to androgen and excreted through the feces. Similarly, it appears that in the human placenta, testosterone and androstenedione are formed from progesterone metabolites.[53]

Pregnancy in Prepuberal Mice

It has been possible to cause young female mice to rear offspring by administering appropriate hormones to induce receptivity to the male, ovulation, implantation, maintenance of pregnancy, parturition, and lactation.[52] In mice and other species it is possible to induce ovulations and to obtain offspring from them by transplanting the early embryos into the uteri of sexually mature recipients, but to induce a sexually immature animal to rear its own young is a more difficult undertaking.

Ovulation and sexual receptivity to the male may be induced in young mice by administering appropriate gonadotrophins. Blastocysts are produced regularly by this procedure, but implantation does not ensue because of improper functioning of the corpora lutea and the consequent absence of a progestational uterus. Viable blastocysts may float free in the uteri for as long as 22 days post coitum without implanting. This shows that blastocysts may survive for relatively long periods in a nonprogestational uterus. In both intact and ovariectomized mice, the blastocysts may be caused to implant by giving small daily injections of progesterone. Larger doses of progesterone are necessary to continue pregnancy.

Progesterone, in the absence of either exogenous or ovarian estrogen, carries pregnancy to completion in mice. The mammary glands of females carrying fetuses to term have developed lobuloalveolar systems that contain secretory products. On the other hand, the mammary glands remain poorly developed in females receiving progesterone treatments in the absence of fetuses and placentae. These facts indicate that endogenous estrogen is being supplied from some source, most likely from the placentae or fetuses.

Parturition can be affected in these animals. Thus, it is possible through hormone manipulations to induce in young, sexually immature mice all of the events of gestation, parturition, and lactation.

Gonadotrophins Peculiar to Pregnancy

The placenta and, in certain species, the endometrium produce gonad-stimulating hormones that are similar in some respects to those produced by the anterior hypophysis but that differ from the latter both physiologically and chemically. The pregnancy gonadotrophins are present in a variety of mammals but are strikingly different in their physiologic properites.[1, 14, 46]

Chorionic Gonadotrophin

This hormone is a glycoprotein and is characteristic of pregnancy in primates, although hormones similar in activity may be present in lower mammals. It is secreted by the chorionic villi of the placenta and appears in the blood and urine during early pregnancy. Human chorionic gonadotrophin (HCG) appears in the urine shortly after implantation and reaches a high peak about one month after the first missed menstrual period (Fig. 15–2). At this time, around 100,000 R.U. (rat units) may be excreted daily. After this peak, the blood and urinary titers of the hormone drop to low levels, which remain fairly constant until a few days after parturition. In the chimpanzee and monkey, chorionic gonadotrophin is produced for a brief period during early pregnancy and disappears thereafter.

Human chorionic gonadotrophin is a glycoprotein with a molecular weight of about 30,000. Its chemical structure and properties are like those of luteinizing hormone (LH); it is composed of at least two sub-units, one of which is common to FSH, LH, and TSH. This chemical similarity undoubtedly accounts for the immunological relatedness of HCG to these pituitary hormones. HCG resembles LH from the anterior hypophysis in most of its actions, and in addition it seems to have the properties of a luteotrophin inasmuch as it prolongs the functional status of the corpus luteum. It converts the corpus luteum of the menstrual cycle into the corpus luteum of pregnancy, thereby prolonging the luteal production of hormones until the placenta becomes capable of secreting the high amounts of gonadal steroids required for the continuation of pregnancy. Although HCG has some ability to cause follicle stimulation in hypophysectomized rodents, its main action in the female is on the corpus luteum.

Although HCG is found normally only in pregnant women, it produces a great variety of gonadal actions in many other vertebrates. When given to the human male, it causes the differentiation of Leydig cells and induces and maintains the production of testicular androgens. When administered to intact animals, it produces follicular growth and ovulation, probably by acting synergistically with the circulating endogenous gonadotrophins of pituitary origin.[61] It causes a release of spermatozoa when given to lower vertebrates, such as amphibians. Thus, HCG may act directly in hypophysectomized animals—or indirectly in the presence of pituitary gonadotrophins of intact subjects—and affect the follicles and corpora lutea of the ovaries and the cells of Leydig or seminiferous tubules of the testis.

Chorionic gonadotrophin may be found in certain pathologic states associated with pregnancy and in others that have no connection with pregnancy. In such conditions as hydatidiform mole and chorioepithelioma of the female, high titers of HCG may be produced. Some neoplastic diseases of the testis may likewise result in the secretion of this substance.

Pregnancy Tests. Since chorionic gonadotrophin is secreted by placental tissue, its presence in the blood or urine has formed the basis for many tests for pregnancy. The Aschheim-Zondek test depends on the capacity of pregnancy urine to induce corpora lutea or "blood points" in the ovaries of mice and rats within 96 hours after treatment. The production of vaginal estrus in the immature rat, 72 to 96 hours after injecting the sample of urine, is a sensitive pregnancy test. In the Friedman test, pregnancy urine causes the formation of corpora lutea within 24 hours after being injected into immature or isolated mature rabbits. The amphibian tests are quicker and perhaps more reliable than those done on mammals. Females of some species of frogs and toads ovulate within 6 to 8 hours after pregnancy urine has been injected into the dorsal lymph sacs. The Galli Mainini test depends on the prompt evacuation of sperms from the testes of frogs. If the injected urine contains HCG, sperms can be identified in the cloacal fluid within 3 hours after the injection. The African frog *(Xenopus laevis)* is about 10 times more sensitive to pregnancy urine than is the female rat. While these various pregnancy tests have been much used in the past, they are time consuming and unwieldy. Nevertheless, they represent interesting applications of the biologic activity of HCG.

A number of immunologic pregnancy tests are now in common use. Most of these are based on the agglutination-inhibition reaction utilizing either erythrocytes or latex particles sensitized with HCG. These methods are accurate and can be completed within an hour or less.[56, 62]

Equine Gonadotrophin

The blood serum of pregnant mares contains a gonadotrophin having biologic properties similar to those of a mixture of pituitary FSH and LH. The predominant effect seems more like that of FSH. The PMS is, however, quite different from human chorionic gonadotrophin and from the hypophysial gonadotrophins. Its molecular weight, about 7000, is greater than that of other gonadotrophins, and it has a high carbohydrate content (49 per cent). Unlike HCG and pituitary FSH and LH, PMS remains in the blood and lymph and is practically absent from the urine. Even when PMS is injected into other animals, it remains in the blood for long periods, not being so rapidly metabolized as the other gonadotrophins. If small doses of PMS are given subcutaneously to hypophysectomized rats, growth of the ovarian follicles ensues. When the subcutaneous injection is followed by intravenous injections, ovulation or luteinization occurs. Since the hormone has high FSH activity, cystic follicles are often produced, especially if large doses are given repeatedly.

The PMS appears in the blood of the mare on about the fortieth day of pregnancy and remains high until about day 120; then it drops and is absent after day 180 (Fig 15–3). The corpus luteum of ovulation has begun to wane by the time that PMS appears in the blood. Under the influence of PMS, the mare's ovaries form large vesicular follicles. Some of these follicles ovulate and form corpora lutea, whereas others undergo luteinization without ovulating. In this manner a crop of accessory corpora lutea is normally formed during pregnancy. The accessory corpora persist until about day 180 of gestation, and from this time until the end of pregnancy, the ovaries contain neither corpora lutea nor large follicles. It is apparent that the ovaries of the mare do not provide a source of progesterone throughout the whole course of gestation. The placenta apparently secretes both estrogen and progesterone during the second half of pregnancy. It appears significant that the formation and persistence of the accessory corpora lutea coincide with the period of high levels of PMS in the blood. The ovaries of the nilgai and African elephant also contain accessory corpora lutea during pregnancy.[47] The gestation period of the elephant is about two years, and accessory corpora are found only between the sixth and ninth months. It is inferred that these animals produce a pregnancy gonadotrophin similar to that of the mare, but its nature remains to be determined.

The gonads of equine fetuses also respond to the circulating hormones of the mother (Fig. 15–3). Under the influence of serum gonadotrophin and estrogen, the fetal ovaries become larger than those of the mother. The fetal testes also are larger than the testes of newborn males.

Whereas human chorionic gonadotrophin is produced by the placenta, specifically by the Langhans cells of the fetal chorion, equine gonadotrophin appears to be formed in the endometrial cups (Fig. 15–4) and hence is uterine in origin.[13] The following evidence indicates that the endometrial cups produce PMS: (1) the hormone can be extracted from the cup areas but not from other parts of the endometrium; (2) the hormone appears in the blood coincident with the development of endometrial cups; and (3) when the endometrial cups first appear, they contain higher concentrations of PMS than are present in the blood.

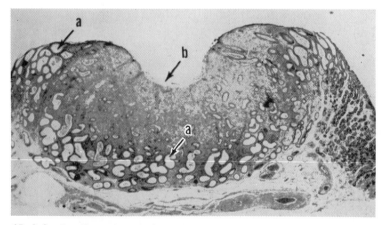

Figure 15–4. Section through an endometrial cup of a pregnant mare. Note the dilated uterine glands (a). The coagulum has been removed from the central region of the cup (b). (From Amoroso, E. C.: Ann. N. Y. Acad. Sci. 75, 1959.)

Mechanisms of Uterine Accommodation

During gestation, a new individual develops inside a hollow, muscular organ, the uterus, and it is apparent that the latter must undergo profound modifications in order to accommodate and support the products of conception (Fig. 15–5). Provision must be made for the nutritional, respiratory, and excretory requirements of the retained embryo. As pregnancy progresses there must be gradual enlargement of the uterus to permit growth of the fetus, but at the same time, its muscular walls must remain quiescent enough to prevent premature expulsion. At parturition, the myometrium must be activated in order to deliver the new individual to the exterior, and in mammals the mammary glands must be called into action for the postpartum nutrition of the young.[49]

The uterus passes through three stages in its adjustments to the products of conception: uterine preparation, growth, and stretching. During the period of *preparation,* before the blastocysts implant, estrogen augments the blood supply to the uterus and causes some increase in the number of cells. With the release of increasing amounts of progesterone there is a decided wave of hyperplasia involving all tissues—particularly the smooth muscle cells. Thus, by the time of implantation, the number of cells has increased tremendously. Since the resulting cells are smaller than those from which they arose by mitosis, the marked hyperplasia produces no significant increase in the size and weight of the uterus. The period of uterine *growth* begins immediately after implantation. As the products of conception enlarge sufficiently to constitute an effective physical stimulus, the uterus adapts itself through hypertrophy of the cells already present. The tremendous degree of hypertrophy occurring in the smooth muscle cells is

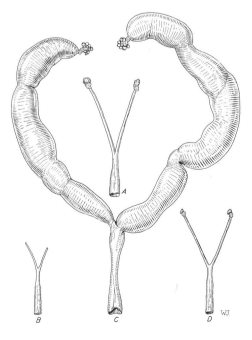

Figure 15–5. Female genitalia of the rat, showing size changes during different natural and experimental conditions. *A,* Tract removed from a normal, adult, virginal animal during diestrus. *B,* Tract from an animal which had been oöphorectomized at 30 days of age and autopsied 6 months later. *C,* Tract removed on the nineteenth day of normal pregnancy. Observe the large corpora lutea of the ovaries and the marked distention of the uteri produced by the products of conception. Compare with *A,* *D,* Tract from an animal which had been hypophysectomized for six months. (All the tracts were dissected out *in toto* and drawn to scale.)

sufficient to account for most of the increase in uterine size during middle and late pregnancy. During the period of uterine *stretching,* the products of conception grow at an accelerating rate, whereas uterine growth diminishes. The period of uterine stretching lasts for only a day and a half in the hamster, but it continues for better than three weeks in the guinea pig.

Distention of the uterine lumen is recognized as an important factor conditioning enlargement of this organ. Clinicians have been aware for many years that in advanced ectopic pregnancy the empty uterus remains much smaller than in normal intrauterine pregnancies. Implantations often occur unilaterally in laboratory rodents having a duplex type of uterus, the equivalent uterus remaining empty or sterile. This condition may be produced experimentally by ligating or sectioning the oviduct on one side. In all these instances, it has been obvious that the sterile uterus does not enlarge to the same degree as the gravid uterus, even though both are exposed to the same circulating hormones. Moreover, it has not been possible through the administration of hormones to modify the size and structure of a nongravid uterus until it is comparable to a gravid one. These observations, as well as many others, indicate that the tension produced by the growing products of conception constitutes a stimulus that enables the uterus to become structurally adapted to its contents. Tension produced by introducing paraffin pellets or rolled rubber dam into the lumen of the uterus exerts a growth-promoting action comparable to that resulting naturally from the products of conception. Pathologic and surgical conditions that enforce the accumulation of uterine secretions within the lumen produce a similar effect. From the foregoing statements one would be justified in conjecturing that the mature uterus is capable of undergoing two types of normal growth: (1) that which occurs periodically during the sexual cycle mainly as a result of chemical stimulation by the ovarian hormones, and (2) that which takes place during pregnancy under the influence of a complex of hormones, together with the added physical stimulus of tension produced by the growing products of conception.

Spacing and Migration of Blastocysts

Little is known about the mechanisms that operate in polytocous mammals to regulate the spacing of embryos in the uterus.[6] In species such as the rabbit, the implantation sites are approximately the same distance apart. Moreover, in mammals having bicornate uteri, the blactocysts may shift from one horn to the other in order to balance the two sides. In the pig, for example, the left ovary produces more eggs than the right one, but the right and left horns of the uterus accomodate approximately the same number of fetuses. In monotocous species, the fetus may be found in the uterine horn opposite to the ovary that gave rise to the egg.

The spacing and implantation of blastocysts have been carefully studied in the rabbit.[7] The three principal mechanisms are muscle activity, adhesion, and invasion. From three to five days post coitum, the blastocysts are moved along the uterus in a random manner and increase rapidly in diameter after this period. It is thought that progesterone conditions the uterus so that muscular contractions arise from both ends and wherever it happens to be stimulated by a blastocyst that has attained a certain size. The contractions emanating from each blastocyst spread in both directions but they lose propulsive strength with increasing distance from the source. In this manner, each blastocyst may repel others above or below it, but remain unaffected by the contractions it has produced. Since the repulsions are mutual and become weaker with distance, the blastocysts become separated from each other by about the same distances. At seven days post coitum, the blastocysts have become so enlarged that they cannot be moved up or down the uterus. The antimesometrial muscle over each blastocyst loses tone and forms a pocket in which the blastocyst is held. The adjacent circular muscle behaves as an incomplete sphincter and holds the blastocyst in the pocket. The adhesion of the rabbit's blastocyst to the uterus is probably alkali induced. The trophoblast penetrates the uterine lining by both displacement and destruction of cells. Adhesion and invasion occur where the epithelium has an underlying capillary and may result from local elevations of pH attendant upon the transfer of carbon dioxide or similar materials to the maternal circulation.

When a silk suture is placed in the antimesometrial wall of one horn of the rat's uterus before mating, blastocysts do not implant in the sutured horn, though they do implant normally in the unsutured horn. Insertion of the suture before estrus does not induce deciduoma, nor does it interfere with fertilization and tubal transport of the ova. The foreign body may produce an unfavorable intrauterine environment which causes death of the blastocysts, or, by interfering with tone and motility of the uterus, it may allow the blastocysts to escape into the vagina before they have had a chance to implant.[23]

Parturition

The mechanisms involved in the onset of labor are very complex and remain poorly understood. It is certain that we cannot think of parturition as being triggered by any single substance but must regard it as the consequence of many synchronized events that have occurred during the course of gestation. The uterus is relatively quiescent during gestation, but as labor approaches there are signs of increasing myometrial irritability and the development of more efficient patterns of contraction. At the end of gestation, the amount of actomyosin, the contractile protein of muscle, increases, and thus facilitates the forceful muscle contractions that are required to expel the fetus. There is increased sensitivity of the uterine muscles to hormones and various kinds of mechanical stimuli.

When the fetuses are removed surgically, the placentae and extraembryonic membranes being left *in situ,* gestation continues for the characteristic period. The placentae and empty membranes are carried to term and delivered at the normal time. This shows that hormones or toxic materials released by the fetus do not give the signal for parturition. The length of the gestation period is genetically determined, although it can be modified by many internal or external environmental factors. In certain genetic strains of cattle, the fetus continues to grow *in utero* during a greatly prolonged gestation. The fetuses become so large that normal delivery is impossible, and they must be removed by caesarean section. On the other hand, some strains may carry abnormally small fetuses for prolonged periods. These considerations indicate that fetal size itself does not determine when labor will begin.

The hormones generated from the placenta and ovaries are known to play key roles in determining the onset of labor. In most mammalian species, progesterone exerts a pregnancy-stabilizing effect, and labor cannot occur until its influence is effectively diminished. In some species, progesterone is produced by the ovary throughout pregnancy but, in others, it arises from both the ovary and placenta. Estrogens promote rhythmic contractility of the uterus. It is probably significant that estrogen increases in amount and effective form as the end of gestation draws near. Oxytocin from the neurohypophysis is also known to have a powerful effect on uterine contractility, and there is circumstantial evidence that it may be involved in the labor mechanism.[40] The fact that totally hypophysectomized animals may deliver young normally does not necessarily prove that oxytocin is not involved in the process; the hypothalamic nuclei that form the hormone may add effective amounts of it to the circulation in the absence of the posterior pituitary. If oxytocin is involved, there is the problem of how it is released at exactly the right time.

Without the proper hormonal balance and timing, labor would be abnormal and would injure the fetus and mother. For example, it is well known that labor may be precipitated by the administration of large doses of oxytocin. However, if the cervical canal has not been softened and the pubic ligaments relaxed by the action of relaxin and other hormones, the violent uterine contractions would probably kill the fetus and rupture the uterus instead of expelling it through the vagina. Whatever the exact mechanism of labor may be, it is certain that all of the events are nicely synchronized and that no single factor can account for the process.[18] The hormones and other factors that tend to stabilize pregnancy are gradually overcome by forces that act in an opposite direction and tend to end it.

The Theory of Progesterone Blockage[19]

Estrogens encourage the muscles of the uterus to contract, whereas progestogens inhibit uterine contractions and thus prevent premature expulsion of the fetus. As long as progesterone is dominant in the uterus, the myometrium is "blocked" and cannot deliver the fetus. Since progesterone does not affect the actomyosin content of muscle, it must act at a higher level of organization. Progesterone has been found to reduce the excitability of uterine muscle, and no excitation wave spreads from the point of stimulation. Many types of experiments prove that the myometrium is unable to respond effectively to stimulants as long as it is under the influence of progesterone. The concept has been advanced that it is the *progesterone block* that maintains pregnancy, and withdrawal of the block is responsible for the onset of parturition.

Some insight into the mechanism of labor has been gained by studying a rare anomaly of human pregnancy. On very rare occasions, a septum divides the human uterus into two horns, and twins having separate placentae may develop in the separate chambers. The fetus in one horn of the uterus may be born prematurely, whereas the other may not be born until as much as two months later. Seemingly, the onset of labor centers around some local effect of the placenta in these cases. It has been proposed that the placenta discharges its progesterone directly into the uterine tissues rather than into the general circulation. If this is true, the highest levels of progesterone would be found at the implantation site, with a diminishing concentration gradient extending into the myometrium from this area. This would explain why little or no progesterone from the placenta of one twin reaches the myometrium of the opposite horn. If placental progesterone is carried by the blood stream, the failure of one placenta should not cause delivery, since the producing placenta would provide enough progesterone to block myometrial contractions in both horns of the uterus. Experiments on laboratory animals indicate that the concentration of progesterone in the uterus during late pregnancy declines with distance from the placenta.

The position of the placenta in the uterus appears to be a very important matter (Fig. 15–6). If the placenta is attached at or below the midline of the uterus one would expect, according to the progesterone block concept, that the fundus would recover first from progesterone inhibition after the

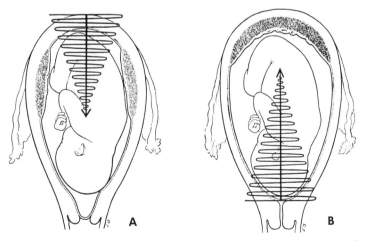

Figure 15–6. Hypothetical illustration of a progesterone gradient in the parturient myometrium determined by the position of the placenta. The normally located placenta *(A)* releases progesterone well down in the uterus. At parturition, the corpus of the uterus recovers first from the progesterone block, and uterine contractions push the fetus toward the vagina. When the placental progesterone is concentrated in the upper end of the uterus *(B)*, the lower end of the uterus recovers first from the progesterone block and uterine contractions push the fetus in the wrong direction (From Csapo, A.: Ann. N. Y. Acad. Sci. *75,* 1959.)

placenta ceases producing this hormone. Thus myometrial contractions would start at the superior end of the uterus and push the fetus through the cervix. If, on the other hand, the placental attachment is at the upper end of the uterus, the activity gradient would start from the cervical end of the uterus and push the fetus in the wrong direction. These theoretical assumptions strongly imply that a local factor, presumably the progesterone block, performs a decisive role in delivery, but they do not rule out the possibility that substances other than progesterone may be important in conditioning myometrial activity.

THE MAMMARY GLAND AND LACTATION

Anatomy

The mammary glands are regarded as homologous with sweat glands since they originate as integumentary ingrowths. The manner of embryonic origin is the same in both sexes. Each mammary gland of the human female is composed of 16 to 25 lobes that radiate from the nipple. Each lobe of the gland is drained by a lactiferous duct that extends toward the areola, the pigmented area around the nipple. At this level, each lactiferous duct dilates into a sinus, again constricts, and opens at the tip of the nipple. The lactiferous ducts branch repeatedly, producing an extensive arborization within the mammary lobe. The resting gland consists mostly of an extensive duct system; however, a few end buds and alveoli may be proliferated from the ducts in the nonpregnant woman (Fig. 15–7). Each lobe is subdivided by connective tissue into lobules of various sizes. At puberty, a rapid and extensive deposition of fat occurs in the breast.

The immature glands consist of a few short ducts radiating from the nipple. The glands of the male do not differentiate much beyond this infantile condition, but a conspicuous growth and branching of the duct system occurs in the prepuberal female under the influence of increasing titers of ovarian hormone. In the postpuberal virginal female, slight fluctuations in the mammae may be correlated with ovarian changes during the reproductive cycle. An extensive and characteristic differentiation of the glands occurs during pregnancy. The duct system becomes extensively arborized, and the terminal twigs end in secretory alveoli. The alveolar lining constitutes a secretory surface from which milk arises. At parturition, the secretion of milk is intensified, and the gland gradually involutes until lactation ceases.[4, 36, 37]

Development of the Mammary Glands (Mammogenesis)

Complete functioning of the mammary glands, like pregnancy and parturition, is an exceedingly complex phenomenon involving the interplay of many hormones as well as nervous factors. It is another example of hormones working in concert rather than in isolation. Mammary gland phys-

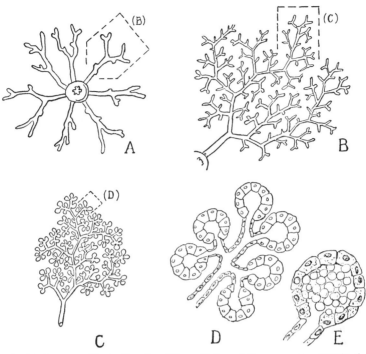

Figure 15–7. Diagrams illustrating the differentiation of the mammary glands. *A,* The gland of prepuberal animals consists of relatively simple ducts radiating from the nipple. *B,* Small segment of *A* enlarged to show the condition of the adult, virginal gland. Under the influence of estrogens the duct system becomes extensively branched. *C,* Small area of *B* enlarged again to show the condition of the gland during pregnancy. Note the great development of terminal alveoli. *D,* Diagram illustrating the cell structure of a few terminal alveoli. *E,* The accumulation of milk globules within an alveolus. (From George W. Corner, 1942.)

iology logically falls into two categories; development of the glands to a functional state, and the formation and evacuation of milk.

Early studies involving the administration of ovarian hormones to intact or ovariectomized animals pointed to the conclusion that estrogen is particularly concerned with growth of the duct system and that progesterone, acting in concert with estrogen, is required for full alveolar growth. In species such as the mouse, rat, and monkey, large doses of progesterone, without estrogen priming, have been shown to evoke the development of both the duct and alveolar systems. There are many species variations in the manner in which the mammary rudiment responds to the ovarian steroids. Without discussing the many species differences, it is sufficient to state that there is general agreement that estrogen and progesterone function synergistically and both are needed for the experimental production of glands structurally comparable to those of midpregnancy. Since the anterior pituitary gonadotrophins (*viz.,* FSH, LH, and prolactin) are essential for the production of ovarian hormones during pregnancy, it is obvious that they are indirectly involved in mammary growth. In addition to pituitary effects mediated by the ovary, it has been shown that prolactin and somatotrophin

(STH) can act directly on mammary tissue and that ACTH and TSH can influence mammary functions through their respective target organs.[28, 29, 42, 44, 60]

The action of pituitary hormones on the mammary glands has remained a live field of experimentation since Stricker and Grueter (1928) demonstrated that crude extracts of the anterior hypophysis have lactogenic effects.[54] It was soon found that estrogen, alone or in combination with progesterone, fails to induce mammary development in hypophysectomized animals. This finding led to the proposal that estrogen and progesterone acted indirectly on the mammary glands by stimulating the pituitary to secrete specific mammogenic hormones in addition to its six well-authenticated protein hormones. Originally it was suggested that one pituitary "mammogen" stimulated duct growth and the other alveolar growth. The mammogen hypothesis has undergone considerable modification by its originators, but it must remain highly questionable since it has not been possible to separate these special substances from pituitary tissue in any state approaching chemical purity. Most workers in the field feel that pituitary-mammary relationships can be accounted for on the basis of the known anterior lobe hormones and that it is not necessary to postulate the existence of other hypophysial factors. With the availability of highly purified anterior pituitary hormones, many aspects of the problem are beginning to be clarified.[21, 38, 59]

Studies on the rat have been systematically pursued by a number of investigators, and, while the results may not be directly applicable to all species, the differences are likely to be in the relative importance of the various hormones rather than in the kinds of hormones required. It appears probable that at least five of the anterior lobe hormones, in addition to ovarian steroids, are involved in the production of a fully developed mammary gland such as is found during late pregnancy. Some of the most pertinent facts may be summarized as follows:

1. When estrogen is administered to castrated male or female rats, it produces mainly growth of the duct system. If larger doses are given for prolonged periods, some alveolar development may appear. Physiologic doses of estrogen plus progesterone produce full mammary growth (pregnancy type) when administered to castrates. Estrogen alone, given to intact females, produces both ductal and lobuloalveolar development. In the latter instance, it is probable that estrogen encourages the hypophysial release of prolactin and this hormone stimulates the secretion of progesterone by the corpora lutea.

2. In hypophysectomized rats, estrogens and progestogens, alone or in combination, fail to induce mammary development. Hormones FSH and LH, administered to hypophysectomized subjects, do not stimulate the mammary glands. This indicates that mammary development requires hormones in addition to FSH, LH, estrogens, and progesterone.

3. In immature rats lacking both pituitaries and gonads, a combination of estrogen and somatotrophin (STH) is necessary to produce growth of the arborescent system of milk ducts. If the adrenal glands, in addition to the pituitaries and ovaries, are removed, ductal growth requires estrogen plus STH plus adrenal corticoids.

4. In order to obtain full lobuloalveolar growth, comparable to that of

late pregnancy, prolactin and progesterone are needed in addition to estrogen, STH, and adrenal corticoids. In the presence of the adrenal glands, ACTH may be used instead of the corticoids. Thus, a quintet of hormones is needed to build up the gland to the prolactational stage.

5. Milk secretion (lactogenesis) may be induced in the prolactational gland by withdrawing or diminishing the estrogen and progesterone and continuing the prolactin and adrenal corticoids (or ACTH). Although STH and TSH are not necessary for lactogenesis in the rat, both hormones probably contribute to the normalcy of the process in the intact animal.

These facts concerning the development of the mammary gland have been derived largely from *in vivo* experiments. Recent studies of mammary tissue in organ culture have given new insight into the development of this gland under the influence of various hormones and growth-promoting substances. First of all, it appears that cell differentiation into functional mammary tissue requires a previous cell division in order to render the cells competent to stimulation by cortisone or hydrocortisone. Subsequently, the action of prolactin or placental lactogen can cause these cells to synthesize milk proteins and to become secretory. Various agents, including insulin, STH, or growth factors such as EGF (epithelial growth factor, a polypeptide derived from mouse submaxillary glands) can cause stem cells of the mammary gland to divide, but these cells do not respond to prolactin until they are converted to secretory cells through the action of adrenal corticosteroids. Undifferentiated cells that have not undergone cell division lack the capacity to become secretory under stimulation by prolactin. In other words, it seems that the chain of events in the differentiation of a mammary stem cell to the functional state is: cell division, preparation by corticosteroids, stimulation by a lactogen, and secretion. Apparently these various steps relate to specific gene activation leading ultimately to the synthesis of specific milk proteins.[58]

Many types of experiments, particularly those involving hypophysectomized animals, suggest that the placenta performs an important role in mammary development during the second half of pregnancy. Ablation of the pituitary gland at midpregnancy does not prevent full mammary growth in the rat and certain other species. There is a tendency to think of milk secretion as beginning at or shortly after parturition but, on the contrary, the transformation from a prolactational to a lactational gland in the rat is very gradual, and there is considerable evidence of secretion during the second half of pregnancy. There is ample evidence that the placenta secretes estrogen, progesterone, and a potent prolactin-like hormone, human placental lactogen (HPL) (see Chapter 4).[26] Placental lactogens have been the subject of several recent investigations, and it appears that lactogenic activity is demonstrable in the placentae of a variety of mammalian species.[55] It is likely that such placental lactogens contribute to maternal mammary gland development. HPL, like its pituitary counterpart, affects two target organs during pregnancy, namely, the corpora lutea of the ovaries and the mammary glands. It may be supposed that these two targets compete for the prolactin present in the system; but, as the corpora lutea wane during the end of pregnancy, the mammary apparatus gains priority. This ascendancy is retained by the mammary glands after parturition, even though a new crop of corpora lutea is formed as a result of the postpartum estrus.

Milk Secretion (Lactogenesis)

The anterior hypophysis is necessary for the initiation and maintenance of milk secretion. The discovery that crude anterior pituitary extracts are lactogenic was followed by the isolation and purification of prolactin. It was found that minute amounts of purified prolactin, injected into an appropriate teat canal of the rabbit, produced lactation in localized sectors of the mammary gland, neighboring untreated sectors remaining unaffected. Since the rabbits were not hypophysectomized, the possibility that other pituitary hormones participated in the response was not ruled out.

The importance of the adrenal cortex in the initiation of lactation in a variety of mammals has been clearly established. Although animals that are adrenalectomized during pregnancy may deliver normal litters, lactation is so meager that they cannot raise their young. Lactation may be induced in the pseudopregnant rat by prolactin plus adrenal cortical hormone, but purified prolactin alone is ineffective. That lactation can be induced in hypophysectomized rats and guinea pigs by giving either prolactin plus adrenal cortical hormone or prolactin plus ACTH has been shown.

After parturition there is a striking increase in milk secretion. The exact mechanisms that operate at this time have not been fully agreed upon. There is evidence that estrogen and progesterone act synergistically to inhibit lactation. At parturition there is a fall in the circulating titers of ovarian and placental steroids, and this operates in some manner to turn the full force of the pituitary and adrenal cortex upon the mammary apparatus. Low levels of estrogen in the blood stimulate the pituitary to increase its output of prolactin, whereas high levels of estrogen tend to inhibit lactation. It is not known whether this inhibitory action of estrogen is effected through the pituitary or at the level of the mammary gland, or both. It may be that at parturition the fall in the relative ratio of progesterone to estrogen allows the latter hormone to exert its positive effect in promoting the release of prolactin from the anterior hypophysis. Whatever the exact mechanism may be, it is reasonably certain that prolactin and adrenal corticoids are the most essential hormones for the initiation of lactation.

The hormones that are involved in mammogenesis and lactogenesis in the rat are summarized in Figure 15–8. Hormones FSH and LH function synergistically to promote the secretion of estrogen by the ovary. ACTH stimulates the adrenal cortex to secrete corticoids. Growth of the duct system is produced by the action of estrogen, STH, and adrenal corticoids. Prolactin stimulates the corpora lutea to secrete progesterone. Full lobuloalveolar (prolactational) development requires a combination of prolactin, STH, estrogen, progesterone, and corticoids. Milk secretion by the developed gland ensues when the influence of estrogen and progesterone is diminished and prolactin and adrenal corticoids attain supremacy. It is probable that lactogenesis is facilitated by STH and TSH, although neither is absolutely necessary in the rat.[39, 48]

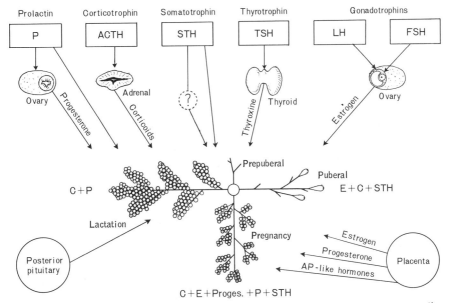

Figure 15–8. A simplified diagram showing the action of hormones on mammary growth and lactation. Upper diagram, rudimentary gland; lower diagrams prolactational gland of pregnancy; right side, prepuberal to puberal gland; left, lactating gland. (From Lyons, W. R., Li, C. H., and Johnson, R. E.: Rec. Prog. Horm. Res., *14,* 1958.)

Maintenance of Lactation (Galactopoiesis)

After delivery of the young, milk yield rises rapidly and then declines slowly until the young are weaned. The hormonal mechanisms involved in galactopoiesis are very similar to those that initiated milk production. Hypophysectomy at any period during lactation terminates the process. The continued production of prolactin is probably essential throughout the period of lactation, and there can be little doubt that ACTH, STH, and TSH are likewise of importance. When milk production begins, pressure develops within the glands and, if it is not relieved by suckling or milking, it rises to the point where milk secretion is retarded. The mammary glands of mice and rats involute quickly after removal of the litters, but the administration of prolactin to such animals tends to maintain the alveolar epithelium and retard involution. When the young are removed from rats on the fourth day of lactation, injections of oxytocin markedly delay mammary involution. Ablation of the neural lobe of the hypophysis of lactating rats abolishes the milkejection reflex, and the young die from starvation unless injections of oxytocin are given the mother. When such operated mothers become pregnant a second time, parturition and lactation are normal, indicating that regeneration of the neural lobe occurs in this species. After removing the litters from postpartum rats, milk production can be maintained for as long as 75 days by injecting a combination of prolactin, oxytocin, and cortisol.

Studies have shown that the stimulus of suckling, either with or without the removal of milk, temporarily lowers the content of prolactin in the anterior pituitaries of rats, guinea pigs, and rabbits. There are also indications that regular applications of the suckling stimulus maintain prolactin secretion at a high level.[43] The rat normally lactates for about three weeks since the young are weaned at this time, but experiments show that the mammary glands are capable of responding for a much longer time. The lactation period has been prolonged for 70 days by providing rats with fresh litters every 10 days.[45] The lobuloalveolar system shows little or no evidence of involution during this extended period, although there is a decline in milk yield as judged by litter weight gains. It is generally agreed that stimulation of the nipple during the act of suckling reflexly prolongs the release of prolactin and other galactopoietic hormones from the animal's hypophysis.

Sectioning of the spinal cord immediately craniad of the first lumbar vertebra in lactating rats completely paralyzes that portion of the body that bears the last three pairs of nipples. If the cranial nipples are covered so as to force the young to suck the denervated nipples, the young rapidly lose weight and succumb from inanition. When other lactating litters are introduced, they die in the same manner. If two of the innervated glands are exposed to suckling litters, lactation continues in all the glands, irrespective of the nerve supply. It may be inferred that this surgical procedure has destroyed nervous pathways that are essential for the stimulus of suckling to prolong the release of galactopoietic hormones from the pituitary gland.

Involution of the mammary glands of mice is delayed when the nipples are irritated by the local application of spirits of turpentine. If this substance is applied to selected nipples, some remaining untreated, lactation from all the glands is prolonged in the absence of nursing litters. Turpentine applied to the skin of the back produces no such effect; such nonirritating materials as water applied to the nipples do not delay mammary involution.

Milk Ejection

For full understanding of lactation, it is necessary to distinguish between milk secretion and milk removal since the two processes appear to be regulated by different neuroendocrine mechanisms.[15, 31] The former, which we have already discussed, centers around the release of prolactin and other hormones from the anterior hypophysis. Milk removal, on the other hand, involves the reflexive release of oxytocin from the neurohypophysis (Fig. 15–9). Oxytocin is conveyed by the circulation and causes milk evacuation by contracting the myoepithelial cells that surround the mammary alveoli. The act of suckling or milking reflexly stimulates both milk secretion and milk ejection. If a young animal is permitted to nurse from an anesthetized mother, only the milk stored in the cistern and larger ducts can be withdrawn without any active participation of the mother. The greater part of the milk in the gland can be obtained only if there is activation of a neurohormonal reflex and a consequent contraction of the mammary alveoli. Within some 30 to 90 seconds after application of the suckling or milking stimulus, intramammary duct pressure suddenly rises and milk begins to flow freely. This results from the onset of the milk-ejection reflex and, in popular language, is called the "let-down" or the "draught."[24, 32]

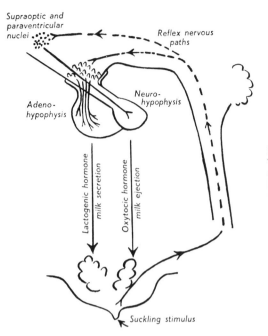

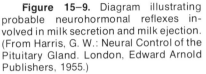

Figure 15–9. Diagram illustrating probable neurohormonal reflexes involved in milk secretion and milk ejection. (From Harris, G. W.: Neural Control of the Pituitary Gland. London, Edward Arnold Publishers, 1955.)

The afferent component of the reflex arc is nervous, whereas the efferent limb is hormonal. The sensory stimuli associated with suckling excite receptors in the mammary glands and impulses are conveyed over spinal and brain stem tracts to the diencephalon and supraoptic nuclei of the hypothalamus. Through the mediation of the supraoptico-hypophysial tracts, the neural division of the hypophysis discharges oxytocin and probably some vasopressin. Oxytocin in the blood forms the efferent component of the arc, and the myoepithelial basket cells around the mammary alveoli constitute the effector tissue. This or a similar mechanism operates in a great variety of laboratory and domestic animals, and there is much evidence that it functions in lactating women as well. The milk-ejection reflex may be excited by various kinds of conditioned stimuli, and it is also subject to inhibition by emotionally stressful situations.

Many factors other than mechanical stimulation of the mammary glands can induce the milk-ejection reflex. The importance of milking cows at a set time every day is well recognized. The sound of buckets, the presence of calves, washing the udder, the sight of food, and so on may all constitute stimuli to which the animals become conditioned. Manipulation of the external genitalia and other events associated with mating, rather than with nursing or milking, may be sufficient to cause the discharge of milk, presumably through the reflexive release of oxytocin.

It had been known for many years that crude extracts of the posterior hypophysis facilitate milk evacuation, but the situation has been clarified since purified and synthetic preparations became available. Although oxytocin is five to six times more effective than vasopressin in eliciting milk ejection, the latter hormone possesses some intrinsic capacity to do so. Milk ejection occurs after the administration of oxytocin to lactating subjects even without mechanical stimulation of the mammary glands, as well as after the glands have been denervated. Suckling does not lead to milk ejection after severance of the pituitary stalk or after certain areas of the hypothalamus are destroyed by electrolytic lesions. Electrical stimulation of the supraoptico-hypophysial tract of goats and rabbits causes a copious discharge of milk. Jugular vein blood drawn from goats thus treated has the capacity of inducing milk ejection when administered to lactating test animals. These and many other types of experiments indicate that the reflexive release of milk is mediated through the hypothalamus and neurohypophysis.[17]

The Myoepithelial Cells

For many years it has been assumed, on rather inadequate evidence, that smooth muscle tissue in connection with the alveoli served the function of squeezing milk from the gland. Histologic studies, however, failed to reveal the presence of this tissue in association with the alveoli, except in very meager amounts. Earlier histologists had identified myoepithelial cells or "basket cells" intimately surrounding the alveoli, but their distribution and structural features remained vague until they were studied after silver impregnation.[50] There is now no reasonable doubt that these cells are the effector contractile tissue of the mammary gland (Fig. 15–10).

Direct microscopic studies of the living gland have shown that the myoepithelial cells are capable of contracting. Direct mechanical or electrical stimulation causes them to contract and evacuate the alveolar contents. They may be caused to contract by the local application of oxytocin or vas-

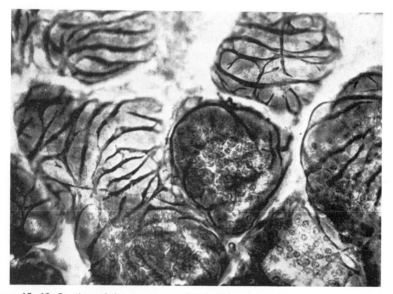

Figure 15–10. Section of the mammary gland of the goat, showing the myoepithelial cells surrounding the alveoli. (From Harris, G. W.: Proc. Roy. Soc., B., *149*, 1958.)

opressin. Various drugs, such as histamine, acetylcholine, pilocarpine, and 5-hydroxytryptamine, also contract the myoepithelial cells after local application. Epinephrine and norepinephrine, on the other hand, have no effect on these cells, though they do not prevent oxytocin from exerting its usual effect.

Inhibition of Milk Ejection

Clinicians are aware that worry, fear, embarrassment, sadness, and other strong emotions at the time of nursing may inhibit the flow of milk in women. In human beings as well as in many other mammals, milk ejection may be blocked by the administration of epinephrine. It is probable that the epinephrine blockade is due to vasoconstriction within the mammary gland since epinephrine does not inhibit the action of oxytocin on mammary alveoli *in vitro*. In the majority of cases, emotional stress seems to block the ejection of milk by preventing the nervous stimulus from reaching the neurohypophysis and causing a discharge of oxytocin. Experiments on laboratory animals have shown that it may also result from a sympatheticoadrenal discharge from the hypothalamus, which produces constriction of the mammary blood vessels.[16]

It is well known that lactation ceases rather promptly if the mammary glands become engorged with milk through absence of suckling or milking or through disturbances in the milk ejection mechanism. Experiments on lactating rats have provided some interesting information on the mechanism of mammary involution after engorgement. On the day after parturition, the teat ducts of some of the mammary glands are ligated subcutaneously, the unoperated teats of the same animal serving as controls. As the animals continue nursing their litters, the operated glands become conspicuously distended by 8 hours and reach a maximum at 24 hours. If the ligatures are loosened at this stage, milk ejection can be elicited by the intravenous injection of oxytocin. If the ducts remain tied for 48 hours, the glands lose their pinkish color and histologic examination reveals that the capillary meshwork of the gland is collapsed and devoid of blood cells. If the sutures are removed at this stage and oxytocin administered intravenously, milk ejection no longer ensues. However, contraction of the myoepithelial cells occurs when minute amounts of oxytocin are topically applied to the surface of the gland. These observations indicate that the failure to eject milk is due to capillary reduction rather than to myoepithelial incompetence. It is not known whether such constriction of the capillary bed occurs naturally in cases of engorgement, although there are suggestions that it does.

REFERENCES

1. Albert, A., and Derner, I.: Studies on the biologic characterization of human gonadotropins. Nature and number of gonadotropins in human pregnancy urine. J. Clin. Endocr. *20*: 1225, 1960.

2. Amoroso, E. C.: De la signification du placenta dans l'évolution de la gestation chez les animaux vivipares. Ann. d'endocrinol. *16*:435, 1955.
3. Amoroso, E. C.: Comparative anatomy of the placenta. Ann. N. Y. Acad. Sci. *75*:885, 1959.
4. Benson, G. K., Cowie, A. T., Folley, S. J., and Tindal, J. S.: Recent developments in endocrine studies on mammary growth and lactation. *In* C. W. Lloyd (ed.): Endocrinology of Reproduction. New York, Academic Press, 1959, p. 457.
5. Bisset, G. W.: Milk ejection. *In* R. O. Greep and E. B. Astwood (eds.): Handbook of Physiology, Section 7, Endocrinology, Vol. IV, Part 1, pp. 493–520. Baltimore, Williams & Wilkins Co., 1974.
6. Blandau, R. J.: Biology of eggs and implantation. *In* W. C. Young (ed.): Sex and Internal Secretions, Vol. 2. Baltimore, Williams & Wilkins Co., 1961, p. 797.
7. Böving, B. G.: Implantation. Ann. N. Y. Acad. Sci. *75*:700, 1959.
8. Bragdon, D. E., Lazo-Wassem, E. A., Zarrow, M. X., and Hisaw, F. L.: Progesterone-like activity in the plasma of ovoviviparous snakes. Proc. Soc. Exp. Biol. Med. *86*:477, 1954.
9. Browning, H. C.: Role of prolactin in regulation of reproductive cycles. Gen. & Comp. Endocrinol., Suppl. *2*:42, 1969.
10. Buchanan, G. D., Enders, A. C., and Talmage, R. V.: Implantation in armadillos ovariectomized during the period of delayed implantation. J. Endocr. *14*:121, 1956.
11. Chang, M.C.: Maintenance of pregnancy in intact rabbits in the absence of corpora lutea. Endocrinology *48*:17, 1951.
12. Chieffi, G.: Endocrine aspects of reproduction in elasmobranch fishes. Gen. Comp. Endocr., Suppl. *1*:275, 1962.
13. Clegg, M. T., Boda, J. M., and Cole, H. H.: Endometrial cups and allantochorionic pouches in the mare with emphasis on the source of equine gonadotrophin. Endocrinology *54*:448, 1954.
14. Cole, H. H. (ed): Gonadotropins: Their Chemical and Biological Properties and Secretory Control. San Francisco, W. H. Freeman & Co., 1964.
15. Cowie, A. T., and Folley, S. J.: Neurohypophysial hormones and the mammary gland. *In* H. Heller (ed.): The Neurohypophysis. London, Butterworth & Co., 1957, p. 183.
16. Cross, B. A.: Neurohormonal mechanisms in emotional inhibition of milk ejection. J. Endocr. *12*:29, 1955.
17. Cross, B. A.: The posterior pituitary gland in relation to reproduction and lactation. Brit. M. Bull. *11*:151, 1955.
18. Cross, B. A.: Neurohypophyseal control of parturition. *In* C. W. Lloyd (ed.): Endocrinology of Reproduction. New York, Academic Press, 1959, p. 441.
19. Csapo, A.: Function and regulation of the myometrium. Ann. N. Y. Acad. Sci. *75*:790, 1959.
20. Cunningham, J. T., and Smart, W. A. M.: Structure and origin of corpora lutea in some of the lower vertebrates. Proc. Roy. Soc., B, *116*:258, 1934.
21. Damm, H. C., and Turner, C. W.: Evidence for the existence of mammogenic hormone. Proc. Soc. Exp. Biol. Med. *99*:471, 1958.
22. Deanesly, R.: Endocrine activity of the early placenta of the guinea-pig. J. Endocr. *21*:235, 1960.
23. Doyle, L. L., and Margolis, A. J.: Intrauterine foreign body: Effect on pregnancy in the rat. Science *139*:833, 1963.
24. Folley, S. J.: The Physiology and Biochemistry of Lactation. London, Oliver & Boyd, 1956.
25. Friesen, H.: Purification of a placental factor with immunological and chemical similarity to human growth hormone. Endocrinology *76*:369, 1965.
26. Friesen, H. G., Suwa, S., and Pare, R.: Synthesis and secretion of placental lactogen and other proteins by the placenta. Rec. Progr. Hormone Res. *25*:161, 1969.
27. Gallien, L.: Endocrine basis for reproductive adaptations in Amphibia. *In* A. Gorbman (ed.): Comparative Endocrinology. New York, John Wiley & Sons, 1959, p. 479.
28. Grosvenor, C. E., and Turner, C. W.: Pituitary lactogenic hormone concentration and milk secretion in lactating rats. Endocrinology *63*:535, 1958.
29. Grosvenor, C. E., and Turner, C. W.: Thyroid hormone and lactation in the rat. Proc. Soc. Exp. Biol. Med. *100*:162, 1959.
30. Hammond, J., Jr.: The rabbit corpus luteum; oestrogen prolongation and the accompanying changes in the genitalia. Acta Endocr. *21*:307, 1956.
31. Harris, G. W.: The central nervous system, neurohypophysis and milk ejection. Proc. Roy. Soc., B, *149*:336, 1958.
32. Haun, C. K., and Sawyer, C. H.: Initiation of lactation in rabbits following placement of hypothalamic lesions. Endocrinology *67*:270, 1960.
33. Healy, M. J. R.: Foetal growth in the mouse. Proc. Roy. Soc., B, *153*:367, 1960.
34. Hisaw, F. L.: Endocrine adaptations of the mammalian estrous cycle and gestation. *In* A. Gorbman (ed.): Comparative Endocrinology. New York, John Wiley & Sons, 1959, p. 533.
35. Hisaw, F. L.: Endocrines and the evolution of viviparity among the vertebrates, *In* F. L. His-

aw, Jr. (ed.): Physiology of Reproduction. Proc. 22nd Ann. Biol. Colloq. Corvallis, Oregon State University Press, 1963, p. 119.

36. Kon, S. K., and Cowie, A. T. (eds.): Milk: The Mammary Gland and Its Secretion, Vol. 1. New York, Academic Press, 1961.

37. Linzell, J.L.: Physiology of the mammary glands. Physiol. Rev. *39*:534, 1959.

38. Lyons, W. R., Johnson, R. E., and Li, C.H.: Local action of pituitary and ovarian hormones on the mammary glands of hypophysectomized-oöphorectomized rats. Anat. Rec. *127*: 432, 1957.

39. Lyons, W. R., Li, C. H., and Johnson, R. E.: The hormonal control of mammary growth and lactation. Rec. Progr. Hormone Res. *14*:219, 1958.

40. Marshall, J. M.: Effects of neurohypophysial hormones on the myometrium. *In* R. O. Greep and E. B. Astwood (eds.): Handbook of physiology, Section 7, Endocrinology, Vol. IV, Part 1, pp. 469–492. Baltimore, Williams & Wilkins Co., 1974.

41. Matthews, L. H.: The evolution of viviparity in vertebrates. Mem. Soc. Endocr., No. 4, 129, 1955.

42. Meites, J., and Shelesnyak, M. C.: Effects of prolactin on duration of pregnancy, viability of young and lactation in rats. Proc. Soc. Exp. Biol. Med. *94*:746, 1957.

43. Meites, J., and Turner, C. W.: Influence of suckling on lactogen content of pituitary of post-partum rabbits. Endocrinology *31*:340, 1942.

44. Moon, R. C.: Growth hormone and mammary gland lobule-alveolar development. Amer. J. Physiol. *201*:259, 1961.

45. Nicoll, C. S., and Meites, J.: Prolongation of lactation in the rat by litter replacement. Proc. Soc. Exp. Biol. Med. *101*:81, 1959.

46. Noble, R. L., and Plunkett, E. R.: Biology of the gonadotrophins. Brit. M. Bull. *11*:98, 1955.

47. Perry, J. S.: The reproduction of the African elephant *(Loxodonta africana)*. Phil. Trans. Roy. Soc., B, *237*:93, 1953.

48. Reece, R. P.: Mammary gland development and function. *In* J. T. Velardo (ed.): The Endocrinology of Reproduction. New York, Oxford University Press, 1958, p. 213.

49. Reynolds, S. R. M.: Gestation mechanisms Ann. N. Y. Acad. Sci. 75:691, 1959.

50. Richardson, K. C.: Contractile tissues in the mammary gland, with special reference to myoepithelium in the goat. Proc. Roy. Soc., B, *136*:30, 1949.

51. Smith, P. E.: Continuation of pregnancy in Rhesus monkeys (*Macaca mulatta*) following hypophysectomy. Endocrinology 55:655, 1954.

52. Smithberg, M., and Runner, M. N.: The induction and maintenance of pregnancy in prepuberal mice. J. Exp. Zool. *133*:441, 1956.

53. Solomon, S., Bird, C. E., Ling, W., Iwamiya, M., and Young, P. C. M.: Formation and metabolism of steroids in the fetus and placenta. Rec. Progr. Hormone Res. 23:297, 1967.

54. Stricker, P., and Greueter, F.: Action du lobe antérieur de l'hypophyse sur la montée laiteuse. Compt. rend. soc. de biol. 99:1978, 1928.

55. Talamantes, F.: *In vitro* demonstration of lactogenic activity in the mammalian placenta. Amer. Zool. 15:279, 1975.

56. Taymor, M. L., Yahia, C., and Goss, D. A.: A three-minute immunologic test for pregnancy. Internat. J. Fertil. *10*:41, 1965.

57. Tindal, J. S.: Stimuli that cause the release of oxytocin. *In* R. O. Greep and E. B. Astwood (eds.): Handbook of Physiology, Section 7, Endocrinology, Vol. IV, Part 1, pp. 257–267. Baltimore, Williams & Wilkins Co., 1974.

58. Turkington, R. W.: Hormone-dependent differentiation of mammary gland *in vitro*. *In* A. A. Moscona and A. Monroy (eds.): Current Topics in Developmental Biology, Vol. 3. New York, Academic Press, 1968, p. 199.

59. Turner, C. W.: Regulation of lactation. Conf. Radioactive Isotopes in Agric., East Lansing, Michigan, 403, 1956.

60. Turner, C. W., Yamamoto, H., and Ruppert, H. L., Jr.: Endocrine factors influencing the intensity of milk secretion: estrogen, thyroxine and growth hormone. J. Dairy Sci. *40*:37, 1957.

61. Velardo, J. T.: Hormonal actions of chorionic gonadotropin. Ann. N. Y. Acad. Sci. *80*:65, 1959.

62. Wide, L., and Gemzell, C. A.: An immunological pregnancy test. Acta Endocr. 35:261, 1960.

CHAPTER 16

Gastrointestinal Hormones and Other Hormone Candidates

As we have pointed out earlier, there is no general agreement as to what constitutes an endocrine gland or as to what cellular products should be accorded hormonal status. Biologists are forced to the conclusion that there are profound gradations within organisms with respect to the degree of differentiation of glands. It appears that cells and tissues may be rather highly differentiated in other directions and still remain capable of releasing special substances into the body fluids. As was pointed out in Chapter 3, this is certainly the case with the nervous system and the neurohormones they produce, and to some extent the same may be true of the digestive tract and its gastrointestinal hormones. Just as we have come to accept neurohormones and neurotransmitters as legitimate hormones, the various gastrointestinal principles are also considered as hormones. In a sense this seems surprising, in view of the fact that secretin was the first compound to which the term "hormone" was applied. However, it belongs to a category of substances, the gut or gastrointestinal hormones, which do not always fit all the criteria that many investigators consider as essential features of a hormone. One of the problems in this regard concerns the overlapping activities of the various gastrointestinal hormones that make it difficult to decide whether the actions of these substances are physiological or pharmacological.

Because of the nebulous definition of the term "hormone," it is difficult to classify substances that are at least analogous to hormones. For example, among a number of substances of external origin that are known to affect the behavioral physiology of animals is a group of compounds called "pheromones." This is an arbitrary grouping of compounds, which are not necessarily related, that have the capacity to affect the behavior or development of receptive organisms. Sex attractants are the most well-known of this group, and because of their endocrine implications they are often thought of as hormones. They are really not hormones, however, and we shall not consider them as such. They fall into the same realm as do embryonic inductors and gamones, the substances produced by eggs and sperms that are so active in the physiology of fertilization.

It is the purpose of this chapter to discuss briefly some of the coordinatory agents that are unique in some respects and which do not coincide exactly with the classic connotations of the term "hormone."

524

GASTROINTESTINAL HORMONES[12, 13, 17]

Localized areas of the alimentary tract form three recognized gastrointestinal hormones, secretin, gastrin, and cholecystokinin. A multitude of activities are attributed to them, and as indicated in Figure 16–1, each of these peptide hormones has several physiological roles. This has often led to confusion, in that an activity thought to be the unique role of a specific hormone has also been called "cholecystokinin-pancreozymin." While the example, it was long thought that a discrete hormone, pancreozymin, was responsible for stimulating secretion of enzymes from the acinar cells of the pancreas. It is now known that this activity is an additional function of cholecystokinin, a peptide known to stimulate gall bladder contraction. This hormone has also been called "cholecystokinin-pancreozymin." While the three gastrointestinal hormones have achieved recognized status, it should not be concluded that others do not exist. Indeed, an array of "candidate hormones of the gut" are under active consideration.[13] Among these candidate hormones is a group of pure peptides with gastrointestinal actions that have been extracted from intestinal mucosa, but which are of uncertain hormone status. The gastric inhibitory peptide (GIP) and urogastrone, an inhibitor of HCl secretion, are among this group. Another major category of candidate hormones includes hormones whose existence is postulated on the basis of physiological evidence but about which little or no chemical information is available. The list of such potential hormones includes bulbogastrin, duocrinin, enterogastrone, enteroglucagon, incretin, villikinin, and vagogastrone. As more information about these substances accumulates, a new system of nomenclature for gastrointestinal hormones will arise.

Of the established gastrointestinal hormones, it is known that they are

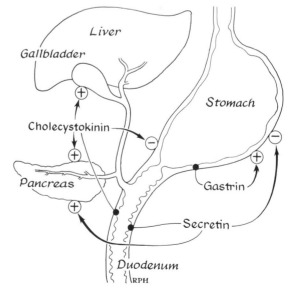

Figure 16–1. Diagram illustrating the source and action of the gastrointestinal principles. The arrows extend from the sources of the hormones and point toward the organs affected. Stimulation indicated by positive sign and inhibition by negative sign.

released into the circulation and their actions supplement those of the autonomic nervous system. One conspicuous feature of the endocrine glands, other than those of the gastrointestinal tract, is that their activities are interrelated in such a manner as to produce a system of checks and balances. No such interrelationship has been clearly demonstrated for the gastrointestinal hormones; they are not known to be influenced by other glands of the endocrine system or to be interrelated among themselves. Their secretion is conditioned largely by the presence or absence of particular food substances in the lumen of the alimentary tract, rather than by other glandular products in the circulation. Little is known about the specific cells responsible for their production. The gastrointestinal hormones produce their effects quickly after the application of appropriate stimuli for their release, and they are quickly destroyed after withdrawal of the stimulus. They are polypeptide in nature and, surprisingly, contain amino acid sequences that resemble not only those of one another, but also those of peptides of other natural sources, such as the hormone glucagon and the amphibian skin secretion, caerulein.[1, 12]

Secretin

After the ingestion of food there is no appreciable release of pancreatic juice until the partially digested food passes through the pyloric sphincter into the duodenum. About the turn of the century it was thought that this release of pancreatic juice was the result of a nervous reflex. However, it was demonstrated in the classic experiments of Bayless and Starling that section of the vagus nerve did not abolish the response, nor could the intravenous administration of acids and secretagogues influence pancreatic activity. It was concluded that some substance must diffuse from the duodenal mucosa into the blood and be thus transported to the pancreas, where it induces release of pancreatic juice. Indeed, injection into the blood of extracts of duodenal mucosa initiated the flow of pancreatic juice. The active substance was considered a chemical messenger and was called secretin. The passage of chyme from the stomach causes the duodenal mucosa to release secretin into the blood, and the hormone stimulates the flow of pancreatic juice but not the release of enzymes; the flow of bile and intestinal juices is stimulated to a lesser extent. The hormone acts directly on the acinar cells of the pancreas. Secretin is most active when given intravenously, and, since it is inactivated by gastric and pancreatic juices, it is totally ineffective when given by mouth. The hormone disappears rapidly from the circulation owing to the destructive action of an enzyme called "secretinase."

Secretin has been obtained in crystalline form from extracts of porcine duodenal and jejunal mucosa. It is a peptide consisting of 27 amino acid residues (Fig. 16–2). There are three other members of the secretin family of peptides: pancreatic glucagon, gastric inhibitory peptide (GIP), and vasoactive intestinal peptide (VIP). While GIP and VIP have been isolated from intestinal mucosa, their hormone status is uncertain. All four members of the secretin family of peptides share many amino acid sequences in com-

mon. The number of identical residues in secretin and glucagon is especially striking, but knowledge about the mechanism of action of secretin is only
now beginning to accumulate because of the availability of the hormone in a
pure state. It has been revealed that its range of physiological properties is
remarkable (Fig. 16–1). In addition to its well known action in the stimulation
of pancreatic secretion, secretin stimulates hepatic bile flow and gastric
pepsin secretion, inhibits gastrointestinal motility and gastric acid secretion, and exerts an influence on insulin release, fat cell lipolysis, renal function, and cardiovascular activities. A distinction can be made between various actions of secretin on the basis of hormone dose. Certain actions, such
as lipolysis and insulin release, can be brought about only by high doses of
hormone; others, such as pancreatic activity and the stimulation of pepsin
and gastrin secretion, require much lower blood concentrations of the hormone. These observations imply the existence of more than one order of
receptor sites on the various cells that are targets of secretin action. Knowledge of the precise mechanisms of action of secretin is fragmentary. In part,
such studies are impeded because the entire molecule is necessary for physiological activity. Even the removal of the N-terminal histidine residue
markedly diminishes the action of secretin. Despite their chemical similarity,
the physical properties of these two molecules are quite different, and while
both molecules share certain physiological properties, there are differences
in activity which are attributable to their structural differences. It is significant that the complete sequence of amino acids is necessary for full biological activity of secretin.

	1	2	3	4	5	6	7	8	9	10	11	12	13	14
Secretin	His	Ser	Asp	Gly	Thr	Phe	Thr	Ser	Glu	Leu	Ser	Arg	Leu	Arg
Glucagon	His	Ser	Gln	Gly	Gly	Phe	Thr	Ser	Asp	Tyr	Ser	Lys	Tyr	Leu
GIP	Tyr	Ala	Glu	Gly	Gly	Phe	Ile	Ser	Asp	Tyr	Ser	Ile	Ala	Met
VIP	His	Ser	Asp	Ala	Val	Phe	Thr	Asp	Asn	Tyr	Thr	Arg	Leu	Arg

	15	16	17	18	19	20	21	22	23	24	25	27	26	28	29
Secretin	Asp	Ser	Ala	Arg	Leu	Gln	Arg	Leu	Leu	Gln	Gly	Leu	Val	NH$_2$	
Glucagon	Asp	Ser	Arg	Arg	Ala	Gln	Asp	Phe	Val	Gln	Trp	Leu	Met	Asp	Thr
GIP	Asp	Lys	Ile	Arg	Gln	Gln	Asp	Phe	Val	Asn	Trp	Leu	Leu	Ala	Gln
VIP	Lys	Gln	Met	Ala	Val	Lys	Lys	Tyr	Leu	Asn	Ser	Ile	Leu	Asn	NH$_2$

Figure 16–2. Structures of the porcine secretin-glucagon family of peptides.

With the availability of purified secretin, it has been possible to utilize
immunological techniques to localize the site of secretin production. The
application of immunofluorescent methods has revealed the presence of
secretin in endocrine cells of the duodenum and the first portion of the je-
junum. Electron microscopy has revealed that these cells possess small
granules of varying degrees of electron density which possess secretin.
They appear to have no immunoreactivity with glucagon antibodies.

Research on the biological nature of secretin is in its infancy. Soon
much new information about the mechanisms of its action will become
available. In addition, considerable knowledge will be derived about the
specific sites and conditions of its synthesis and release. Studies on lower

forms are now underway, and this will contribute not only to our knowledge of the evolution of secretin, but to our understanding of how all the gastrointestinal hormones evolved.

Gastrin

On the basis of many physiological experiments, it has long been suggested that the pyloric region of the stomach produces gastrin in response to mechanical distension and the local action of secretagogues contained in the food. Gastrin was postulated to be absorbed into the blood and carried to the fundic cells, causing them to secrete hydrochloric acid. In the early 1960's, two pure polypeptides having the ability to stimulate gastric secretion were isolated from porcine mucosa. Both peptides contained identical sequences of 17 amino acids; however, one, designated gastrin II, differed from the other, gastrin I, in that its tyrosine residue was sulfated (Fig. 16–3). Subsequently, similar pairs of peptides were isolated from the antral mucosa of several other species, including man. These molecules are very similar to one another and differ only in trivial amino acid substitutions in the body of the molecule. In the process of the synthesis of porcine gastrins, various fragments were obtained and were tested for physiological activity. It was learned that the C-terminal tetrapeptide amide Trp-Met-Asp-Phe-NH_2, common to all the known gastrins, is capable of all the physiological activities of the complete molecule. This fragment possesses about one-tenth the activity of the whole molecule, but this is markedly reduced by even one amino acid substitution. Currently, much interest concerns the existence of several molecular forms of gastrin. While 17-amino acid gastrins predominate in the antral mucosa, both smaller and larger forms are present in other tissues. In the Zollinger-Ellison tumor (a pancreatic islet cell tumor), a minigastrin of 13 amino acids and several larger molecules have been found. A gastrin of 34 amino acids has been found in the blood. This large molecule, known as big gastrin, consists of the gastrin heptadecapeptide amide covalently linked to an additional sequence of 17 amino acids. Also present in some tissues is a big big gastrin, which is considered to be a macromolecular form of the molecule.

Gastrin exhibits a broad spectrum of action. At low concentrations these include: secretion of water and electrolytes by stomach, pancreas, liver and Brunner's glands; inhibition of water and electrolyte absorption from the ileum; stimulation of enzyme secretion from stomach and pancreas; stimulation of the lower esophageal sphincter and stomach muscle; inhibition of the tone of the sphincter of Oddi; increase of blood flow in the gastric mucosa; and stimulation of amino acid incorporation into proteins in the gastric mucosa. At high doses, gastrin stimulates the growth of gastric mucosa, stimulates the release of insulin, inhibits gastric secretion, and stimulates smooth muscle of gut, gall bladder, and uterus. While structure-activity relations of gastrin polypeptides have been under intensive investigation, and some knowledge about binding sites is available, relatively little is known about the precise mechanism of action of gastrin.

CAERULEIN
Pyr—Gln—Asp—Tyr(SO_3H)—Thr—Gly—Trp—Met—Asp—Phe—NH_2

PORCINE GASTRIN II
Pyr—Gln—Pro—Trp—Met—$(Glu)_5$—Ala—Tyr(SO_3H)—Gly—Trp—Met—
Asp—Phe—NH_2

PORCINE CHOLECYSTOKININ
Lys—Ala—Pro—Ser—Gly—Arg—Val—Ser—Met—Ile—Lys—Asn—
Leu—Gln—Ser—Leu—Asp—Pro—Ser—His—Arg—Ile—Ser—Asp—
Arg—Asp—Tyr(SO_3H)—Met—Gly—Trp—Met—Asp—Phe—NH_2

Figure 16–3. Structures of three related polypeptides having gastrointestinal activities. The five amino acid sequences at the C-terminal are identical.

With the availability of pure gastrin preparations, it has been possible to utilize immunological procedures in studying the physiology of these polypeptides. Radioimmunoassay techniques have been developed, and their use has increased our understanding of the relationships between the various gastrin peptides. Immunological techniques have revealed that gastrin is localized in secretion granules of specific gastrin or G-cells prevalent in the antral glands. The release of hormone from these cells is promoted by vagal stimulation or by acetylcholine. The presence of various amino acids in the stomach serves to stimulate gastrin release, and the presence of hydrochloric acid in the stomach inhibits this release through a negative feedback mechanism.

Cholecystokinin

Another member of the gastrin family, but nevertheless a discrete hormone, is cholecystokinin. The existence of this hormone was deduced from the fact that contraction could be induced in the denervated gallbladder by the presence in the duodenum of such substances as fat, fatty acids, dilute acids, and peptides. Moreover, the presence of a cholecystic agent was found in porcine duodenal extracts. Because these extracts also had the ability to stimulate pancreatic enzyme secretion, they were thought to contain another hormonal principle, pancreozymin. As these extracts were further purified, both physiological activities were retained and it was finally realized that these two different physiological properties were two discrete functions of the same hormone. The hormone has been referred to as cholecystokinin-pancreozymin, but recent publications commonly use its simpler designation, cholecystokinin.

Purification of cholecystokinin from porcine duodenal and jejunal preparations has revealed it to be a linear peptide consisting of 33 amino acid residues. The C-terminal pentapeptide is identical to that of gastrin, and the tyrosyl residue is sulfated just as in gastrin (Fig. 16–3). Because of this structural similarity, cholecystokinin and gastrin have many functions in common. For example, both hormones can promote pancreatic secretion and stimulate gastric secretion. The structure of caerulein, a decapeptide isolated from the skins of an Australian tree frog *Litoria (Hyla) caerulea,* also resembles those of gastrin and cholecystokinin.[6] The C-terminal octapeptide sequence of caerulein differs from that of cholecystokinin only by the substitution of threonine for methionine. The resemblance is remarkable at the C-terminus not only with respect to the amino acid sequence, but also with regard to the presence of a sulfated tyrosyl residue. The question of why frog skin secretions contain a molecule like caerulein is an interesting one that cannot yet be answered; however, studies of such secretions hold the promise of making interesting contributions to our knowledge of biochemical evolution.

Phylogenetic Considerations

As we look back at the structures and functions of the various gastrointestinal hormones, it is obvious that there are at least two distinct families, secretin-glucagon-VIP-GIP and gastrin-cholecystokinin. How these molecules and the endocrine gut evolved provide interesting and challenging questions. It is likely that the endocrine gut is phylogenetically old, for obviously, the problems of digestion have been with animals for a long time. Possibly, these problems were solved early and this could account for the relative primitive organization of the present-day endocrine gut. For example, endocrine cells are scattered throughout the gut epithelium rather than arranged as circumscribed endocrine glands. Some evidence for the condensation of endocrine cells is seen in the stomach, where gastrin cells are concentrated in the antrum. Whether this represents a late evolutionary development is unknown. Another manifestation of what might be a primitive feature of the gut is the fact that gastrointestinal hormones regulate the same organs in which they are produced.

Secretin probably predates the other gastrointestinal hormones, for it has been found in the intestine of molluscs, including a sea hare and an octopus. Moreover, together with cholecystokinin it has also been found in the lamprey intestine. Probably, primitive vertebrates had no stomach; thus it seems reasonable to hypothesize that these two intestinal polypeptides evolved before gastrin. However, this is pure speculation and much more work is needed on comparative aspects of gastrointestinal endocrinology before we can reasonably understand the evolution of this system.

ANGIOTENSIN[33]

Since the early publications of Bright (1827), it has been known that chronic disease of the human kidney is frequently correlated with high blood pressure, or hypertension. As early as the turn of the century it was shown that extracts of kidney tissue raised the blood pressure of experimental animals. By regulating heart action and the caliber of blood vessels, the nervous system brings about rapid changes in blood pressure and the flow of blood through tissues. Various hormones and other chemical agents, in addition to the nervous system, have important roles in the regulation of blood pressure. For instance, certain tumors of the adrenal medulla, called *pheochromocytomas,* secrete large amounts of epinephrine and norepinephrine and thus cause a profound elevation of blood pressure. Since the kidneys process a large volume of blood and function in the maintenance of a relatively constant internal environment, it is not surprising to find that they are involved in a humoral mechanism that influences blood pressure. Two methods have been found whereby permanent hypertension may be experimentally produced with regularity: (1) sectioning of the modulator nerves produces *neurogenic* hypertension, and (2) mechanical alteration of the hemodynamics of the kidneys produces *renal* hypertension.

Although various workers devised experimental procedures for modifying kidney functions in attempts to produce renal hypertension, Goldblatt and his collaborators were the first to work out a technique that produces permanent hypertension consistently enough to be used in systematic studies.[10] Their method was to produce a deficient flow of blood through the kidneys (ischemia) by applying an adjustable clamp to the renal artery. By this method, hypertensive states have been produced in a variety of mammals, *e.g.,* dogs, sheep, goats, rats, and monkeys. There is conclusive proof that localized ischemia of the kidneys produces a persistent hypertension; some workers have followed up such animals for seven years or longer. In dogs having an ischemic kidney on one side only, the contralateral kidney remaining normal, removal of the damaged kidney is followed by a rapid return of blood pressure to normal levels. The same type of hypertension may be produced by ligation of the ureters or by the injection of such nephrotoxic substances as mercury, bismuth, and lead. It appears that almost any procedure that results in a deficiency of oxygen in the renal tissues can cause the blood pressure to rise.

Persistent hypertension in a variety of mammals results from procedures that induce perinephritis. For example, when the kidneys are encapsulated by collodion, cellophane, or silk, they react to the foreign substance by forming a fibrocollagenous shell around the organ that compresses the renal parenchyma and does not permit the natural expansion of the kidney while it is functioning. This technique may be used advantageously in small animals in which difficulties would be encountered in applying a clamp to the renal arteries. Renal hypertension results from these procedures after denervation of the kidneys; after bilateral section of the splanchnic nerves; after total sympathectomy, including total denervation of the heart; after subdiaphragmatic splanchnicectomy, the celiac and upper ganglia being removed; after bilateral section of the ventral roots of the spinal nerves; and even after the destruction of the spinal cord below the fifth cervical vertebra.

The hypertensive state is not prevented or modified by ablation of the adrenal medullae. If a kidney is transplanted into the neck by uniting the renal artery with the carotid and the renal vein with the jugular, the intact kidney being removed and the transplanted kidney being made ischemic by clamping the renal artery, typical hypertension ensues. Under these circumstances, the ischemic kidney, completely devoid of nervous control, releases a substance that is responsible for the elevation of the blood pressure. Certain types of hypertension in the human subject appear to be due to arteriosclerotic plaques or other obstructions to the flow of blood through the kidneys. In other cases, there appears to be no obstruction of renal blood flow, and the precise mechanism that causes the release of renin by the kidneys remains obscure.

Much progress has been made in defining the mechanism whereby the kidneys influence blood pressure (Fig. 16–4).[23] *Renin* is an enzyme produced by the juxtaglomerular cells of the kidney and released into the circulation. Apparently this release is triggered by the detection of changes in sodium concentration by receptors in the macula densa and in the vasculature of the kidney.[7] Renin acts on *renin-substrate,* a globular protein that the liver frees into the blood stream, and produces a substance which is called "angiotensin I." (This substance was originally called "angiotonin" and "hypertensin" by different workers; the hybrid term "angiotensin" is now in general use.) Another blood protein, called "converting enzyme," acts on angiotensin I to split off a pair of amino acids from one end of the peptide chain, thus producing the active substance, angiotensin II. The latter is conveyed to the capillary beds, where it causes constriction of the arterioles.

Apparently, angiotensin II also acts on the zona glomerulosa of the adrenal, leading to the production of aldosterone, which in turn affects the distal tubules of the kidney, causing an increase in sodium and water resorption. The resulting changes in sodium concentration and the blood pressure-blood volume changes ensuing from the principal actions of angiotensin provide the juxtaglomerular cells with cues for the production of renin.

The amino acid sequence in the angiotensin molecule has been deter-

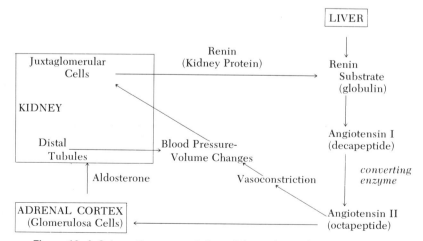

Figure 16–4. Schematic representation of the renin-angiotensin system.

mined and the substance has been produced synthetically.[28] Angiotensin I is a peptide chain consisting of 10 amino acids:

$$Asp—Arg—Val—Tyr—Ile—His—Pro—Phe—His—Leu$$

Angiotensin II, the active form, is identical with the inactive form except for the absence of the terminal amino acids, histidine and leucine. Angiotensins from different species are generally similar, but slight variations are known to occur. Synthetic angiotensin elevates the blood pressure of man and laboratory animals and causes the contraction of uterine muscle. It is probably the most potent vasopressor substance known. Angiotensin I elevates the blood pressure only because it is rapidly converted in the bloodstream to angiotensin II; it has no effect on uterine muscle in vitro since the converting enzyme is not present in the tissue. It thus appears that the organism can convert renin-substrate to angiotensin I and store it in this inactive form, converting it to the active octapeptide as the need arises. It is a well-known fact that certain enzymes are similarly stored as inactive proteins. All tissues exhibit some peptidase activity capable of destroying angiotensin II, but kidney and intestine are especially active in this respect.

It is interesting that several other peptides present in the organism exert the same physiologic effects as angiotensin II. For example, vasopressin, a hormone of the neurohypophysis, causes an elevation of blood pressure, and oxytocin has a strong effect on uterine contractility. The neurohypophysial hormones, like angiotensin II, are octapeptides, but no other structural similarities between the two types of substances have been detected. Hydrolysis of blood serum or of certain of its proteins by proteolytic enzymes yields various polypeptides, and some of these exert pharmacologic actions simulating those of vasopressin, oxytocin, and angiotensin II.

The role of the angiotensin system in stimulating aldosterone secretion has been the subject of considerable attention.[9] It began with the discovery that the kidney is the source of a powerful aldosterone-stimulating substance, and subsequently it was shown that angiotensin II duplicates the action of these renin preparations. Angiotensin II acts directly on the zona glomerulosa of the adrenal cortex and leads to the specific stimulation of aldosterone secretion without leading to an appreciable rise in glucocorticoid secretion. Numerous experiments involving the use of low sodium diets and nephrectomy confirm the view that the action of angiotensin II on the zona glomerulosa is much like that of ACTH on the zona fasciculata. Whether the action of angiotensin on the glomerulosa is mediated by cyclic AMP, as in the action of ACTH, has not been established.

Most early work on the renin-angiotensin system has been carried out on mammals; however, it is now known that renin is a constituent of the kidney of several fishes. Moreover, it has recently been demonstrated that vasopressor activity attributable to the corpuscles of Stannius of teleosts has the characteristics of renin.[29] It appears that the renin-angiotensin system is present among most vertebrates.[21] While neither renin activity nor juxtaglomerular cells have been found in cyclostomes and elasmobranchs, they have been detected in primitive bony fishes.[20] Angiotensin-like substances are present in fishes; however, their chemical properties differ from those of mammalian and other tetrapod angiotensins. How these substances are involved in the evolution of the renin-angiotensin system is as yet unknown.

UROTENSINS

The caudal end of the spinal cord of fishes including teleosts, elasmobranchs, holosteans, and chondrosteans contains secretory cells that are part of a neurohemal organ known as the urophysis. Over the years morphological evidence has suggested a possible endocrine role for this organ; this inference has been substantiated, more recently, by the results of pharmacological studies.[5] Several active principles have been isolated from the teleost urophysis, and these have been referred to as urotensins. Some of these extracts influence blood pressure, especially in mammalian systems, and others stimulate smooth muscle contraction, affect Na^+ movement, stimulate hydrosmotic activity, or play a role in the reproduction of both male and female teleosts. Evidence is now available that one of the urotensins is identical to arginine vasotocin and that the other active principles of urophysial extracts are peptides having molecular weights of about a thousand. Their amino acid compositions have not yet been established. In physiological studies, urotensins I and II have received the most attention. It appears that urotensin I is primarily associated with pressor effects and that urotensin II is fundamentally involved in the contraction of smooth muscle. Probably, the effects of urotensin II on reproductive tissue are based upon the ability of this principle to stimulate smooth muscle. While the physiologic status of the urophysis has long been enigmatic, recent studies have begun to clarify its role as an endocrine gland, and it seems likely that the urotensins will soon assume a legitimate hormonal status.

PROSTAGLANDINS

During the past few years, a new class of compounds has made a profound impact on endocrine physiology.[4] These are the prostaglandins, a family of lipids discovered in human semen in the early 1930's. Attention was attracted to these compounds because of the ability of seminal fluid to stimulate contraction or relaxation of the human uterus. Probably the term "prostaglandin" is a misnomer, for even though semen represents one of the richest sources of these compounds, they have been discovered in a number of other tissues, and their uterine effects represent only a small fraction of their total spectrum of action.

The chemical structure of prostaglandins is unusual. They are all 20-carbon fatty acids having the same basic "skeleton," prostanoic acid, and are derived from essential fatty acids by cyclization and oxidation. The first two prostaglandins to be isolated in pure crystalline form, PGE_1 and PGE_{1a},

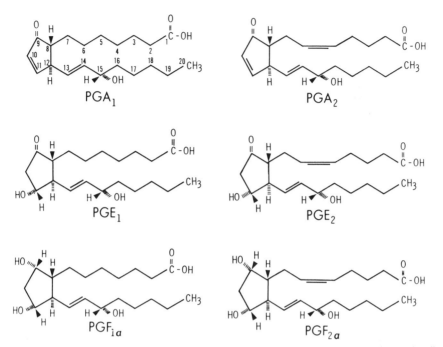

Figure 16–5. Structures of the most commonly occurring biologically active prostaglandins. (From Williams, R. H.: Textbook of Endocrinology, 5th Ed. W. B. Saunders Company, Philadelphia, 1974.)

were obtained from sheep seminal vesicles. A variety of other prostaglandins have been discovered in various mammalian tissues, such as lung, thymus, brain and spinal cord, kidney, iris, and placenta. They are suspected of being present and physiologically active in a number of other tissues.

The naturally occurring prostaglandins have been divided into four groups that have been designated by the letters E, F, A, and B. These groups are distinguished by differences in the cyclopentyl group of the basic 20-carbon skeleton of the prostanoic acid (Fig. 16–5). Unsaturations and substitutions in side chains provide an array of compounds in each series. Prostaglandins have been produced both biosynthetically from appropriate polyunsaturated fatty acids and by total chemical synthesis. The synthesis of a variety of analogs has been accomplished, and many of these hold promise of incorporating desirable properties of naturally occurring prostaglandins. Synthesis of the various prostaglandins is difficult because of the numerous asymmetric centers and the relative positions of functional groups. In tissues, prostaglandin synthesis from polyunsaturated fatty acids is catalyzed by prostaglandin synthetase. This enzyme is present in virtually all tissues, but its activity is particularly high in the renal medulla and in the seminal vesicles. Prostaglandins may be inactivated and degraded in tissues by enzymes such as prostaglandin isomerases, dehydrogenases, and reductases.

Prostaglandins have a wide spectrum of activities, and individual compounds differ in their actions. They act in smooth muscle stimulation as well as in relaxation; they affect the cardiovascular system, acting as pressor agents under some circumstances and as depressor agents under others. Other manifestations of prostaglandin effects on smooth muscle are represented by their oxytocic actions on the gravid uterus and by their abilities to stimulate intestinal motility. Prostaglandin effects on reproduction are quite pronounced. High levels of prostaglandins are associated with a breakdown of the corpus luteum and a depression in progesterone secretion. They are also implicated in the release of LH by mediating the release of LRF in the hypothalamus. It is striking that these reproductive effects are specifically brought about by the E and F series of prostaglandins. Prostaglandins are implicated in the inflammatory response, in various aspects of the immune response, in the hematopoietic system, in gastrointestinal secretion, and in the central nervous system, where certain prostaglandins have been implicated as neurotransmitters.

Perhaps the most important activities of prostaglandins concern their involvement with the actions of cyclic AMP, the second messenger in so many trophic hormone activities.[4] It has been known for some time that prostaglandins are implicated in the mediation of lipolysis by the second messenger, and it is now thought that they function through an activation of adenylate cyclase. How this is accomplished is not known; however, one view considers prostaglandins to act as transducers between the trophic hormone receptor and adenylate cyclase in the cell membrane.[16] Whatever the specific function of prostaglandins is in the adenylate cyclase system, there can be no doubt that its involvement is widespread. This is evidenced by the fact that prostaglandins increase the tissue content of cyclic AMP in so many tissues and organs including lung, spleen, diaphragm, adipose tissue, blood platelets, liver, pituitary, aorta, bone, gastric mucosa, kidney, heart, corpus luteum, thyroid, and erythrocytes. PGE_1 is the prostaglandin most active in this regard.[33]

THE PINEAL BODY

Clinicians have known for many years that pineal tumors are sometimes associated with precocious puberty, and this aroused the suspicion that some kind of a pineal-gonadal relationship might prevail at the human level. A review of clinical literature, made in 1954, suggests that true parenchymatous pinealomas correlate with depressed gonadal function, whereas tumors resulting in destruction of the pineal are frequently associated with precocious puberty.[14] This suggests that if the pineal is the source of a hormone affecting the gonads, it would probably exert an inhibitory effect. Reports of the inhibitory effects on the gonads in all vertebrate classes by substances associated with the pineal have filled the literature and are currently being analyzed. Important in this analysis is the consideration that the pineal of the intact organism functions in a circadian rhythm (24 hour cycle) presumably correlated with photoperiod. Accordingly, variations in the biochemical constitution of the pineal must be considered in relation to the photoperiod to which the animal is exposed. Since most animals are seasonal breeders, the circannual (12 month) cycle must also be considered.

Most studies on the physiological role of the pineal have involved melatonin and related indoles, and since the mid-sixties melatonin has been considered a pineal hormone. We noted earlier that the pineal has a high content of serotonin and an enzyme which converts this compound to melatonin and methoxytryptophol. This enzyme, hydroxyindole-O-methyl transferase (HIOMT), was thought to be present in only the pineal body. It has since been found in the brain and lateral eyes (see Chapter 5). The activity of the HIOMT in the rat follows a circadian rhythm, more melatonin being produced at night than during the day. Similar observations have been made on the pineals of chickens and quail. During the estrous cycle of the rat, HIOMT activity in the pineal is greatest at diestrus and falls appreciably during proestrus and estrus. The methoxyindoles of the pineal have been reported to depress the incidence of vaginal smears showing estrous phases in the rat. Denervation of the rat pineal by superior cervical ganglionectomy, like removal of the eyes, prevents the "early" response of the rat ovary to light.

It has been proposed that one function of the pineal in the rat is to serve as a neuroendocrine transducer, mediating the effects of environmental lighting on the gonads. Accordingly, information about lighting is perceived by the retina and nervous impulses are conveyed to the pineal by way of sympathetic nerves. The pineal responds by altering its production of methoxyindoles; these are thought to enter the bloodstream and influence physiological events. Melatonin has been identified in the blood of the chicken, where it exhibits a diurnal variation; melatonin content is highest in darkness. Similarly, studies on the melatonin content of the blood of humans reveals that while none can be detected during the day, measurable quantities can be found at night.

The inhibitory actions of melatonin on reproductive functions include a range of effects. By both injections and subcutaneous implantation, melatonin has been shown to retard gonadal growth in both males and females of a variety of mammals. It has also been shown to be an effective inhibitor of ovulation and of LH release. Possibly, the latter represents an action of melatonin at the level of the brain, for it has been reported that direct application of melatonin to neural structures leads to a reduction in gonadotrophic levels of both pituitary and plasma.

Because of the lack of emergence of a unifying concept concerning the pineal and reproductive phenomena, the possibility arises that some of the organisms that have been most studied in this regard may represent exceptions. For example, the laboratory rat has been so widely inbred that some of its responses are no longer the same as those of its wild counterpart. With this in mind, attention was given to the hamster which, because of its shorter history as a laboratory animal, is less removed from animals in the wild state. Results of experimental studies with hamsters revealed that in this species the antigonadotrophic activity of the pineal is more convincing than in any other so far studied.[26] Reduction of the amount of light to which hamsters are exposed not only leads to an involution of their sexual organs, but is accompanied by a reduction in circulating gonadotrophins. These effects can be abolished by interruption of nervous input to the pineal. These findings are especially significant because, in their natural habitat, hamsters are seasonal breeders, hibernating in the winter and breeding only during the summer months. Convincing arguments have been presented that the quiescent winter period results from a response of the pineal to a short photoperiod such that pineal activity inhibits reproductive function. During the summer, reproductive activity would be high because the inhibitory function of the pineal would be precluded by the effects of increased day length. It has been presumed that melatonin is the pineal agent responsible for these reproductive effects in the hamster. However, convincing evidence now excludes the possibility that melatonin is the causative agent.[27] It has been shown that the testicular involution and regression of accessory sex organs occurring in male hamsters exposed to only one hour of light and 23 hours of darkness can be abolished either by pinealectomy or by administration of melatonin. In view of all that has been said about melatonin, this observation is a real paradox.

The suggestion that melatonin is not the pineal antigonadal factor in the hamster (and probably other mammals) is not surprising to a number of investigators who have championed the candidacy of polypeptides as dominant pineal secretory products.[3, 8] Thieblot and colleagues have been principal proponents of the view that the pineal produces and releases a polypeptide hormone of relatively low molecular weight.[31] Other laboratories have also isolated antigonadal inhibitory peptides from pineal extracts, and the chemical elucidation of these agents is underway. In the meantime, the problem of the biochemical nature of the antigonadal principles remains unresolved, with both indoles and peptides remaining as principal candidates. Possibly, both types of compounds are involved.

Despite the fact that there is still no clearly elucidated role of the pineal as a vertebrate endocrine organ, the indirect evidence in support of this contention is overwhelming,[26] and its role in reproductive events will surely be soon understood. Probably, the role of the pineal in the blanching reactions of amphibian larvae is the clearest example of its function as an endocrine gland (see Chapter 5); however, this is such a limited physiologic event that other functions must be sought. The prominence of this organ in so many vertebrates is surely indicative of its basic importance, and the many demonstrations of changes in its physiology corresponding with external stimuli emphasize its probable role as a physiologic coordinator. The time has probably arrived when it is justifiable to consider the pineal as an endocrine gland.

THE THYMUS

It is known that the thymus glands are essential for the establishment and maintenance of immunologic competence in neonatal rodents. When mice are thymectomized soon after birth, their ability to form antibodies in response to particulate antigens and skin homografts is greatly reduced.[18] Thymectomy of adult rodents is accompanied by a fall in lymphocytes, but does not result in any impairment of their immune functions. Two general theories have been advanced to explain the action of the thymus: (1) it may be an essential and exclusive source of immunologically competent cells which leave the organ and populate peripheral lymphoid tissues, and (2) it may be the source of a thymic hormone which conditions the proliferation and maturation of potential immunologically competent cells in many other tissues.

Studies have shown that liver cells from embryonic mice become immunologically competent when passed through the body of a host possessing its thymus gland, but not when passed through thymectomized hosts. The diminished ability of mice to form antibodies after neonatal thymectomy can be restored to normal by implanting into them thymus tissue enclosed in cell-tight Millipore filter chambers. This indicates the presence of a noncellular, diffusible material which is probably conveyed by the blood. If a neonatally thymectomized mouse is allowed to become pregnant when mature, the pregnancy repairs the mother's ability to form antibodies. This has been interpreted as meaning that a hormone or similar substance is produced by the thymus glands of the fetuses *in utero*, and this traverses the placenta and acts to restore immunologic competence to the mother.[22] These and many other experiments suggest that the thymus is the source of a blood-borne factor which induces the differentiation of lymphoid precursor or stem cells, rendering them capable of participating in immune reactions.

The search for a thymic hormone has resulted in the isolation and purification of a polypeptide that has been designated "thymosin."[11] This substance is free of lipid and carbohydrate and appears to be a straight chain peptide having a molecular weight of about 12,000. Administration of thymosin preparations to thymectomized mice stimulated the proliferation of lymphocytes and restored the spectrum of immunological properties absent in such animals. The development of T-lymphocytes, recognizable by their surface antigens, occurs; and cell-mediated immunological responses are restored. Induction of T-lymphocyte differentiation *in vitro* from competent precursor cells of spleen and bone marrow has also been demonstrated.[15] Of additional significance, it has been shown that T-cell differentiation can be induced in lymphocytes of the bursa of Fabricius by thymosin preparations.[30] The immunological role of the bursa is clearly established. With the availability of purified thymosin, radioimmunoassay techniques for its detection have been developed and their application has revealed the presence of thymosin in the blood. Altogether, it would seem that thymosin can now be considered to be a legitimate hormone.

Among the evidence for endocrine activity of the thymus is the fact that it is sensitive to steroid hormones. The diminution of the size of the thymus as sexual maturity approaches is at least partially due to an inhibition provided by gonadal steroids. Adrenal steroids also inhibit the thymus, and this effect was once used as a parameter for the assay of corticosteroids. This phenomenon is not limited to mammals, for even the amphibian thymus is sensitive to endocrine changes. The thymus glands of hypophysectomized tadpoles are more than twice the size of those of intact siblings. Whether these are indirect effects resulting from the lack of development of the adrenal cortex or whether they are due directly to the lack of some hypophysial factor is not known.[2]

Studies on the role of the thymus in poikilotherms are now underway and have been important in the development of the new field of comparative immunology. It can be expected that our knowledge of the endocrine implications of this organ will be augmented greatly in the near future.

PHYTOHORMONES[24]

Phytohormones are biologically active materials of plant origin that are effective in minute concentrations at sites remote from the tissues in which they are formed.[32] The term includes auxins, wound hormones, flowering hormones, some of the B vitamins, carotenoids, and steroids. The term *auxin* is now used to designate materials that induce the longitudinal growth of shoots; this growth is accomplished by cell elongation rather than by cell division. The variety of growth effects attributable to the various phytohormones includes: root and shoot initiation, vascular induction in callus, wound regeneration and vascular induction in intact plants, induction of secondary thickening, mobilization of cereal endosperm, and stem and coleoptile extension.

Growth Regulators in Plants

The best known auxin is indole-3-acetic acid (IAA). It is a true, naturally occurring auxin that has been isolated from *Rhizopus* cultures and from a number of different species of higher plants (Fig. 16–6). It is considered to be the principal auxin of most plants. The auxins are produced most abundantly by regions of active growth, such as coleoptile tips, apical buds, root tips, and young leaves, and are rapidly translocated to other regions of the plant where they exert their actions. Several routes of IAA synthesis occur in plants, but all start from the amino acid tryptophan. Leaves contain an enzyme that is capable of converting tryptophan into IAA. It is known that plant tissues contain auxin in both the free and bound forms. Some of the IAA is loosely adsorbed on the surface of protein fractions; the auxin is active in this state but is not capable of free movement within the plant. Indoleacetaldehyde has been extracted from plant tissues and is an inactive precursor of IAA. Auxin precursors may form complexes with certain growth inhibitors; this is often found in storage tissues such as seeds and tubers. Plant tissues contain an enzyme system, IAA oxidase, which attacks IAA and converts it into a compound that is without growth-promoting properties. Some tissues contain an inhibitor of IAA oxidase. In addition to an oxidative breakdown of IAA, conjugates may be formed with other molecules yielding products that may be either physiologically active or inert.

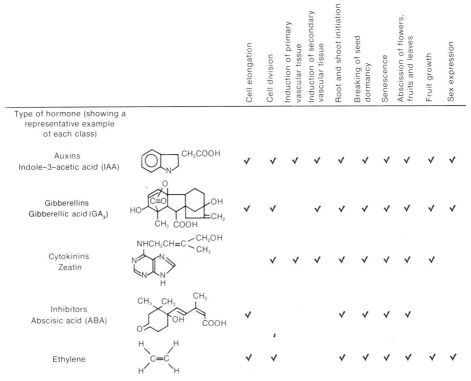

Figure 16–6. Some major plant hormones. A check indicates the involvement of the hormone in the process indicated. (From Graham, C. F., and Wareing, P. F., The Developmental Biology of Plants and Animals. Blackwell Scientific Publications, Ltd., Oxford, 1976.)

Auxins are involved in various aspects of plant growth and development (Fig. 16–6). Natural auxin promotes the growth of shoots by stimulating both cell enlargement and cell division, but the growth of roots is generally inhibited. However, at extremely low levels of concentrations, root growth is usually promoted. In assessing different growth-promoting activities of IAA, attention must be given to the rate and degree of translocation of the hormone from its site of production to its place of action. While much is unknown about the mode of translocation of auxins, it has long been known that polar transport is involved. Generally, this movement is from the apical to basal regions; however, the reverse has been demonstrated in roots. Such polar translocations were first discovered by Went in 1928 in his classic studies on shoot (coleoptile) growth that became the basis for the *Avena* (oat) coleoptile assay for auxins. It is known from such work that if the apical bud is removed from a shoot and a small quantity of IAA is applied to the stump, the lateral buds cease growing. Thus, the same concentration of auxin that promotes growth of the shoots inhibits growth of the lateral buds. As the terminal bud grows away from the lateral buds, the auxin supply is weakened by distance and the lateral buds at a lower level on the stem begin to grow out. A large number of synthetic auxins have been prepared; however, their specific activities vary greatly relative to those of IAA.

Some of the synthetic compounds, though not growth-promoting in them-selves, may potentiate the action of auxin; they may act as synergists in low concentrations but as inhibitors when present in larger amounts. 2,3,5-Triiodobenzoic acid is an auxin synergist that behaves in this manner. It is possible that the synergistic effect may be associated with a facilitation of auxin transport, whereas the inhibitory effect may be due to competition with auxin for an enzyme system. Structure-activity studies on auxins and their analogs have been valuable in understanding the mechanism of action of auxins. Various theories are now available concerning the interaction of IAA with appropriate receptor sites in target tissues.

Recent studies have shown that the basic mechanism of action of auxin is not unlike that of animal hormones, in that it appears to operate at the level of gene-controlled protein synthesis. Apparently, auxin stimulates the synthesis of both RNA and the specific enzymes involved in the growth of the cell wall, for it is known that cell enlargement can be inhibited by acti-nomycin, puromycin, and chloramphenicol.

Many of the synthetic auxins have become useful tools in plant culture. They have been employed for the rooting of cuttings, induction of flowering and fruit setting, prevention of preharvest dropping of fruits, production of parthenocarpic fruits, and the killing of weeds. All of these varied responses are related to the general function of growth.

Gibberellins. A rice disease, called "baka-nae" (foolish seedling), was first reported in Japan in 1898. The disease is due to a fungus, *Gibberella fujikuroi,* which causes the seedlings to grow unusually tall and then to die. Several growth-stimulating compounds, called "gibberellins," have been isolated from the causative fungus.[19, 25] Extracts from certain flowering plants have been found to give gibberellin-like responses. The gibberellins produce a wide variety of growth responses in flowering plants (Fig. 16–6). Among these may be mentioned stimulation of shoot growth, root elonga-tion in maize, resumption of normal growth in certain genetically dwarfed phenotypes of maize, and the transformation of bush beans to the pole type. The gibberellins also promote flowering in certain plants. Gibberellic acid is a tetracyclic dihydroxylactonic acid having the composition $C_{19}H_{22}O_6$ (Fig. 16–6).

Young leaves, embryos, and the apices of roots have been shown to be centers of gibberellin production. Thus, it seems that both auxins and gib-berellins are synthesized in the same regions of the plant. The biosynthesis of gibberellins is much like that of various terpenoids which are found in plants. These include such substances as carotenoids and steroids which are built from isoprene units. Relatively little is known about the catabolism of gibberellins. While auxin transport is polar, translocation of gibberellins is less ordered; it is known that these substances can pass in all directions in the plant. Relatively little is known about the mechanism of action of gib-berellins.

Cytokinins. Stimulation of cell division in cultured plant tissues or in young embryos requires, in addition to various nutrients, the presence of growth factors known as cytokinins. Knowledge of the necessity of such factors in growth stimulation evolved from the early classic experiments which utilized coconut milk and other liquid endosperms in the culture of plant tissues and cells. It was observed that the need for coconut milk could be overcome by the addition of adenine and other purine bases to the medium. Later it was observed that kinetin, a 6-substituted derivative of adenine first obtained from yeast extracts, could increase the formation of buds in seedlings. Kinetin does not naturally occur in plants; however, several other chemically related substances that have growth-promoting properties like those of kinetin have been isolated from plants. These are designated as *cytokinins*. The first naturally occurring cytokinin to be identified, zeatin (Fig. 16–6), was isolated from corn. Cytokinins are not usually found in the free state in plants, but are normally bound to pentose. Thus, they are found in the riboside or even in the ribotide form. There is evidence that cytokinins in the nucleotide form are constituents of transfer RNA, and it is possible that their mechanism of action involves translational control of protein synthesis. Relatively little is known about the metabolism and transport of cytokinins in plant tissues.

Growth Inhibitors. While it is usual to consider hormones as agents of stimulation, several naturally occurring plant substances are considered to be hormones even though their principal activities are inhibitory. The best known of these is *abscisic acid* (Fig. 16–6), a sesquiterpenoid first isolated from the leaves and buds of a sycamore. This substance promotes dormancy in plants and induces leaf abscission. It is also thought to play a role in senescence and in flower initiation. While relatively little is known about the translocation of abscisic acid, there is evidence that it is produced in the leaves of woody plants and is transported to the shoot apex via the phloem.

Ethylene. Considerable evidence has accumulated to support the view that ethylene is a true plant hormone. This is indeed unique in view of the fact that it is a gas. Ethylene is present in plants in low concentrations, dissolved in the aqueous phase of cells. The fact that it is active in plants at low concentrations supports its candidacy as a hormone. Ethylene plays an important role in the ripening of fruits and seems to duplicate many of the effects that are induced by relatively high concentrations of auxins.

REFERENCES

1. Anastasi, A., Erspamer, V., and Endean, R.: Isolation and amino acid sequence of caerulein, the active decapeptide of the skin of *Hyla caerulea*. Arch. Biochem. Biophys. *125*:57, 1968.
2. Bagnara, J. T.: Hypophyseal control of anuran thymus. Anat. Rec. *137*:336, 1960.
3. Benson, B., Matthews, M. J., and Hruby, V. J.: Characterization and effects of a bovine pineal antigonadotropic peptide. Amer. Zool. *16*:17, 1976.
4. Bergström, S., Carlson, L. A., and Weeks, J. R.: The prostaglandins: A family of biologically active lipids. Pharmacol. Rev. *20*:1, 1968.
5. Berlind, A.: Caudal neurosecretory system: A physiologist's view. Amer. Zool. *13*:759, 1973.
6. Bertaccini, G., DeCarlo, G., Endean, R., Erspamer, V., and Impicciatore, M.: The action of caerulein on pancreatic secretion of the dog and biliary secretion of the dog and the rat. Brit. J. Pharmacol. *37*:185, 1969.
7. Davis, J.: The control of renin release. Am. J. Med. *55*:333, 1973.
8. Ebels, I., Isolation of avian and mammalian pineal indoles and antigonadotropic factors. Amer. Zool. *16*:5, 1976.
9. Ganong, W. F., Biglieri, E. G., and Mulrow, P. J.: Mechanisms regulating adrenocortical secretion of aldosterone and glucocorticoids. Rec. Progr. Hormone Res. 22:381, 1966.

10. Goldblatt, H., Lynch, J., Hanzel, R. F., and Summerville, W. W.: The production of persistent elevation of systolic blood pressure by means of renal ischemia. J. Exp. Med. *59*:347, 1934.
11. Goldstein, A. L., and White, A.: Thymosin and other thymic hormones: Their nature and roles in the thymic dependency of immunological phenomena. *In* A. J. S. Davies and R. L. Carter (eds.): Contemporary Topics in Immunobiology, Vol. 2, New York, Plenum, 1973, 339 p.
12. Gregory, R. A.: The gastrointestinal hormones: A review of recent advances. J. Physiol. *241*: 1, 1974.
13. Grossman, M. I.: Gastrointestinal hormones: Spectrum of actions and structure-activity relations. *In* W. Y. Chey and F. P. Brooks (eds.): Endocrinology of the Gut. Charles B. Slack, Inc., Thorofare, N. J., 1974.
14. Kitay, J. L.: Pineal lesions and precocious puberty: A review. J. Clin. Endocr. *14*:622, 1954.
15. Komuro, K., and Boyse, E. A.: *In-vitro* demonstration of thymic hormone in the mouse by conversion of precursor cells into lymphocytes. Lancet *1*:740, 1973.
16. Kuehl, F. A., Jr., Humes, J. L., Ham, E. A., and Cirillo, V. J.: Cyclic AMP and prostaglandins in hormone action. Intra-Science Chem. Rept. *6*:85, 1972.
17. Makhlouf, G. M.: The neuroendocrine design of the gut: The play of chemicals in a chemical playground. Gastroenterology *67*:159, 1974.
18. Miller, J. F. A. P.: The thymus and the development of immunologic responsiveness. Science *144*:1544, 1964.
19. Nickell, L. G.: Production of gibberellin-like substances by plant tissue cultures. Science *128*:88, 1958.
20. Nishimura, H., and Ogawa, M.: The renin-angiotensin system in fishes. Amer. Zool. *13*:823, 1973.
21. Ogawa, M., Oguri, M., Sokabe, H., and Nishimura, H.: Juxtaglomerular apparatus in the vertebrates. Gen. Comp. Endocrinol. Suppl. *3*:374, 1972.
22. Osoba, D.: Immune reactivity in mice thymectomized soon after birth. Normal response after pregnancy. Science *147*:298, 1965.
23. Peart, W. S.: The functions of renin and angiotensin. Rec. Progr. Hormone Res. *21*:73, 1965.
24. Phillips, I. D. J.: Introduction to the Biochemistry and Physiology of Plant Growth Hormones. McGraw-Hill Book Co., New York, 1971, 173 pp.
25. Phinney, B. O., West, C. A., Ritzel, M., and Neely, P. M.: Evidence for "gibberellin-like" substances from flowering plants. Proc. Nat. Acad. Sci. *43*:398, 1957.
26. Reiter, R. J.: Endocrine rhythms associated with pineal gland function. *In* L. W. Hedlund, J. M. Franz, and A. K. Kenny (eds.): Biological Rhythms and Endocrine Function. Plenum Press, New York, 1975.
27. Reiter, R. J., Vaughan, M. K., Blask, D. E., and Johnson, L. Y.: Pineal methoxyindoles: New evidence concerning their function in the control of pineal-mediated changes in the reproductive physiology of male golden hamsters. Endocrinology *95*:206, 1975.
28. Skeggs, L. T., Jr., Lentz, K. E., Kahn, J. R., Shumway, N. P., and Woods, K. R.: The amino acid sequence in hypertensin II. J. Exp. Med. *104*:193, 1956.
29. Sokabe, H., Nishimura, H., Ogawa, M., and Ogure, M.: Determination of renin in the corpuscles of Stannius of the teleost. Gen. Comp. Endocrinol. *14*:510, 1970.
30. Teodorczyk, J. A., and Potworowski, E. F.: Induction of T-cell differentiation in the bursa of Fabricius by a soluble thymus factor. Immunology *28*:711, 1975.
31. Thieblot, L., Alassimone, A., and Blaise, S.: Étude chromatographique et électrophorétique du facteur antigonadotrope de la glande pinéale. Ann. Endocrinol. *27*:861, 1966.
32. Thimann, K. V.: Toward an endocrinology of higher plants. Rec. Progr. Hormone Res. *21*: 579, 1965.
33. Williams, R. H.: Textbook of Endocrinology, 5th ed. W. B. Saunders Co., Philadelphia, 1974, 1138 pp.

CHAPTER 17

Endocrine Mechanisms in the Invertebrates

Neurosecretory cells, producing chemical messengers (neurohormones) for prolonged action at a distance, are the first elements of this kind to appear during the phylogeny of animal organisms. These glandlike neurons function together with purely nervous elements to adjust the organism to environmental changes. Epithelial endocrine glands appear to be absent in coelenterates and annelids, neurosecretory mechanisms operating alone to control such processes as growth and reproduction. The same is probably true of flatworms, nemerteans and nematodes, though these groups have not been explored in sufficient detail. The cephalopod molluscs appear to be the first organisms to achieve a structural organization requiring the presence of endocrine glands. Circumscribed endocrine glands increase in complexity through the arthropod and vertebrate classes, but neurosecretory cells continue to be of great importance.

SOME INVERTEBRATE PHYLA

Echinodermata

The radial nerves of starfish are the source of a gonad-stimulating peptide. This neural hormone acts upon the ovary to initiate the secretion of a second substance, identified as 1-methyladenine, which leads to spawning and the maturation of oocytes. This second substance is not a peptide, but is a small molecule insoluble in organic solvents such as ether, benzene, or acetone. It is likely that 1-methyladenine may be produced by the follicle cells of the ovary in response to the neural peptide. It has been reported that echinoid radial nerves produce a factor which induces spawning in both starfish and sea urchins.[5, 28]

Neuroendocrine Mechanisms in Annelida

Neurosecretory cells are present in the central nervous systems of all three major classes of annelids, and neurohemal organs have been identified in some species. The neuroendocrine complexes of polychaetes and oligochaetes appear to be involved in the control of three processes: (1) maturation of the gonads, (2) somatic transformations related to reproduction, and (3) the regeneration of posterior segments. The presence of true, non-neural endocrine glands in this phylum has not been established.

Polychaeta

As many polychaetes become sexually mature, they undergo somatic modifications which equip them to swim at the surface of the sea and engage in spawning activity. This transformation of an immature individual (atoke) into a reproductive individual (epitoke) is called *epitoky,* and involves changes in the parapodia, chaetae, musculature, eyes, size of the segments, etc. (Fig. 17–1).

Much evidence indicates that neurosecretory cells within the brain of

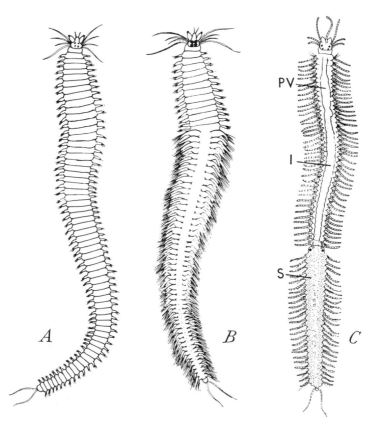

Figure 17–1. Metamorphosis in polychaete annelids. *A,* The immature or atokous stage of *Nereis. B,* The adult or epitokous stage of *Nereis. C,* Stolonization in a syllid polychaete. I, intestine; PV, proventriculus; S, stolon. (From Charniaux-Cotton, H., and Kleinholz, L. H.: *In* Pincus, G., Thimann, K. V., and Astwood, E. B. [eds.]: The Hormones, Vol. 4. New York, Academic Press, 1964; after Durchon, 1960.)

nereids are the source of a neurohormone that inhibits gonadal maturation and epitoky. By analogy with insects, this is sometimes called "juvenile hormone" since it acts to keep the animals sexually immature. Surgical removal of the cerebral ganglia, in nereids, with or without natural epitoky, results in premature and accelerated development of the gametes. In species in which epitoky occurs, decerebration of the atokous worms causes the premature attainment of the same metamorphic transformations as normally occur when the worms become sexually mature. All these changes that follow decerebration can be prevented by implanting ganglia from atokous donors; ganglia contributed by epitokous donors do not prevent the precocious epitoky and sexual maturation. The onset of normal epitoky can be delayed in intact individuals by the implantation of ganglia from atokous donors. Production or liberation of the inhibitory brain neurohormone apparently ceases after the onset of sexual maturity. Certain species and races of nereids normally reproduce in the atokous condition (without epitoky) and, in these forms, decerebration does not induce epitoky; the operation, however, does result in the precocious maturation of male germ cells. It is not known what factors operate to shut off the production of brain neurohormone as the nereids approach sexual maturity.[22]

Ablation and implantation experiments indicate that neurosecretory cells in the posterior portions of the cerebral ganglia of nereids are the source of a neurohormone that controls the regeneration of posterior segments. Little or no posterior regeneration occurs if the cerebral ganglia are removed at the time of segment amputation. Intracoelomic implants of the ganglia into decerebrate hosts restore the ability to replace excised posterior segments. Studies on Nereis have shown that both normal growth and regenerative capacity decline as the worms age, and that neurosecretions from the cerebral ganglia are apparently involved in both processes. It is not known whether the growth-promoting and regeneration-promoting neurohormones are identical or distinct secretions.[8, 24]

Some polychaetes of the non-nereid type are capable of caudal regeneration even after excision of the brain. Gonadotrophic hormones affecting vitellogenesis do not occur in the absence of the prostomium.[34, 35]

Oligochaeta

Neurosecretory cells within the supraesophageal ganglia of Lumbricus are the probable source of a secretion that governs the maintenance of external sex characters (e.g., clitellum), and possibly the differentiation of gametes. This neurohormone has an inhibitory effect on gonad maturation and is probably involved in the process of egg laying. In some species, the brain is essential for the regeneration of posterior segments.

Hirudinea

The central nervous system of the leech is rich in cells that are obviously neurosecretory. Testicular development is hormonally controlled by certain neurosecretory cells. Decerebration of the leech leads to a striking reduction of gamete clusters; the injection of brain extracts into such animals brings about the restoration of germ cells to a normal level. It is believed that the brain of the leech secretes a gonadotrophic hormone which regulates spermatogenesis.[23]

Neuroendocrine Mechanisms in Mollusca

Neurosecretory cells are found within the brains of all mollusca that have been studied and, in addition, appear in connection with many of the ganglia. The epithelial vesicles of cephalopods (squids and octopuses) show some structural evidence of neurosecretory competence, though this has not been proved. The epistellar body of the octopus is such a structure, and the indications are that it is a rudimentary photoreceptor.[26]

The genital ducts and accessory glands of slugs (e.g., Limax) undergo functional development at the time of gonadal maturation. Precocious development of these sex accessories may be induced by transplanting pieces of mature gonads into young recipients. The accessory sex organs involute following the castration of adults, and these changes are repaired by gonadal transplants. Accordingly, there is reason to believe that the gonads of pulmonate gastropods are the source of a hormone which is essential for the development and functioning of the accessory genital complex. In addition to neurosecretory complexes, true endocrine glands are present in the Mollusca.[6]

The optic glands of cephalopods are small *endocrine* organs lying on the optic stalks on either side of the brain (Fig. 17–2). Such glands have been found in all cephalopods examined, with the exception of *Nautilus,* and have been most carefully studied in *Octopus.*[48, 49] They contain no neurosecretory cells and are the source of a gonadotrophin which induces ovarian and testicular enlargement. The production of gonadotrophin by the gland is regulated by an inhibitory nerve supply extending to it from the subpedunculate lobe of the brain. The inhibitory centers in this portion of the brain seem to be governed by changes in photoperiod. Thus, light stimuli received by the eyes activate nerve centers in the brain and these hold the optic glands in check, and the gonads are inhibited through a lack of gonadotrophin. After blinding or excision of the subpedunculate lobes, the optic glands enlarge and the ovaries develop precociously. These procedures have no effect on the gonads after removal of the optic glands (Fig. 17–2). Functioning of the brain-optic gland-gonadal system of *Octopus* is suggestive of the regulation of sexual maturity in vertebrates by the hypothalamic-pituitary-gonadal axis. It should be noted, however, that neurosecretory cells seem not to be involved in the case of *Octopus.*

After excision of the optic glands of *Octopus,* the oocytes develop normally but follicle cells do not, and yolk deposition fails to occur. The gonadotrophin from the optic gland of the male appears to promote spermatogenesis. Ablation of the subpedunculate lobes of very young males results in enlargement of the optic gland, increased testicular weight, and the precocious appearance of spermatophores in the testis.

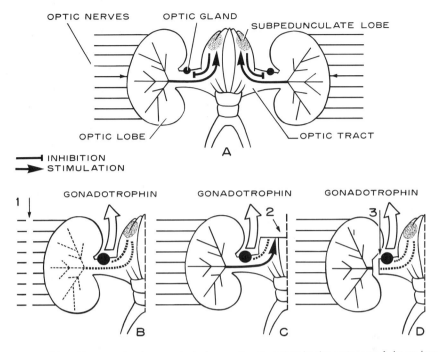

Figure 17–2. Neuroendocrine control of gonad maturation in the octopus. *A,* In an immature animal, unoperated upon, the production of gonadotrophin by the optic glands is held in check by an inhibitory nerve supply originating in the subpedunculate lobe of the brain. Activation of this brain center appears to depend upon changes in photoperiod. *B,* Section of the optic nerves (point 1) prevents activation (broken lines) of the inhibitory nerve center; the optic glands enlarge and secrete gonadotrophin, which induces hypertrophy of the gonads. The same result may be accomplished by ablation of the subpedunculate lobes *(C,* at point 2*)* or by section of the optic tract *(D,* point 3*).* (Modified from figures by Wells and Wells.)

There is no information on the chemical nature of the optic gland hormone. Experiments on the transplantation of optic glands and the effectiveness of fractionated organ extracts would probably yield interesting results.

NEUROENDOCRINE MECHANISMS IN THE CRUSTACEA

Location of Structures

The regulatory mechanisms of crustaceans are extremely complex and are very closely related to the central nervous system. The principal endocrine structures of a generalized crustacean are shown in Figure 17–3. Neurosecretory cells are abundant in the brain and in practically all of the other ganglia. The endocrine organs in crustaceans, as in insects, fall into three categories: (1) aggregations of neurosecretory cells that produce neurohormones and discharge them from their axonic terminals, (2) neurohemal organs for the storage, possible modification, and liberation of neurohormones, and (3) true endocrine glands (non-neural) that release hormones into the blood.

Important neurosecretory centers are found in connection with the optic ganglia which lie within the eyestalks. Best known of these are the "X organs" which are present in the eyestalks of most stalk-eyed species, or in the head when stalked eyes are absent (Fig. 17–3). Two kinds of X organs are now recognized: the *ganglionic X organ* and the *sensory pore X organ*. The two X organs fuse to form a single structure on the medulla terminalis of brachyurans but, in natantians, they are separated groups of neurosecretory cells. Clusters of secretory neurons are also found within the brain, the thoracic ganglia, the esophageal connective ganglia, and the tritocerebral commissure.

The sinus gland was early recognized as a potent source of hormones, and it was assumed initially that the secretions arose from glandular elements comprising the structure. Since the sinus glands do not show the

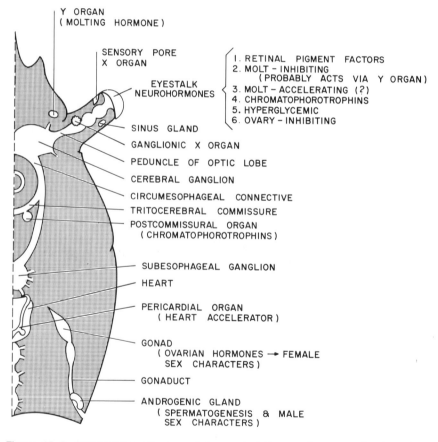

Figure 17–3. Summarizing diagram of the cephalothorax of a generalized crustacean, showing the locations of the best-known endocrine glands and neuroendocrine areas. The active principles from these structures are listed or shown in parentheses. Neurosecretory cells are present in all components of the central nervous system, and no attempt has been made to show them.

histologic characteristics of a typical gland of internal secretion, it became apparent that their products probably arose elsewhere. As surgical procedures improved, it was possible to remove this small organ alone without resorting to ablation of the entire eyestalk. It became apparent that these two surgical procedures result in different physiologic effects, and this led Bliss and Welsh (1952) to conclude that the sinus glands are essentially reservoirs for the storage and discharge of neurohormones derived from the axons of neurosecretory neurons. This concept has been amply confirmed and is now generally accepted. Like other neurohemal organs, the sinus glands consist chiefly of axonic terminals and are closely associated with rich vascular channels. In addition to discharged secretions, they contain nonglandular cells that seem comparable to the pituicytes present within the pars nervosa of the vertebrate neurohypophysis. These glia-like elements often appear to be wrapped around the bulbous terminals of the secretory axons. While it is possible that the sinus glands may possess some inherent secretory ability, like the corpora cardiaca of insects, they are chiefly storage-release centers for neurohormones.

The postcommissural and pericardial organs also appear to be essentially neurohemal in nature. The secretion-charged axons from cells within the brain and esophageal connective ganglia terminate in the postcommissural organs, which store and discharge the neurohormones. Neurosecretory cells, having their perikarya within the ganglia of the ventral chain, deliver their products to the pericardial organs located near the openings of the large veins into the pericardial sac (Fig. 17–3).

Three endocrine glands, not composed of secretory neurons, are found in the Crustacea: the Y organs, the androgenic glands, and the ovaries. The Y organs are located in the antennary or maxillary segment and resemble, in some respects, the prothoracic, molt-regulating glands of insects. They appear to be devoid of direct innervation, and are probably regulated by neurosecretions derived from the eyestalk complex. Androgenic glands have been found in a variety of crustaceans, and in a few species of insects. They are generally located outside the testes and are typically found along the vas deferens (Fig. 17–3). Although rudimentary androgenic glands are present in females, they develop only in males. These masculinizing glands are probably controlled by neurohormones from the X organ–sinus gland complex. The crustacean ovary, unlike the testis, serves in an endocrine capacity.[3, 4]

Retinal Pigment Migration

The compound eyes of higher crustaceans are composed of a large number of units called *ommatidia*. Three functionally distinct groups of pigments are possessed by each ommatidium: distal retinal pigment, proximal retinal pigment, and reflecting white pigment. The distal and proximal pigments screen the sensory component of the ommatidium, the rhabdome, in bright light, and migrate away from the rhabdome in darkness. The white pigment increases the effectiveness of dim light as a stimulus by reflecting

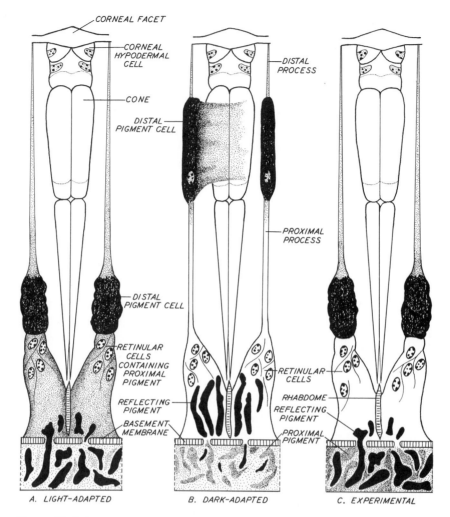

Figure 17–4. Ommatidia from the eyes of the shrimp *Palaemonetes vulgaris,* showing general morphology and the positions of the pigments under different conditions. *A,* The light-adapted condition. The distal pigment has migrated inwardly and is concentrated near the retinular cells. Most of the proximal pigment, contained within the retinular cells, lies distad to the basement membrane. The reflecting pigment moves through the basement membrane, *i.e.,* away from the rhabdome. *B,* The dark-adapted state. The distal pigment surrounds the distal end of the cone; the reflecting pigment surrounds the rhabdome, and the proximal pigment migrates into the portions of the retinular cells which lie below the basement membrane. *C,* An ommatidium from an animal which had been adapted to darkness and then had an injection of an extract of the eyestalks (sinus glands). The extract causes the distal and reflecting pigments to assume the positions characteristic of light adaptation; the proximal pigment apparently is not influenced in this species. (Modified after Kleinholz, L. H.: Amer Zool. *6*:161, 1936.)

the light that enters the eye over adjacent receptors. When the eye is adapted to darkness, the distal pigment migrates distally to enclose the dioptic apparatus, the proximal pigment moves to a position below the basement membrane, and the reflecting pigment surrounds the rhabdome. In the light-adapted eye, the distal pigment disperses proximally as far as the retinula cells, the proximal pigment moves distally to meet the distal retinal pigment, and the reflecting pigment moves away from the rhabdome and assumes a position below the basement membrane. Eyestalk extracts, prepared from light-adapted prawns, result in light adaptation of the distal and reflecting pigments when injected into dark-adapted recipients; the proximal pigment remains unchanged (Fig. 17–4).

The distal retinal pigment hormone from the eyestalks of *Pandalus borealis* is an octadecapeptide and has the following composition: Ala-Arg-Asp$_2$-Glu-Gly$_2$-Ileu$_3$-Leu-Met$_2$-Pro-Ser$_2$-Thr-Val.[27]

Chromatophorotrophins and Color Change

The chromatophores, or pigment cells, of crustaceans may contain white, red, yellow, black, brown, and blue pigments. By appropriate condensation or dispersal of particular pigments within the chromatophores, crustaceans can approximate rather accurately the colored backgrounds upon which they rest. It is known that crustacean pigment cells are devoid of nerves and are adjusted by regulatory agents present in the blood (chromatophorotrophins). Studies involving eyestalk or X-organ ablation, coupled with the testing of extracts made from different regions of the nervous system, have demonstrated that the chromatophorotrophins are products of neurosecretory cells. Some of these factors are abundant in the tritocerebral commissure and the postcommissural organs. Multiple chromatophorotrophins have been extracted from the nervous systems of decapod crustaceans, but the exact number has not been agreed upon. It is possible that the effective agents obtained through the extraction of neurosecretory aggregations (*e.g.,* ganglionic X organ) are not of the same chemical form as the finished products liberated by neurohemal organs (*e.g.,* sinus gland).[9, 10, 11, 12]

The red pigment-concentrating hormone, purified from *Pandalus borealis,* is an octapeptide with the following amino acid sequence: Asp-Glu-Gly-Leu-Phe-Pro-Ser-Trp.[27]

Though barnacles have neither compound eyes nor chromatophores, extracts of their nervous systems have chromatophore-activating properties when tested on decapod crustaceans. Blind cave crayfishes possess no retinal pigments and no chromatophores, yet their nervous systems contain both the distal pigment, light-adapting principle and another principle affecting integumentary chromatophores.

Molting

Growth is a discontinuous process in arthropods, increase in size being restricted to the period between loss of the old exoskeleton and the production of a new one. Molting may be seasonal or continuous, and is influenced by a great variety of environmental conditions. Loss and replacement of the exoskeleton are an outward expression of a whole complex of major metabolic adjustments occurring within. Four periods are recognized in the crustacean molt cycle: (1) During *premolt,* inorganic constituents of the old exoskeleton are resorbed and stored in gastroliths or hepatopancreas. Oxygen consumption increases, glycogen is deposited in the hypodermis, and lost limbs are regenerated rapidly. (2) *Molt* is the sloughing of the old cuticle, and this is accompanied by a marked increase in size. The immediate increase in size results from a rapid absorption of water, which thus reserves enough space to permit growth even after the new cuticle has hardened. (3) *Postmolt* is the period during which a new exoskeleton is formed through the redeposition of chitin and inorganic salts. (4) *Intermolt* is characterized by relative quiescence, but there is generally some storage of reserves in preparation for the next molt. Some crustaceans eventually cease molting and consequently undergo no further growth, a condition called *anecdysis.*

In most species of crustaceans, the ablation of both eyestalks results in accelerated molting and precocious growth. Extracts of the ganglionic X organ–sinus gland complex act to prevent molting. These and other observations led to the conclusion that neurosecretory cells in the ganglionic X organ secrete a molt-inhibiting neurohormone that is stored and released from the sinus gland. Studies on the formation of gastroliths in crayfish indicate that the molt-inhibiting factor is derived from components of the eyestalk. These concretions normally form in the stomach wall during premolt, but may be induced at any period of the molt cycle by ablating both eyestalks or by excision of the X organ–sinus gland complex. Gastrolith formation in eyestalkless animals can be prevented by the implantation of sinus glands. Profound quantitative shifts in the metabolism of carbohydrate, protein, lipid, and inorganic materials occur in relation to the molt cycle. As might be expected, these biochemical adjustments are facilitated by the endocrine factors that control molting.[30, 38]

Whether the components of the eyestalk produce a second factor, a molt-accelerating principle, remains unresolved. Under certain conditions, and in certain species, molt inhibition may follow eyestalk ablation; but certain workers feel that this can be explained on other grounds, and hence there is not sufficient evidence for a molt-accelerating neurohormone. On the other hand, it has been suggested, from studies on the crayfish *(Orconectes virilis),* that both molt-inhibiting and molt-accelerating factors from the eyestalk are involved in regulating the cyclic changes which characterize metabolism of the hepatopancreas.

The Y organs were discovered by Gabe (1953), and it is certain that they produce a hormone which performs a positive role in the molting process. Young crabs are prevented from molting by bilateral removal of the Y organs, but molting cycles may be restored in these animals by implanting several Y organs. These organs normally degenerate after puberty in the crab *Maia,* and no further molting occurs. It seems probable that the molt-inhibiting neurohormone from the ganglionic X organ–sinus gland complex may exert its effects by regulating the functional status of the Y organs. It would follow that the molt-inhibiting neurosecretion is continuously produced during postmolt and intermolt periods to stall the production of molting hormone by the Y organs; during premolt, the production of neurosecretion ceases, or diminishes, and the Y organs are allowed to secrete molting hormone.

The Y organs are analogous (and possibly homologous) to the prothoracic glands of insects. It is interesting that both endocrine glands secrete hormones that control molting, and that both are regulated by neurosecretions from the central nervous system. The prothoracic glands degenerate in adult insects, following the last molt, and the Y organs are greatly reduced in crabs during anecdysis.

Reproduction

There is more evidence for the existence of sex hormones in the malacostracans, the higher crustaceans, than in the other invertebrates. Hormones regulating the differentiation of male and female sexual characters arise from the ovaries and the androgenic glands; the testis itself probably has no endocrine function. Neurosecretions of the ganglionic X organ – sinus gland complex have inhibitory effects on ovarian maturation and secretory activity of the androgenic glands. There is evidence that the molting hormone from the Y organs is also essential for normal differentiation of both the ovary and the testis. After bilateral ablation of Y organs in very young crabs *(Carcinus),* mitotic processes are impaired in both the ovary and testis. In the ovary, oogonial mitoses cease and follicles are not formed around the oocytes; vitellogenesis, or yolk deposition, does not occur in the oocytes that lack follicles. Spermatogonial mitoses are arrested, and the testes become depleted of mature germ cells.

Bilateral removal of the ovaries in certain crustaceans *(e.g., Orchestia)* results in the loss of specific secondary sex characters. Secondary characters of the female type may be induced in genetic males by removing the androgenic glands and implanting ovaries. Two ovarian hormones have been postulated, with good evidence, but neither is known chemically.

It has been shown in many species of crustaceans that ablation of the eyestalks, during periods of sexual quiescence, is followed by enlargement of the ovaries and by a precocious deposition of yolk in the oocytes. Extracts prepared from eyestalks, ganglionic X organs, or sinus glands effectively prevent ovarian enlargement when administered to females that are entering the period of reproductive activity. Such extracts are without effect when given to very immature females or to females immediately after the end of the reproductive period. It appears that the primary action of this ovarian-inhibiting neurohormone is to prevent vitellogenesis. The production of this factor is apparently regulated by environmental stimuli that impinge on sensory receptors.

The important androgenic glands were discovered by Charniaux-Cotton (1954) in the amphipod *Orchestia gammarella,* and have since been found in quite a variety of crustacean species. The following observations indicate that the androgenic gland hormone regulates spermatogenesis and the secondary sex characters of the male: (1) In *O. gammarella,* ablation of the

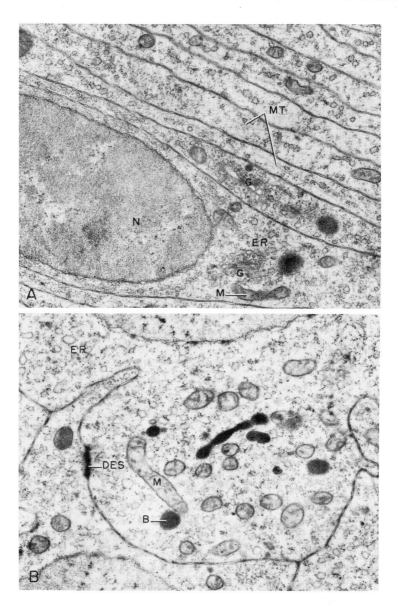

Figure 17–5. Electron micrographs of the androgenic glands of the amphipod *Orchestia gammarella*. The cells of these glands are characterized by a well-developed granular endoplasmic reticulum, long mitochondria with transverse cristae, and frequent Golgi bodies. These ultrastructural features make it very probable that the androgenic gland hormone is a polypeptide or protein, rather than a steroid. *A,* × 15,300; *B,* × 21,780. B, probably a lysosome; DES, desmosome; ER, endoplasmic reticulum; G, Golgi body; M, mitochondrion; MT, microtubules; N, nucleus. (Courtesy of Mr. Jean-Jacques Meusy, Centre National de la Recherche Scientifique, Paris.)

androgenic glands causes spermatogenic activity in the testis to wane, and regenerated appendages develop neither the male nor the female sex characteristics; in *O. montagui,* oogenesis ensues in the testis. (2) If androgenic glands are grafted to intact female hosts, the ovaries eventually transform into testes and proliferate spermatocytes, spermatids, and functional spermatozoa. The appendages progressively assume male form, and masculine sexual behavior is acquired. The bipotentiality of the primordial germ cells is clearly indicated. (3) Castration of normal males, the androgenic glands remaining intact, has no effect other than to remove the source of germ cells. (4) If ovaries are grafted into males that have been deprived of androgenic glands, they persist as functional ovaries. When grafted into males possessing androgenic glands, with or without host testes, the ovaries quickly acquire testicular structure. (5) Aqueous extracts of androgenic glands, injected into males deprived of these organs, effectively prevent changes in the testes and secondary sex characters. In certain species, blood plasma from males, injected into female recipients, causes the ovary to assume testicular structure and function (Fig. 17–5).

It follows from these observations that the differentiation of germ cells of crustaceans is reversible, regardless of their genetic constitution: In the absence of androgenic gland hormone, the gonads can become ovaries, but testicular differentiation requires the presence of this hormone. Several species of decapod crustaceans are protandric hermaphrodites, and it is known that androgenic glands are present during the male phase and are lost before the onset of the female phase. The androgenic glands of some species are closely applied to the testes, and it is probable that the sex reversals formerly attributed to destruction of the gonads by parasites actually result from destruction of or damage to the androgenic glands.

Heart Acceleration

The pericardial organs are neurohemal in nature and release a neurohormone which increases the frequency and amplitude of the heartbeat. Although extracts of pericardial organs contain 5-hydroxytryptamine, it is believed that the major activity of the extracts comes from one or two peptides of neurosecretory origin.

Metabolism

Striking variations in tissue metabolism occur during the molting cycle in Crustacea, and eyestalk factors, presumably neurosecretions, are known to be involved. Identity of the active principles and the manner in which they interact are problems that require further elucidation. Molt-inhibiting and molt-accelerating factors from the eyestalk, and molting hormone from the Y organs, are apparently implicated in these cyclical changes in metabolism. After removal of the eyestalks, the blood sugar concentration decreases, whereas the glycogen content of the hypodermis increases. The metabolic changes following eyestalk removal are comparable to those that occur in the intact animal in preparation for a molt. Hyperglycemia may be induced by administering extracts of the eyestalk or X organ–sinus gland complex to normal animals. Since the same effect is induced by subjecting intact animals to stressful stimuli, it appears that the response is normally mediated by the neuroendocrine system of the eyestalk. The importance of carbohydrate metabolism in the molting process is indicated by the fact that chitin is one of the major constituents of the exoskeleton and is derived from glycogen.

Evidence for a hyperglycemic neurohormone has been adduced. It appears to be a protein and thus differs from the chromatophorotrophins and the light-adapting retinal pigment principle.

NEUROENDOCRINE MECHANISMS IN THE INSECTA

Among the Insecta, as among the Crustacea, the key position in the endocrine system is held by neurosecretory centers that elaborate neurohormones acting directly on target tissues or indirectly on endocrine glands. Since insects are a very diversified group, many kinds of microsurgical procedures have been employed for the study of hormonal mechanisms. Among these may be mentioned transplantation, ablation of organs, parabiosis, isolation of larval parts by constriction, tissue cultures, the fusion of individuals by capillary tubes, and the isolation of pupal parts by fusion to glass plates. Methods are being perfected for the bioassay of insect hormones, and several hormones have been isolated in pure form. Certain unifying concepts of hormone action have emerged, making it clear that the same general principles operate in both hemimetabolous and holometabolous insects. It has become apparent that the various hormones interact with one another, just as in vertebrates, and this makes it difficult to assign definite actions to a specific hormone. What a particular hormone accomplishes often depends upon other hormones that are present with it, upon the hormone titer in the body fluids, and upon the competence of the target tissues to respond.

Insect Life Cycles

In hemimetabolous development, illustrated by the locust, the cockroach, and the blood-sucking bug *Rhodnius*, the newly hatched young resemble the adults in many respects; the most important differences are size, the absence of wings, and immature genitalia (Fig. 17–6). The young nymph, as it is called, undergoes a series of molts, during which it gradually acquires adult characters, the most profound metamorphic changes occurring at the final molt. The number of nymphal instars varies with the species and may be altered by environmental conditions. All instars are capable of feeding, and there is generally no cessation of development during this type of cycle; however, growth occurs mostly between the nymphal molts.

Moths and butterflies are examples of holometabolous insects. Their eggs hatch into wormlike larvae that bear practically no resemblance to the adult (Fig. 17–6). These caterpillars feed and undergo a series of molts, and, since growth occurs at molting, each succeeding instar is somewhat larger

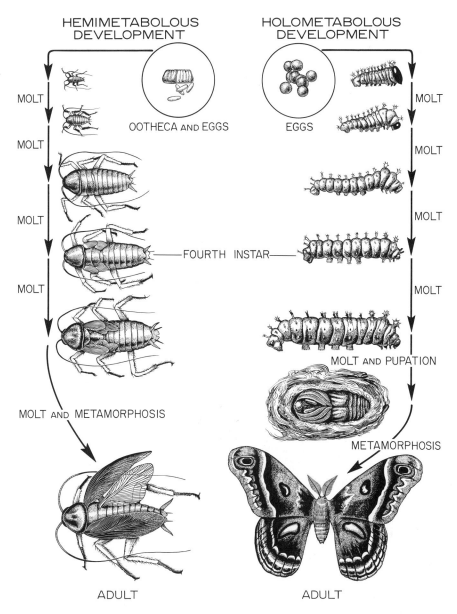

HEMIMETABOLOUS
DEVELOPMENT

HOLOMETABOLOUS
DEVELOPMENT

MOLT

MOLT

MOLT

MOLT

MOLT

MOLT AND METAMORPHOSIS

OOTHECA AND EGGS

EGGS

——FOURTH INSTAR——

MOLT

MOLT

MOLT

MOLT AND PUPATION

METAMORPHOSIS

ADULT

ADULT

Figure 17–6. Two contrasting types of life cycles among insects. In those exhibiting direct or hemimetabolous development, the last nymphal instar molts and metamorphoses into the adult. In forms undergoing indirect or holometabolous development, the last larval instar passes through a pupal stage before metamorphosing into the adult. The cockroach *(Periplaneta americana)* is taken as an example of hemimetabolous development; the giant silkworm moth *(Hyalophora cecropia)* is used as an example of holometabolous development. The instars are drawn to scale.

than the preceding one. The larval instars, though differing in size, usually do not undergo profound structural changes. Eventually, the last instar molts and transforms into a chrysalis or pupa, a quiescent stage which is incapable of feeding. During pupation, the individual undergoes a rather complete structural reorganization, so that it resembles the adult much more closely than did the preceding larval stages. Eventually, the pupal case is burst, and an imago emerges; it may feed, but it undergoes no further growth or profound modification in structure.

Though certain organs may be transmitted from the larva to the adult without much change, many must undergo a complete reorganization. These changes involve the destruction of larval tissues (histolysis) and the differentiation of adult tissues and organs (histogenesis and organogenesis) from larval anlagen called imaginal discs. All these postembryonic changes must be timed and coordinated properly in order to produce the normal adult.

Metamorphosis includes the changes in form normally undergone by an animal during its life cycle, and these events are genetically determined. Since the cells of the larva, pupa, and adult contain the same genetic information, it appears that different sets of genes are sequentially brought into action during the life cycle. There is increasing evidence that the genetic switch, or activation of an alternative set of genes, is triggered by neuroendocrine adjustments. The establishment of differential hormone environments, known to prevail during particular periods of the life cycle, may often be effected by external changes such as photoperiods, temperature, food, etc.[20, 52]

Diapause

The life cycles of many insects include a period of dormancy, called *diapause,* during which growth and differentiation are almost in complete abeyance. The diapause may result from the direct effects of adverse environments, or it may appear regularly under the most favorable conditions as a phase of the life cycle. Depending upon the species, such periods of suspended development may occur at any time in the life cycle—egg, nymph, caterpillar, pupa, or adult. These periods of dormancy may have the net effects of producing young at a time when their chances for survival are maximal, and of enabling the individual to survive hazardous environmental conditions.

Periods of developmental arrest in the egg are characteristic of certain insects. Some silkworm *(Bombyx mori)* races are single-brooded or univoltine, each generation appearing in the spring following a period of arrested embryonic development during the winter. Other races are divoltine or multivoltine, the nondiapausing summer eggs producing one or more generations before the winter generation of diapausing eggs is produced. The diapausing eggs can be distinguished by the appearance of pigment in the serosa. Whether a female produces diapause or nondiapause eggs depends upon the photoperiod to which she was exposed while in the egg stage or as a very young larva. In the case of the divoltine race, the diapause eggs survive the winter and produce adults in spring. Females of the first generation produce nondiapause eggs because of their exposure to short days. Females of the second generation, derived from nondiapause eggs of spring, produce their eggs during midsummer, under the influence of long days and high temperatures. These eggs are of the diapause type and do not develop until spring. The necessary information for the production of diapause eggs by these moths is derived from the long hours of daylight, and this photoperiodic mechanism provides the basis for winter survival.

It has been shown that the immediate stimulus for the production of diapause eggs by *Bombyx* is a neurohormone derived from a pair of neurosecretory cells in the subesophageal ganglion of the mother, and this secretion is released only in mothers that were exposed to long periods of daylight when they themselves were eggs, or more precisely, developing embryos. The neurohormone of the mother acts upon the eggs (embryos) before they are released from the genital tract. When the ovaries of a univoltine race (diapause eggs only) are transplanted into larvae of a divoltine race (diapause or nondiapause eggs), the eggs produced by the grafted ovary, after the host attains adulthood, always show the voltinism of the host. There are indications that the brain exerts an inhibitory effect, by way of the esophageal connectives, on the release of diapause neurohormone by the subesophageal ganglion.[17, 18]

In certain butterflies *(e.g., Araschnia levana),* the photoperiod to which the young larvae are exposed determines whether or not a pupal diapause occurs. The adults emerging from diapausing and nondiapausing pupae may be quite different in appearance, and occasionally, spring and summer varieties have been mistaken for different species (Fig. 17-7).

The Cecropia moth *(Hyalophora cecropia)* undergoes a pupal diapause in nature, and the individual passes the winter in this condition. Mating occurs in the spring, and in about two weeks, the eggs hatch to give rise to the first larval instars. There are four larval molts, and the fifth instar spins a silken cocoon in which it pupates. With the rising temperatures of spring, the diapause ends and the adult emerges from the old pupal cuticle and escapes from the cocoon. Adult Cecropia do not feed, and between 25 and 33 per cent of the pupal weight is utilized in the production of about 300 yolk-laden eggs. Pupal dormancy in this species normally lasts for about eight months, but it has been found that the length of the diapause may be materially shortened by chilling the pupae and then returning them to room temperatures.

With the onset of pupal diapause, there is a sudden and complete cessation of growth, and few if any mitotic divisions occur during this long dormancy. The heart continues to beat and the animal utilizes oxygen and produces carbon dioxide, but all metabolic processes are reduced to a very low level. The rate of oxygen consumption in diapausing Cecropia is only 1.4 per cent that of the mature larva, and 5 per cent that of the adult moth just before the last molt. Just prior to the spinning of the cocoon, the larva ceases the intake of substances other than atmospheric oxygen; henceforth until its death as a mature moth 8 to 10 months later, the materials of its own body are reworked as a source of energy. The metabolism of an adult moth in flight is approximately 2000 times that of a diapausing pupa.

The destructive larvae of the European corn-borer *(Ostrinia nubilalis)* enter pupal diapause in response to falling temperatures and short daily photoperiods.[1]

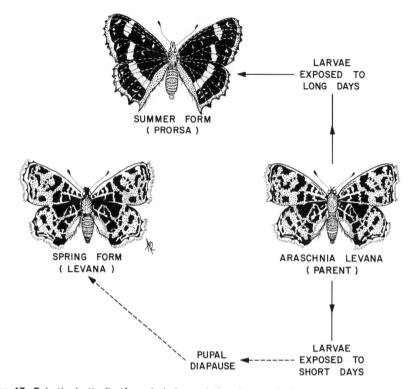

Figure 17-7. In the butterfly *(Araschnia levana)*, the photoperiod to which the young larvae are exposed determines whether or not a diapause will occur at the pupal stage. Larvae exposed to short days undergo a pupal diapause; those exposed to long days do not. Diapausing pupae produce the spring form and nondiapausing pupae produce the summer form. The spring and summer varieties are so different in appearance that they have been mistaken for separate species. (Redrawn and modified from Wigglesworth, V. B.: Endeavour, 1965).

Some insects undergo diapause in the adult stage, and this generally takes the form of arrested reproduction in the female. In the Colorado potato beetle *(Leptinotarsa)*, for example, the females begin to burrow into the soil during autumn and become quiescent; the metabolic rate falls, thoracic muscles degenerate, and egg maturation ceases. All these diapausal changes can be reversed in this beetle by implanting active corpora allata into their bodies. This suggests that the reproductive arrest is brought about by environmental factors which act via the corpora allata to inhibit the production of juvenile hormone.

Control of Postembryonic Development

The endocrine mechanism regulating growth and differentiation in all insects centers in the neurosecretory system of the brain. The extrinsic stimulus varies from species to species: In the bloodsucking bug *Rhodnius*, stretching of the larval abdomen by a meal of blood provides a nervous

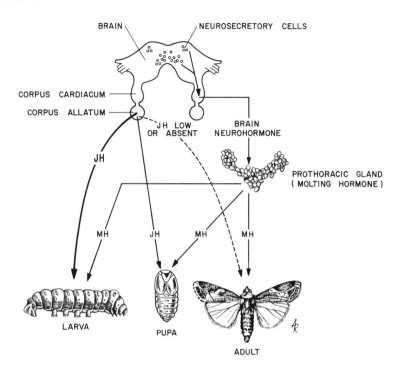

BRAIN   NEUROSECRETORY CELLS

CORPUS CARDIACUM

CORPUS ALLATUM

JH LOW
OR ABSENT

JH

BRAIN
NEUROHORMONE

PROTHORACIC GLAND
(MOLTING HORMONE)

MH   JH   MH   MH

LARVA

PUPA

ADULT

Figure 17–8. Diagram illustrating the neural and endocrine control of growth and molting in a moth. Neurosecretory cells of the brain release a principle which stimulates the prothoracic glands to secrete molting hormone (MH or ecdysone). Juvenile hormone (JH) arises from the corpora allata and promotes the retention of larval characters. Adult differentiation occurs when MH acts in the absence of JH.

stimulus to the brain; in locusts, the act of chewing and swallowing may accomplish the same effect; in Cecropia, temperature changes activate the brain. The activated neurosecretory cells of the brain produce a brain hormone (BH) which their axons discharge into the corpora cardiaca, where it is stored and from where it is liberated into the blood. The BH probably acts through the prothoracic glands to produce a hormone that has been variously named molting hormone (MH), growth and differentiation hormone, prothoracic gland hormone, and ecdysone. The MH acts directly upon the tissues of the body, causing them to differentiate in the direction of adult structures. A second hormone, called juvenile hormone (JH), is secreted by the corpora allata, and its action is to encourage the laying down of larval or nymphal structures. In other words, JH suppresses pupal and imaginal differentiation (Fig. 17–8). The secretory activity of the corpora allata is also regulated by the nervous system, and the amount of JH present in the blood diminishes progressively with successive molts. Imaginal differentiation occurs under the influence of MH, when very little, if any, JH is present.

The body form attained by organisms depends upon the genetic control of developmental processes. It appears that multiple sets of genes are present in insect species, and that these sets can be called into expression successively during the life cycle. As these genic complexes are activated (or suppressed), larval, pupal, and imaginal characters differentiate.

Endocrine Structures and Their Secretions

Organs of Nervous Origin

Neurosecretory cells are numerous in insects and have important functions. Medial and lateral groups of such cells are present in the brain (protocerebrum); other aggregations are found in the subesophageal ganglion, and in all other ganglia of the ventral chain.

The corpora cardiaca arise from the nervous system and are situated behind the brain in close association with the dorsal aorta. They are paired in some species, but are fused in others. The corpora cardiaca are neurohemal organs and are composed of four cellular elements: (1) the bulbous endings of neurosecretory axons whose perikarya are located in the dorsum of the brain, (2) the perikarya of neurosecretory cells that send axons into nerves that supply various peripheral organs, (3) glia-like cells, and (4) intrinsic corpus cardiacum cells. Although the corpora cardiaca are storage-release centers, there is increasing evidence that their own cells are capable of producing secretions.

Organs of Epithelial Origin

The best known endocrine glands of the insect originate from ectodermal cells proliferated from the surface epithelium in the vicinity of the mouth parts. Aggregations of such cells approach the posterior margin of the brain and become the corpora allata (Fig. 17–9). These glands are commonly paired and laterally placed *(Periplaneta)*, or they may fuse to form a single structure *(Rhodnius)*. Other clusters of cells, derived in the same manner, may come to rest in the head or be carried farther back into the thorax. These anlagen form the *ventral glands* of the head in certain species, or the thoracic or *prothoracic glands* in others. The ventral and

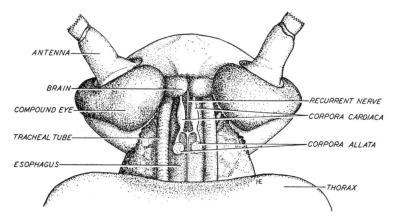

Figure 17–9. A dissection of the head of the roach *(Periplaneta americana)*, showing the paired corpora allata and corpora cardiaca and the relations of these glands to other structures of the head.

prothoracic glands are structurally and functionally comparable, differing only in location. The prothoracic glands are circumscribed and can be surgically removed in some species, such as the roach, but in others, the tissue is so scattered that ablation is difficult or impossible. These glands undergo autolysis shortly after completion of metamorphosis, and hence are not present in adult insects. Their ultrastructure does not resemble that of other glands known to secrete steroid or peptide hormones.[32]

The prothoracic glands were described in the goat moth by Lyonet as early as 1762, and Toyama followed their embryonic development in the silkworm in 1902. The functional significance of these ductless glands was not fully appreciated until the classic studies of Fukuda on the larvae of *Bombyx mori* in 1940.[17] Through ingenious ligation and transplantation experiments, he proved that the prothoracic glands are essential for the larvae of this moth to undergo pupation. The clear-cut experiments of Williams on the isolated pupal abdomens of the Cecropia moth demonstrated that the prothoracic glands are incapable of promoting the production of molting hormone unless they are activated by a principle from the brain.

In some of the Diptera, the corpus cardiacum, corpus allatum, and prothoracic gland fuse to form a structure surrounding the aorta. This retrocerebral complex is called the *ring gland* of Weismann.

Epithelial cells of the hindgut are known to be the source of a hormone (proctodone) which is required to activate the neurosecretory system of the brain. The hormone has been found in two species of Lepidoptera in which it plays a role in photoperiodism and diapause.[1]

Neurohormones of the Brain

Kopec (1917) correctly concluded that the brain is the source of a blood-borne factor which is required for pupation (Fig. 17–10).[31] Wigglesworth (1940), working on *Rhodnius,* traced the source of this brain principle to collections of neurosecretory cells present in the pars intercerebralis.[51] He accomplished this by excising the pars intercerebralis regions of brains from nymphs that had fed a few days previously (during the critical period), and implanting these into nymphal hosts that had been decapitated immediately after feeding (before the critical period). The decapitated hosts could live 6 to 10 months, but never molted; the activated neurosecretory cells contained in the brain implants induced them to molt. He found that no other part of the nervous system would stimulate molting when implanted into the same recipients. For the first time, it was possible to assign a functional role to particular neurosecretory cells.

Pupae of the Cecropia moth remain in diapause for 5 to 6 months when they are kept at a temperature of 25° C. After surgical removal of the brain, such pupae never metamorphose, though they may live for approximately a year. The intact pupae may be induced to metamorphose precociously by chilling them at 3 to 5° C. for about 6 weeks and then returning them to room temperatures. Implanted brains from chilled pupae induce metamorphosis when implanted into unchilled pupae. When chilled pupae are para-

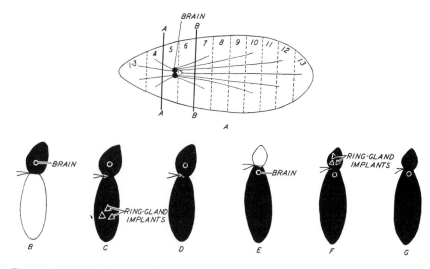

Figure 17–10. Ligation experiments upon the larvae of dipterans. Studies of this type indicate that the brain, or some closely associated structure, releases one or more blood-borne agents that are essential for pupation. *A,* Diagram of a muscid larva, showing the position of the brain. Ligatures may be placed in front of the brain (line *A–A*) or behind it (line *B–B*). In diagrams *B* to *G,* the pupated regions of the body are indicated in black. *B,* Larva ligated behind the brain before the critical period. Only the portion of the body containing the brain undergoes pupation. It is presumed that the posterior part of the body fails to pupate because the ligature prevents the dissemination of an essential substance (ecdysone) contained in the body fluid. *C,* Same as *B,* with ring glands implanted into the body posterior to the ligature. The ring glands induce pupation in that portion of the body isolated from the brain. *D,* Same as *B,* but the ligature was placed after the critical period, *i.e.,* after the essential endocrine substances had attained effective concentrations in the body fluid. The entire body pupates. *E,* Larva ligatured in front of the brain before the critical period. Pupation is accomplished only by the segment of the body containing the brain. *F,* Same as *E,* but with ring glands implanted into the fragment lacking the brain. This procedure produces pupation of the anterior region. *G,* Same as *E,* but the ligature was placed after the critical period. All the body pupates.

biotically united with unchilled pupae, both molt synchronously in a little less than 2 months. These experiments indicate that pupal diapause in Cecropia results from a failure of the brain to produce BH, brain activation depending upon a temperature stimulus. Different mechanisms are undoubtedly involved in other species of Lepidoptera.

While it is common practice to refer to the prothoracic gland–stimulating factor as "brain hormone" or "prothoracotrophin," it must be recognized that the neurosecretory cells of the brain produce additional secretions that have other actions. The medial neurosecretory cells in the brain of the blowfly *(Calliphora)* supply a neurohormone that stimulates egg maturation in this species. This is accomplished by evoking the formation of proteases in the gut, thereby facilitating the breakdown of proteins to supply amino acids for the synthesis of egg proteins.[43]

Bursicon (Tanning Hormone)

Studies on blowflies have shown that neurosecretory cells within the brain produce a blood-borne hormone which triggers the "tanning" or "darkening" of the adult cuticle. This was later termed bursicon, a protein hormone with a molecular weight of about 40,000. Bursicon is produced by the cerebral neurosecretory cells and is released into the fused thoraco-abdominal ganglia; it is definitely distinct from the brain neurohormone which stimulates the prothoracic gland. Bursicon is released after the emerged fly has dug its way out of the soil, but in some insects the hormone may be secreted slightly before or during the loss of the old skin. The tanning factor is found in a variety of insect species. A substance originating in the eyestalks of crayfishes plays some role in tanning of the newly formed exoskeleton.[13, 15, 16, 46]

The Eclosion Hormone

Silkmoths and other insects switch over from pupal to adult emergence consequent upon a rich variety of hormones which regulate the central nervous system and thereby trigger the regulated behaviors. Median neurosecretory cells of the brain produce the eclosion hormone, which collects in the corpora cardiaca and is released into the blood at the proper time. In most species of insects, the hormone acts upon neurons within the abdominal ganglia to initiate the pre-eclosion behavior. The hormone "turns on" the kind of behavior which requires adult emergence; many of the neurons which evoked pupal behavior then die, since many cannot survive during adulthood.

In moths and other insects, adult eclosion is "turned on" only during a specific period of day or night. The environmental photoperiod may interact with the internal biological clock within the brain, and this may be referred to as the "eclosion gate." If the insect is ready for adult development, nothing can happen since the gate has closed for that particular day; the only opportunity for eclosion is the next gate on the succeeding day. In the life history of moths, the eclosion hormone is absent during larval and pupal stages. In preparation for adult emergence, the hormone is released from neurosecretory cells in the brain and may enter the blood from the corpora cardiaca.[44, 45]

Hormones of the Corpora Cardiaca

Aqueous extracts of the corpora cardiaca of the roach *Periplaneta* elevate the blood concentration of trehalose, the main circulating carbohydrate of insects. The effective substance, reported to be a polypeptide, acts upon the enzyme system of the fat body (where glycogen is stored) to promote glycogenolysis.[40]

Efferent nerve activity in *Periplaneta* is inhibited by the subesophageal ganglion. Extracts of the corpora cardiaca mimic the surgical removal of this inhibitory system, but it is not known whether the effective substance arises *in situ* or is merely stored there.

The corpora cardiaca of the cockroach appear to secrete a peptide hormone that acts indirectly to increase the heart rate. It apparently stimulates the pericardial cells, scattered along the heart, to produce a pharmacologically active factor, which in turn acts upon the heart to increase its rate of beating. The differential centrifugation of extracts from corpora cardiaca of the roach has yielded neurosecretory particles that accelerate the heart. Studies on the roach indicate that many cardioregulatory substances, probably small peptides, can be isolated from various tissues such as the nervous system, gastrointestinal tract, heart, utricles, and hemolymph.[36]

Molting Hormone (Ecdysone)

In saturniid moths, activation of the brain and consequent termination of pupal diapause depend upon exposure to low temperatures. The classical experiments of Williams on Cecropia moths demonstrated conclusively that brain hormone (BH) does not act directly upon the tissues, but rather, that it exerts a trophic effect upon a specific target—the prothoracic glands.[53] Brainless pupae survive for long periods, but never terminate diapause. When a brainless, diapausing pupa was grafted to a chilled pupa, the two animals metamorphosed simultaneously. The pupae of these moths could be transected anterior to the sixth abdominal segment, and the cut surfaces sealed over with coverslips; these parts were viable for 8 months or longer and made some instructive experiments possible. Chilled anterior parts, or brainless anterior parts that had received implants of chilled brains, metamorphosed into adults. The isolated abdomens (lacking prothoracic glands) did not metamorphose even after receiving multiple implants of chilled brains. The isolated abdomens could be induced to metamorphose by introducing both chilled brains and prothoracic glands; unactivated prothoracic glands alone were not adequate. It has been shown in a great variety of insects that metamorphosis depends upon two factors: brain hormone and molting hormone from the prothoracic glands. The prothoracic glands quickly regress after the final molt that gives rise to the adult stage. The molting hormone is a steroid called *ecdysone;* it has been synthesized and is now available in large quantities (Fig. 17–16).[42, 50]

The life cycle of the flagellate *Trichonympha,* living symbiotically in the gut of the wood-eating roach *Cryptocercus,* undergoes modifications in response to endocrine fluctuations in the insect. The administration of ecdysone to adult roaches, themselves incapable of molting in response to the hormone, induces encystment and gametogenesis in the flagellates. It is probable that this is a direct effect of the host hormone upon the protozoa, and that it has adaptive value in their survival.

Juvenile Hormone

The tissue reactions to molting hormone (MH) are modulated by juvenile hormone (JH), which is a product of the corpora allata. The tropical bug *Rhodnius,* used so extensively by Wigglesworth and his colleagues, was a convenient insect for the experimental elucidation of the factors involved in molt and metamorphosis. There are five nymphal instars in *Rhodnius,* and molting occurs a definite number of days after a meal of blood; abdominal distention is the stimulus that activates the neurosecretory complex of the brain. The elongated head of *Rhodnius* made it possible to cut transversely at different levels and obtain animals deprived of brain (corpus allatum intact), or animals deprived of both brain and corpus allatum. The decapitated animals survive six to 10 months. It was possible to join decapitated animals by means of capillary tubes, or to graft instars and adults in many telobiotic and parabiotic combinations.

Two grafting experiments in *Rhodnius* may be mentioned to illustrate the action of JH. If a fourth-stage nymph is decapitated after the critical period and is telobiotically grafted to a fifth-stage nymph also decapitated after the critical period, both individuals molt, but the fifth-stage nymph becomes a giant, supernumerary nymph instead of an adult. Though adult *Rhodnius* normally does not molt, it may be induced to do so by grafting nymphal stages. When fourth-stage nymphs, possessing their corpora allata as a source of JH, are united with an adult, the latter molts and shows a partial return to the nymphal condition (Fig. 17–11).

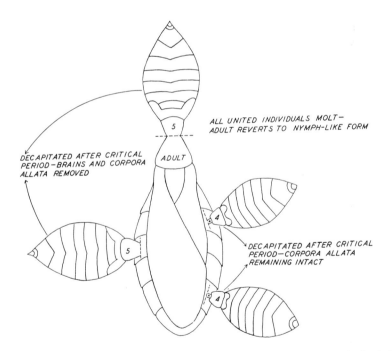

Figure 17–11. The induction of molt in adult *Rhodnius.* The broken lines indicate the level of decapitation; the blackened dot in the proximal end of the head represents the corpus allatum, and the number of the nymphal instar is indicated on the thorax. The decapitated adult is coupled with two fifth-stage nymphs, totally decapitated after the critical period, and with two fourth-stage nymphs partially decapitated after the critical period. The fifth-stage nymphs provide the adult with ecdysone, whereas the fourth nymphs, having their corpora allata, provide juvenile hormone in addition to ecdysone. All the combined individuals molt; the fifth nymphs become supernumerary nymphs (sixth stage), the fourth nymphs become fifth instars, and the adult reverts to a nymphlike form.

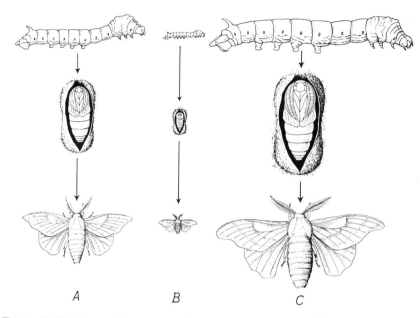

A B C

Figure 17–12. Effects of the corpora allata on postembryonic development of *Bombyx mori*. *A,* Normal fifth instar, pupa, and adult. *B,* Allatectomized third instar, diminutive pupa, and diminutive adult. *C,* Supernumerary larva produced from fifth instar by transplanting corpora allata of young larvae, giant pupa, and giant adult. (Drawn from figures of C. M. Williams.)

In the roach *Leucophaea maderae,* the adult stage is preceded by an average of eight nymphal instars. Removal of the corpora allata (allatectomy) of the fifth, sixth, or seventh instars produces an abbreviation of development, the final molt being accomplished at an earlier stage than in the unoperated controls. Fifth and sixth instars, deprived of JH by allatectomy, develop characters that are intermediate between nymph and adult (preadultoids) and must molt again before attaining adult characters to a conspicuous extent (adultoids).

Walking sticks *(Dixippus)* are neotenic insects, the females beginning to reproduce parthenogenetically before they are fully adult. If third-stage larvae are allatectomized, two more molts ensue before egg laying begins. By implanting corpora allata into the semimature adults of *Dixippus,* they may be caused to molt two more times and to become giant insects. After implanting corpora allata from young donors into sixth-stage larvae, as many as four extra molts may be produced, and the insects become about twice the normal size.

Allatectomized caterpillars of the commercial silkworm undergo no further molts; they metamorphose prematurely into normally formed but miniature adults. The earlier the corpora allata are removed, the smaller the resulting adult. On the other hand, implantation of corpora allata produces supernumerary larval molts and giant caterpillars that metamorphose into giant adults (Fig. 17–12).

When pupae of the Cecropia moth are grafted to a decapitated adult male moth, the pupae undergo a second pupal molt rather than metamorphosing into adults. In other words, these pupae develop as though they had received a heavy dose of JH. Studies on these moths have shown that the corpora allata of adult males produce large quantities of JH and that it is stored in the abdomen. The tissues of the adult female abdomen contain only traces of this hormone.

It is apparent from experiments of this type that three endocrine factors are involved in the growth and metamorphosis of insects: BH from neurosecretory cells of the pars intercerebralis initiates the production of MH by the prothoracic glands; MH acts upon the cells to promote growth and differentiation to the adult stage; and if the third hormone, JH, is present, MH and JH act in concert to retard metamorphosis. When high titers of JH are present with MH, the animal grows but remains immature: imaginal differentiation results when MH is unopposed by JH (Fig. 17–8).

The feasibility of using insect hormones as insecticides was confirmed quite accidentally a few years ago. Slama transferred a stock of *Pyrrhocoris apterus* from Charles University in Prague to the laboratory of Williams at Harvard University, but found that the European bugs would not metamorphose into adults in the American environment. The fifth-instar larvae molted into supernumerary larvae and these died during the adult molt (Fig. 17–13). Since implanted corpora allata cause the retention of larval characteristics, it became apparent that the bugs were inadvertently being exposed to JH activity from some source. It was finally determined that the paper towels used in the culture jars were the source of a substance called "paper factor" that mimics the action of JH and shows some chemical resemblance to

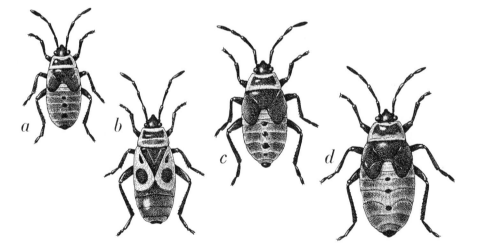

Figure 17–13. Effect of *paper factor* on the development of the bug *Pyrrhocoris apterus*. The fifth and final instar *(a)* normally molts to form the winged adult *(b)*. After exposure to paper factor, the fifth instar molts to form a sixth-stage larva *(c)*, and this sometimes molts to form a giant seventh-stage larva *(d)*. The supernumerary instars grow but they die without becoming adults. (From Third-generation pesticides, by C. M. Williams. Copyright © 1967 by Scientific American, Inc. All rights reserved.)

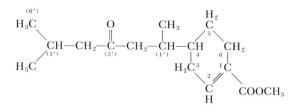

Methyl 4-[1',5'-dimethyl-3'-oxo]hexyl cyclohex-1-enoate

Figure 17–14. Chemical structure of the paper factor found in balsam fir. The compound mimics the action of juvenile hormone in only one family of insects, exemplified by *Pyrrhocoris apterus*. In this European bug, it prevents the attainment of adult characters and leads to death.

it (Fig. 17–14). Newspapers of American origin had the same effect, whereas papers from Europe and Japan had no effect. The balsam fir *(Abies balsamea)* is the main source of wood pulp in the United States, and extracts of this tree have very potent JH activities when assayed on *Pyrrhocoris.* The paper factor present in the trees is carried through to the paper products; it is not added during the manufacturing process.[39]

Juvenile hormone is essential for normal insect development, but it must be present in correct amounts at precisely determined periods. In *Pyrrhocoris,* for example, JH analogues applied directly to the eggs disturb development and render the embryos inviable. Minute amounts applied topically to a mature female cause her to lay inviable eggs for the remainder of her life. The males of *Pyrrhocoris* can tolerate relatively large amounts of topically applied JH analogues, but they pass on to females during mating sufficient amounts to sterilize them permanently.

It is known that certain parasites are capable of influencing the growth and development of their insect hosts by liberating a substance that has the same effects as JH from the corpora allata. The larvae of *Tribolium* (Coleoptera), when infected with the sporozoan parasite *Nosemba*, undergo supernumerary molts to produce giant larvae which weigh twice as much as the uninfected controls. These infected larvae seldom pupate: The infection mimics JH in prolonging larval life at the expense of pupal and imaginal differentiation. Studies indicate that the parasite itself produces a substance with JH activity, rather than acting upon the host's corpora allata to stimulate the production of intrinsic JH.[14]

Proctodone

Larval diapause in the European corn borer *(Ostrinia nubilalis)* is induced by short-day photoperiods and terminated by long-day photoperiods. When diapausing larvae are ligatured between the sixth and seventh abdominal segments, thus cutting off circulation in the two terminal segments of the abdomen, exposure to long-day photoperiods fails to terminate diapause. Cutting the ventral nerve cord at the level of the sixth abdominal segment does not prevent diapause termination in response to long days.

These observations indicated that some endocrine mechanism, necessary for brain activation and consequent termination of diapause, might be located in the terminal abdominal segments. Glandular cells were found in the proctodeal epithelium, and because of its source, the name *proctodone* was applied to the hormone. It is blood-borne and participates in diapause termination by activating the neurosecretory complex of the brain.[1, 2]

Endocrines in Insect Reproduction

The belief prevailed for many years that sexual differentiation in insects was entirely genetic, hormones not being involved. Recent studies on the firefly, *Lampyris noctiluca,* show that this is not true, at least in this species, and suggest that similar observations ought to be extended to other insects. In *Lampyris* the apical tissue of the testis is the source of an androgenic hormone that induces masculine differentiation of the gonads and secondary sex characters. Transplantation of apical testes to female larvae causes the gonads of the hosts to differentiate as testes and induces male secondary characters to appear. Ovaries transplanted to male larvae are without effect. The capacity of *Lampyris* testes to masculinize genetic females is reduced after pupation and is lost in the adult.[33]

Gonadal functions are conditioned by several internal secretions. Juvenile hormone from the corpus allatum is essential for yolk deposition in the eggs and for formation of spermatophores in many species of insects. In *Rhodnius,* for example, removal of the corpus allatum prevents the production of ripe eggs: The oocytes grow as long as they are attached to the nurse cells, but degenerate at the period when yolk deposition should occur. Allatectomy and ligation experiments on the milkweed bug, *Oncopeltus fasciatus,* indicate a similar relationship, corpora allata being necessary for yolk deposition and secretion by the oviducts. Full production of eggs in *Oncopeltus* also depends on the medial neurosecretory cells of the brain. Among certain flies *(e.g., Calliphora),* the medial neurosecretory cells are of special importance inasmuch as their products promote the formation of amino acids to be used by the eggs for the synthesis of proteins.

Reproduction in the cockroach *Byrsotria* depends upon the release of a volatile sex attractant by the female, this pheromone being essential for attracting males and releasing their courtship behavior. Gonadectomy does not impair the mating behavior of either sex. Allatectomy of the female, shortly after the imaginal molt, prevents the production of sex pheromone; the production of pheromone is reinstated by the implantation of corpora allata. In this species of roach, secretions from the corpora allata are essential not only for oocyte maturation and accessory gland secretion, but also for production of the sex attractant which makes mating behavior possible. Allatectomy of the male does not impair reproductive behavior.

In *Bombyx* as well as the Cecropia silkworm, the corpora may be removed from the pupae of either sex without disturbing the sexual functions of mature moths; the organs are not necessary for the maturation of gametes and the production of normal young. Molting hormone of the pro-

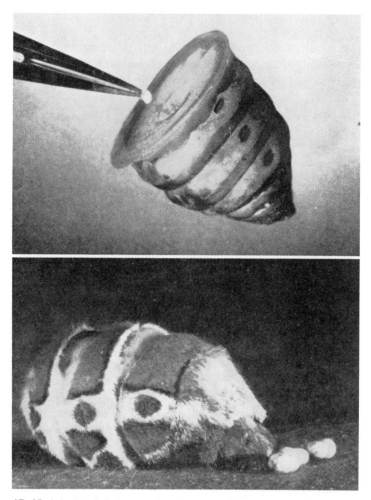

Figure 17–15. *A,* Isolated abdomen of a diapausing Cecropia pupa sealed to a plastic cover slip. Prothoracic glands from postdiapausing pupae are being introduced into the abdomen through a central hole in the slip. *B,* The same abdomen after differentiating adult characters; eggs are being deposited. Corpora allata are not necessary for gamete maturation in these moths. (From Williams, C. M.: Biol. Bull. *103,* 1952.)

thoracic gland appears to be the only one necessary for sexual maturation of both sexes in these moths (Fig. 17–15). Pupae deprived of their brains, corpora cardiaca, and corpora allata become sexually mature adults after the administration of crystalline ecdysone. Thus, in these Lepidoptera, the corpora allata are highly active in the adults, but no function has as yet been ascribed to them at this stage of the life cycle. It may be significant, however, that the silkworms that have been studied most carefully are short-lived moths which lack functional mouth-parts in the adult. The adult stage is greatly abbreviated, and ripe eggs are ready for oviposition soon after the individual emerges from the pupa. It may be that the lack of functional mouth-parts in the adult correlates with a precocious maturation of the gonads, which can occur in the absence of any gonadotrophic function of the corpora allata. The corpora allata of feeding, long-lived species of adult Lepidoptera may possibly exert gonadotrophic effects similar to those described for numerous other orders of insects.

In *autogenous* mosquitoes of the genus *Culex,* ovarian development does not depend upon the consumption of food in the adult stage, but the ovaries of *anautogenous* species do not develop beyond a resting stage until a blood meal of adequate size has been consumed. The implantation of corpora allata from autogenous donors into anautogenous recipients enables the ovaries to mature without the consumption of a meal. When anautogenous ovaries are transplanted to autogenous hosts, egg maturation occurs in the grafts even though the host does not feed. Ovaries from autogenous donors do not mature after being transplanted to anautogenous hosts. In addition to a hormone from the corpus allatum, a factor from the brain is also involved in these phenomena.

Studies on several species of insects show that the functional status of the corpora allata is regulated by the brain. In the milkweed bug and some of the roaches, the corpora allata are supplied by inhibitory nerves from the brain: Sectioning these nerves releases the corpora allata from inhibition, and egg maturation and ovulation occur. Distention of the gut appears to be the effective signal for egg development and ovulation in anautogenous mosquitoes; in certain roaches, it is the act of mating that is the signal.

Water Balance in Insects

Some insects that feed upon fluids have evolved mechanisms for the quick elimination of excessive water (diuresis). Rapid elimination of fluid occurs in *Rhodnius* following the consumption of a blood meal, and it has been reported that the fused thoracic ganglia are the source of a diuretic neurohormone which acts upon the Malpighian tubules to promote the loss of fluid. The response can be evoked in isolated Malpighian tubules by exposing them to blood taken from recently fed *Rhodnius.*

Evidence for an antidiuretic principle in the roach *Periplaneta americana* has been obtained through studies on the rate of indigo carmine uptake by Malpighian tubules, tested *in vitro,* following subjection of the animals to different osmotic conditions. Since the diet of these insects consists of solids or semisolids, there is little likelihood that excessive fluid intake would constitute a problem; however, periods of desiccation might require a diminished excretion of fluids and withdrawal of water from the gut. The Malpighian tubules from dehydrated and salt-loaded animals showed lower than normal levels of dye uptake, indicating that they had been exposed to a factor inhibiting excretion. Extracts of corpora allata from normal animals, in contrast to those from dehydrated animals, reduced the rate of dye uptake by the tubules. Brain extracts, prepared from dehydrated subjects, also reduced dye uptake. The experiments were interpreted as indicating that an antidiuretic factor is produced by the brain and conveyed to the corpora allata, where it is stored and released when the organism needs to conserve water.[47]

THE CHEMISTRY OF ARTHROPOD HORMONES

Steroid Hormones

The isolation and chemical characterization of molting hormones in insects and crustaceans have been facilitated by the availability of a satisfactory bioassay method for estimating activity. Larvae of the blowfly, *Calliphora*, are generally used for this purpose. When the larvae are ligatured behind Weismann's ring, endogenous hormone causes puparium formation to proceed anterior to the ligature, but the portion of the body behind the ligature does not pupate. Extracts containing ecdysones induce pupation when injected into the body posterior to the ligature. As little as 0.01 μgm of crystalline ecdysone is uniformly effective and this quantity of hormone is called a *Calliphora* unit.

Using 500 kg of silkworm *(Bombyx)* pupae, Butenandt and Karlson (1954) extracted about 25 mg of crystalline molting hormone, which they called *ecdysone.* About 10 years later, enough α-ecdysone was obtained from 4 tons of pupae (wet weight) to determine the chemical structure of this steroid (Fig. 17–16). When tested on various insects, it is found to duplicate all the known effects of the natural hormone. It is obvious that steroid hormones are not an innovation peculiar to the vertebrates. Ecdysone has the same carbon skeleton as cholesterol and probably is derived from it. When radioactive cholesterol is administered to *Calliphora* larvae, much of the radioactivity becomes incorporated in the ecdysone molecule. It has been observed that cholesterol can be converted to ecdysone in the abdominal segments of some insects. The secretion of α-ecdysone is produced *in vitro* by the prothoracic glands.[7, 19, 29] Insects cannot synthesize cholesterol from acetate, but phytophagus species can convert plant sterols to cholesterol. Carnivorous insects would obtain cholesterol and various steroids from their food. Fifteen or more phytoecdysones have been isolated from the leaves and roots of plants, and more are certain to be found (Fig. 17–17).

Several ecdysones in addition to α-ecdysone can be isolated from

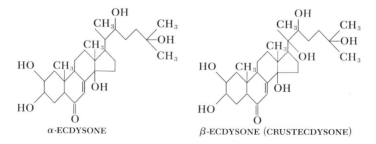

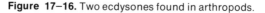

Figure 17–16. Two ecdysones found in arthropods.

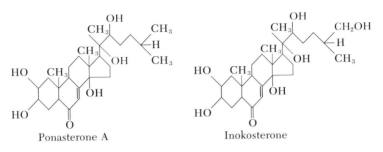

Figure 17–17. Two plant steroids having ecdysone activity.

Bombyx pupae, the most important one probably is β-ecdysone (20-hydroxyecdysone). The latter steroid differs from α-ecdysone only by the presence of a hydroxyl group at position 20 (Fig. 17–16). Both steroids are found in many insects and, in some species, the β-ecdysone predominates. After finding that homogenates of crustacean tissues have some activity in the *Calliphora* test and that crystalline ecdysone accelerates molting in certain Crustacea, it became apparent that the crustacean molting hormone is a steroid similar to α-ecdysone. These experiments led to the isolation of the crustacean steroid, called *crustecdysone;* the present indications are that it is identical with β-ecdysone of insects. A second crustacean molting hormone, called *deoxycrustecdysone*, has been isolated from certain marine species. The presence of multiple ecdysones in insects and crustaceans is interesting but hard to explain: The different steroids might have different physiologic effects, or they might actually be precursors or breakdown products of a single hormonally effective molecule. One might wonder why certain plants have become specialized in the synthesis of phytoecdysones. It has been suggested that this forcing of insects to metamorphose at unpropitious seasons might be a method employed by the plant to protect itself against harmful insects.[54]

Although the ecdysones are recognized as the molting hormones of crustaceans and insects, there is insufficient information about their origin and metabolism within the body. The Y organs and prothoracic glands seem to be essential for the production of these steroids, but there are reasons for believing that their synthesis may occur at sites peripheral to these organs. It has been suggested that these glands may provide enzymes, the actual synthesis of hormones occurring in the blood.

The nature of the hormone from crustacean androgenic glands remains uncertain. It was originally regarded as proteinaceous, but there is circumstantial evidence that the gland may be a source of steroids. The administration of testosterone to certain crabs causes the ovary to differentiate as a testis, but does not induce secondary sex characters of the male type. Tissues of the lobster possess the necessary enzymes for converting certain precursors to testosterone. It is conceivable that the androgenic gland could produce both a protein and a steroid hormone.[21]

Juvenile Hormone of Insects

The abdomens of adult male Cecropia *(Hyalophora)* moths are especially rich in juvenile hormone (JH), and the first active extracts were prepared from this source.[87] When extracts containing the hormone are injected into pupae, they molt into second pupae instead of becoming adults, an effect identical to that of implanted corpora allata. Allatectomized animals do not contain JH. The hormone may be assayed in various species by applying it locally to the last larval instar or to the pupa: The epidermal cells below the point of application secrete another larval or pupal cuticle, whereas the remaining parts of the body form a normal cuticle of adult type. Rapid progress was made in purifying *Hyalophora* extracts, but isolation and chemical characterization of the hormone were a difficult and elusive undertaking. Complications arose from the fact that an extremely large number of compounds and extracts from many sources gave positive results when assayed for JH activity (Fig. 17–18). The feces of the mealworm *(Tenebrio)* were found to exhibit JH activity in bioassays, and further studies showed the active ingredients in feces to be terpenoid compounds, particularly farnesol and its oxidation product, farnesal. These and related compounds produced all the effects attributable to JH and, after finding farnesol in extracts of male *Hyalophora* abdomens, it seemed certain that farnesol was JH. However, purified extracts were many times more potent in the various tests than farnesol and related derivatives. Furthermore, surgical removal of the corpora allata from *Hyalophora* pupae was found to eliminate JH from the adult males, but did not diminish the content of farnesol in them. Thus, it was apparent that terpenoid compounds mimic the actions of JH to varying extents in different species, but they themselves are not the hormones.

Röller and his colleagues established the definitive structure of JH iso-

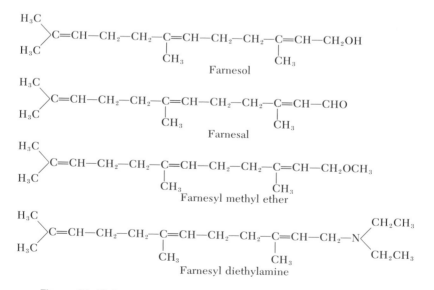

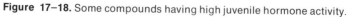

Figure 17–18. Some compounds having high juvenile hormone activity.

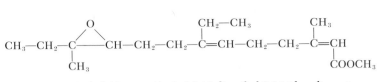

Methyl 10-epoxy-7-ethyl-3,11-dimethyl-2,6-tridecadienoate

Figure 17–19. Structure of the juvenile hormone of the moth, *Hyalophora cecropia*.

lated from *Hyalophora cecropia* in 1967 (Fig. 17–19). Chemically, the hormone is methyl 10-epoxy-7-ethyl-3,11-dimethyl-2,6-tridecadienoate. The molecule can take 16 different stereoisomeric forms, but only one of these can be the authentic hormone. A number of analogues have been prepared that have more or less activity. It is likely that considerable species variability may be found in chemistry of the hormone since the corpora allata vary in functional importance.[37]

Arthropod Neurohormones

While the neurohormones of invertebrates have not been isolated and chemically characterized, evidence from arthropods strongly supports the belief that they are proteins or polypeptides. Though current evidence is against this, the possibility should be recognized that the hormone might be a relatively small molecule combined with some kind of a carrier macromolecule.

The X organ–sinus gland complex of the crustacean eyestalk contains a variety of hormones, including a family of chromatophorotrophins that regulate the integumentary pigment cells, and hormones that control the light and dark-adaptation of retinal pigment cells. It is generally agreed that these neurosecretory products are relatively small peptides. Probably the large number of pigmentary-effector hormones, claimed on the basis of extracts tested on many different species, will be reduced as the chemistry of the molecules becomes known.

The hyperglycemic hormones as well as the diuretic hormones are inactivated by chymotrypsin and are likely to be polypeptides. The hormones affecting heart rate in cockroaches and locusts exhibit many of the properties of polypeptides. The brain hormone of *Bombyx* is water soluble and is inactivated by incubation with bacterial proteases. It has many properties of a protein, and this is in accord with what is known of neurohormones in other animals. The *Bombyx* brain hormone appears to be a complex molecule, and determination of its chemistry is not an easy task.[25]

Insect Hormones as Pesticides

There is currently much interest in the possibility of controlling harmful insects by exposing them to their own hormones, or to synthetic analogues thereof, at wrong periods of the life cycle or in wrong concentrations. Pesticides such as DDT are too broad in their effects: They kill all insects indiscriminately and may increase in concentration as they are passed along the food chain, endangering other animals, including man. Moreover, a number of harmful insects have become resistant to common insecticides. For example, the *Anopheles* mosquito, the vector that transmits human malaria, is entirely resistant to DDT. It is not likely that insects could survive if they developed immunity to their own secretions, which are essential for development. The insect hormones are often quite specific and are not known to be harmful to other organisms.

The effectiveness of juvenile hormone analogues in controlling agricultural pests has already been demonstrated. For example, by treating stored grain with such compounds, infestations of *Tribolium castaneum* and other insects can be reduced or prevented.[41] In terms of controlling the pests that transmit diseases to man and domestic animals, increasing the production of field crops, and diminishing the wastage of food, hormone mimics may be of incalculable value as they become more widely applied.

REFERENCES

1. Beck, S. D., and Alexander, N.: Proctodone, an insect development hormone. Biol. Bull. *126*:185, 1964.
2. Beck, S. D., Shane, J. L., and Colvin, I. B.: Proctodone production in the European corn borer, *Ostrinia nubilalis*. J. Insect Physiol. *11*:297, 1965.
3. Bliss, D. E., and Boyer, J. R.: Environmental regulation of growth in the decapod crustacean *Gecarcinus lateralis*. Gen. Comp. Endocr. *4*:15, 1964.
4. Carpenter, M. B., and deRoos, R.: Seasonal morphology and histology of the androgenic gland of the crayfish, *Orconectes nais*. Gen. Comp. Endocr. *15*:143, 1970.
5. Chaet, A. B.: Neurochemical control of gamete release in starfish. Biol. Bull. *130*:43, 1966.
6. Charniaux-Cotton, H., and Kleinholz, L. H.: Hormones in invertebrates other than insects. *In* G. Pincus, K. V. Thimann, and E. B. Astwood (eds.): The Hormones. New York, Academic Press, p. 135.
7. Chino, H., Sakurai, S., Ohtaki, T., Ikekawa, N., Miyazaki, H., Ishibashi, M., and Abuki, H.: Biosynthesis of α-ecdysone by prothoracic glands *in vitro*. Science *183*:529, 1974.
8. Clark, R. B.: Endocrine influences in annelids. Gen. Comp. Endocr., Suppl. *2*:572, 1969.
9. Fingerman, M.: Behavior of chromatophores of the fiddler crab *Uca pugilator* and the dwarf crayfish *Cambarellus shufeldti* in response to synthetic *Pandalus* red pigment-concentrating hormone. Gen. Comp. Endocr. *20*:589, 1973.
10. Fingerman, M.: Neurosecretory control of pigmentary effectors in crustaceans. Amer. Zool. *6*:169, 1966.
11. Fingerman, M.: Chromatophores. Physiol. Rev. *45*:296, 1965.
12. Fingerman, M., Fingerman, S. W., and Hammond, R. D.: Comparison of red pigment-concentrating hormones from the eyestalks of the fiddler crab, *Uca pugilator*, and the prawn, *Palaemonetes vulgaris*, with synthetic red pigment-concentrating hormone of *Pandalus borealis*. Gen. Comp. Endocr. *23*:124, 1974.
13. Fingerman, M., and Yamamoto, Y.: Endocrine control of tanning in the crayfish exoskeleton. Science *144*:1462, 1964.
14. Fisher, F. M., Jr., and Sanborn, R. C.: *Nosema* as a source of juvenile hormone in parasitized insects. Biol. Bull. *126*:235, 1964.
15. Fraenkel, G.: Interactions between ecdysone, bursicon, and other endocrines during puparium formation and adult emergence in flies. Amer. Zool. *15* (Suppl. 1):29, 1975.
16. Fraenkel, G., and Hsiao, C.: Bursicon, a hormone which mediates tanning of the cuticle in the adult fly and other insects. J. Insect Physiol. *11*:513, 1965.
17. Fukuda, S.: Induction of pupation in silkworm by transplanting the prothoracic gland. Proc. Im. Acad. Tokyo *16*:414, 1940.
18. Fukuda, S., and Takeuchi, S.: Studies on the diapause factor-producing cells in the suboesophageal ganglion of the silkworm, *Bombyx mori* L. Embryologia *9*:333, 1967.
19. Gersch, M., and Stürzebecher, J.: Über eine Synthese von Ecdyson-3H und Ecdysteron-3H in abgeschnürten Abdomina von *Mamestra brassicae*-Rauper. Experientia *27*:1475, 1971.
20. Gilbert, L. I.: Endocrine action during insect growth. Rec. Progr. Horm. Res. *30*:347, 1974.
21. Gilgan, M. W., and Idler, D. R.: The conversion of androstenedione to testosterone by lobster (*Homarus americanus* Milne Edwards) tissues. Gen. Comp. Endocr. *9*:319, 1967.

22. Golding, D. W.: Studies in the comparative neuroendocrinology of polychaete reproduction. Gen. Comp. Endocr., Suppl. *3*:580, 1972.

23. Hagadorn, I. R.: Neurosecretion in the Hirudinea and its possible role in reproduction. Amer. Zool. *6*:251, 1966.

24. Highnam, K. C., and Hill, L.: The Comparative Endocrinology of the Invertebrates. London, Edward Arnold, 1969.

25. Ishizaki, H., and Ichikawa, M.: Purification of the brain hormone of the silkworm *Bombyx mori.* Biol. Bull. *133*:355, 1967.

26. Joosse, J.: Endocrinology of reproduction in molluscs. Gen. Comp. Endocr., Suppl. *3*:591, 1972.

27. Josefsson, L.: Structure and function of crustacean chromatophorotropins. Gen. Comp. Endocr. *25*:199, 1975.

28. Kanatani, H., and Shirai, H.: On the maturation-inducing substance produced in starfish gonad by neural substance. Gen. Comp. Endocr., Suppl. *3*:571, 1972.

29. King, D. S.: Ecdysone metabolism in insects. Amer. Zool. *12*:343, 1972.

30. Kleinholz, L. H.: A progress report on the separation and purification of crustacean neurosecretory pigmentary-effector hormones. Gen. Comp. Endocr. *14*:578, 1970.

31. Kopec, S.: Studies on the necessity of the brain for the inception of insect metamorphosis. Biol. Bull. *42*:323, 1922.

32. Moriyama, H., Nakanishi, K., King, D. S., Okauchi, T., Siddall, J. B., and Hafferl, W.: On the origin and metabolic fate of α-ecdysone in insects. Gen. Comp. Endocr. *15*:80, 1970.

33. Naisse, J.: Contrôle endocrinien de la différenciation sexuelle chez les insects. Arch. Anat. Micro. Morphol. Exp. *54*:417, 1965.

34. Olive, P. J. W.: A vitellogenesis-promoting influence of the prostomium in the polychaete *Eulalia viridis* (Müller) (Phyllodocidae). Gen. Comp. Endocr. *26*:266,1975.

35. Olive, P. J. W., and Moore, F. F.: Hormone independent regeneration in *Eulalia viridis* (Polychaeta-Phyllodocidae). Gen. Comp. Endocr. *26*:259, 1975.

36. Ralph, C. L.: Heart accelerators and decelerators in the nervous system of *Periplaneta americana* (L). J. Insect Physiol. *8*:431, 1962.

37. Röller, H., Bjerke, J. S., Holthaus, L. M., Norgard, D. W., and McShan, W. H.: Isolation and biological properties of the juvenile hormone. J. Insect Physiol. *15*:379, 1969.

38. Scudamore, H. H.: Sinus gland and O_2 consumption in crayfishes: Hormonal control of gastrolith formation in crayfishes. Physiol. Zool. *20*:187, 1947.

39. Slama, K., and Williams, C. M.: The sensitivity of the bug, *Pyrrhocoris apterus,* to a hormonally active factor in American paper-pulp. Biol. Bull. *130*:235, 1966.

40. Steele, J. E.: The site of action of insect hyperglycemic hormone. Gen. Comp. Endocr. *3*:46, 1963.

41. Thomas, P. J., and Bhatnager-Thomas, P. L.: Use of juvenile hormone analogue as insecticide for pests of stored grain. Nature *219*:949, 1968.

42. Thompson, M. J., Svoboda, J. A., Kaplanis, J. N., and Robbins, W. E.: Metabolic pathways of steroids in insects. Proc. Roy. Soc. London B. *180*:203, 1972.

43. Thomsen, E., and Moller, I. B.: Influence of neurosecretory cells and of corpus allatum on intestinal protease activity in the adult *Calliphora erythrocephala* Meig. J. Exp. Biol. *40*: 301, 1963.

44. Truman, J. W.: Physiology of insect ecdysis. II. The assay and occurrence of the eclosion hormone in the Chinese oak silkmoth, *Antheraea pernyi.* Biol. Bull. *144*:200, 1973.

45. Truman, J. W.: How moths "turn on": a study of the action of hormones on the nervous system. Amer. Scientist *61*:700, 1973.

46. Truman, J. W.: Physiology of insect ecdysis. III. Relationship between the hormonal control of eclosion and of tanning in the tobacco hornworm, *Manduca sexta.* J. Exp. Biol. *58*: 821, 1973.

47. Wall, B. J., and Ralph, C. L.: Evidence for hormonal regulation of malpighian tubule excretion in the insect *Periplaneta americana* L. Gen. Comp. Endocr. *4*:452, 1964.

48. Wells, M. J.: Optic glands and the ovary of *Octopus.* Symp. Zool. Soc. Lond. *2*:87, 1960.

49. Wells, M. J., and Wells, J.: Hormonal control of sexual maturity in *Octopus.* J. Exp. Biol. *36*: 1, 1959.

50. Wigglesworth, V. B.: The breakdown of the thoracic gland in the adult insect, *Rhodnius prolixus.* J. Exp. Biol. *32*:485, 1955.

51. Wigglesworth, V. B.: The determination of characters at metamorphosis in *Rhodnius prolixus* (Hemiptera). J. Exp. Biol. *17*:201, 1940.

52. de Wilde, J.: An endocrine view of metamorphosis, polymorphism, and diapause in insects. Amer. Zool. *15* (Suppl. 1):13, 1975.

53. Williams, C. M.: Ecdysone and ecdysone-analogues: Their assay and action of diapausing pupae of the cynthia silkworm. Biol. Bull. *134*:344, 1968.

54. Williams, C. M., and Robbins, W. E.: Conference on insect-plant interactions. BioScience *18*(8):791, 797, 1968.

Index

Note: In this index, page numbers in *italic* type refer to illustrations; page numbers followed by (t) refer to tables.